MEDICAL RADIOLOGY

Diagnostic Imaging and Radiation Oncology

Springer
Berlin
Heidelberg
New York
Barcelona
Budapest
Hong Kong
London
Milan
Paris
Santa Clara
Singapore
Tokyo

Carcinoma of the Prostate

Innovations in Management

With Contributions by

T.E. Ahlering · L. Baert · M.A. Bagshaw · P. Bertrand · L.W. Brady · S.-C. Chen
G.A. Coetzee · B.J. Costleigh · R.S. Cox · P. Dal Cin · D. De Ridder · A.A. Elgamal
J.A. Freeman · J.E. Freire · H. Goethuys · G.D. Grossfeld · S.L. Hancock · B.S. Hill
D. Kahn · W.J. Kirkels · G. Lieskovsky · M.A. Lockett · W.A. Longton · G. Luxton
E. Mazeman · B. Micaily · J. Michalski · C.T. Miyamoto · P. Montemaggi
A.M. Nissar Syed · B.J. Norlén · B. Norouzi · R.H. Oyen · C.A. Perez · Z. Petrovich
N. Piotrkowicz · R.K. Ross · J.D. Schmidt · D.G. Skinner · B. Stawarz · S. Szmigielski
W.M. Van de Voorde · H. Van Den Berghe · H. Van Poppel · R.D. Williams · H. Zielinski

Edited by

Zbigniew Petrovich, Luc Baert, and Luther W. Brady

Foreword by

Luther W. Brady and Hans-Peter Heilmann

Preface by Donald G. Skinner

Springer

Zbigniew Petrovich, MD
Professor, Department of Radiation Oncology and Urology
Chairman, Department of Radiation Oncology
University of Southern California School of Medicine
1441 Eastlake Avenue
Los Angeles, CA 90033
USA

Luther W. Brady, MD
Professor and Chairman
Department of Radiation Oncology and Nuclear Medicine
Medical College of Pennsylvania and Hahnemann University
230 N. Broad Street
Philadelphia, PA 1902–1192
USA

Luc Baert, MD
Department of Urology
St. Pieter's Hospital
University of Leuven
Brusselsestraat 69
B-3000 Leuven
Belgium

MEDICAL RADIOLOGY · Diagnostic Imaging and Radiation Oncology

Continuation of
Handbuch der medizinischen Radiologie
Encyclopedia of Medical Radiology

With 124 Figures in 190 Separate Illustrations, Some in Colour

ISSN 0942-5373
ISBN-13:978-3-642-64627-0 e-ISBN-13:978-3-642-60956-5
DOI: 10.1007/978-3-642-60956-5

Library of Congress Cataloging-in-Publication Data. Carcinoma of the prostate: innovations in management/[edited by] Z. Petrovich, L. Baert, L.W. Brady: with contributions by T. Ahlering . . . [et al.]; foreword by L.W. Brady and H.-P. Heilmann; preface by D.G. Skinner. p. cm. – (Medical radiology) Includes bibliographical references and index.

ISBN-13:978-3-642-64627-0 (hardcover: alk. paper)

1. Prostate – Cancer. I. Petrovich, Zbigniew. II. Baert, L. (Luc) III. Brady, Luther W., 1925– . IV. Series. [DNLM: 1. Prostatic Neoplasms – diagnosis. 2. Prostatic Neoplasms – therapy. 3. Tumor Markers, Biological – blood. 4. Prostatectomy. 5. Radiotherapy – methods. 6. Brachytherapy – methods. WJ 752 C265 1996] RC280.P7C37 1996 616.99'463–dc20 DNLM/DLC for Library of Congress 95-52110

Softcover reprint of the hardcover 1st edition 1996

Cover design: Springer-Verlag, E. Kirchner

Typesetting: Best-set Typesetter Ltd., Hong Kong

SPIN: 10487547 21/3135/SPS – 5 4 3 2 1 0 – Printed on acid-free paper

This book is dedicated
to Zofia Petrovich, MD, and Bea Baert

Foreword

The American Cancer Society anticipates that during 1995, 244 000 new cases of cancer of the prostate will have been diagnosed in the United States, with 40 400 deaths from the disease process. The rapid increase in the actual number of new cases in the United States is directly related to more regularized digital rectal examinations and the more frequent and widespread use of prostate-specific antigen (PSA) screening programs. As a consequence, major controversies have emerged in how best to manage the patient with cancer of the prostate. These include the necessity of PSA screening programs, how to interpret PSA values, what imaging studies are most appropriate for definition of the true extent of the disease process, the value of pretreatment surgical staging of the disease process, and the value of different treatments. The latter encompass a wide range of options: observation, radical prostatectomy, the Walsh-type prostatectomy procedure, definitive external beam radiation therapy, local interstitial implantation using iodine-125, iridium-192, or palladium-103, orchiectomy, cryosurgery, hyperthermia, and various antitestosterone agents such as estrogens or LH,RH agonists.

The present volume deals with the major parameters of controversy with regard to cancer of the prostate and will enable the reader to acquire a better understanding of the disease and how best it might be managed to achieve an optimal outcome with a minimum of complications.

This book attempts to address a wide audience which includes: epidemiologists, pathologists, basic scientists, diagnostic radiologists, radiation oncologists, and urologists. Additionally, we hope that it will be a useful reference for medical students, physicians in training, and other physicians interested in the management of prostate cancer.

The authors have done an excellent job in bringing into contemporary focus the widely diverse opinions with regard to the overall management of the man with cancer of the prostate.

Philadelphia
Hamburg
October 1995

LUTHER W. BRADY
HANS-PETER HEILMANN

Preface

The incidence of newly diagnosed cancer of the prostate has increased dramatically over the past decade, and it presents a growing health problem in Western societies. The number of patients diagnosed each year has continued to increase, largely due to increase in patient awareness, increasing life expectancy, and in particular the widespread use of the blood test to measure prostate-specific antigen (PSA). Considerable controversy exists as to whether it is appropriate to use PSA as a screening tool and many question whether earlier detection of this disease will translate into a reduced mortality. To date, the age-adjusted mortality for cancer of the prostate has not declined for nearly half a century, yet studies by the American College of Surgeons have demonstrated a dramatic increase in the percentage of newly diagnosed patients with cancer of the prostate who have organ-confined disease. Most urologic oncologists believe it will be only a matter of time before age-adjusted mortality rates decline, but it may require nearly 15 years of follow-up before definitive therapy of early-stage disease translates into prolonged survival.

Strategies to reduce death from prostate cancer include prevention, early detection, use of effective and acceptable therapeutic modalities for localized disease, and improved innovative approaches for management of those unfortunate patients who present with or develop advanced metastatic disease. The purpose of this book is to review current knowledge regarding the epidemiology, development, and natural history of untreated cancer of the prostate, and the available therapeutic options; with regard to the latter, morbidity of therapy and potential impact on survival are fully considered.

Although the organ site of origin of prostate cancer is within the traditional domain of the urologist, it is clear that a single modality-oriented approach to therapy – surgery versus radiation versus chemotherapy versus hormone therapy – is outmoded. Drs. Petrovich, Baert, and Brady have brought together an impressive array of experts representing various medical, surgical, epidemiological, and basic science disciplines. Their vast personal experience in all areas of prostate cancer – causes, prevention, detection, and management – will help the clinician to acquire a better understanding of all management options and alternatives.

This book is a comprehensive and authoritative review of current concepts regarding etiology, detection, and management and should have relevance for all physicians concerned with the diagnosis and treatment of cancer of the prostate.

Donald G. Skinner, M.D.
Professor and Chairman
USC/Department of Urology

Preface

Contents

1 The Epidemiology and Etiology of Prostate Cancer

R.K. Ross and G.A. Coetzee

CONTENTS

1.1 Introduction

Prostate cancer is the most frequently diagnosed cancer in the United States. Until recently most attempts by epidemiologists to identify risk factors and understand the etiology of prostate cancer were unfocused, searching for clues which could lead to more definitive and detailed evaluations. In the past few years epidemiologic studies have increasingly centered around three main themes – family history, diet, and hormones – although a few additional risk factors seem to be reproducible across studies and among different target populations, so that these also have received substantial recent attention.

We believe that all of these factors, including at least part of the familial risk, might be explicable by a unifying hypothesis related to hormonal influences on prostatic epithelium. We begin this chapter by discussing briefly some of the interesting demographic characteristics of prostate cancer. We then present a central hypothesis related to prostate cancer etiology. We discuss each of the areas listed above around which recent epidemiologic attention has focused, attempting to incorporate observations made in each of these areas into an underlying hormonal hypothesis. We complete our review with a discussion of prostate cancer genetics, which includes sections on both germline and somatic genetic changes that might contribute to prostate cancer development or progression.

1.2 Demographic Risk Factors

In 1994 prostate cancer surpassed female breast cancer to become the leading cancer in the United States (American Cancer Society 1994). An estimated 200 000 men were diagnosed with prostate cancer in 1994. Prostate cancer is the second leading cause of cancer deaths in men, exceeded only by lung cancer; it accounted for 38 000 deaths in 1994.

Prostate cancer in the United States demonstrated a small but steady increase in incidence and mortality during the 1970s and the 1980s, averaging about 5% per year in incidence and 1% per year in mortality (Ries et al. 1990). During the late 1980s the rate of increase in incidence rapidly escalated, so that in some areas of the country incidence rates more than doubled in only a 5-year period (Table 1.1). This increase in incidence was not accompanied by any increase whatsoever in mortality from prostate cancer. Thus, it is plausible that this increase is, in a sense, artifactual, resulting from increased utilization of newly available tools for finding prostate cancer when it is clinically inapparent. In particular, use of serologic testing for prostate-specific antigen (PSA), a protein produced specifically by prostate epithelium, is likely to have contributed to this increase. If this test is detecting progressive prostate cancer and is leading to earlier diagnosis and curative therapy, then the increase in prostate cancer incidence occurring now should be followed by a reduction in prostate cancer mortality in the near future.

R.K. Ross, MD, Professor, Department of Preventive Medicine, USC School of Medicine, Kenneth Norris Jr. Cancer Hospital and Research Institute, Los Angeles, CA 90033-0804, USA
G.A. Coetzee, PhD, Associate Professor, Department of Urology, USC School of Medicine, Kenneth Norris Jr. Cancer Hospital and Research Institute, Los Angeles, CA 90033-0804, USA

Table 1.1. Age-adjusted prostate cancer incidence and mortality rates (per 100000) in Los Angeles County, California, 1988–1993: non-Latino whites and African-Americans only

	Incidence		Mortality	
	Whites	African-Americans	Whites	African-Americans
1988	99	136	23	50
1989	104	148	22	50
1990	123	166	21	41
1991	168	208	22	45
1992	190	248	24	44

Like all cancer, prostate cancer risk is strongly related to age; in fact, prostate cancer is the most age-related of all epithelial cancers (Ross et al. 1979). Prostate cancer incidence begins to increase for men in their early 40s, and then continues to increase logarithmically at about the 8th to 9th power of age throughout the remainder of life.

The other well-established demographic characteristic of prostate cancer is its strong international and racial/ethnic variation in incidence. African-American men have by far the highest prostate cancer rate in the world, whereas Asian men, including Japanese, Chinese, and probably other Asian ethnicities, have the lowest (Muir et al. 1987). Historically, the difference in incidence between these high- and low-risk populations has been reported to be on the order of 50- to 100-fold. Part of this historical difference is likely to be due to differences in detection strategies used for finding prostate cancer in different populations (Shimizu et al. 1991). With the increased utilization of PSA as a detection method it has become increasingly difficult to determine the true range of prostate cancer incidence around the world. Nonetheless, examining differences in prostate cancer mortality, which are much less sensitive to such detection biases, there remains substantial international and racial/ethnic variation (Zaridze et al. 1984).

1.3 The Role of Androgens in Prostate Cancer Development

In the last decade, it has been established that for a normal cell to change into a malignant phenotype requires a series of genetic changes. Cell division is an absolute requirement for these genetic changes, even though they can occur via several mechanisms, so that cell division becomes an essential part of the mechanism of carcinogenesis. Cell division in the prostate is under androgen control (Coffey 1979). Testosterone, the major circulating human androgen, freely diffuses into prostate epithelium, where it is rapidly and irreversibly converted to its reduced and metabolically more active form, dihydrotestosterone (DHT). DHT binds to the androgen receptor (testosterone also binds to the androgen receptor but with lower affinity) and the androgen/receptor complex translocates to the nucleus for transactivation of androgen responsive genes, including those which control cell division (Parker and Schimmer 1994). Thus, given the probable importance of cell division on prostate cancer pathogenesis, it is reasonable to explore genetic and environmental influences on androgen secretion and metabolism as potential contributors to prostate cancer etiology.

1.4 External Factors

1.4.1 Diet

1.4.1.1 Fat

Although a variety of dietary factors have received attention as possibly related to prostate cancer risk enhancement or reduction, recent attention has focused particularly around consumption of fat or its subcomponents, vitamin A or its precursors, vitamin D metabolites, and phytoestrogenic foods.

Interest in the possible role of dietary fat in prostate carcinogenesis began at least 2 decades ago with the observation that prostate cancer mortality rates correlated very strongly with per capita fat consumption on an international basis (Armstrong and Doll 1975). Although such an observation provides at best very weak evidence of a causal relationship, a series of epidemiologic studies, both case-control and cohort in design, have subsequently been conducted, providing a more direct test of this hypothesis. Although these studies have varied considerably in quality, they have rather consistently demonstrated an association between high fat consumption and prostate cancer risk. Of the seven case-control studies with reasonable statistical power to determine an overall relationship between fat consumption and prostate cancer risk, six found that the prostate cancer patients tended to consume more fat than the controls (Ross and Schottenfeld, in press). These six studies have involved populations with a wide range of underlying prostate cancer risk, but have utilized a variety of strategies for selecting controls, some based more on convenience than representativeness. Overall, these studies do not suggest any systematic differences in risk by type of fat intake (animal vs vegetable or saturated vs unsaturated).

There have also been three prospective studies which have reported on the possible association between fat consumption and prostate cancer risk (Severson et al. 1989; LeMarchand et al. 1994; Giovannucci et al. 1993). This type of study design has the important potential advantage over case-control studies of not being subject to recall bias, as the dietary history is collected prior to disease development.

Two of these prospective studies were conducted in Hawaii with different results. One involved 8000 Japanese-Americans and included 174 men who had developed prostate cancer during follow-up; this study found no association with fat consumption (Severson et al. 1989). The second study was larger (more than 20 000 participants with 198 incident prostate cancers) and multiethnic, but was limited by an incomplete dietary history (LeMarchand et al. 1994). Nonetheless, those men in the highest tertile of a summary index of consumption of foods high in animal fat had a 60% increase in prostate cancer risk. The most comprehensive prospective study to date to examine this relationship was the Health Professionals Follow-up Study of 47 855 men aged 40–75 years who completed a 131-item food frequency questionnaire (Giovannucci et al. 1993). After 4 years of follow-up, 300 prostate cancers had occurred. Men in the highest quartile of estimated fat intake had an elevated risk of prostate cancer. This association was limited to men with advanced disease, who had an 80% increase in risk, relative to men in the lowest quartile, and the relationship was primarily due to fat from animal sources, especially red meat.

A relationship between at least certain components of dietary fat and prostate cancer is also supported by a prospective study which measured certain essential fatty acids in plasma among men who developed prostate cancer and those who did not (Gann et al. 1994). Plasma concentrations of α-linolenic acid were elevated in the 120 men with prostate cancer. Men in the highest quartile had a threefold excess risk compared to men in the lowest quartile. Red meat is a major source of α-linolenic acid.

Although an association between fat consumption and prostate cancer is not fully established, published studies certainly support the existence of such a relationship. Berg proposed in 1975 that dietary fat might affect prostate cancer occurrence by altering the hormonal environment (Berg 1975). Two small studies, one a trial in which men were given an isocaloric low fat diet (Hill and Wynder 1979) and the second of Seventh Day Adventists who either adhered to a lacto-ovo vegetarian diet or did not (Ellis and Nyberg 1992), both suggested that a reduction in fat, especially from animal sources, might result in a reduction in circulating testosterone levels.

1.4.1.2 Vitamin A/Beta Carotene

Beta carotene is a provitamin A antioxidant which can deactivate free radicals which damage DNA, potentially causing mutations or other genetic changes involved in carcinogenesis. The parent compound, vitamin A, has also generated considerable interest as a cancer chemopreventive agent because of its important role in cellular differentiation and in enhancing cell membrane permeability. Interest in these compounds related to prostate cancer risk specifically was stimulated by a report by Hirayama in 1979 (Hirayama 1979). In a prospective study of 265 000 Japanese men and women, daily consumption of green-yellow vegetables, a principal source of beta carotene, was associated with a 60% reduction in prostate cancer mortality. There have been a large number of subsequent studies which have evaluated some aspect of the relationship between vitamin A compounds and prostate cancer risk (Ross and Schottenfeld, in press). However, as many studies have found an increased risk of prostate cancer with increasing intake of vitamin A as have found a decreased risk. The literature is somewhat more supportive of a protective influence of beta carotene but again study results are not highly consistent. In addition to the dietary studies, there have been four prospective studies and one case-control study of serum levels of vitamin A compounds and prostate cancer risk (Kark et al. 1981; Willett et al. 1984; Hsing et al. 1990; Reichman et al. 1990; Hayes et al. 1988). These studies rather consistently observed lower retinol levels in prostate cancer patients than in controls, but none had substantial statistical power. The totality of epidemiologic evidence for a role of vitamin A compounds in altering risk of prostate cancer is not compelling.

1.4.1.3 Vitamin D

Although there are limited data on the relationship between vitamin D and prostate cancer risk currently, this possible association has received increased attention in the past few years. 1,25-dihydroxyvitamin D (1,25-D), the active human vitamin D metabolite, inhibits cells proliferation in cultured normal and malignant prostatic epithelium and plays a role in differentiation of prostate cells (SKOWRONSKI et al. 1993). There are no adequate studies of vitamin D and prostate cancer related to either dietary or sunlight sources; in fact, the relationship between these vitamin D sources and circulating levels of 1,25-D is not fully known. A prospective serologic study of 1,25-D found that levels were substantially and significantly lower among men who developed clinically apparent prostate cancer than those who did not (CORDER et al. 1993).

1.4.1.4 Phytoestrogens

Phytoestrogens, for example isoflavonoids found in soy products, are estrogens with weak biologic activity, which have been suggested as possibly playing a role in the low risk of Asian men of developing prostate cancer. Circulating levels of phytoestrogen metabolites are, as predicted, much higher on average in Asian men than in whites (ADLERCREUTZ et al. 1993). These estrogenic compounds may reduce androgenic action in the prostate by weakly competing for androgen receptor binding sites or perhaps via other mechanisms.

1.4.2 Sexually Transmitted Diseases

There have been a substantial number of studies over the past 25 years which have evaluated the relationship between sexual activity factors (age at first intercourse, frequency of intercourse, number of sexual partners, history of sexually transmitted diseases, etc.). Studies of most of these factors have produced highly inconsistent results, perhaps in part because of the difficulty in ascertaining accurate self-reported information on these matters (ROSS and SCHOTTENFELD, in press). Nonetheless, a fairly consistent finding in epidemiologic studies of prostate cancer is an increased risk associated with a past history of sexually transmitted diseases, especially gonorrhea, the elevation in risk across all such studies being two- to threefold among men reporting such a history (ROSS and SCHOTTENFELD, in press). As there is minimal additional experimental or epidemiologic support that prostate cancer is caused directly by a sexually transmitted agent, an alternative explanation has been proposed for this association; namely, the possibility that a sexually transmitted disease history is an index of sexual activity, which, in turn, might be an index of an individual's underlying androgen profile.

1.4.3 Vasectomy

Honda and colleagues first suggested that a positive relationship exists between vasectomy and prostate cancer (HONDA et al. 1988). Although they did not find a statistically significant association between vasectomy and prostate cancer risk overall, among the relatively young (<age 60) men they studied, the risk level clearly increased with interval from vasectomy, and that relationship was statistically significant. As 15% of all U.S. men over age 40 have had a vasectomy (HUBER 1986), it is clearly important to establish definitively this possible relationship. GIOVANNUCI et al. (1993) conducted a meta-analysis of the six better designed studies (five case-control and one cohort study) which had addressed this hypothesis. They found a 50% overall increase in risk of prostate cancer associated with vasectomy ($P < 0.05$); risk became more pronounced with interval since vasectomy. Another large well-designed case-control study was reported after the publication of this meta-analysis (JOHN et al. 1995). This study involved multiple racial/ethnic groups but among none of these was there strong evidence of a vasectomy/prostate cancer risk association.

Despite the absence of totally consistent data, the bulk of the evidence supports an association. The most frequently suggested mechanism involves an indirect, rather than a causal, relationship; i.e., that vasectomy is related to sexual practices and to underlying hormonal influences (HONDA et al. 1988). There are some data for example, that vasectomized men have higher testosterone levels than men of similar age who have not undergone this procedure (HONDA et al. 1988; JOHN et al. 1995).

1.5 Internal Factors

1.5.1 Hormonal Influences

Because of the important role played by hormones in controlling growth and proliferation of prostate epithelium, it is reasonable that the same hormones might be intimately involved in abnormal prostate growth, including carcinogenesis.

Although a number of studies have compared circulating and intraprostatic levels of androgens and other hormones in men with and without prostate cancer, the results of these studies are inconsistent and, in any event, are difficult if not impossible to interpret because of the potential confounding influence of the disease process itself on the hormonal milieu.

Studies which have compared cross-sectionally hormonal patterns among healthy men at varying risk of prostate cancer have proven more valuable and have offered substantial, albeit indirect, evidence that androgens might be involved in prostate cancer development. Ross and colleagues, for example, found that young adult African-American men, with an expected lifetime incidence of prostate cancer roughly twice that of young adult white American men, have an approximately 15% higher level of circulating testosterone than whites, a difference that was not explicable on the basis of differences in other known determinants of circulating testosterone (Ross et al. 1986). Others have also found higher testosterone levels in African-American than in white men, but have found that the absolute difference tends to dissipate with age (Howie and Schultz 1985). In fact, the study by Ross and colleagues predicted this phenomenon. They conducted calculations based on assumptions about the effects of changing testosterone levels on prostate cell kinetics and tissue aging and determined that a 15% difference in testosterone between African-Americans and whites sustained over a lifetime was too large to explain the actual difference in prostate cancer incidence between these two groups.

While Asian men at low risk of prostate cancer do not have abnormally low levels of circulating testosterone, there exist cross-sectional data suggesting that such men metabolize testosterone intraprostatically differently than whites and African-Americans. As noted above, testosterone is metabolically activated to its reduced form, DHT, through the activity of 5α-reductase. Although some DHT enters the circulation from the prostate, the majority of DHT is further metabolized to other 5α androgens, androstanediol and to a lesser extent androsterone, by the enzyme 3α-hydroxysteroid dehydrogenase, and these androgens enter the circulation as their glucuronide conjugates. Ross and colleagues have shown that young adult native Japanese men have at least a 25% lower level of these hormones than whites or African-Americans (Ross et al. 1992), whereas Lookingbill et al. (1991) showed similar differences among Hong Kong Chinese men compared to whites.

These combined data suggest that some of the racial/ethnic difference in prostate cancer incidence might be due to a combination of racial/ethnic differences in testosterone secretion and intraprostatic activity of 5α-reductase.

Experimental evidence also supports a role of androgens in prostate carcinogenesis. Historically, it has proven difficult to produce adenocarcinomas of the prostate in any experimental animal model. In the 1970s Noble demonstrated that testosterone administration could produce such tumors in one strain of rats (Noble 1977). Subsequently others have produced adenocarcinomas experimentally in different systems, but there is not yet a highly reproducible animal model for adenocarcinoma of the prostate without an androgen requirement as a primary or adjuvant agent.

1.5.2 Genetics

Conceptually it is possible to distinguish between two types of genetic alterations that are associated with cancer, namely *germline* and *somatic*. Although the two might be linked mechanistically in certain cases, the latter type is often acquired as the result of environmental effects (possibly with genetic interactions) and is specifically confined to the organ in question. In most cases, cancer appears to develop and progress through a well-demarcated sequence of multiple such genetic changes (Vogelstein and Kinzler 1993). Some germline genetic loci associated with cancer simply predispose to the disease. However, such single inherited genetic traits that are necessary and sufficient to cause cancer are rare and have low population attributable risks. Much more common are susceptibility genes with low absolute risk, but with potentially high population attributable risks (Caporaso and Goldstein 1995). Such genes do not directly "cause" cancer, but affect risk of developing cancer indirectly. They probably influence cancer risk in concert with each other, to create what can be viewed as the "polygeric" etiology of the particular cancer in question.

1.5.2.1 Germline Predisposition

There can be no doubt that prostate cancer is a familial disease. A series of epidemiologic studies, mostly case-control in design, have shown that first-degree relatives of men with prostate cancer have themselves a two- to threefold excess risk of developing the disease (Ross and SCHOTTENFELD, in press). Steinberg and colleagues have reported that with two first-degree relatives with prostate cancer, risk is elevated fivefold, while with more than two, risk is more than tenfold higher than in men with no family history (STEINBERG et al. 1990). It is important to distinguish between the terms "hereditary" and "familial" when referring to prostate cancer occurring in families (CARTER et al. 1993). Hereditary prostate cancer is a more specific term and refers to a distribution of cancer cases within a family that is consistent with mendelian inheritance of a single gene. One specific form of hereditary prostate cancer is consistent with an autosomal dominant mode of inheritance in which it has been determined that the putative unknown locus might be responsible for about 9% of all prostate cancer cases (CARTER et al. 1992). This type of prostate cancer is distinguished by an early age of onset. On the other hand, prostate cancer that occurs more commonly in relatives of an affected individual than in the general population is defined as "familial." This type of cancer is likely to be multifactorial, involving more than one gene as well as environmental exposures, in addition to perhaps complex gene-gene and gene-environmental interactions. The well-known androgen dependence of prostate cancer has led to the postulate that androgens and genes associated with the androgen response of prostate epithelial cells might contribute to the development of this form of familial disease.

How does one sort out the genetic predisposition of a complex trait like the susceptibility to prostate cancer? As summarized by LANDER and SCHORK (1994), four major approaches have been successfully employed to address this problem in other complex diseases. These are linkage analysis using pedigrees, allele-sharing methods using sibs (twins or otherwise), association approaches (case-control studies) of candidate genes, and experimental crosses using laboratory animals. Potentially all four can be used to dissect the etiology of prostate cancer, but for at least the first three the identification of candidate genes would be most helpful.

Some of the possible candidate genes predisposing to prostate cancer, their alleles, and potential roles are listed in Table 1.2.

The candidacy of the androgen receptor (AR) as a predisposition gene for prostate cancer has received legitimacy due to different lines of evidence. In two separate studies, HAYES et al. (1995) and NAROD et al. (1995) reported that the relative risks for developing prostate cancer associated with a history of prostate cancer were significantly higher in men reporting affected brothers versus affected fathers. These results not only emphasize the possible presence of a genetic component in prostate cancer risk in the general population, but also suggest a possible genetic association between brothers with the disease, not shared to the same degree by their fathers. In a recent study (MONROE et al. 1995), we obtained similar results in 7272 males among four racial/ethnic groups; the prevalence rate of prostate cancer in subjects with affected brothers was about two or

Table 1.2. Candidate genes for prostate cancer predisposition

Candidate (function)	Alleles	Possible role in prostate carcinogenesis	Reference
Androgen receptor (translates androgen effects)	CAG/GGC micro-satellites	? Variation in transactivation; ? subsequent effects on growth	COETZEE and ROSS (1994)
5α-Reductase (conversion of testosterone to DHT)	TA repeat 3′-UTR	? Variation in enzyme activity	ROSS et al. (1995)
17α-Hydroxylase (CYP17) (catalyzes rate-limiting step in androgen biosynthesis)	MspA1 RFLP 5′ promoter	Creates additional SP1 transcription site; ? increased expression	CAREY et al. (1994)
Vitamin D receptor (translates vitamin D effects)	Bsm 1 RFLP 3′-UTR	? Variation in mRNA stability; ? variation in promotion of differentiation	MORRISON et al. (1994)

more times that in subjects reporting affected fathers, in each of the four racial/ethnic groups under study. As a control for potential confounders in screening practices that could account for these differences, we evaluated the affected sister/mother risks of breast cancer in 13 865 female subjects of the same populations. No mother versus sister differences in risk were observed. These studies suggest the possible involvement of an X-linked genetic component in the etiology of prostate cancer, although rare recessive traits cannot be excluded at this time. A candidate on the X chromosome is the AR, each man inheriting a single allele with his maternal X chromosome. Although the AR was excluded (negative lod score) as a candidate gene in the "hereditary" form of the disease in seven Utah families (Cannon-Albright and Eeles 1995), the data to date do not exclude the AR gene from being one among many genes contributing to the "familial" predisposition of the disease, especially among men in the general population. In fact, we have recently hypothesized (Coetzee and Ross 1994), and have subsequently provided evidence (Irvine et al. 1995), that the two microsatellites located in exon 1 of the AR gene are associated with the development of prostate cancer. We have further postulated that these satellites are not simply silent polymorphisms, but affect receptor activity directly, and in this way predispose certain men to the disease. The AR gene, therefore, seems to be one among several genes participating in prostate cancer risk.

A second candidate for the genetic predisposition to prostate cancer is the steroid 5α-reductase type II gene which is expressed in the prostate (Thigpen et al. 1993). The enzyme product of this gene catalyzes the conversion of testosterone to the physiologically important prostate androgen, DHT (Coffey 1993). Clearly it is conceivable that the levels of intracellular DHT and subsequent downstream events will be affected by the level and activity of this enzyme. We have recently reported on the ethnic allelic differences of this gene and preliminary results indicate that among African-Americans, serum levels of 5α-androgens correlate with the presence of certain variants at this locus (Ross et al. 1995).

A third candidate for the genetic predisposition to prostate cancer is the gene for CYP17 (17α-hydroxylase; 17/20 lyase). This enzyme is rate-limiting in androgen biosynthesis. The gene contains a single base-pair polymorphism in its 5′ promoter region, and two alleles have been described that can be conveniently assayed for due to the creation/destruction of an Msp A1 site. Furthermore, it is possible that this polymorphism is not a silent one, since the C to T transition creates an additional SP-1 type *cis* site, possibly increasing expression of the gene (Carey et al. 1994). In families where female members suffer from polycystic ovaries and males from premature male pattern baldness, the C-containing allele (creating the SP-1 site) is associated with these phenotypes although the locus was excluded as the primary genetic defect (Carey et al. 1994).

Finally, a fourth member of the list of candidates for the predisposition to prostate cancer is the gene for the vitamin D receptor (VDR). As described above, vitamin D metabolites may play an important role in prostate physiology. Recently the exciting finding was reported that allelic variation at the VDR locus accounted for as much as 75% of the total genetic effect on bone density in healthy individuals (Morrison et al. 1994; Yamagata et al. 1994). The allelic variants analyzed (found in introns at this locus) were in strong linkage disequilibrium with several other polymorphisms in the 3′-untranslated region (3′-UTR) of the mRNA, and the authors demonstrated that two of the 3′-UTRs associated with the two most frequent alleles caused a nearly twofold difference in the steady state expression of a reporter gene in in vitro transfection assays (Morrison et al. 1994). This indicates that allelic variation at this locus might affect the quantitative expression of VDR, possibly through differences in mRNA stability. It is therefore possible that variation at the VDR locus will affect prostate cancer in a manner similar to the way it affects bone mineral density. In unpublished results from our group, we observed a deficit in certain VDR alleles among men with prostate cancer (Coetzee, La Pera, Ross and Yu, unpublished observations), substantiating the case for this gene as a candidate in prostate cancer predisposition.

The above-mentioned candidates were chosen for the present discussion simply because of their likely link with prostate cancer and to illustrate the principle of polygeric etiology. Undoubtedly, other genes at other loci will contribute to this disease process as well. We predict that such genes contribute to prostate cancer risk in subtle ways and that a lifelong "exposure" to their effects is needed to increase the risk of the disease. Although important, it will be particularly challenging to characterize the effects of the genes which contribute to subtle risk changes and to determine the modulating potential of life-style variables on risk, so that ultimately risk profiles can be assembled for individual men.

1.5.2.2 Somatic Changes

The most widely held paradigm for cells to change from a normal to a malignant phenotype is the activation of one or several proto-oncogenes and/or the inactivation of one or several tumor suppressor genes. Activation of proto-oncogenes (often genes that promote cellular growth) and/or inactivation of tumor suppressor genes (often genes that normally act to restrict or regulate cellular growth) can occur through a number of somatic mechanisms, including mutation, amplification, and translocation. A model for the sequential changes leading to the progression of prostate cancer has been proposed (Isaacs et al. 1995), and possibly involves chromosomes 8, 10, and 16, perhaps in addition to changes at the sites also found in many other tumors (chromosomes 17 and 13, for example). It is possible, however, that multiple pathways exist for prostate tumor development with respect to sequential genetic changes. Molecular genetic studies support at least two alternate pathways for bladder tumor development, for example (Spruck et al. 1994). Recently described somatic genetic changes specific to prostate cancer include mutations in the MXI1 gene (its product competes with the Myc oncoprotein and inhibits transcription of Myc-activated genes) (Eagle et al. 1995) and methylation (with associated silencing) of the gene for the detoxifying enzyme, glutathione *S*-transferase π (Lee et al. 1994).

Another type of genetic change unique to prostate cancer might be a set of "gain-in-function" somatic mutations in the hormone binding domain (HBD) of the androgen receptor (AR) leading to a selective growth advantage to cells harboring these changes and, thus, to the progression of the disease. One such mutation was first observed in the HBD of the AR in a prostate cancer cell line, LNCap (codon 877), and was responsible for the conversion of antiandrogen (such as flutamide) effects from antagonistic to agonistic (Harris et al. 1990; Veldscholte et al. 1990). Subsequently, the same codon 877 mutation was identified in prostate cancer specimens. Suzuki et al. (1993) reported the mutation in one (of eight) specimens, whereas Gaddipati et al. (1994) selected 24 transurethral resected specimens of prostate cancer and found the mutation in six cases (25%). This strikingly high incidence suggests that the codon 877 mutation may represent a mutational "hot spot" due to its functional consequences. More recently, investigators in The Netherlands (Sharief et al. 1995) identified a mutation in codon 874 in a human prostate cancer specimen. The mutation was recreated and expressed in CV-1 cells conferring growth responsiveness to testosterone, DHT, estradiol, and most importantly also to hydroxyflutamide in a manner similar to the LNCap codon 877 mutation. In another study, Taplin et al. (1995), recently analyzed the AR mRNA for expression and mutations in ten metastatic prostate tumors. All ten patients had received some form of hormone deprivation treatment for periods of 1–48 months. Point mutations (all in the HBD of the receptor) were found in five of these samples and interestingly, three of these patients received flutamide as part of their prior treatment regimen. In the two cases the authors could analyze, the mutations were not found in the primary tumors, and were confined to the metastatic lesions. Functional studies also revealed that two of the mutant receptors could be activated by progesterone or estrogen. The situation regarding ligand specificity in the remaining three is not known. These types of "gain-in-function" mutations have been implicated to explain the clinical phenomena of tumor regression upon flutamide *withdrawal* after prolonged treatment, and subsequent failure, with flutamide (Dupont et al. 1993; Scher and Kelly 1993; Sartor et al. 1994).

Another genetic alteration at the AR locus associated with advanced prostate cancer is gene amplification. As in the case of gain-in-function point mutations, these amplifications are possibly also selected for as a result of hormone deprivation treatments. Such amplifications were in fact observed in men who had received and failed hormone therapy of various kinds (Visakorpi et al. 1995). These authors suggested that "AR amplification emerges during androgen deprivation therapy by facilitating tumor cell growth in low androgen concentrations."

It is possible, therefore, to view the AR gene as a kind of proto-oncogene that functions normally during the development and differentiation of the prostate, but during carcinogenesis can undergo gain-in-function mutations and/or gene amplification contributing to the development of certain cancer cell clones with a selective advantage to grow under conditions that preclude normal prostate epithelium from proliferating (for example during hormone deprivation treatment).

From the above one can draw the conclusion that "hormone refractory" prostate cancer is an operational phrase reflecting the clinical activity of the disease but not the genetic characteristics of the advanced tumor itself. In many cases the hormone "refractile" tumor remains dependent on androgens

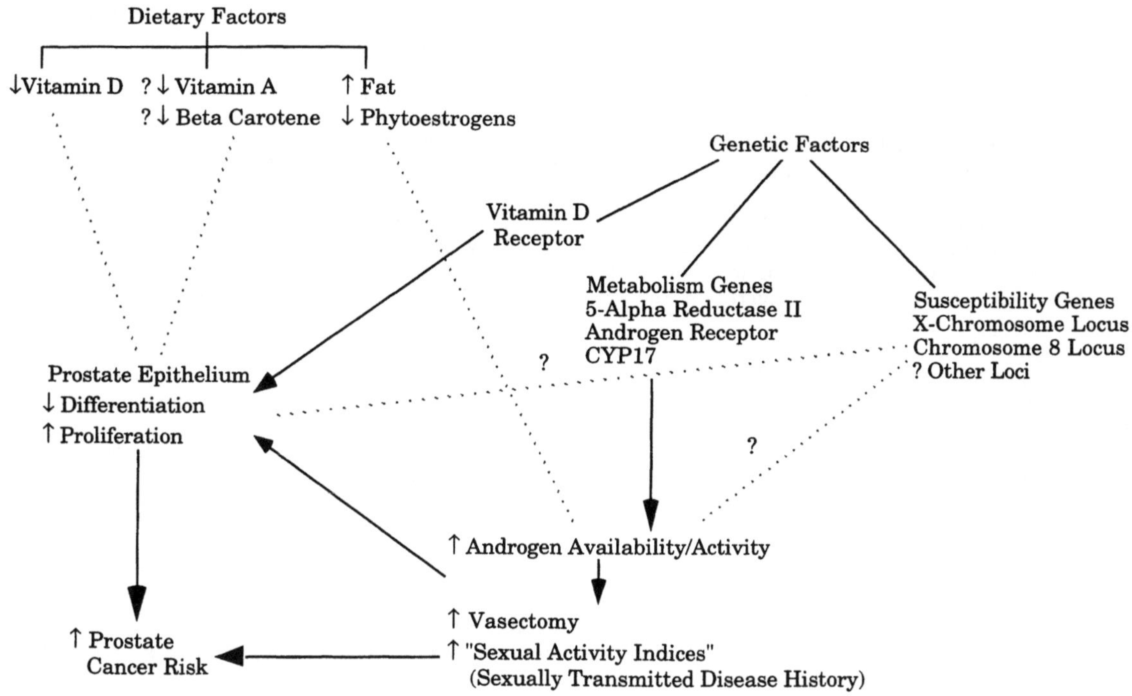

Fig. 1.1. Model overview of prostatic carcinogenesis

(albeit in an altered way) for growth. This recognition might lead to the development of new treatment strategies.

1.6 Conclusion

Figure 1.1 attempts to summarize our current conceptualization of prostate cancer etiology and to tie together in a meaningful way the apparently disparate risk factors for the disease. We believe that all of these risk factors, internal and external, can ultimately be related back to hormonal influences on prostate cell proliferation and differentiation.

References

Adlercreutz H, Markkanen H, Watanabe S (1993) Plasma concentrations of phytoestrogens in Japanese men. Lancet 342:1209–1210

American Cancer Society: Cancer Facts and Figures (1994)

Armstrong B, Doll R (1975) Environmental factors and cancer incidence and mortality in different countries, with special reference to dietary practices. Int J Cancer 15:617–631

Berg JW (1975) Can nutrition explain the pattern of international epidemiology of hormone-dependent cancers? Cancer Res 35:3345–3350

Cannon-Albright L, Eeles R (1995) Progress in prostate cancer. Nature Genet 9:336–338

Caporaso N, Goldstein A (1995) Cancer genes: single and susceptibility: exposing the difference. Pharmacogenetics 5:59–63

Carey AH, Waterworth D, Patel K et al. (1994) Polycystic ovaries and premature male pattern baldness are associated with one allele of the steroid metabolism gene CYP17. Hum Mol Genet 3:1873–1876

Carter BS, Beaty TH, Steinberg GD et al. (1992) Mendelian inheritance of familial prostate cancer. Proc Natl Acad Sci USA 89:3367–3371

Carter BS, Bova S, Beaty TH et al. (1993) Hereditary prostate cancer: epidemiologic and clinical features. J Urol 150:797–802

Coetzee GA, Ross RK (1994) Prostate cancer and the androgen receptor. J Natl Cancer Inst 86:872–873

Coffey DS (1979) Physiological control of prostatic growth. An overview. In: Prostate Cancer. UICC Technical Report Series, vol 48. International Union Against Cancer, Geneva

Coffey DS (1993) The molecular biology of the prostate. In: Lepor H, Lawson RK (eds) Prostate Disease. Saunders, Philadelphia, pp 28–56

Corder EH, Guess HA, Hulka BS et al. (1993) Vitamin D and prostate cancer: a prediagnostic study with stored sera. Cancer Epidemiol Biomarkers Prev 2:467–472

Dupont A, Gomez JL, Cusan L, Koutsilieris, Labrie F (1993) Response to flutamide withdrawal in advanced prostate cancer in progression under combination therapy. J Urol 150:908–913

Eagle LR, Yin X, Brothman AR et al. (1995) Mutation of the MXI1 gene in prostate cancer. Nature Genet 9:249–255

Ellis L, Nyberg H (1992) Racial/ethnic variations in male testosterone levels: a probable contribution to group differences in health. Steroids 57:72–75

Gaddipati JP, McLeod DG, Heidenberg HB et al. (1994) Frequent detection of codon 877 mutation in the androgen

receptor gene in advanced prostate cancers. Cancer Res 54:2861–2864
Gann PH, Hennekens CH, Sacks FM et al. (1994) Prospective study of plasma fatty acids and risk of prostate cancer. J Natl Cancer Inst 86:281–286
Giovannucci E, Rimm EB, Colditz GA et al. (1993) A prospective study of dietary fat and risk of prostate cancer. J Natl Cancer Inst 85:1571–1579
Harris SE, Rong Z, Harris MA, Lubahn DD (1990) Androgen receptor in human prostate carcinoma LNCaP/ADEP cells contains a mutation which alters the specificity of the steroid-dependent transcriptional activation region. Endocrinology 126 (Suppl):93
Hayes RB, Bogdanovicz FAT, Schroeder FH et al. (1988) Serum retinol and prostate cancer. Cancer 62:2021–2026
Hayes RB, Liff JM, Pottern LM et al. (1995) Prostate cancer risk in US Blacks and Whites with a family history of prostate cancer. Int J Cancer 60:361–364
Hill PB, Wynder EL (1979) Effect of vegetarian diet and dexamethasone on plasma prolactin, testosterone and dehydroepiandrosterone in men and women. Cancer Lett 7:273–282
Hirayama T (1979) Epidemiology of prostate cancer with special reference to the role of diet. NCI Monogr 53:149–155
Honda GD, Bernstein L, Ross RK, Greenland S, Gerkins V, Henderson BE (1988) Vasectomy, cigarette smoking, and age at first sexual intercourse as risk factors for prostate cancer in middle-aged men. Br J Cancer 57:326–331
Howie BJ, Schultz JD (1985) Dietary and hormonal interrelationships among vegetarian Seventh-Day Adventists and nonvegetarian men. Am J Clin Nutr 42:127–134
Hsing WA, Comstock GW, Abbey H et al. (1990) Serologic precursors of cancer, retinol, carotenoids, and tocopherol and risk of prostate cancer. J Natl Cancer Inst 82:941–946
Huber DR, Hong S, Ross JA (1986) The international experience with vasectomy. In: Zatuchni GI, Goldsmith A, Spieler JM (eds) Male contraception: advances and future prospects. Harper and Row, Philadelphia, pp 7–18
Irvine RA, Yu MC, Ross RK, Coetzee GA (1995) The CAG and GGC microsatellites of the androgen receptor gene are in linkage disequilibrium in men with prostate cancer. Cancer Res 55:1937–1940
Isaacs WB, Bova GS, Morton RA et al. (1995) Molecular genetics and chromosomal alterations in prostate cancer. Cancer 75:2004–2012
John EM, Whittemore AJ, Wu AH et al. (1995) Vasectomy and prostate cancer: results from a multiethnic case-control study. J Natl Cancer Inst 87:662–669
Kark JD, Smith AH, Switzer BR et al. (1981) Serum vitamin A (retinol) and cancer incidence in Evans County, Georgia. J Natl Cancer Inst 66:7–16
Lander ES, Schork NJ (1994) Genetic dissection of complex traits. Science 265:2037–2048
Lee W-H, Morton RA, Epstein JI et al. (1994) Cytidine methylation of regulatory sequences near the p-class glutathione S-transferase gene accompanies human prostatic carcinogenesis. Proc Natl Acad Sci USA 91:11733–11737
LeMarchand L, Kolonel LN, Wilkens LR et al. (1994) Animal fat consumption and prostate cancer: a prospective study in Hawaii. Epidemiology 5:276–282
Lookingbill DP, Demers LM, Wang C et al. (1991) Clinical and biological parameters of androgen action in normal healthy Caucasian versus Chinese subjects. J Clin Endocrinol Metab 72:1242–1248
Monroe KR, Yu MC, Kolonel LN et al. (1995) Evidence of X-linked genetic component to prostate cancer risk. Nature Med 1:827–829
Morrison NA, Jian CQ, Tokita A et al. (1994) Prediction of bone density from vitamin D receptor alleles. Nature 367:284–287
Muir C, Waterhouse J, Mack T et al. (eds) (1987) Cancer incidence in five continents, vol V. IARC, Lyons
Narod SA, Dupont A, Cusan L et al. (1995) The impact of family history on early detection of prostate cancer. Nature Med 1:99–101
Noble RL (1977) The development of prostatic adenocarcinoma in Nb rats following prolonged sex hormone administration. Cancer Res 37:1929–1933
Parker KL, Schimmer BP (1994) The role of nuclear receptors in steroid hormone production. Semin Cancer Biol 5:317–325
Reichman ME, Hayes RB, Ziegler RG et al. (1990) Serum vitamin A and subsequent development of prostate cancer in the First National Health and Nutrition Examination Survey Epidemiologic Follow-up Study. Cancer Res 50:2311–2315
Ries LAG, Hankey BD, Edwards BK (eds) (1990) Cancer Statistics Review, 1973–87. NIH, Bethesda, MD. NIH Publ 90:2789
Ross RK, Schottenfeld D (1996) Prostate. In: Schottenfeld D, Fraumeni J (eds) Cancer epidemiology and prevention, 2nd edn. W.B. Saunders, Philadelphia (in press)
Ross RK, McCurtis JW, Henderson BE et al. (1979) Descriptive epidemiology of testicular and prostatic cancer in Los Angeles. Br J Cancer 39:284–292
Ross RK, Bernstein L, Judd H et al. (1986) Serum testosterone levels in young black and white men. J Natl Cancer Inst 76:45–48
Ross RK, Bernstein L, Lobo RA et al. (1992) 5-alpha-reductase activity and risk of prostate cancer among Japanese and U.S. white and black males. Lancet 339:887–890
Ross RK, Coetzee GA, Reichardt J, Skinner E, Henderson BE (1995) Does the racial-ethnic variation in prostate cancer risk have a hormonal basis? Cancer 74:1778–1782
Sartor O, Cooper M, Weinberger M et al. (1994) Surprising activity of flutamide withdrawal, when combined with aminoglutethimide, in treatment of "hormone-refractory" prostate cancer. J Natl Cancer Inst 86:222–227
Scher HI, Kelly WK (1993) Flutamide withdrawal syndrome: its impact on clinical trials in hormone-refractory prostate cancer. J Clin Oncol 11:1566–1572
Severson RK, Nomura AMY, Grove JS et al. (1989) A prospective study of demographics, diet, and prostate cancer among men of Japanese ancestry in Hawaii. Cancer Res 49:1857–1860
Sharief Y, Wilson EM, Hall SH et al. (1995) Androgen receptor gene mutations associated with prostatic carcinoma. Proc AACR 36:269
Shimizu H, Ross RK, Bernstein L (1991) Possible underestimation of incidence rate of prostate cancer in Japan. Jpn J Cancer Res 82:483–485
Skowronski RJ, Peehl DM, Feldman D (1993) Vitamin D and prostate cancer: 1,25-dihydroxyvitamin D3 receptors and action in human prostate cancer cell lines. Endocrinology 132:1952–1960
Spruck CH, Ohneseit PF, Gonzalez-Zulueta M et al. (1994) Two molecular pathways to transitional cell carcinoma of the bladder. Cancer Res 54:784–788
Steinberg GD, Carter BS, Beaty TH et al. (1990) Family history and the risk of prostate cancer. Prostate 17:337–347

Suzuki H, Sato N, Watabe Y et al. (1993) Androgen receptor gene mutations in human prostate cancer. J Steroid Biochem Mol Biol 46:759–765
Taplin M-E, Bubley GJ, Shuster TD et al. (1995) Mutation of the androgen-receptor gene in metastatic androgen-independent prostate cancer. N Engl J Med 332:1393–1398
Thigpen AE, Silver RI, Guileyardo JM, Casey ML, McConnell JD, Russell DW (1993) Tissue distribution and ontogeny of steroid 5α-reductase isoenzyme expression. J Clin Invest 92:903–910
Veldscholte J, Ris-Stalpers C, Kuiper GGJM et al. (1990) A mutation in the ligand binding domain of the androgen receptor of human LNCaP cells affects steroid binding characteristics and response to anti-androgens. Biochem Biophys Res Commun 173:534–540
Visakorpi T, Hyytinen E, Koivisto P et al. (1995) In vivo amplification of the androgen receptor gene and progression of human prostate cancer. Nature Genet 9:401–406a
Vogelstein B, Kinzler KW (1993) The multistep nature of cancer. Trends Genet 9:138–141
Willett WC, Polk BF, Underwood BA et al. (1984) Relation of serum vitamins A and E, and carotenoids to the risk of cancer. N Engl J Med 310:430–434
Yamagata Z, Miyamura T, Iijima S, Asaka A, Sasaki M, Kato J, Koizumi K (1994) Vitamin D receptor gene polymorphism and bone mineral density in healthy Japanese women. Lancet 344:1027
Zaridze DG, Boyle P, Smans M (1984) International trends in prostatic cancer. Int J Cancer 33:223–230

2 Natural History of Prostate Cancer

W.J. KIRKELS

CONTENTS

2.1 Introduction

Knowledge of the natural history of prostate cancer is needed to give an indication of the prognosis once the tumor is diagnosed. The patient requires information about the expected course of the disease before a decision can be made about treatment. Several treatment options are available in the case of localized disease. Radical prostatectomy and radiotherapy are advocated for local treatment with curative intention. There is extensive debate over whether treatment is necessary in prostate cancer patients in whom it is possible, and on the other hand whether treatment is possible in those in whom it is needed (WHITMORE 1988).

From autopsy studies it is known that over the age of 50 in the general male population the prevalence of occult prostate cancer is high (FRANKS 1954, 1973), i.e., up to 33% depending upon the step sectioning technique used. BOSTWICK (1989) described a number of steps that can be identified in the pathogenesis of prostate cancer in humans by the use of morphologic and functional criteria. It must be realized that each of these morphologic changes probably reflects genetic events of unknown nature. According to BOSTWICK (1989) the development of prostate cancer can be characterized as follows:

- Normal epithelium
- Prostatic intraepithelial neoplasia (PIN)
- Focal carcinoma
- Adenocarcinoma, hormonally dependent
- Adenocarcinoma, hormone independent

SAKR et al. (1993) found low-grade PIN as early as the third decade of life. High-grade PIN was first found in the fifth decade of life, and all five prostates examined also showed histologic carcinoma. The investigators concluded that the initiating events leading to clinically relevant prostate cancer likely occur at a remarkably young age. CUMMING (1990) showed that there is dedifferentiation of prostatic carcinoma with time. WHITMORE (1988) described the possibilities in stage progression (Fig. 2.1), and recently adapted this model to the TNM system (WHITMORE et al. 1994).

It is clear from Fig. 2.1 that the development of prostate cancer can be expected to follow a strict stepwise pattern, but on the other hand several steps in the development can unexpectedly be omitted or go by undetected. Furthermore, in some cases it has been shown that no disease progression from one stage to another occurs with time, indicating the limited growth potential of some prostate cancers.

The observation that many men die with prostate cancer but do not die from prostate cancer was the basis for the debate about the necessity of treatment of patients with localized tumors. An attempt will be made to elucidate the natural history of prostate cancer based upon data from the literature describing the progression rate, metastasis-free survival, disease-free survival, disease-related mortality and overall mortality in patients treated expectantly.

2.2 Prognosis by Stage

2.2.1 Stage T1a and T1b (A1, A2) Prostate Cancer

Stages T1a and T1b are not palpable on rectal examination. The tumors are usually found in the tissue

W.J. KIRKELS, MD, PhD, Department of Urology, Erasmus University and Academic Hospital Dijkzigt, Dr. Molewaterplein 40, 3015 GD Rotterdam, The Netherlands

```
Stage A ---------> B --------->C ----------> D
Stage A ---------- -- ----------- — ----------> D
Stage A ---------- -- --------->C
Stage A ---------> B ---------------------> D
        time ---------->
```

Fig. 2.1. Possibilities in stage progression of prostate cancer, according to WHITMORE (1988)

removed at the time of transurethral resection or during open prostatectomy for presumably benign disease. The categories T1a and T1b are comparable with stages A1 and A2 in the American staging system. The incidence of these stages depends on: the extent of the surgical removal of the benign prostatic hyperplasia tissue, the age of the patient, and the thoroughness of the pathologic review of the specimen.

Tumors of these stages are commonly referred to as "incidental carcinomas." Such tumors are found in 8%–12% of the patients undergoing surgery for benign disease. This percentage can be expected to decrease with the widespread use of prostate-specific antigen (PSA) determination in patients presenting with micturition complaints. More prostate biopsies can be expected to be performed preoperatively, revealing prostate cancer before surgery is performed because of the complaints of obstruction. Prostate cancer detected by needle biopsy because an elevated PSA was determined is termed stage T1c disease if no abnormality is palpable or visible with transrectal ultrasonography (TRUS) of the prostate. The clinical behavior of stage T1a and T1b prostate cancer has been investigated in longitudinal studies of untreated patients. According to Jewett (1975), a different prognosis can be expected from focal as against extensive incidental carcinoma. The difference between stages T1a and T1b lies in the amount of slide surface positive for cancer (Cantrell et al. 1981). Table 2.1 summarizes the results of the aforementioned longitudinal studies. Most authors have reported higher progression rates for T1b lesions. However, owing to the competing causes of death in the age group included in the studies, patients with T1a and T1b disease rarely die from prostatic cancer. Lowe and Liström (1988) found median times to tumor progression of 162 months for A1 lesions and 54 months for A2 lesions. Five-year progression rates for A2 lesions have been reported to be in the range of 25%–30%. These data rely heavily on the accuracy of the digital rectal examination (DRE). TRUS and determination of PSA may be helpful in excluding extensive disease. Adolfsson et al. (1990) and George (1988) reported progression rates separately for local and systemic disease. It seems that local progression occurs more frequently than progression to metastatic disease. Many clinicians follow patients with A1 (T1a) disease clinically without active treatment. Epstein et al. (1986) and Blute et al. (1986) indicated that younger patients might deserve a different approach because the period of time that they are at risk for progression may be considerably longer. As was reported by Aus et al. (1995), if diagnosis of prostate cancer is made at a younger age, the probability of death from prostate cancer increases. It is agreed that with rates of progression in the order of 25% within 5 years, some kind of treatment is warranted.

2.2.2 Stage T2a and T2b (B1, B2, B3) Prostate Cancer

In stage T2a and T2b (B1, B2, B3) disease there are palpable nodules in the prostate that are organ confined, without extension through the capsule. This category of prostate cancers is considered potentially curable; radical prostatectomy and radiotherapy are competing forms of therapy. In patients with these clinical stages of disease, lymph node dissection detects lymph node metastasis in 10%–25% of cases.

Limited information is available about the natural history of T2 prostate cancer. Warner and Whitmore (1990) presented a retrospective series of patients in respect of whom the "wait and see approach" was adopted for some specific reason (the patients were eligible for radical prostatectomy). With a mean follow-up of almost 10 years, local progression occurred in 52 out of 75 (69%) patients, and progression to metastatic disease occurred in 25 (33%). The 20 patients reported by Byar et al. (1981) represented the control arm of an incomplete randomized study of the Veterans Administration Cooperative Urological Research Group (VACURG). The patients were identified with TUR or biopsy. Those with metastasis were excluded by acid phosphatase determinations and bone radiographs. Seven patients (35%) showed tumor progression with a mean follow-up of 91 months. Of the six patients who died, only one died of prostate cancer. Johansson et al. (1989) reported on patients with stage T1 and T2 prostate cancer, almost excluding grade III tumors. Time to progression was in the order of 7–8 years and progression rates were 30%–35% at 5 years and 56%–70% at 10 years. In all the reported series local progression was more frequent than distant metastasis, and death rates from prostate cancer

Table 2.1. Progression rates (progressive disease: PD), median time to PD, and prostate cancer death rates in patients with untreated, incidental prostate cancer

Reference	No.	Stage	PD n (%)	Median time to PD (months)	Death rate
BLACKARD et al. (1971)	45		13 (28%)	62	2
CANTRELL et al. (1981)	48	A1	1 (2%)	>48	0
	34	A2	11 (32%)	>48	5/23
EPSTEIN et al. (1986)	50	A1	8 (16%)	>96	6/26
BLUTE et al. (1986)	15	A2	4 (26.6%)	134	1/8
Age <60	8	A2	2 (25.0%)	134	1/8
LOWE and LISTRÖM (1988)	143	A1	(50%)	162	3
	55	A2	(50%)	54	12/38
JOHANSSON et al. (1989)	72	T1a	7 (10%)		3/22
	34	T1b	11 (32%)	78	5/10
AUS et al. (1995)	23	T1a			2/20
	80	T1b			26/56

were low. Local progression can be prevented with radical prostatectomy or radiotherapy at the price of side-effects related to treatment. Prostate cancer seems to be a slowly progressing disease, and competing causes of death in the relevant age category are overruling. The advantage in survival to be expected in a randomized study will be only small, considering the small number of patients dying of prostate cancer. However, the predominant opinion is that there is no correlation of younger age or older age with more or less aggressive prostate cancer. Against this background it seems sensible to consider more aggressive and active treatment in the younger patients with a longer life expectancy. Progression rates are high for 5- and 10-year periods of follow-up. The impact of uncertainty and the amount of suffering due to progression are difficult to judge. If effective and well-tolerated treatment modalities without side-effects were available, the balance would be positive for treatment with potentially curative properties.

Recently, SCHELLHAMMER (1994) reviewed the contemporary series of patients managed expectantly. All of the reported studies were nonrandomized. Knowledge of inclusion criteria is of critical importance in order to assess the study outcome. The selection criteria represented a spectrum of exclusionary requirements, like: (a) absence of clinical symptoms (HANDLEY et al. 1988), (b) absence of metastasis (GEORGE 1988), (c) a defined period of nonprogression (WHITMORE et al. 1991), (d) low stage, (e) low grade (JOHANSSON et al. 1992; ADOLFSSON et al. 1992), (f) stage, grade and age suitable for radical prostatectomy (JOHANSSON et al. 1992; ADOLFSSON and CARSTENSEN 1991), and (g) stage A prostate cancer, not palpable before prostatic surgery (ZHANG et al. 1991; EPSTEIN et al. 1986; CANTRELL et al. 1981; BLUTE et al. 1986; STILWELL et al. 1989; THOMPSON and ZEIDMAN 1989).

Two studies described the Swedish experience with expectant management of localized prostate cancer. ADOLFSSON and CARSTENSEN (1991) reported on 122 patients with T1 and T2 disease evaluated in a retrospective study. More than 90% of patients had T2 disease. Tumor grade was equally divided between I and II, and no patients with grade III tumors were included. The median age of the patients was 68 years. Of the 122 study patients, 45% required subsequent treatment. At 5 years the risk of local progression was 57%, progression to metastatic disease, 8%, and progression to death from prostate cancer, 1%. At 10 years the risk of local progression was 69%, progression to metastasis, 28%, and progression to death from prostate cancer, 16%. Deaths from non-prostate cancer-related causes represented 31%. The authors concluded that "the natural history of low grade, localised prostate cancer seems to be a slow but steady local progression with low rate of metastatic disease and lower rate of fatal disease within the first 10 years after diagnosis." Therefore deferred treatment may be a reasonable alternative to active treatment in patients with clinically localized prostate cancer and in those with a life expectancy of less than 10 years.

The second Swedish study evaluated was a prospective population-based study, in which in the region of Orebro, Sweden, all patients with grade I prostate cancer were included (JOHANSSON et al.

1992). In later years some patients with grade II and III prostate cancers were also entered into this study. Only nine had grade III tumors; 33% (76 of 233) of the tumors were stage A1 and 50% were stage B. JOHANSSON showed that patients with grade I cancer selected for expectant therapy (25% were not selected) experienced a very low rate of progression. There was an increase in the incidence of local progression in those with higher initial tumor stage and there was an increase in the incidence of progression to metastasis and death with increasing tumor grade. The most important findings of the Johansson study were the very low death rate of 9% at 10 years from prostate cancer versus 47% from other causes.

The differences between the local progression rate (22% vs 69%), rate of progression to metastatic disease (12% vs 28%), death rate from other causes (47% vs 31%) and death rate from prostate cancer (9% vs 16%) in the Johansson and the Adolfsson series might be explained by selection of the patients included in these studies. The median age of patients in the Johansson study was 72 years, 4 years more than the age of the patients in the Adolfsson study. A higher death rate from non-prostate-related causes can be expected in older patients, which in turn decreases the risk of death from prostate cancer. Another factor responsible for the differences could be the stage of the disease. One-third of the patients in the Johansson series were stage A1, while 90% of Adolfsson's patients were stage B. Higher stage is consistent with greater likelihood of local and metastatic progression. Longer follow-up to 12 years reported by JOHANSSON (personal communication, 1993) showed a rate of progression to metastasis increasing from 12% to 22% and a local progression rate increasing from 22% to 35%. It can be concluded that even with a lower initial stage of disease, with longer follow-up, progression will occur. Reviewing the Swedish experience with expectant management of locally confined prostate cancer, the favorable outcome is paradoxical given that the death rate from prostate cancer in Sweden is the highest in the world. The selection bias might arise not only from physician identification of grade I localized prostate cancer but also from a cultural perspective that favors no active therapy and results in a high threshold for any diagnostic studies. In this setting, a higher percentage of patients would likely have advanced disease when eventually diagnosed. Those tumors still localized at eventual diagnosis would more likely be without metastatic potential (SCHELLHAMMER 1994).

A meta-analysis of data from six series reported on expectant management of prostate cancer patients (CHODAK et al. 1994) and established the relatively long natural history of grade I prostate cancer. The 10-year disease-specific survival was 87% and the 10-year metastasis-free survival was 81%. With grade II tumors the disease-specific survival was also 87%; however, the metastasis-free survival rate dropped to 58%. For patients with grade II prostate cancer, after progression to metastasis, death from prostate cancer occurs with a median interval of 36 months. For grade III tumors the 10-year disease-specific survival was only 44% and the metastasis-free survival only 26%. Patients with grade III prostate cancer are thus unlikely to be candidates for expectant management.

To remove uncertainties about selection bias in the comparison of different series describing any form of active treatment or expectancy, prospective randomized trials are necessary. Such studies are under way in Sweden, where radical prostatectomy or radiotherapy will be compared with expectant management. In Denmark, radiotherapy is being compared with expectant management, and in the large study of the U.S. Veterans Affairs and the National Cancer Institute 2000 men will be randomized between radical prostatectomy and expectant management (PIVOT, Prostate Intervention versus Observation Trial). In the United Kingdom, the Medical Research Council plans to start a randomized trial of 1800 men to compare the efficacy of active treatment (radical prostatectomy or radiotherapy) and expectant management of localized prostate cancer.

2.2.3 Stage T1c Prostate Cancer

As indicated earlier, information is lacking about the natural history of T1c prostage cancer. These prostate cancers are detected because of an elevated PSA level. By definition, they are not palpable and are not visible with TRUS. Concern has arisen that with a liberal biopsy regimen based on PSA determination, extensive numbers of insignificant prostate cancers will be detected. In the series of stage T1c prostate cancers reported by EPSTEIN et al. (1994), pathologic parameters were compared with preoperative clinical parameters. Sixteen percent of the tumors (26 out of 157) were insignificant (less than 0.2 cc and confined to the prostate, with a Gleason sum <7), 10% (15 of 157) were minimal (0.2–0.5 cc and confined to the prostate, with a Gleason sum

<7), 37% (58 of 157) were moderate (>0.5 cc or capsular penetration, with a Gleason sum <7) and 37% (58 of 157) were advanced (capsular penetration, with a Gleason sum of 7 or higher or positive margins, seminal vesicles or lymph nodes). These findings are intermediate between those seen in clinical stage T1a and stage T2 disease. The best model predicting insignificant tumor was: PSA density of less than 0.1 ng/ml per gram and no adverse pathologic findings on needle biopsy, or PSA density of 0.1–0.15 ng/ml per gram, with a low to intermediate grade cancer smaller than 3 mm found in only one needle biopsy core specimen. The positive predictive value of the model was 95%, with a negative predictive value of 66%. Seventy-three percent of the cases of insignificant tumor were accurately predicted. The conclusion was that 84% of impalpable prostate tumors diagnosed by screening techniques are significant tumors and warrant definitive therapy.

Douglas et al. (1995) analyzed 71 patients with T1c prostate cancer. Twenty-nine (41%) had positive margins, and 21 (30%) had either a Gleason sum of 7 or more or poorly differentiated tumor in the surgical specimen. Insignificant tumors were found in 2 of 33 cases in which tumor volume could be assessed; of these two patients, one had extensive high-grade PIN and the other had multifocal disease. These authors also concluded that T1c prostate cancer is rarely insignificant. It has to be determined whether it is reasonable to follow up some of the patients whose tumors are most likely insignificant. Serial PSA determinations and repeated biopsies are thought to be useful for follow up of such tumors. The natural history of impalpable prostate cancer has still to be defined.

2.2.4 Stage T3M0 Prostate Cancer

T3 prostate cancer extends through the capsule of the prostate or is localized in the apex of the prostate. These tumors are at the limit of potential surgical curability or already have passed this stage. It is known that lymph node metastases occur in 50% of these cases. In the event of lymph node involvement, prognosis is determined by the N status rather than by the T category. T3 tumors without lymph node metastasis have a prognosis that is clearly poorer compared with that of smaller intraprostatic lesions. Bosch et al. (1987) showed that cure rates with surgery alone are not to be expected to exceed 30%. Little is known about the natural history of T3 prostate cancer. If lymph node metastases are present, these are of overriding significance for prognosis. Progression rates of lymph node-negative disease have never been determined. In Vacurg study II, the median time to progression was 48 months in the placebo group; however, in this study no attempt was made to rule out or to confirm the presence of lymph node metastasis. In prospective studies the median survival of T3 patients has been found to be approximately 4 years. If effective treatment were available, aggressive management of this disease would be appropriate, particularly in younger patients. However, many patients fail the local treatment and progress with time to develop metastatic disease (Schroder et al. 1989).

2.2.5 N+ and M+ Disease

At the time of surgical staging lymphadenectomy, lymph node metastases are frequently identified. Often the patients are asymptomatic and treatment is deferred. Median time to progression in this group is in the order of 11–24 months. In terms of survival, it seems to be of no importance whether hormonal treatment is deferred or started immediately. Although it has been reported by van Aubel et al. (1985) and Bosch et al. (1987) that the median time to progression can be prolonged to up to 5 years with early hormonal treatment, this is achieved at the cost of side-effects (decreased libido, impotence, and gynecomastia) of sufficient importance to contraindicate such early treatment. Furthermore, the general consensus is that, despite some reports of prolonged survival in patients with minimal lymph node involvement, cure is impossible or at least highly unlikely. In older series, positive lymph nodes were present at diagnosis in up to 53% of all patients with clinical stage A2 tumors (Grossman et al. 1980) and 42% of those with stage B2 tumors (Hackler and Texter 1980; Flanigan et al. 1985). Recently Petros and Catalona (1992) reported that the incidence of unsuspected lymph node metastases in patients with clinically localized prostate cancer fell from 20% before 1986 to 4% after 1986. A higher index of suspicion in the urologic community, earlier cancer detection, more aggressive intervention to establish the diagnosis, use of ultrasound-guided prostate biopsies and more widespread screening for prostate cancer may have contributed to the lower incidence of occult lymph node metastases in patients with localized prostate cancer.

The natural history of M+ disease (patients with distant metastasis beyond the regional lymph nodes) is unknown. Many patients are treated endocrinologically. Following endocrine treatment, median times to progression are in the range of 1–1.5 years and median survival is 2–3 years. After the stage of hormone independence of metastatic disease has been reached, independent of the type of treatment, the mean life expectancy is in the range of 1 year.

2.3 Conclusions

The information available for T1a and T1b prostate cancer is gathered in highly selected patients. Expectant management of these patients can be considered in those with a limited life expectancy. In younger patients and in those with higher grade tumors, more aggressive treatment must be considered.

T2 disease is potentially curable. Preoperative staging is unreliable, which makes estimation of the prognosis difficult.

T1c disease represents a new category of prostate cancer patients; it is occurring with increasing frequency due to the wide implementation of PSA testing for screening purposes. The natural history has still to be elucidated. It is suggested that based upon the tumor volume, determined in surgical specimens, most tumors are of clinical significance. Longer follow-up will be necessary to assess the natural history in this important group of patients.

T3 disease is in many cases beyond cure at diagnosis, owing to unsuspected lymph node metastases or positive surgical margins that result from the fact that the local extent of the tumor has not been appreciated preoperatively.

The prognosis of N+ and M+ disease remains generally poor.

Given all the above-discussed uncertainties we still have no definitive answer to the question: "Is cure necessary in those in whom it is possible and is cure possible in those in whom it is needed?"

References

Adolfsson J, Carstensen J (1991) Natural course of clinical localised prostate adenocarcinoma in men less than 70 years old. J Urol 146:96–98

Adolfsson J, Ronstrom SO, Carstensen J (1990) The natural course of low grade, non metastatic prostatic carcinoma. Br J Urol 65:611–614

Adolfsson J, Carstensen J, Löwhagen T (1992) Deferred treatment in clinically localized prostatic carcinoma. Br J Urol 69:183–187

Aus G, Hugosson J, Norlén L (1995) Long term survival and mortality in prostate cancer treated with non curative intent. J Urol 154:460–465

Blackard CE, Byar DP, Jordan WP (1971) Treatment of stage 1 carcinoma of the prostate: a preliminary report. J Urol 106:729–733

Blute ML, Zincke H, Farrow GM (1986) Long term follow up of young patients with stage A adenocarcinoma of the prostate. J Urol 136:840–843

Bosch R, Kurth KH, Schröder FH (1987) Surgical treatment of locally advanced (T3) prostatic carcinoma – early results. J Urol 138:816–822

Bostwick DG (1989) Prostatic intraepithelial neoplasia (PIN). Urology 34 (Suppl):16–22

Byar DP, Corle DK, Veterans Administration Cooperative Urological Research Group (1991) VACURG randomized trial of radical prostatectomy for stages I and II prostate cancer. Urology 17:7–11

Cantrell BB, De Klerk DP, Eggleston JC (1981) Pathological factors that influence prognosis in stage A prostatic cancer: the influence of extent versus grade. J Urol 125:516–520

Chodak GW, Thisted RA, Gerber GJ et al. (1994) Results of conservative management of clinically localized prostate cancer. N Engl J Med 330:242–248

Correa RJ Jr, Anderson RG, Gibbons RP, Mason J (1974) Latent carcinoma of the prostate-why the controversy? J Urol 111:644–646

Cumming JA (1990) Dedifferentiation with time in prostate cancer and the influence on the course of the disease. Br J Urol 65:271–274

Douglas TH, Sesterhen IA, Moul JDN, McLeod DG (1995) The significance of PSA detected, nonpalpable adenocarcinoma of the prostate (stage T1c). J Urol 153 (Suppl):251A

Epstein JL, Paul LG, Eggleston JC, Walsh PC (1986) Prognosis of untreated stage 1 prostatic carcinoma: a study of 94 cases with extended follow up. J Urol 136:837–839

Epstein JL, Walsh PC, Marué C, Brendler CB (1994) Pathologic and clinical findings to predict tumor extent of nonpalpable (stage T1c) prostate cancer. JAMA 271:368–374

Flanigan RC, Mohler JL, King CT, Atwell JR, Umer MA, Loh FK, McRoberts JW (1985) Preoperative lymph node evaluation in prostatic cancer patients who are surgical candidates: the role of lymphangiography and computerized tomography scanning with directed fine needle aspiration. J Urol 134:84

Franks LM (1954) Latent carcinoma of the prostate. J Pathol Bacteriol 68:603–616

Franks LM (1973) Etiology, epidemiology and pathology of prostatic cancer. Cancer 32:1092–1095

George NJR (1988) Natural history of localised prostatic cancer managed by conservative treatment alone. Lancet I:494–497

Grossman IC, Carpiniello V, Greenberg SH, Malloy TR, Wein AJ (1980) Staging pelvic lymphadenectomy for carcinoma of the prostate: review of 91 cases. J Urol 124: 632

Hackler RH, Texter JH Jr (1980) Evaluation and management of early stages of carcinoma of prostate. Urology 15:329

Handley R, Carr TW, Travis D, Powell PM, Hall RR (1988) Deferred treatment of prostate cancer. Br J Urol 62:249–253

Jewett HJ (1975) The present status of radical prostatectomy for stage A and B prostate cancer. Urol Clin North Am 2:105–124
Johansson JE, Adami MO, Andersson SO, Bergstrom R, Krusemo M, Kraaz W (1989) Natural history of localised prostatic cancer. Lancet I:799–803
Johansson JE, Adami MO, Andersson SO, Bergstrom R, Holmberg L, Krusemo M (1992) High 10 year survival rate in patients with early, untreated prostatic cancer. JAMA 267:2191–2196
Lowe BA, Liström MB (1988) Incidental carcinoma of the prostate: an analysis of the predictors of progression. J Urol 140:1330–1344
Petros JA, Catalona WJ (1992) Lower incidence of unsuspected lymph node metastases in 521 consecutive patients with clinical localized prostate cancer. J Urol 147:1574–1575
Sakr WA, Haas GP, Cassin BF, Pontes JE, Crissman JD (1993) The frequency of carcinoma and intraepithelial neoplasia of the prostate in young male patients. J Urol 150:379–389
Schellhammer PF (1994) Contemporary expectant therapy series: a viewpoint. Urology 44:47–52
Schröder FH, Blom JHM, Bosch JLHR (1989) Considerations on surgical management of locally advanced prostatic carcinoma In: Paulson DF (ed) Prostatic disorders. Lea and Febiger, Philadelphia, p 330
Stilwell TJ, Malch RS, Enger DE, Farrow GM (1989) Incidental adenocarcinoma after open prostatic adenomectomy. J Urol 141:76–78
Thompson IM, Zeidman EJ (1989) Extended follow up of stage A1 carcinoma of the prostate. Urology 33:455–458
van Aubel OGJM, Hoekstra WJ, Schröder FH (1985) Early orchiectomy for patients with stage D1 prostatic carcinoma. J Urol 134:292–294
Warner W, Whitmore WF Jr (1990) Expectant management of localized prostatic cancer. Abstract and oral communication, Canadian Urological Association, Vancouver
Whitmore WF (1994) Localised prostatic cancer: management and detection issues. Lancet 343:1263–1267
Whitmore WF (1988) Overview: historical and contemporary. NCI Monogr 7:7–11
Whitmore WF, Warner JA, Thompson IM (1991) Expectant management of localised prostatic cancer. Cancer 67:1191–1196
Zhang G, Wasserman NF, Ami Sidi A, Reinberg J, Reddy PK (1991) Long term follow up results after expectant management of stage A1 prostatic cancer. J Urol 146:99–103

3 Screening for Prostate Cancer

W.J. KIRKELS

CONTENTS

3.1 Introduction

Screening for prostate cancer is still controversial. With the introduction of screening tools like transrectal ultrasonography (TRUS) and more importantly the use of prostate specific antigen (PSA) determination, increasing numbers of prostate cancer are diagnosed. Nevertheless, digital rectal examination (DRE) is still the keystone of the physical examination of men for prostatic disease.

There are two mainstreams of thinking about prostate cancer screening. One extreme is represented by those who are against screening for prostate cancer because they are concerned about the increasing number of prostate cancer patients coming for treatment. Given the natural history of the disease, however, it is still unclear whether all these patients need treatment (GERBER and CHODAK 1991; HINMAN 1991; CHODAK 1993). In discussions about the natural history it should be realized that most of the knowledge about the natural history is derived from series of highly selected patients who were expectantly managed. Another argument against screening is the fact that treatment-related morbidity may outweigh the probable benefit to be expected from early detection and treatment. ADAMI et al. (1994) even called prostate cancer screening unethical. In their opinion PSA determination should not be offered to men as a screening method – not even to those treated in a prospective randomized study. Their most important argument was that treatment of prostate cancer only causes morbidity and mortality, without any benefit to be expected for the patient in terms of survival.

The opposite view is represented by those investigators who argue that with the tests available to detect prostate cancer at an early stage, men should not be denied the opportunity of early detection and treatment (CATALONA 1993; WALSH 1994). A yearly prostate cancer screening with DRE and PSA is recommended by the American Cancer Society and the American Urological Association (American Urological Association 1992). Up to now more than 50% of men diagnosed with prostate cancer have locally advanced or metastatic disease. However, with the introduction of PSA determination for screening purposes, followed by ultrasound-guided prostate biopsies if suspicion arises, more early-stage prostate cancers are being detected. While this phenomenon was to be anticipated, there is no proof of benefit to patients in terms of survival. It is reasonable to suggest that initially the wide availability of screening for prostate cancer will increase the costs of health care substantially. Treatment of all the patients detected with prostate cancer will cause morbidity and occasional mortality: results in patients treated in centers of excellence are often used to judge the risk of treatment-related morbidity and mortality, but the treatment results can be rather different in the general health care system. A possible solution to this problem can be expected from ongoing prospective randomized screening trials (SCHRÖDER and BOYLE 1993; SCHRÖDER 1993; SCHRÖDER 1995; GOHAGAN et al. 1994). Due to the specific characteristics of prostate cancer, the differences to be detected in a randomized screening trial are relatively small. As a result, extensive studies have to be designed to obtain sufficient statistical power. Because prostate cancer is rather slowly growing, results of such studies are not to be ex-

W.J. KIRKELS, MD, PhD, Department of Urology, Erasmus University and Academic Hospital Dijkzigt, Dr. Molewaterplein 40, 3015 GD Rotterdam, The Netherlands pected until after 10 or more years of follow-up and only then may definitive conclusions be reached. It is unrealistic to expect, however, that screening of prostate cancer can be stopped until the results of randomized studies become available. With the increasing use of PSA determination in the general population, it becomes more difficult to conduct a meaningful prospective randomized study. This is because such PSA-based screening results in the removal of suspicious cases, thus decreasing the prevalence and substantially increasing the sample size needed to obtain sufficient statistical power. Widespread population screening can even make it impossible to reach the projected study endpoints.

3.2 What Is the Goal of Screening?

The basic purpose of screening for a given disease is to separate from a large group of apparently healthy persons those who have a high probability of having the disease under study. These individuals may be given a diagnostic workup and if the diagnosis is established, they can be brought to treatment (Thorner and Remein 1961). Screening is performed in the belief that detection of a disease in its early stages, when cure is possible, will lead to treatment that will result in less morbidity or mortality than had the disease gone undetected (Seay and Thompson 1993). If the diagnosis is made fortuitously, the patient presents with unrelated problems and the examination reveals a prostate cancer; this is called case-finding, which does not meet the objectives for screening. Certain conditions must be met by the screening process that reflect the basic goals of screening:

1. The disease must have a high prevalence.
2. The biologic behavior of the disease must be known (natural history).
3. The screening test applied must have a high sensitivity and specificity.
4. The screening test must be acceptable for the population screened, and should be rapid and ideally noninvasive.
5. Treatment for early-stage disease must be available (Thompson and Fair 1989).

3.3 Definitions

Several terms will be used regarding a disease or the evaluation of the screening tests used for diagnosing prostate cancer. *Incidence* refers to the number of patients developing a disease under study, compared to the number of individuals at risk, per unit of time ("*x*% of patients develop disease *y* per year"). *Prevalence* is the number of cases in the population at risk at a point in time ("the prevalence of disease *y* in the population is *x*%").

Sensitivity and *specificity* are used to evaluate the performance of a diagnostic test. Sensitivity is defined as the proportion of those who truly have the disease and when examined with that test, will have a positive test result. Specificity is defined as the proportion of those patients who are known to be free of the disease and who will be test negative. A positivity criterion can influence the sensitivity and specificity of a test. If the positivity criterion is moved up, the specificity increases but the sensitivity decreases. The number of false-positives would decrease, but the number of false-negatives (those with the disease, but missed by the given test) increases. Also to be considered in the evaluation of a screening test is the *positive predictive value* (PPV), which reflects the probability that if the test is positive, the patient has the disease in question. The best test for screening would be one with a high sensitivity (identifying as many tumors as possible), and a high specificity (to identify all those who truly do not have the disease). The major goal is to increase specificity, because all those with a positive test need further workup (prostate biopsy), causing mental stress in this group of patients and generating costs and morbidity. It is important to be aware of the impact of the prevalence of the disease being sought: screening becomes more efficacious if the prevalence of the disease is high. There is a discrepancy between the clinical prevalence of prostate cancer and the histologic prevalence (autopsy studies). The clinical incidence is in the order of 88/100000. If all those are included who had the disease for a period of time, the prevalence is between 400 and 1300/100000. In autopsy studies, however, the histologic prevalence is in the order of 40%. It is clear that the majority of men with histologic prostate cancer will never present with clinical prostate cancer and even those who do present with clinical but asymptomatic disease may have a low statistical chance of dying from the disease.

Several effects can be observed in prostate cancer screening:

1. *Length time bias*: the differences in tumor biology observed in tumors detected with screening versus those tumors detected due to patients'

complaints. The latter tumors tend to be more aggressive. Patients found with prostate cancer in a screening situation generally do better than those with clinically apparent disease. This is not a result of screening but because of the selection process: men without complaints related to the presence of prostatic carcinoma probably harbor less aggressive tumors, with different growth potential.

2. *Lead time bias*: If as an endpoint survival is used to evaluate screening, an important bias occurs. Survival is defined as the period of time between diagnosis and death. In the case of screening the tumor will be detected earlier than when clinical complaints lead to the diagnosis. It is very well possible that the moment that death occurs is not influenced by early detection. To exclude lead time bias, duration of survival is not to be used as an endpoint of prostate cancer screening studies.

3. *Overdetection*: The prevalence of histologic prostate cancer (latent or "histologic-only" prostate cancer) is much higher than the clinical prevalence and incidence of prostate cancer. If many of the insignificant, small prostate cancers are detected, which would never be life-threatening for the patient, overdetection occurs. This is one of the major concerns of those who argue against systematic prostate cancer screening (CHODAK and SCHOENBERG 1989). In a randomized study it may be possible to evaluate the length time bias and the lead time bias. And if overdetection occurs this can be determined.

3.4 Screening Tests

3.4.1 Digital Rectal Examination

Of the several tests available for screening, DRE is the most widely used. Initially screening was only based on the results of DRE (JENSEN 1960; FAUL 1982; WAALER et al. 1988; MUELLER et al. 1988). In a review of DRE as a screening method (BENTVELSEN and SCHRÖDER 1993) it was concluded that the detection rate is low in several reported studies, with a variation between 0.13% (FAUL 1982) and 1.65% (MUELLER et al. 1988). CHODAK et al. (1989) reported a detection rate of 1.45% and a positive predictive value of 25%. Others reported positive predictive values between 6% and 39% (BENTVELSEN and SCHRÖDER 1993). It can be concluded that DRE has a low sensitivity and specificity for the detection of prostate cancer. There is a tendency to detect the larger tumors with DRE, and the risk of detecting clinically insignificant tumors with DRE is low. On the other hand, small multifocal lesions with an aggressive biologic potential are not detected with DRE alone.

The general belief is that DRE is highly subjective, although VARENHORST et al. (1993) found good correlation between different observations of examiners when assessing the prostate in a systematic way.

3.4.2 Transrectal Ultrasonography

Transrectal ultrasonography (TRUS) of the prostate can also be used for screening for prostate cancer. In most centers TRUS is used if PSA is elevated or DRE raises suspicion. With TRUS, prostate cancer is often seen as a hypoechoic lesion in the peripheral or central zone of the prostate. The structure of the transition zone is difficult to evaluate because of the marked inhomogeneity on sonograms. The volume of the prostate can be assessed accurately and reproducibly. This can be a valuable test for determination of PSA density (PSA value divided by the volume of the prostate). TRUS is very important for guidance of the biopsy in combination with modern springloaded devices. The procedure can easily be performed on an outpatient basis. Representative material can be collected from suspicious lesions and/or in a systematic manner (sextant biopsies). The positive predictive value for a suspicious TRUS is highly dependent on the patient selection and on the experience of the investigator. TERRIS et al. (1991) evaluated preoperative TRUS in patients who subsequently underwent a radical cystoprostatectomy for bladder cancer. Of the 51 patients examined, 27 (53%) showed no abnormality on TRUS and were without prostate cancer (27/51 patients). In eight patients (16%), TRUS demonstrated a hypoechoic lesion that proved to be a prostate cancer; seven patients (14%) with a normal ultrasound scan had prostate cancer and nine (18%) had lesions on TRUS but no cancer. The investigators concluded that the sensitivity was 53%, and the specificity, 75%. Additional analysis showed that TRUS is more accurate in the detection of tumors with a volume of 0.2 cc or more. TRUS is more accurate in the detection of peripheral zone tumors than in the detection of transition zone tumors. The reported PPV varies between 10% and 56%. The highest PPV was reported in patients investigated in a urologic outpatient department. COONER et al. (1990) reported a detection rate of 15% and a PPV of 31%. The predictive value for the combination of abnormal TRUS with abnormal DRE was 43%. For the combination of an abnormal TRUS and PSA levels higher than 4 ng/ml, it was 49%. An abnormal PSA predicted cancer in 35%. If PSA and DRE were both abnormal, the PPV was 60%. In a randomly selected population, GUSTAFSSON et al. (1992) reported the PPV in relation to the PSA value. The overall PPV for DRE was 22%, for TRUS-positive and DRE-negative cases, 14%, and for TRUS-positive and DRE-positive cases, 38%. In the case of a combination of PSA <4 ng/ml and positive DRE the PPV was only 6%; it was also 6% for PSA <4 ng/ml, negative DRE, and positive TRUS. The PPV was 12% for PSA <4 ng/ml, positive DRE, and positive TRUS. With PSA >4 ng/ml the PPV increased for the combinations with DRE- and TRUS-positive results.

3.4.3 PSA Determination

The most important characteristics of PSA determination for screening are the acceptance of a blood test by the general population, and the facts that the result is objective and the test is easy to perform. The problem with PSA testing is the choice of the cutoff value. PSA is not prostate cancer specific; rather, it is only prostate specific. Benign prostatic hyperplasia also can cause elevated PSA values, so the volume of the prostate is of importance for the PSA value. CATALONA et al. (1991) were the first to report on PSA screening for prostate cancer. A cutoff of 4 ng/ml was chosen; with a PSA above 4 ng/ml, DRE and TRUS was performed. In this study no information could be obtained about the detection rate with a low PSA. Of the study patients, showed normal PSA, 10% had a PSA between 4 and 10 ng/ml and 2% had a PSA >10 ng/ml. Among those with a PSA >10 ng/ml, 60% had a prostate cancer. Of the 304 men with a PSA between 4 and 10 ng/ml, 58 (19%) had prostate cancer. The detection rate in this study was 2.44%. The PPV was 33%. Catalona reported that 21% of men in a control group had prostate cancer with a PSA of <4 ng/ml. In the American Cancer Society National Prostate Cancer Detection Project, 33% of 88 prostate cancers would have been missed if screening had been applied using a cutoff value of 4 ng/ml (METTLIN et al. 1991).

LABRIE et al. (1992) found, in a screening study, that the best balance between sensitivity (80.7%) and specificity (84.6%) for PSA determination was at a cutoff value of 3 ng/ml. With a lower cutoff value the sensitivity increases, but the specificity decreases. As a result the number of men to be biopsied increases enormously. In conclusion, PSA is a valuable screening tool for prostate cancer detection. The test characteristics depend on the cutoff value taken as normal. For screening, PSA is not advisable as a single test, and most screening studies utilize PSA testing in combination with DRE.

3.5 Randomized Screening Studies

There are several reasons for performing prospective randomized screening trials:

1. It is possible to detect prostate cancer at an early stage.
2. The public is aware of the possibilities of screening.
3. The patterns of care are already changing, without proof of a benefit from screening.
4. Scientific proof is needed that prostate cancer screening is beneficial.

The most important question that should be addressed in such studies is: Will prostate cancer mortality decrease due to prostate cancer screening (early detection and treatment)? As was discussed earlier, to answer this question, extensive studies are needed. Sample size calculations have been done. For screening of men in the age category between 55 and 70 years old, in each arm of the study 67 500 men must be included. The mortality reduction to be achieved is 20%, with a statistical power of 90%, taking into account that 20% of the men in the control arm will go for screening on their own initiative (cross-over). As proposed, a prospective randomized trial of screening for prostate cancer also can be useful to determine the test characteristics of the screening studies (DRE, TRUS, and PSA). Another secondary endpoint will be the assessment of life years gained and the cost at which this result has been obtained.

In the Rotterdam region (The Netherlands), pilot studies have been done to assess the feasibility of a large randomized screening study. Such pilot studies were also performed in the Antwerp region (Belgium). The results were reported recently (SCHRÖDER et al. 1995). The conclusions were that a randomized screening study is feasible and acceptable. From these pilot studies a protocol for a larger international study was formulated, with proposals being made in respect of the important issues of randomization, prostate cancer mortality as an endpoint, age at screening (50–70 years), biopsy policy, rescreening interval, treatment policies, and follow-up.

To illustrate the organization of the randomized screening study in the Rotterdam region, some features will be listed:

1. Men between 55 and 70 years of age are identified in the population register.
2. A letter of invitation is sent to all of these men, together with a health questionaire, a WHO-PPS score, and an informed consent form to be sent back if the man wants to participate.
3. Response = returning the informed consent form with the health questionnaire and the WHO-PPS.
4. Randomization into control group (no screening tests, only follow-up) and screening group (testing with PSA, DRE, and TRUS).
5. Invitation of the screening group to attend for the screening; explanation of the procedures; drawing of blood for PSA determination and storage for future use; DRE and TRUS reported independently.
6. Biopsy in the event of suspicious DRE and/or TRUS independently of PSA (to include biopsy of the lesion and sextant biopsies). If DRE and TRUS are normal but PSA exceeds 4 ng/ml, then sextant biopsies are taken.
7. The result of the biopsy is discussed with the participant by a staff urologist. If prostate cancer is detected, the participant is referred to the regional health care system.
8. Follow-up will be done with the help of the Comprehensive Cancer Center, where all the diagnoses of prostate cancer will be registered. For detailed follow up patient charts and doctors reports will be used.
9. Rescreening will be done after 4 years and all those men in whom a biopsy was taken and no cancer detected will be reinvestigated after 1 year.

In the first year of the study approximately 87% of the men screened had a PSA below 4 ng/ml, and 67% had a PSA below 2 ng/ml. Due to the low PPV of DRE and TRUS many biopsies were taken from men with a PSA below 4 ng/ml. The number of cancers is very limited. For the future it is expected that the protocol will be slightly altered. Those men with a PSA below a certain cutoff (still to be determined) will not be investigated with DRE and TRUS. With this policy, many men will not need to be examined, and more importantly, fewer biopsies will need to be taken. A very small number of cancers will not be detected if this screening strategy is implemented.

It is felt that the prerequisites for a screening study are fulfilled and that prospective randomized screening studies are feasible. International cooperation is necessary, so the study designs need to be comparable. The major endpoint is the effect of screening and early treatment on prostate cancer-related mortality, but quality of life assessment is an important secondary endpoint of screening studies.

References

Adami H-O, Baron JA, Rothman KJ (1994) Ethics of prostate cancer screening trial. Lancet 343:958–960

American Urological Association (1992) Executive Committee Report. American Urological Association, Baltimore, MD

Bentvelsen FM, Schröder FH (1993) Modalities available for screening for prostate cancer. Eur J Cancer 29A:804–811

Catalona WJ (1993) Screening for prostate cancer: enthusiasm. Urology 42:113–115

Catalona WJ, Smith DS, Ratliff TL (1991) Measurement of prostate specific antigen in serum as a screening test for prostate cancer. N Engl J Med 321:1156–1161

Chodak GW (1993) Questioning the value of screening for prostate cancer in asymptomatic men. Urology 42:116–118

Chodak GW, Schoenberg HW (1989) Progress and problems in screening for carcinoma of the prostate. World J Surg 13:60–64

Chodak GW, Keller P, Schoenberg HW (1989) Assessment for screening for prostate cancer using the digital rectal examination. J Urol 141:1136–1138

Cooner WH, Mosley BR, Rutherford CL et al. (1990) Prostate cancer detection in a clinical urological practice by ultrasonography, digital rectal examination and prostate specific antigen. J Urol 143:1146–1154

Faul P (1982) Experience with the German annual preventive check-up examination. In: Jacobi GH, Hohenfellner R (eds) Prostate cancer. Williams and Wilkins, Baltimore, pp 57–70

Gerber GS, Chodak GW (1991) Routine screening for cancer of the prostate. J Natl Cancer Inst 83:329–335

Gohagan JK, Prorok PC, Kramer BS, Cornett JE (1994) Prostate cancer screening in the prostate, lung, colorectal and ovarian cancer screening trial of the National Cancer Institute. J Urol 152:1905–1909

Gustafsson O, Norming U, Almgard LE, Fredriksson A, Gustavsson G, Harvig B, Nyman CR (1992) Diagnostic methods in the detection of prostate cancer: a study of a randomly selected population of 2400 men. J Urol 148:1827–1831

Hinman F Jr (1991) The value of screening for prostatic carcinoma: a commentary. Urol Int 46:275–278

Jensen CB, Shahon DB, Wangensteen OH (1960) Evaluation of annual examinations in the detection of cancer: special reference to cancer of the gastrointestinal tract, prostate, breast and female reproductive tract. JAMA 174:1783–1788

Labrie F, Dupont A, Suburu R et al. (1992) Serum prostate specific antigen as pre-screening test for prostatic cancer. J Urol 147:846–852

Mettlin C, Lee F, Drago J, Murphy GP and the investigators of the American Cancer Detection Project (1991) The American Cancer Society National Prostate Cancer Detection Project. Findings on the detection of early prostate cancer in 2425 men. Cancer 67:2949–2959

Mueller EJ, Crain TW, Thompson IM, Rodrigues FR (1988) An evaluation of serial digital rectal examinations in screening for prostate cancer. J Urol 140:1445–1447

Schröder FH (1993) Prostate cancer: to screen or not to screen? BMJ 306:407–408

Schröder FH (1995) Detection of prostate cancer. Screening the whole population has not yet been shown to be worthwhile. BMJ 310:140–141

Schröder FH, Boyle P (1993) Screening for prostate cancer – necessity or nonsense? Eur J Cancer 29A:656–661

Schröder FH, Denis LJ, Kirkels W, de Koning HJ, Standaert B (1995) European randomized study of screening for prostate cancer. Progress report of Antwerp and rotterdam pilot studies. Cancer 76:129–134

Seay TM, Thompson IM (1993) Screening for carcinoma of the prostate. Progress and problems. In: Das S, Crawford ED (eds) Cancer of the prostate. Marcel Dekker, New York, pp 119–146

Terris MK, Freiha FS, McNeal JE, Stamey TA (1991) Efficacy of transrectal ultrasound for identification of clinically undetected prostate cancer. J Urol 146:78–84

Thompson IM, Fair WR (1989) Screening for carcinoma of the prostate: efficacy of available screening tests. World J Surg 13:65

Thorner RM, Remein QR (1961) Principles and procedures in the evaluation of screening for disease. In: Public Health Monograph 67, US Department of Health Education and Welfare

Varenhorst E, Berglund K, Löfman O, Pedersen K (1993) Interobserver variation in assessment of the prostate by digital rectal examination. Br J Urol 72:173–176

Waaler G, Ludvigsen TC, Runden TO, Stenehjem E, Ogreid P, Schei OM (1988) Digital rectal examination to screen for prostatic cancer. Eur Urol 15:34–36

Walsh PC (1994) Prostate cancer kills: strategy to reduce deaths. Urology 44:463–466

4 Pathology of Prostatic Carcinoma

W.M. Van de Voorde

CONTENTS

4.1 Introduction

The prostate is the largest accessory reproductive gland in the male, and exhibits a marked propensity for pathologic behavior. However, little is known about its specific function. The importance of the prostate gland to pathologists is constantly increasing. Prostate surgery is the most common surgical procedure performed on American males, most often because of prostatic hyperplasia. Radical prostatectomy is now widely used in the attempt to cure clinically localized prostate cancer. Many efforts of urologists, oncologists, and pathologists are concentrated on the diagnosis of premalignant lesions and early prostate cancer and the search for reliable prognostic parameters (Chiarodo 1991; Bostwick et al. 1992b; Ware 1994).

W.M. Van de Voorde, MD, PhD, Professor, Department of Pathology, University Hospitals (K.U. Leuven), Minderbroedersstraat 12, 3000 Leuven, Belgium

4.2 Applied Morphology

4.2.1 Embryologic and Fetal Development

The development of the genital system is intimately related with that of the urinary system. Androgen-dependent stromal–epithelial interactions are essential, with stroma having an inductive role in epithelial differentiation during embryogenesis (Cunha et al. 1980) and an essential role in growth and function, designated as the so-called prostatic functional unit (Aumüller 1983). The development of the prostate starts in the 10th week of gestation and is regulated by androgens, the secretion of which depends on testicular function (Siiteri and Wilson 1974).

The prostate is derived from the endodermal urogenital sinus or pelvic urethra, at the junction with the mesonephric (wolffian) ducts adjacent to the bladder, due to the action of dihydrotestosterone. Testosterone, which is secreted by testicular Leydig cells, is reduced to dihydrotestosterone by the enzymatic action of 5α-reductase (Kellokumpu-Lehtinen et al. 1980). Two zones can be distinguished in fetal prostates, i.e., an inner (submucosal) zone and a peripheral zone (Xia et al. 1990).

Testosterone itself stimulates the mesonephric (wolffian) duct to transform into an epididymis, vas deferens, and seminal vesicle.

The antimüllerian hormone, secreted by the testicular Sertoli cells, causes the paramesonephric (müllerian) ducts to regress rapidly between 8 and 10 weeks of embryonal development (Larsen 1993). A müllerian remnant exists in the adult prostate as an expansion of the prostatic urethra, i.e., the prostatic utricle. It now seems evident that in normal adult men the epithelium of this embryonic müllerian vestige has undergone prostatic differentiation, with epithelium showing strong diffuse cytoplasmic immunostaining for prostate specific antigen (PSA) and prostate specific acid phosphatase (PSAP).

4.2.2 Topographic and Applied Anatomy

4.2.2.1 Topography

The prostate is situated at a low level in the lesser pelvis, behind the inferior border of the symphysis pubis and the pubic arch, and anterior to the ampulla of the rectum, through the wall of which it may be palpated. It is somewhat conical in shape, resembling a chestnut, and thus presents for examination a base or vesical aspect, an apex, and posterior, anterior, and two posterolateral surfaces. The convex anterior surface is covered by the superficial and deep venous plexus (Santorini's labyrinth) (Myers 1991a). Substantial bleeding during retropubic surgery may occur if care is not exercised in the control of these veins. The flattened posterior surface is covered by Denonvilliers' fascia, which separates the prostate from the rectum. The base of the prostate is contiguous with the bladder neck. This "strategic" position at the bladder outlet, surrounding the most proximal part of the urethra, is the direct cause of much mischief in cases of prostatic hyperplasia. The prostatic urethra runs from the base to the apex through the prostate. A 35° anterior angulation at the verumontanum divides the prostatic urethra into a proximal and a distal half. The verumontanum tapers distally to form the crista urethralis. The utricle, the ejaculatory ducts, and the majority of the prostatic ducts join the prostatic urethra at the level of the verumontanum. The seminal vesicles and vasa deferentia are implanted at the posterior aspect of the base.

4.2.2.2 Applied Anatomy

Three notions are of major importance in the surgical anatomy and pathology of the prostate, i.e., the anatomic shape of the apex, the neurovascular bundles, and the capsule. The *prostatic configuration* at radical prostatectomy especially is influenced by the presence or absence of benign prostatic hyperplasia. Most enlarged prostates appear to have a "doughnut" configuration with a well-developed anterior commissure of fibromuscular and hyperplastic glandular tissue that provides a relatively long commissural bridge of tissue between the lateral lobes of the prostate anterior to the urethra. Less common is the smaller gland with a diminutive anterior commissure that results in an anterior apical notch between the lateral lobes, within which sits a portion of the membranous urethra and striated muscle urethral sphincter (Myers et al. 1987). In this latter "croissant" configuration, apical dissection is much more difficult, and transection of the urethra at a more cranial level can result in a portion of the posterior apical prostate being left behind (Van Poppel et al. 1992).

The autonomic nerves supplying the seminal vesicles, prostate, urethra, and penile corpora cavernosa arise from the pelvic plexus and travel together with the vascular supply in the paired neurovascular bundles (Lepor et al. 1985). These *neurovascular bundles* extend vertically along the pelvic wall in close proximity to the posterolateral aspects of the prostate. Nerve-sparing radical prostatectomy may overcome postoperative impotence (Walsh et al. 1983; Eggleston and Walsh 1985), but also may jeopardize surgical margins, particularly in the case of capsular penetration (Van Poppel et al. 1992). Indeed, nerve and arterial branches leave the neurovascular bundles at the superior and inferior pedicle insertion areas to supply the prostate, and most examples of capsule penetration by cancer represent tumor extension through the capsule along perineural spaces (Villers et al. 1989).

The evaluation of surgical margins of radical prostatectomy specimens is essential and positive resection margins most often are related to capsular penetration. The *prostate capsule* is in fact a laminated structure of dense connective tissue located between the gland and the loose periprostatic tissue, especially at the posterolateral and lateral aspects of the prostate. It is not a true capsule since it cannot be separated from the prostate and is incomplete (Ayala et al. 1989). This (pseudo-)capsule is largely absent at the apex and anterior aspect of the prostate (personal observation).

4.2.3 Histology

4.2.3.1 McNeal's Zonal Concept of the Prostate

The prostate is composed of tubuloalveolar glands without recognizable differences between ducts and acini. The folded, distensible glands guarantee a large storage capacity for a slow and continuous secretion. The glands are surrounded by fibromuscular stroma, facilitating an occasional, rapid expulsion of prostatic fluid into the urethra during ejaculation.

Different concepts concerning the anatomic organization of prostatic parenchyma have been used during the past century (McNEAL 1980; BENOIT et al. 1993). The most accurate exploration of adult prostate morphology has been performed by McNeal. A global description (McNEAL 1988a) correlates well with pathologic anatomy (McNEAL 1983), and distinguishes a nonglandular and a glandular compartment, the latter being subdivided into several regions. The urethra and ejaculatory ducts, piercing the prostate in different planes, represent the major anatomic reference points. The ejaculatory ducts together with the utricle form the ejaculatory complex, which is in direct contact with the seminal vesicles. The concept of McNeal currently is applied in the transrectal ultrasonographic evaluation of the prostate (see Chap. 7).

4.2.3.1.1 Nonglandular Compartment. The nonglandular part of the prostate, containing the preprostatic sphincter, striated sphincter, anterior fibromuscular stroma, and prostatic capsule, is responsible for much of the anterior convexity of the organ.

The *anterior fibromuscular stroma* is an apron of tissue that extends downward from the bladder neck over the anteromedial surface of the prostate, narrowing to join the urethra at the apex. It is composed of randomly orientated large compact bundles of smooth muscle cells, merging with those of the bladder neck. Anteriorly it is close to the *external striated urethral sphincter* (personal observation). This vertical sphincter complex extends from the bladder neck to the corpus spongiosum, anteriorly and laterally (MYERS 1991b). Because of the absence of the (pseudo-)capsule at the apex, no strict delineation between apical prostatic tissue and periapical soft tissue with striated sphincter can be seen (personal observation).

A second so-called *preprostatic sphincter* is represented by a sleeve of smooth muscle fibers surrounding the proximal urethral segment between the bladder neck and the base of the verumontanum (McNEAL 1988a). It is thought to prevent retrograde ejaculation and possibly to maintain closure of the proximal urethral segment.

4.2.3.1.2 Glandular Compartment. The prostate contains three major glandular regions (Fig. 4.1) that differ histologically and biologically: the peripheral zone, the central zone, and the transition zone (Table 4.1).

The *transition zone* surrounds the proximal prostatic urethra and is the exclusive site of origin of benign prostatic hyperplasia (BPH), which starts as early as the fourth decade of life, due to the reawakening of embryonic capabilities in this part of the adult prostate (McNEAL 1983). The hyperplastic transition zone can be removed surgically by transurethral resection (TURP) or simple (subtotal) prostatectomy, leaving behind the peripheral zone. The "surgical capsule," which develops between the

Table 4.1. Histology of the glandular zones of the human prostate

	Transition zone	Peripheral zone	Central zone
1. Volume of normal prostate	5% (increasing with BPH)	70%	25%
2. Anatomic localization	Surrounding the proximal prostatic urethra	Posterior and lateral to TZ and surrounding distal prostatic urethra	Surrounding ejaculatory complex
3. Urethral orifices of ducts	Posterolateral wall at distal end of proximal urethra	Posterolateral wall of distal prostatic urethra	Verumontanum, adjacent to ejaculatory ducts
4. Histologic features			
Glands	Simple, small rounded glands	Simple, small rounded glands	Complex, large polygonal glands with intraluminal ridges
Stroma	Compact	Loose	Compact
5. Proposed embryologic origin	Urogenital sinus	Urogenital sinus	Wolffian duct
6. Pathology	BPH, BCH, AAH 25% of carcinomas	PIN 70% of carcinomas Prostatitis	Rare (problem in differential diagnosis)
7. Sampling	TURP, SP, (NCB)	NCB	Difficult

BPH, Benign prostatic hyperplasia; BCH, basal cell hyperplasia; AAH, atypical adenomatous hyperplasia; PIN, prostatic intraepithelial neoplasia; TURP, transurethral resection of prostate; SP, simple prostatectomy; NCB, needle-core biopsy; TZ, transition zone

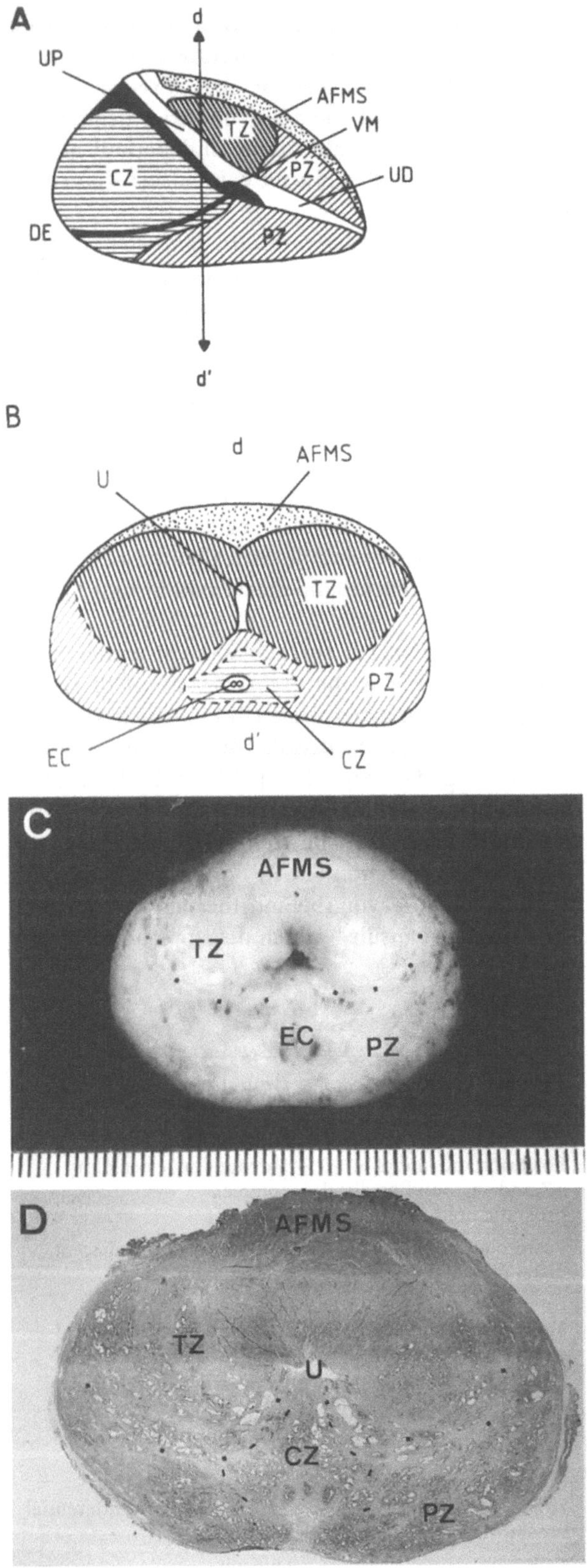

compressed glandular tissue of the peripheral zone and the hyperplastic nodules, serves as a plane of cleavage in the surgical removal.

The *peripheral zone* is localized posterior and lateral to the transition zone and surrounds the distal prostatic urethra. The glands of the transition zone and peripheral zone have a similar caliber, spacing, and histologic appearance; only, the stroma in the peripheral zone is loosely woven with randomly arranged muscle bundles, in contrast to the compact interlacing smooth muscle bundles of the transition zone. The peripheral zone is the region most susceptible to prostatitis, and most carcinomas of the prostate (CaP) originate in the peripheral zone (McNeal 1983).

The *central zone*, surrounding the ejaculatory complex, is best developed at the base and diminishes towards the verumontanum. The branching of the duct systems is more elaborate and the larger glands are subdivided by prominent intraluminal partitions. In contrast to the other zones, the epithelium in the central zone is exuberant, and the cells appear crowded with nuclei lying at different levels. This histologic pattern resembles ejaculatory ducts and seminal vesicles, and can be confused with prostatic intraepithelial neoplasia. It is difficult to identify the central zone on transverse sections, especially in enlarged prostates with BPH. Furthermore, little pathology is encountered in the central zone, and when it is, it does not have distinct histologic features. In pathology practice, the central zone is taken together with the peripheral zone.

4.2.3.2 Prostatic Epithelium

In normal and hyperplastic prostate glands two cell layers can be distinguished, namely, an outer basal cell layer surrounded by the basal membrane and an inner columnar secretory cell layer lining the lumen. Recently, the existence of a third cell type, i.e., the neuroendocrine cell, has been recognized (Fig. 4.2).

4.2.3.2.1 The Secretory Cell. Secretory cells are tall columnar cells (10–20 μm), and secrete enzymes

◄

Fig. 4.1A–D. Prostatic zones. Median (**A**) and transverse (**B–D**) sections proximal to the verumontanum (*VM*), illustrate the location of the proximal (*UP*) and distal (*UD*) prostatic urethra (*U*), the ejaculatory duct (*DE*) and ejaculatory complex (*EC*), the anterior fibromuscular stroma (*AFMS*), the transition zone (*TZ*), the central zone (*CZ*), and the peripheral zone (*PZ*). *d*, Anterior; *d'*, posterior

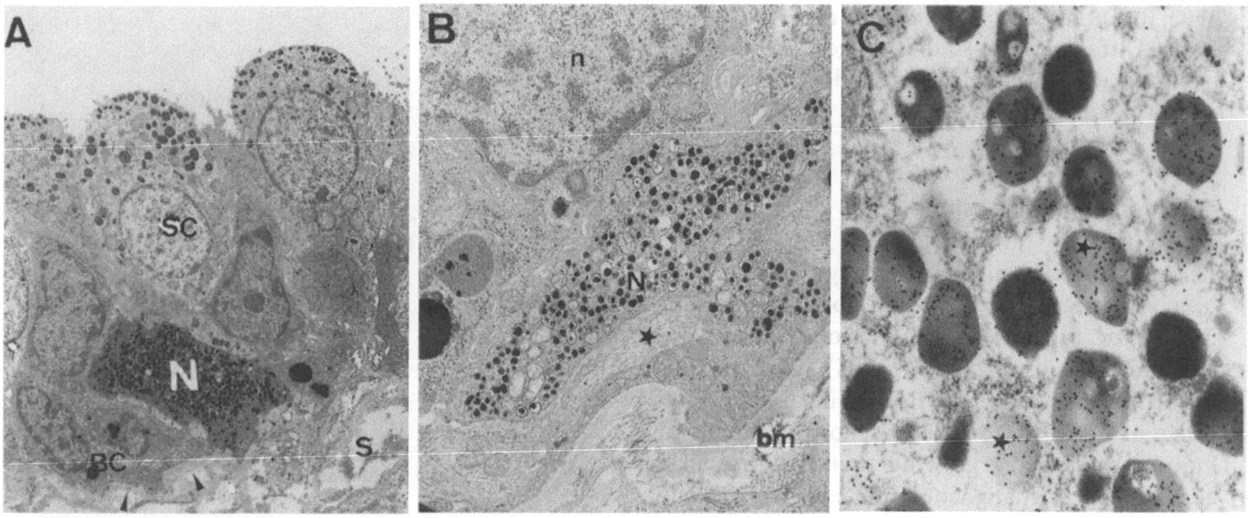

Fig. 4.2A–C. Ultrastructure of prostatic epithelium. **A** Overview (×4750) of glandular epithelium lining a lumen with secretory cells (*SC*), basal cells (*BC*), and a neuroendocrine cell (*N*) filled with dark neurosecretory granules; the basal membrane (*arrowheads*) separates the epithelium from the stroma (*S*). **B** Neuroendocrine cell (*N*) in close contact with a nerve ending (*asterisk*). *n*, Nucleus; *bm*, basal membrane (×17 300). **C** Neurosecretory granules (*asterisk*) contain gold-labeled (*black dots*) serotonin (×73 450)

such as PSA and PSAP. Only secretory cells of the central zone produce pepsinogen II and tissue plasminogen activator (McNeal 1988a). They are terminally differentiated and express cytokeratins 8, 18, and 19, a profile typical of secretory cells. The secretory epithelium is composed of androgen-dependent cells as documented by their sensitivity to androgen withdrawal and the presence of nuclear androgen receptors (Bonkhoff and Remberger 1993).

4.2.3.2.2 The Basal Cell. Basal cells are much smaller and contain an oval-shaped nucleus, the long axis of which is oriented parallel to the basal membrane. They express a basal cell-specific monoclonal antibody 34βE12 (Hedrick and Epstein 1989). Most basal cells do not express PSA or nuclear androgen receptor (Ware 1994). Nuclear receptor for both estrogen and progestagen are only expressed in the basal cell layer (Bonkhoff and Remberger 1993).

Basal cells in human prostate most probably are reserve cells capable of proliferation (Bonkhoff et al. 1994b) and differentiation towards secretory cells (Bonkhoff et al. 1994a). Basal cells may demonstrate immunophenotypic myoepithelial differentiation in related benign proliferative conditions, such as sclerosing adenosis and florid basal cell hyperplasia, in spite of the absence of this feature in the normal prostate (Van de Voorde et al. 1994a).

4.2.3.2.3 The Neuroendocrine Cell. Neuroendocrine cells occur in all areas of the prostate but tend to be more abundant in the major ducts and are more irregularly distributed throughout acinar tissue (Abrahamsson et al. 1986). Our morphometric investigations indicate that the prostatic glandular epithelium in the peripheral zone, with a neuroendocrine–epithelial cell ratio of 12/1000, seems to harbor a higher proportion ($P \leq 0.0001$) of neuroendocrine cells than the epithelium in the transition zone, with a 6/1000 ratio (unpublished data). The morphology of these prostatic neuroendocrine cells (di Sant'Agnese and de Mesy Jensen 1984) strongly resembles that of the cells belonging to the diffuse neuroendocrine or APUD system (Pearse 1969), demonstrating neurosecretory granules that contain chromogranin A and serotonin (Fig. 4.2C), and expressing immunohistochemically several neuroendocrine markers such as chromogranin A (Abrahamsson et al. 1989), neuron-specific enolase (NSE; di Sant'Agnese et al. 1985), serotonin (di Sant'Agnese et al. 1985), synaptophysin, N-CAM, and protein gene product 9.5 (personal observations). It is hypothesized that these prostatic neuroendocrine cells, producing several biogenic peptides such as calcitonin, TSH, and gastrin-releasing peptide, may be involved in an autocrine/paracrine pathway of regulation of growth, differentiation, secretion, and neuroendocrine-immune interactions (Abrahamsson and di Sant'Agnese

1993; REICHLIN 1993; DI SANT'AGNESE and COCKETT 1994). Ultrastructural studies suggest the possibility of innervation of single neuroendocrine cells (Fig. 4.2B) (DI SANT'AGNESE 1992).

4.3 Premalignant Lesions

Recently, the existence of premalignant lesions has been widely recognized. These lesions can be divided into two categories, i.e., lesions of atypical adenomatous hyperplasia (AAH) and prostatic intraepithelial neoplasia (PIN). While the real significance of AAH (or so-called adenosis) remains unknown, evidence is growing that PIN has to be considered a premalignant lesion, at least in relation to carcinomas localized in the peripheral zone (International Society of Urologic Pathology: Prostatic Intraepithelial Neoplasia and the Origins of Prostatic Carcinoma - First International Consultation Meeting, Ancona, Italy, September 1994). Both these lesions may be the subject of challenging differential diagnostic problems in daily uropathology practice (JONES and YOUNG 1994).

4.3.1 Atypical Adenomatous Hyperplasia

Atypical adenomatous hyperplasia (adenosis) is a focal proliferation of new glandular units showing a variety of architectural deviations from normal but usually not accompanied by significant cytologic changes (MCNEAL 1988b). AAH mostly forms a well-circumscribed nodule of tightly packed small acinar structures, often with a back-to-back arrangement (Fig. 4.3).

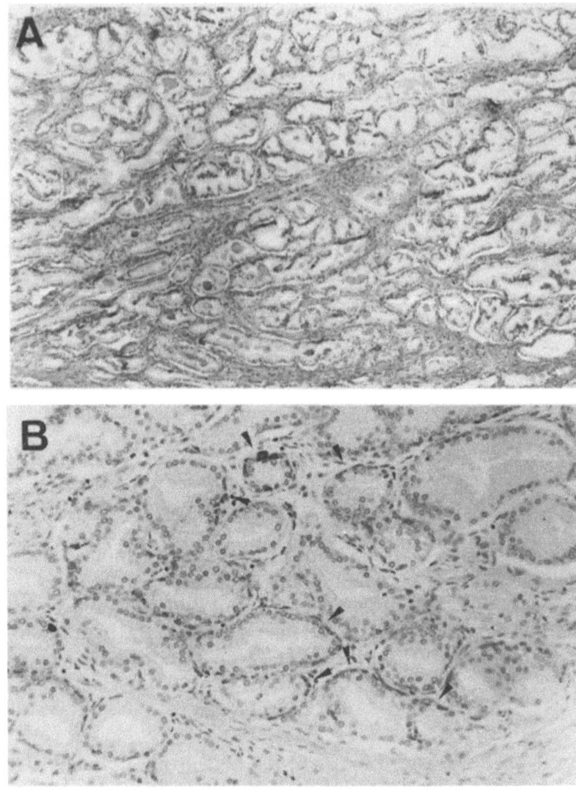

Fig. 4.3A,B. Atypical adenomatous hyperplasia (AAH). **A** Low-power view of densely packed acini (×40). **B** The majority of acini are surrounded by a discontinuous layer of basal cells immunoreacting with CK 34βE12 (*arrowheads*) (×100)

The biologic sense and, consequently, possible premalignant potential of this lesion is not well known. AAH most commonly is found in association with BPH. In 44% of 50 consecutive step-sectioned radical prostatectomies, performed for clinically localized CaP, we found AAH that was localized in the transition zone (82%) or in both the transition and the peripheral zone (18%). Also, AAH occurred more frequently and more extensively in the specimens with a primary transition zone carcinoma (data presented at the First International Consultation Meeting: Prostatic Intraepithelial Neoplasia and the Origins of Prostatic Carcinoma, 1994). If AAH is a premalignant (or a coexisting) lesion, it probably is associated with a subset of cancers arising in the transition zone (BOSTWICK et al. 1992a). The recognition of AAH mainly is important because AAH may cause considerable trouble in the differential diagnosis with well-differentiated CaP (BOSTWICK et al. 1993c; GAUDIN and EPSTEIN 1994; EPSTEIN 1995).

4.3.2 Prostatic Intraepithelial Neoplasia

Prostatic intraepithelial neoplasia is defined as cytologic, particularly nuclear, changes resembling those of invasive cancer in the lining epithelium of preexisting glands whose architecture is only minimally distorted (MCNEAL 1988b). Three different degrees of increasing severity were originally described (MCNEAL and BOSTWICK 1986). High-grade PIN, corresponding to grade II and III lesions, is characterized by multilayering and irregular crowding of the epithelium of involved glands together with markedly increased nuclear size, nuclear pleomorphism, and presence of one to multiple large, prominent nucleoli (Fig. 4.4). Four common patterns have been identified, usually with multiple patterns in each case: tufting, (micro)papillary, cribriform and flat (BOSTWICK et al. 1993a). A basal cell layer is present but mostly disrupted or discontinuous. The cribriform pattern of PIN has to be differentiated from, for example, clear cell cribriform hyperplasia, invasive carcinoma (Gleason grade III), and central zone gland, particularly in needle biopsies directed towards the base of the prostate (Fig. 4.5).

High-grade PIN has been postulated to be the main precursor of invasive carcinoma, and mainly is encountered in the peripheral zone (DE LA TORRE et al. 1993). High-grade PIN was present in all 50 radical prostatectomy specimens with CaP, and in 82% it was located exclusively in the peripheral zone, against 18% in both the peripheral and the transition zone. Furthermore, lesions were found in close proximity to a peripheral zone cancer in more than 80% of the cases (data presented at the First International Consultation Meeting: Prostatic Intraepithelial Neoplasia and the Origins of Prostatic Carcinoma, 1994). Studies indicate that PIN is mostly multicentric, and is strongly associated with a carcinoma in the peripheral zone. Consequently, the finding of high-grade PIN on needle biopsy often represents a sampling problem with carcinoma nearby (in more than 70% of cases). Thus, the presence of high-grade PIN on needle biopsy merits vigorous follow-up, including rebiopsy. In particular, patients with increased serum PSA appear to be at greater risk of harboring CaP (WEINSTEIN and EPSTEIN 1993). Since CaP is not always present, no aggressive therapy for PIN is warranted (BOSTWICK et al. 1993a; WEINSTEIN and EPSTEIN 1993).

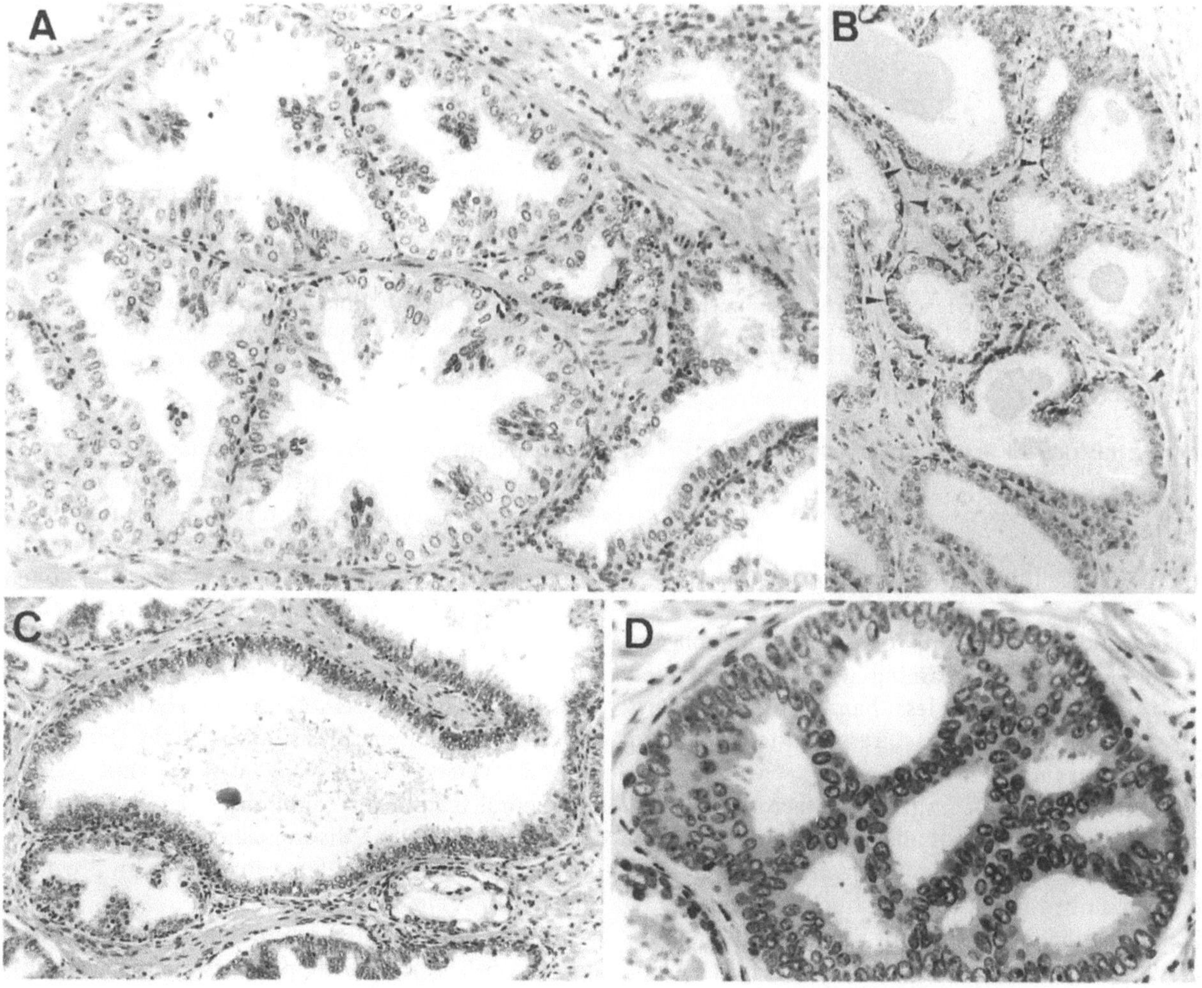

Fig. 4.4A–D. Prostatic intraepithelial neoplasia (high-grade PIN). **A** PIN lesion demonstrating the most common "tufting" pattern with obvious cytologic atypia of the lining epithelium (×100). **B** The presence of an interrupted basal cell layer is shown with immunostaining for CK 34βE12 (*arrowheads*) (×100). **C** PIN: "flat" type (×100). **D** PIN: "cribriform" type (×200)

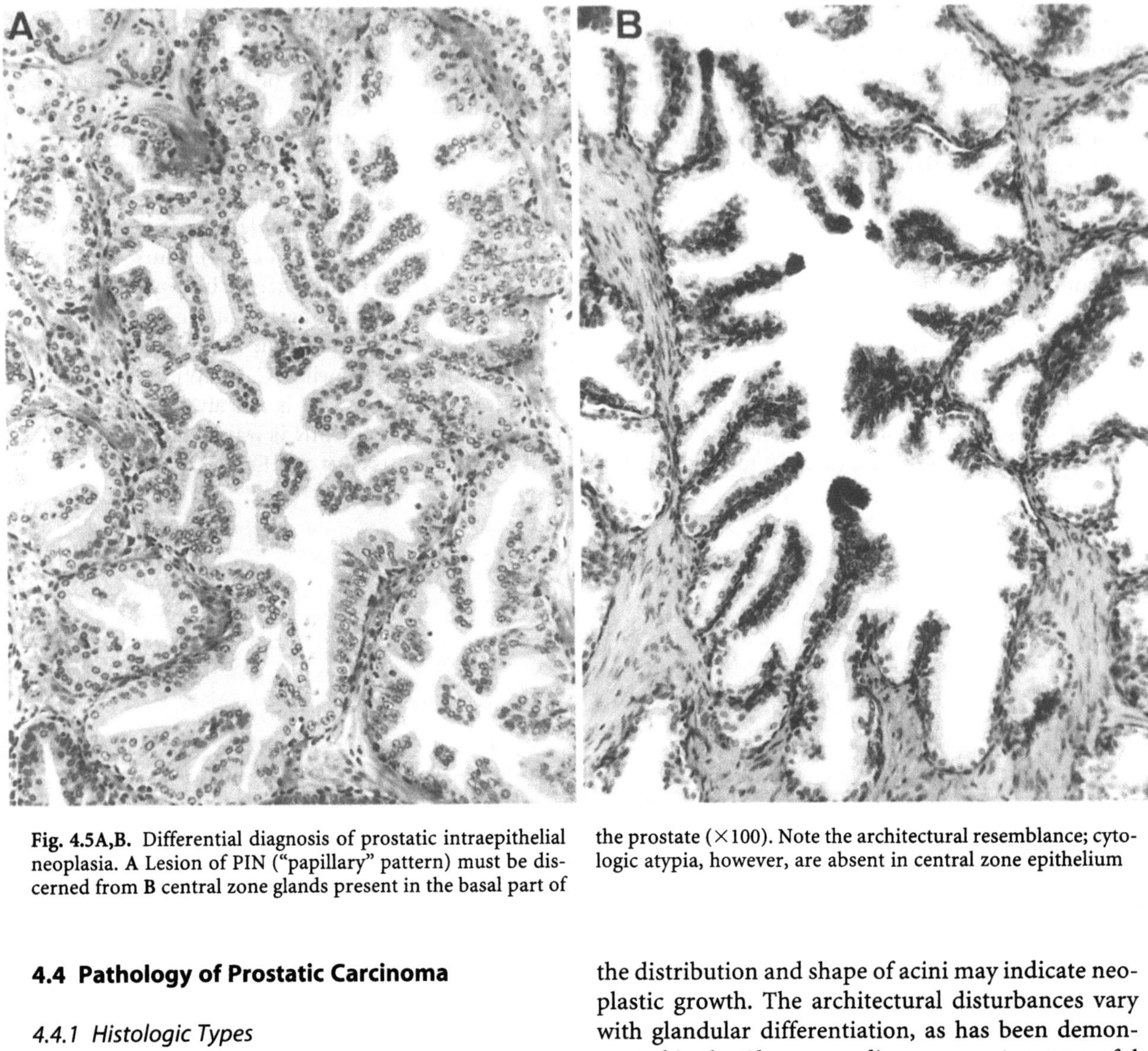

Fig. 4.5A,B. Differential diagnosis of prostatic intraepithelial neoplasia. **A** Lesion of PIN ("papillary" pattern) must be discerned from **B** central zone glands present in the basal part of the prostate (×100). Note the architectural resemblance; cytologic atypia, however, are absent in central zone epithelium

4.4 Pathology of Prostatic Carcinoma

4.4.1 Histologic Types

4.4.1.1 Classic (Acinar) Adenocarcinoma

Adenocarcinoma accounts for almost all neoplasms of the prostate, the remaining histologic types such as sarcomas composing less than 2% of cases. Most prostatic adenocarcinomas are gland-forming, and the size and uniformity of glands vary with the degree of tumor differentiation. Macroacinar and small-acinar subtypes of adenocarcinoma are mentioned. Histologic criteria for diagnosis of CaP have been described in detail (MOSTOFI and PRICE 1973). Pathologic diagnosis is mainly based on nuclear anaplasia and architectural disturbances (Fig. 4.6). Enlarged round and vesicular nuclei with one or more macronucleoli are a hallmark of malignancy, but nuclear morphology may appear innocuous in well-differentiated tumors. Crowding and irregularity of the distribution and shape of acini may indicate neoplastic growth. The architectural disturbances vary with glandular differentiation, as has been demonstrated in the Gleason grading system. A most useful diagnostic criterion of invasive tumor is the complete absence of basal cells in malignant acini. Therefore, immunohistochemical staining with cytokeratin 34βE12 may be very helpful in distinguishing CaP from resembling benign lesions such as AAH, basal cell hyperplasia, and atrophy (HEDRICK and EPSTEIN 1989; WOJNO and EPSTEIN 1995). Perineural invasion is commonly seen in CaP (Fig. 4.6A), but has to be distinguished from the rarely occurring perineural indentation of benign prostate glands (EPSTEIN 1992).

In less differentiated carcinomas, papillary, ductal, and cribriform growth patterns are regularly encountered, most often in association with typical acinar carcinoma. Sometimes a variable amount of signet ring cells (Fig. 4.6B) may be seen in moderately to poorly differentiated CaP (GUERIN et al.

1993), and the comedo type of necrosis (Fig. 4.6C) invariably signifies a high-grade CaP (CURRIN et al. 1988).

4.4.1.2 Ductal Adenocarcinoma (with Endometrioid Features)

Prostatic adenocarcinomas originating in the primary prostatic ducts at the verumontanum most often demonstrate a papillary (Fig. 4.7A) and complex ramifying growth pattern (Fig. 4.7B). They exhibit a striking histologic similarity to endometrial adenocarcinoma of the female genital tract, and may present as polypoid masses in the prostatic urethra (ELGAMAL et al. 1994b). It is now widely accepted that this variant of CaP has nothing to do with the müllerian duct; rather it is of prostatic origin (Ro et al. 1988a). CaP with a dominating ductal component also may occur in a peripheral location, and it seems that duct cancers are at an advanced pathologic stage by the time of presentation and have a much higher short-term failure rate after radical prostatectomy than do acinar cancers (CHRISTENSEN et al. 1991).

4.4.1.3 Mucinous Carcinoma

Although focal mucinous differentiation is observed in some 35% of cases of CaP, the diagnosis of mucinous carcinoma of the prostate requires that at least 25% of the tumor be composed of lakes of extracellular mucin (Fig. 4.7C) (Ro et al. 1990; McNEAL et al. 1991).

Clinical presentation and prognosis are similar to those of the usual CaP. An extraprostatic, e.g., gastrointestinal origin of this tumor variant must be excluded (EPSTEIN and LIEBERMAN 1985).

4.4.1.4 Small Cell Undifferentiated Carcinoma

While dispersed neuroendocrine differentiated tumor cells frequently are found in conventional prostatic adenocarcinoma (see Sect. 4.4.4.5), the specific type of neuroendocrine tumor, i.e., small cell undifferentiated carcinoma, is only sporadically encountered (Fig. 4.7D). This type is morphologically indistinguishable from its counterpart in the lung (Ro et al. 1987). The small anaplastic tumor cells immunohistochemically express epithelial membrane antigen and NSE, but remain unstained with PSA and PSAP, except for individual tumor cells (CHRISTOPHER et al. 1991). One has to exclude the possibility of metastasis of a primary lung carcinoma to the prostate, which is an infrequent occurrence.

Patients with small cell carcinoma of the prostate may present with a paraneoplastic syndrome. It must be emphasized that small cell anaplastic carcinoma

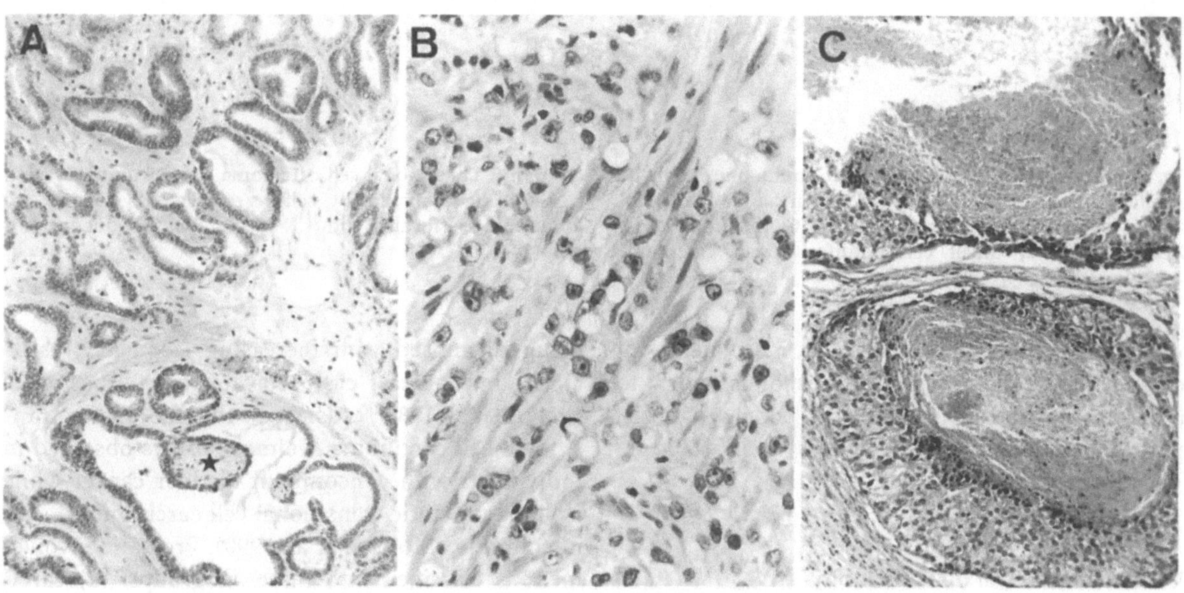

Fig. 4.6A–C. Prostatic adenocarcinoma (CaP). **A** Conventional adenocarcinoma (Gleason grade III) with perineural invasion (*asterisk*) (×100). **B** Poorly differentiated CaP (Gleason grade V) with signet ring cells (×200). **C** Comedo-type CaP (Gleason grade V) (×100)

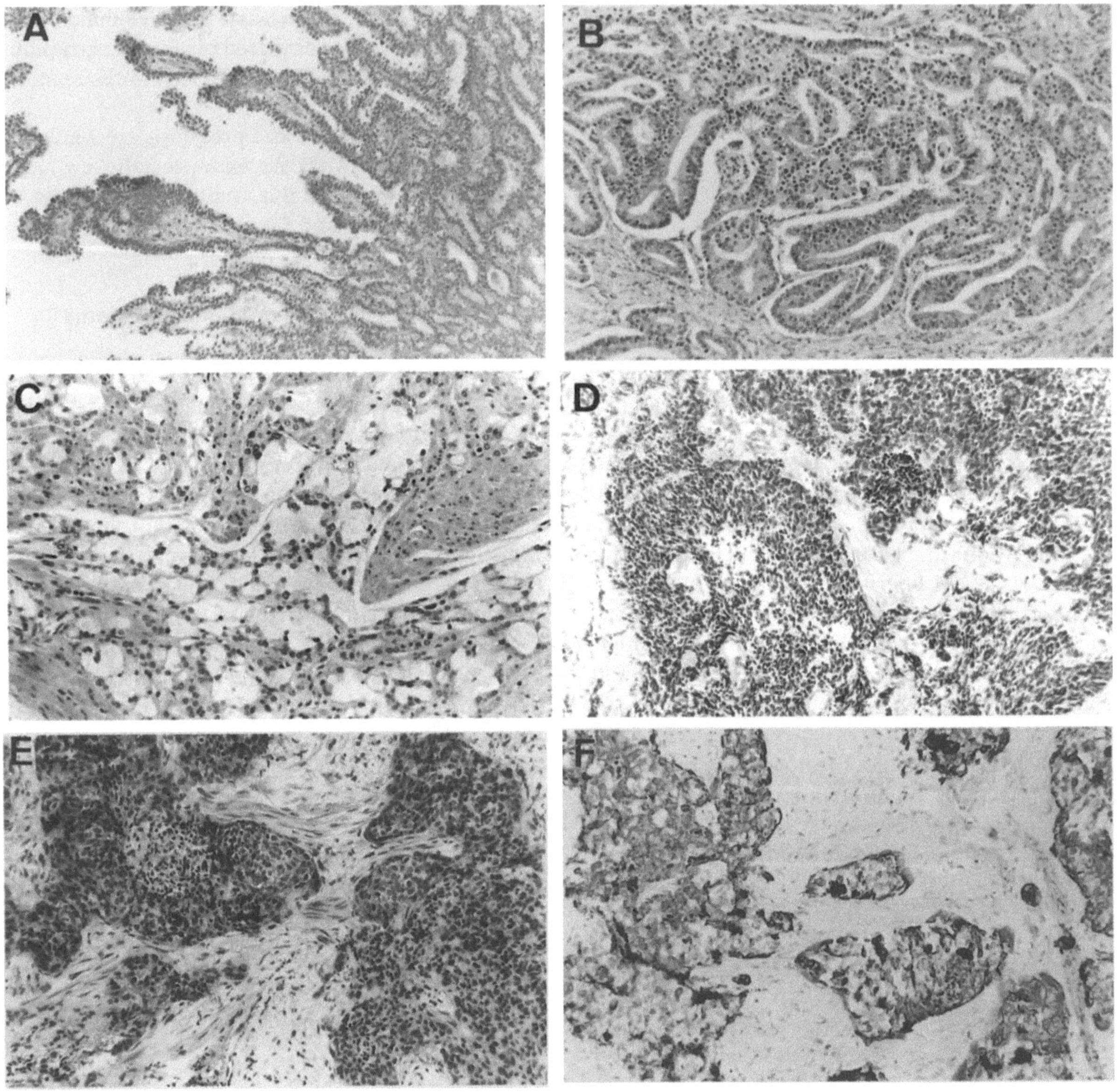

Fig. 4.7A–F. Variants of CaP. **A** Ductal carcinoma: exophytic papillary growth pattern (×100). **B** Ductal carcinoma: endophytic "endometrioid" pattern (×100). **C** Mucinous carcinoma (×100). **D** Small cell undifferentiated carcinoma (×100). **E** Transitional cell carcinoma with stromal invasion (×100). **F** Transitional cell carcinoma is shown to immunoreact (focally) with CK 34βE12 (back-stained tumor cells) (×100)

of the prostate is highly malignant, is frequently of advanced stage at presentation, responds poorly to antiandrogen therapy, and has a poor prognosis, with a median survival of less than 2 years (Oesterling et al. 1992).

4.4.1.5 Transitional Cell Carcinoma

Transitional cell carcinoma of the prostate is histologically indistinguishable from bladder cancer. It is being diagnosed with increasing frequency, especially in radical cystoprostatectomy specimens (Wood et al. 1989; Reese et al. 1992). Prostatic transitional cell carcinoma is almost always observed in individuals with concomitant bladder cancer while isolated prostatic transitional cell carcinoma is very uncommon (Montie et al. 1990). Prostatic involvement is classified into three subgroups: (a) carcinoma in situ of the prostatic urethra, (b) spread into prostatic ducts and acini, and (c) invasion of prostatic stroma (Fig. 4.7E) (Matzkin et al. 1991). This uncommon form of CaP must be considered in the evaluation of patients with bladder cancer (MONTIE et al. 1990). It is of major help in the differential diagnosis that transitional cell carcinomas do not immunoreact with antisera against PSA and PSAP, as is seen in CaP (Fig. 4.7F).

4.4.2 Grading, Staging, and Tumor Volume

4.4.2.1 Grading

Histologic tumor grade is a strong predictor of outcome for men with CaP (BOSTWICK 1994b). Several grading systems have been proposed, and the WHO has accepted the criteria of Mostofi with evaluation of both glandular differentiation and nuclear anaplasia (MOSTOFI et al. 1980). The Gleason system, however, is preferred and is the most commonly used system internationally. This grading system, the de facto standard for grading (BOSTWICK 1994b), identifies histologic patterns by the degree of architectural glandular differentiation (Table 4.2). Five different patterns (Fig. 4.8), i.e., Gleason grades I–V, are recognized as defined in a standardized drawing (GLEASON 1990). Tumor heterogeneity is accounted for by using the histologic score, i.e., Gleason (sum) score ranging from 2 to 10; this score is the sum of the two dominant grade numbers (if only one grade is present, that grade is multiplied by 2).

The Gleason score is a strong predictor of survival (GLEASON et al. 1974; SOGANI et al. 1985), recurrence after radical prostatectomy (HUMPHREY et al. 1993), and pathologic stage (BOSTWICK 1994b). Prognosis is unfavorable for patients with a Gleason score of 7 or greater (EPSTEIN et al. 1993c).

4.4.2.2 Staging

Multicentricity of CaP has been known for many years (BYAR et al. 1972). As many as five separate tumors may be found in the same prostate. Most frequently, one dominant tumor can be identified and associated with one or more microscopic small independent lesions. Considering the natural history of CaP (MCNEAL et al. 1986), the dominant or largest tumor can be considered the primary, clinically most important, or best detectable (index) tumor.

Pathologic stage translates the extent of tumor, and reflects the state of its progression. The modified TNM classification (SCHRÖDER et al. 1992) is used in the evaluation of tumor extent in surgical specimens (Table 4.3). T1 represents *incidental carcinoma*, found upon TURP, subtotal prostatectomy, or needle biopsy; T2 corresponds to *organ-confined CaP* while *non-organ-confined disease* can be divided into (a) capsular penetration only with extraprostatic extension (= T3a–3b), (b) extension into adjacent organs, i.e., seminal vesicles (T3c) and bladder (T4a), and (c) distant metastases (T4b).

Metastases to (regional) lymph nodes are separately staged (pN), and are found in 5%–10% of lymphadenectomy specimens (VAN POPPEL et al. 1994). CaP with nodal metastases invariably shows tumor progression within 5 years following radical prostatectomy, irrespective of therapy. Regional lymph nodes in CaP are involved slightly more frequently than bones. Metastases to other organs are less common. Most commonly the obturator lymph nodes are involved, followed in order of frequency by the presacral, presciatic, and internal and external iliac nodes. Even spread to supradiaphragmatic lymph nodes may occur. Bone metastases are most frequently osteoblastic, and primarily occur in the axial skeleton.

4.4.2.3 Tumor Volume

Tumor volume has been shown to correlate well with Gleason grade, pathologic stage, and surgical resection margins (MCNEAL 1992). It has not yet been

Table 4.2. Gleason grading system: histologic patterns

Grade	Appearance of glands	Size of glands	Architecture of glands
I	Simple, round, little variation	Medium, regular	Closely packed, rounded masses
II	Simple, round, some variation	Medium, less regular	Loosely packed, rounded masses
III	Angular, papillary, or cribriform marked variation	Small to irregular	Variably packed, mostly irregular masses
IV	Microacinar, papillary, or cribriform	Irregular	Fused, trabecular, "hypernephroid"
V	Comedo or absence of lumina	Irregular or single tumor cells	Fused sheets or diffuse infiltrative

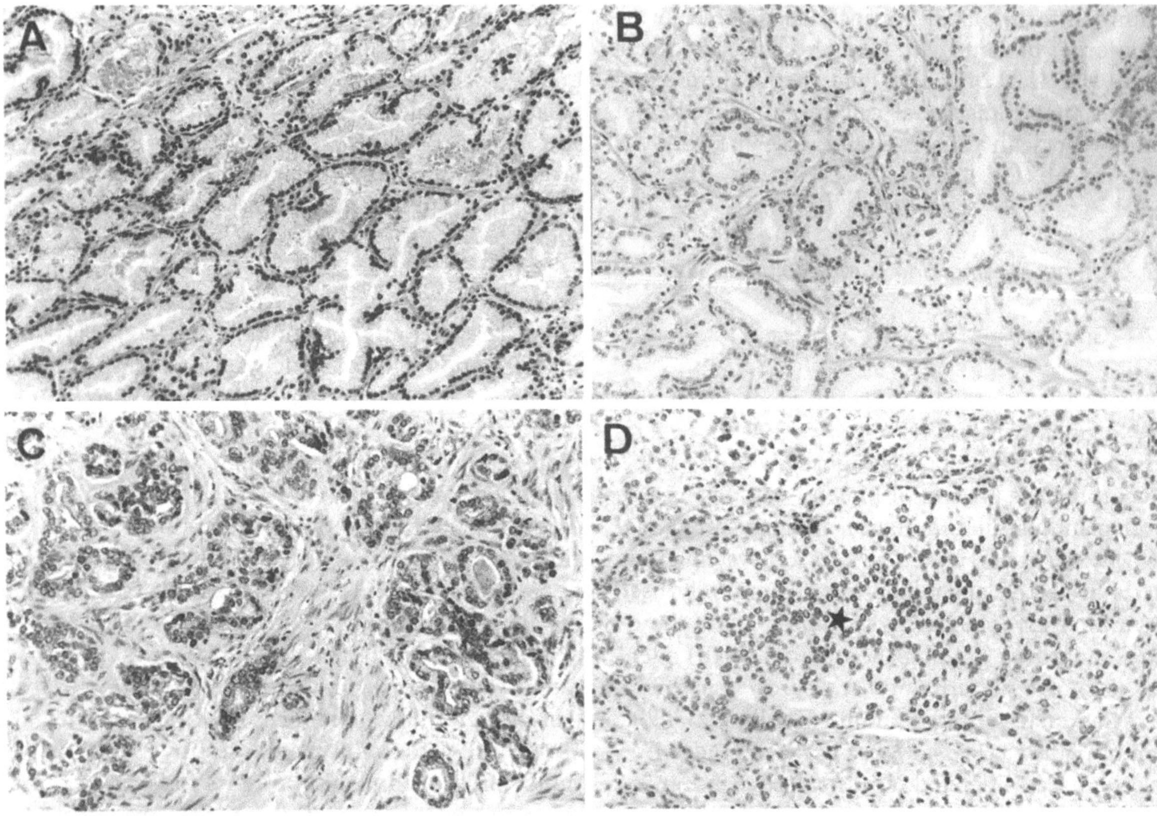

Fig. 4.8A–D. Gleason grading of CaP. **A** Grade I (×100). **B** Grade II (×100). **C** Grade III (×100). **D** Grade IV (*asterisk*) and V (×100)

clearly established which of these important variables provides independent prediction of prognosis in CaP. EPSTEIN et al. (1993a) have recently addressed this problem. In their multivariate analysis, Gleason score was the best predictor of clinical progression, and tumor volume did not provide independent prognostic information.

It is now thought that a patient with a clinically discovered cancer less than 0.5 cm^3 in volume is a comfortable number of years away from any likelihood of metastases, particularly if the Gleason score does not reach 4 or 5 (MURPHY et al. 1994). The capacity to metastasize is probably expressed only in tumor larger than 1 cm^3. This is a manifestation of tumor progression. Tumors larger than 12 cm^3 are nearly always incurable (MCNEAL et al. 1986). Tumor volume is also a good positive predictor of tumor extension. There is a 10% probability of capsular invasion in tumors of 0.3 cm^3, a 10% probability of seminal invasion in tumors of 4.0 cm^3, and a 10% probability of lymph node metastases in tumors of 5.0 cm^3 (BOSTWICK et al. 1993b).

4.4.3 Anatomic Localization of the Primary Tumor

It has been established that 70% of CaP originate in the peripheral zone; only approximately 25% arise in the transition zone, and the remaining 5% are located in the central zone (MCNEAL et al. 1988b). It is not necessary to distinguish carcinomas arising in the peripheral and central zones (GREENE et al. 1991) because of the rare occurrence of the latter and the difficulties in recognizing the central zone on transverse planes of histologic sections. Transition zone cancers seem to display morphologic features different from those of peripheral zone carcinomas (MCNEAL et al. 1988b; GREENE et al. 1991).

Tumor location in the prostate (Fig. 4.9) is responsible for differences in clinical presentation (Table 4.4). Because of the tumor location in the anteromedial part of the prostate, most transition zone carcinomas remain "silent" unless incidentally detected at pathologic examination of prostate specimens. The majority of impalpable, stage cT1 cancers are in fact transition zone carcinomas (MCNEAL

Table 4.3. Staging of prostatic cancer

Whitmore 1956 (with modifications) Stage		TNM 1978–82 Category		TNM 1992	
A	Not palpable on rectal exam.	T0pT1–3	No tumor palpable	T0	No evidence of primary tumor
A1	Focal cancer (<3 chips)	T0pT1	<3 foci	T1	Clinically inapparent tumor, not palpable and not visible by imaging
				T1a	Tumor an incidental histologic finding in ≤5% of tissue resected
A2	Diffuse (>3 chips)	T0pT2–3	>3 foci	T1b	Tumor an incidental histologic finding in >5% of tissue resected
				T1c	Tumor identified by needle biopsy (e.g., because of elevated serum PSA)
B B1	Unilobar, <2 cm	T1	Tumor intracapsular; surrounded by palpable normal gland	T2	Tumor confined within the prostate[a]
				T2a	Tumor involves half of a lobe or less
B2	Unilobar, >2 cm	T2	Tumor confined to gland; smooth nodule deforming contour	T2b	Tumor involves more than half a lobe but not both lobes
B3	All other, intracapsular			T2c	Tumor involves both lobes
C	Extending through capsule	T3	Tumor extending beyond capsule with or without involvement of lateral sulci and/or seminal vesicles	T3	Tumor extends through the prostatic capsule[b]
C1	Sulcus or sulci not free			T3a	Unilateral extracapsular extension
C2	>Base of seminal vesicles ±sulci			T3b	Bilateral extracapsular extension
				T3c	Tumor invades seminal vesicle(s)
C3	>Base of seminal vesicles ±other adjacent organs	T4	Tumor fixed or infiltrating neighboring structures	T4	Tumor fixed or invades adjacent structures other than seminal vesicles
				T4a	Tumor invades bladder neck and/or external sphincter and/or rectum
				T4b	Tumor invades levator muscles and/or is fixed to pelvic wall
D	Any local extension				
D1	Lymph node involvement				
D2	Other metastases				

[a] Tumor found in one or both lobes by needle biopsy, but not palpable or visible by imaging, is classified as T1c
[b] Invasion into the prostatic apex or into (but not beyond) the prostatic capsule is not classified as T3 but as T2

Table 4.4. Differences between transition zone cancers (TZCa) and peripheral zone cancers (PZCa)

	TZCa	PZCa
1. Incidence	25%	75%
2. Clinical stage	T1	≥T2
3. Localization	Central part (anterolateral to the urethra)	Peripheral part (posterolateral to the urethra)
4. Clinical detection	Incidental	Palpable nodules (DRE) Echopenic lesion (TRUS)
5. Pathologic diagnosis	TURP, SP (systematic random NCB)	NCB
6. Tumor extension	Base and apex AFMS PZ (late in evolution)	Through posterolateral capsule (often at apex) Into NVB Ejaculatory complex and seminal vesicles TZ (late in evolution)

DRE, Digital rectal examination; TRUS, transrectal ultrasonography; TURP, transurethral resection of prostate; SP, simple prostatectomy; NCB, needle-core biopsy; AFMS, anterior fibromuscular stroma; NVB, neurovascular bundle; TZ, transition zone

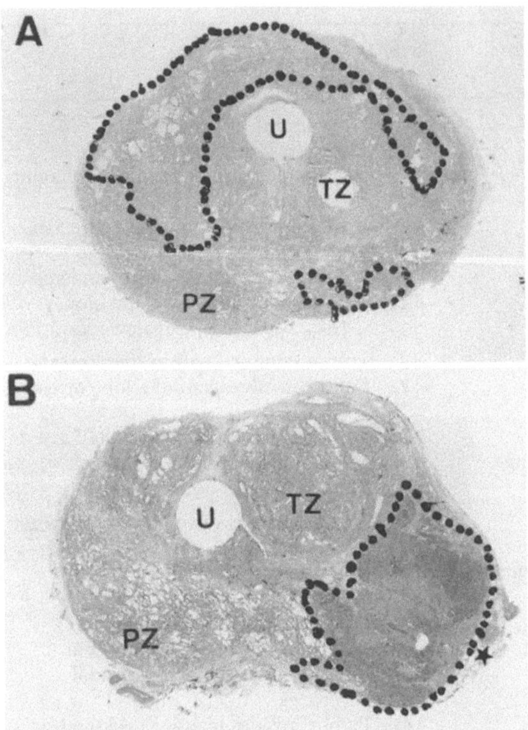

Fig. 4.9A,B. Localization of CaP. **A** Transition zone cancer: the largest tumor is located anteriorly, in the transition zone (*TZ*) surrounding the urethra (*U*); a small secondary tumor is present in the left peripheral zone (*PZ*). **B** Peripheral zone cancer: the left peripheral zone (*PZ*) is expanded by a tumoral mass just beneath the capsule, in close vicinity to the neurovascular bundle (*asterisk*)

1988a; CHRISTENSEN et al. 1990; GREENE et al. 1991) and are not visible on transrectal ultrasonography. The transition zone is not adjacent to the prostatic capsule at any point (see Sect 4.2.2) or to the ejaculatory complex, which explains the lower rates of capsular penetration, positive surgical margins, and seminal vesicle invasion in transition zone cancers (MCNEAL et al. 1988b, 1990; GREENE et al. 1991; VAN DE VOORDE et al. 1995b).

It is still a matter of debate whether transition zone cancers and peripheral zone cancers are biologically similar malignancies, distinguished only by their site of origin (MCNEAL et al. 1988b), or whether they have a different histogenesis, with more favorable pathologic features and a less malignant potential in the case of transition zone cancers (GREENE et al. 1991, 1995). The latter conclusion may be supported by the finding of a significant lower average Gleason score in transition zone carcinomas (CHRISTENSEN et al. 1990; GREENE et al. 1991; VAN DE VOORDE et al. 1995b). Furthermore, surgically treated patients with a primary transition zone carcinoma tend less often to have lymph node metastases (MCNEAL 1992; VAN DE VOORDE et al. 1995b). DNA ploidy analysis shows a significantly higher rate of nondiploidy in cancers of peripheral zone origin compared to transition zone cancers (GREENE et al. 1995). Our investigation of 213 patients with untreated primary CaP (164 cases originating in the peripheral zone and 49 in the transition zone) also indicated a lower proliferative activity, considering mitotic figure counts ($P = 0.02$) and proliferating cell nuclear antigen (PCNA) labeling indices ($P = 0.001$), as well as a generally smaller number of neuroendocrine differentiated tumor cells (chromogranin A labeling index; $P = 0.005$) in the 49 patients with tumors in the transition zone than in the 164 with tumors in the peripheral zone (unpublished data).

4.4.4 Pathobiologic Parameters

4.4.4.1 Secretion

A variable degree of *mucin* secretion is commonly seen in CaP (MCNEAL et al. 1991; ALLSBROOK and SIMMS 1992). Periodic acid-Schiff stained neutral mucins are secreted by benign and malignant epithelial cells, but alcian blue-positive (pH 2.5) acid mucins mainly are found in the lumina of malignant acini (RO et al. 1988b). The latter rarely may be encountered in, for example, AAH and basal cell hyperplasia (VAN DE VOORDE et al. 1994a).

Prostate-specific antigen is a 33-kDa glycoprotein that has been identified as a kallikrein-like serine protease (ALLSBROOK and SIMMS 1992; BOSTWICK 1994a). It is secreted by both benign secretory cells into the prostatic ductal system, where it catalyzes the liquefaction of seminal coagulation after ejaculation, and malignant cells. Any process that disrupts the normal architecture of the prostate allows diffusion of PSA into the stroma, where it gains access through the microvasculature to the bloodstream. Elevated serum PSA levels are seen with prostatitis, prostatic infarcts, BPH, and transiently after manipulations such as biopsy, digital rectal examination, or prostatic massage. It is of importance that serum levels correlate well with volume of both CaP and BPH. Cancer produces less PSA per cell than benign epithelium, but the greater number of malignant cells, the stromal disruption, and probably the neovascularization associated with cancer account for a greater elevation of PSA level. One gram of cancer on average produces 3.5 ng/ml of PSA elevation, in contrast to only 0.3 ng/ml in the case of BPH (STAMEY et al. 1987). Immunohistochemical staining of normal and hyperplastic prostatic epithelium is uniform and strong, while the same staining of CaP is more heterogeneous. Staining intensity seems to decrease with increasing grade and stage. Immunohistochemical expression of PSA in tissue sections allows determination of the prostatic origin of (metastatic) adenocarcinomas, although extraprostatic expression has been reported in several tissues (BOSTWICK 1994a; ELGAMAL et al. 1994a).

Prostate specific acid phosphatase is a 100-kDa sialoglycoprotein produced by benign secretory cells and malignant prostatic epithelial cells. PSAP is considered less useful than PSA because of the problem with its measurement and a lack of specificity (ALLSBROOK and SIMMS 1992; BOSTWICK 1994a). Serum PSAP now has little utility, but PSAP is valuable for immunohistochemical tissue staining technique when used in combination with stains for PSA. Immunohistochemical reactivity of CaP for PSAP seems to decrease with increasing grade and stage of the tumor.

4.4.4.2 Proliferation

Tumor proliferation rate in CaP (using DNA labelling index) often correlates well with tumor aggressiveness.

Mitotic activity may reflect tumor cell proliferation rate. Our studies have shown that the mitotic index strongly correlates with tumor volume and tumor grade, and increases with advancing stage of the tumor. The mitotic index may be a useful prognostic parameter in evaluating the long-term prognosis of CaP patients (VESALAINEN et al. 1995).

Immunohistochemical cell cycle markers recently have been described. Monoclonal antibodies to these antigens, e.g., PCNA and Ki-67, present in the nucleus, allow quantification of cells expressing the antigens and can be used as a measure of cellular proliferation (CHER et al. 1995). Few reports have mentioned a significant correlation between increasing *PCNA labeling* (Fig. 4.10A) and increasing (Gleason) grade (HARPER et al. 1992; SPIRES et al. 1994). In their study, HARPER et al. found that the group of patients with the lower PCNA score survived significantly longer than those with the higher PCNA score (HARPER et al. 1992).

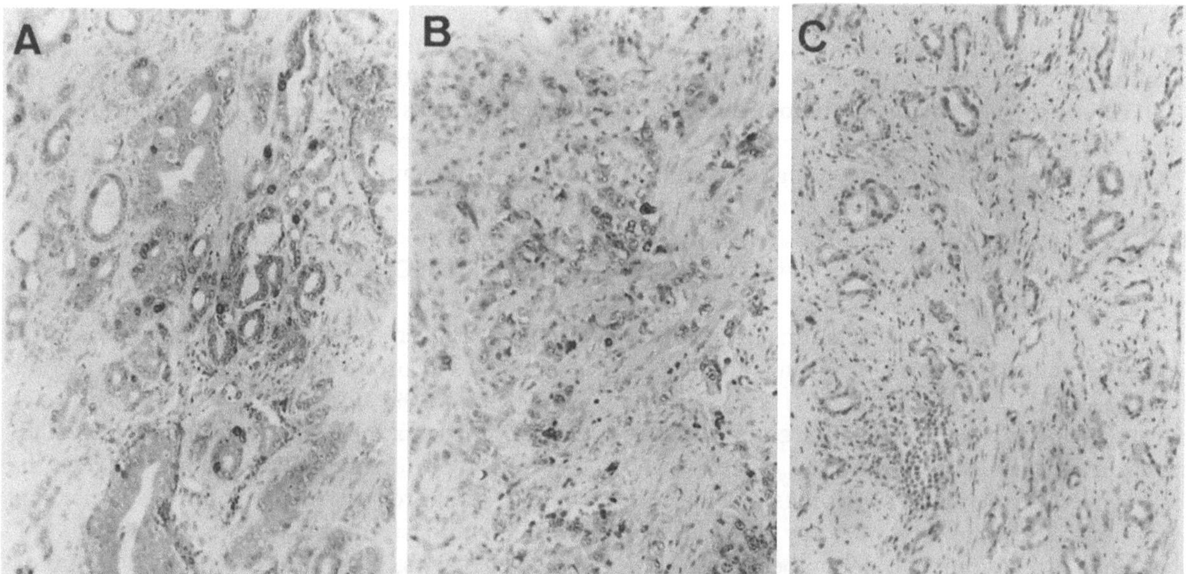

Fig. 4.10A–C. Immunohistochemistry. **A** Proliferating tumor cells express PCNA (black nuclei) (×100). **B** A minority of cells express nuclear p53 protein (black nuclei) (×100). **C** Most cells demonstrate nuclear androgen receptor reactivity (dark-stained nuclei) (×100)

The usefulness of *DNA measurements* by flow cytometry and image analysis is currently under investigation. It seems that an aneuploid tumor has a poor prognosis and is expected to respond poorly to either irradiation or endocrine therapy (SCHRÖDER et al. 1994).

4.4.4.3 p53 Protein

Genetic alterations or mutations are a required process of carcinogenesis involving oncogenes and tumor-suppressor genes such as p53 and retinoblastoma gene (BOOKSTEIN and ALLRED 1993). The p53 tumor suppressor gene, so-called guardian of the genome, prevents the development of cancer by blocking the division of cells that have sustained DNA damage and possibly triggering cell death by apoptosis (LANE 1994). Inactivation of p53 is one of the most common molecular steps in the development of cancer (HOLLSTEIN et al. 1991). Located on chromosome 17p, the p53 gene encodes a 53-kDa phosphoprotein (wild type) that appears to play an important role in controlling cell proliferation (ULLRICH et al. 1992). Several types of mutation in p53 have been shown to occur in human malignancies (VOGELSTEIN and KINZLER 1992). The study of these alterations needs molecular biologic techniques and they are most probably infrequent in clinically localized CaP (ITTMANN et al. 1994).

Missense mutations in exons 5–8 of the p53 gene, however, result in increased stability and accumulation of the p53 protein (mutant type), permitting p53 protein detection by immunohistochemical techniques (Fig. 4.10B). The frequency of p53 mutation in CaP is low, with a reported range of immunohistochemical expression of 13%–20% (THOMPSON et al. 1992; BOOKSTEIN et al. 1993; THOMAS et al. 1993; KALLAKURY et al. 1994; APRIKIAN et al. 1994b).

Compiled data indicate correlations between p53 nuclear immunostaining and increasing tumor grade (KALLAKURY et al. 1994; APRIKIAN et al. 1994b), tumor stage (BOOKSTEIN et al. 1993; MYERS et al. 1994), androgen independence (BERNER et al. 1993), and possibly decreased survival (THOMAS et al. 1993). Examining 191 radical prostatectomy specimens we have found a significant correlation between p53 labeling and mitotic index ($r = 0.3712$; $P \leq 0.0001$) (unpublished data). It has been postulated that p53 gene mutation may be a late event in the progression of CaP (NAVONE et al. 1993), and may occur prior to development of metastasis. It may be difficult, however, to identify a subclass of CaP that expresses a high potential for metastasis (MYERS et al. 1994). The p53 labeling index does seem to be significantly higher in CaP patients with lymph node involvement (personal observation).

4.4.4.4 Androgen Receptor

The androgen dependency of CaP has been apparent for several decades (HUGGINS and HODGES 1941). A number of methods of androgen deprivation are currently being used as the primary therapy of advanced CaP (SCOTT et al. 1980) and in the neoadjuvant treatment of localized cancer prior to surgery (FAIR et al. 1993). Hormonal therapy, however, has been found to be effective for only a limited time because of the presence and/or development of hormone-resistant tumor cell clones (ISAACS and COFFEY 1984). It is thought that androgen receptor expression may be used to predict clinical response to antiandrogenic treatment, and antibodies are raised against human androgen receptor.

The gene that codes the androgen receptor is on the X chromosome, and the coding sequence for the protein is divided into eight exons that, via mRNA transcription, are translated into a 110-kDa protein consisting of 910 amino acids (BRINKMAN et al. 1992). This androgen receptor protein has a strong affinity for nuclear binding under conditions of androgen stimulation. The binding of, for instance, dihydrotestosterone to the androgen receptor is regulated by the level of phosphorylation of the receptor. It has been suggested that PSAP, for example, may play a role in dephosphorylation and, consequently, inactivation of androgen receptors.

Immunohistochemical reactive androgen receptor (Fig. 4.10C) has been detected in CaP (RUIZEVELD DE WINTER et al. 1990; LODA et al. 1994). It has been established that the androgen receptor content correlates inversely with tumor grade (MASAI et al. 1990; CHODAK et al. 1992) and stage (personal observation). However, the reported studies have failed to reveal a correlation between the content of androgen receptor-positive nuclei and patients' responsiveness to therapy (SADI et al. 1991; VAN DER KWAST et al. 1991; SADI and BARRACK 1993). Recently, it has been suggested that point mutations and consequent androgen receptor structural alterations may have significance in tumor progression (KLOCKER et al. 1994).

4.4.4.5 Neuroendocrine Differentiation

Several published reports have shown that a majority of conventional prostatic adenocarcinomas demonstrate (focal) neuroendocrine differentiation (CAPPELLA et al. 1981; DI SANT'AGNESE and DE MESY JENSEN 1987; ABRAHAMSSON et al. 1987; COHEN et al. 1990; APRIKIAN et al. 1993; BOSTWICK et al. 1994; VAN DE VOORDE et al. 1995b).

Neuroendocrine cells in prostatic adenocarcinoma are demonstrable with histochemical and immunohistochemical staining techniques (Fig. 4.11A,B). Tumoral neuroendocrine cells most commonly express NSE, chromogranin A, and serotonin, as well as eutopic and ectopic neuropeptides such as thyroid-stimulating hormone, calcitonin, gastrin-releasing peptide, and adrenocorticotropic hormone (DI SANT'AGNESE and COCKETT 1994). Besides the immunohistochemical localization of these products in CaP neuroendocrine cells, different hormones have been found in serum and urine, and paraneoplastic syndromes have also occurred in patients with CaP (DI SANT'AGNESE 1992). CaP neuroendocrine cells may coexpress PSA and/or PSAP (APRIKIAN et al. 1993; BONKHOFF et al. 1994a).

In 10% (ADLAKHA and BOSTWICK 1994) to 13% (unpublished data) of CaP, neuroendocrine differentiation is revealed by the presence of so-called Paneth-like cells (Fig. 4.11C,D) that are in fact neuroendocrine differentiated tumor cells with prominent eosinophilic cytoplasmic granules (ADLAKHA and BOSTWICK 1994; VAN DE VOORDE et al. 1994c).

There is contradictory evidence regarding the prognostic significance of neuroendocrine differentiation in prostatic adenocarcinoma. Some studies have indicated that this feature is related to more aggressive tumor behavior (COHEN et al. 1990), and that as the prognosis worsens the larger is the neuroendocrine cell fraction (DAUGE and DELMAS 1987). A recent study has shown a statistically significant correlation between neuroendocrine differentiation and the development of metastases (CASAMENTO et al. 1992). Neuroendocrine tumor cells have also been detected in lymph node and bone

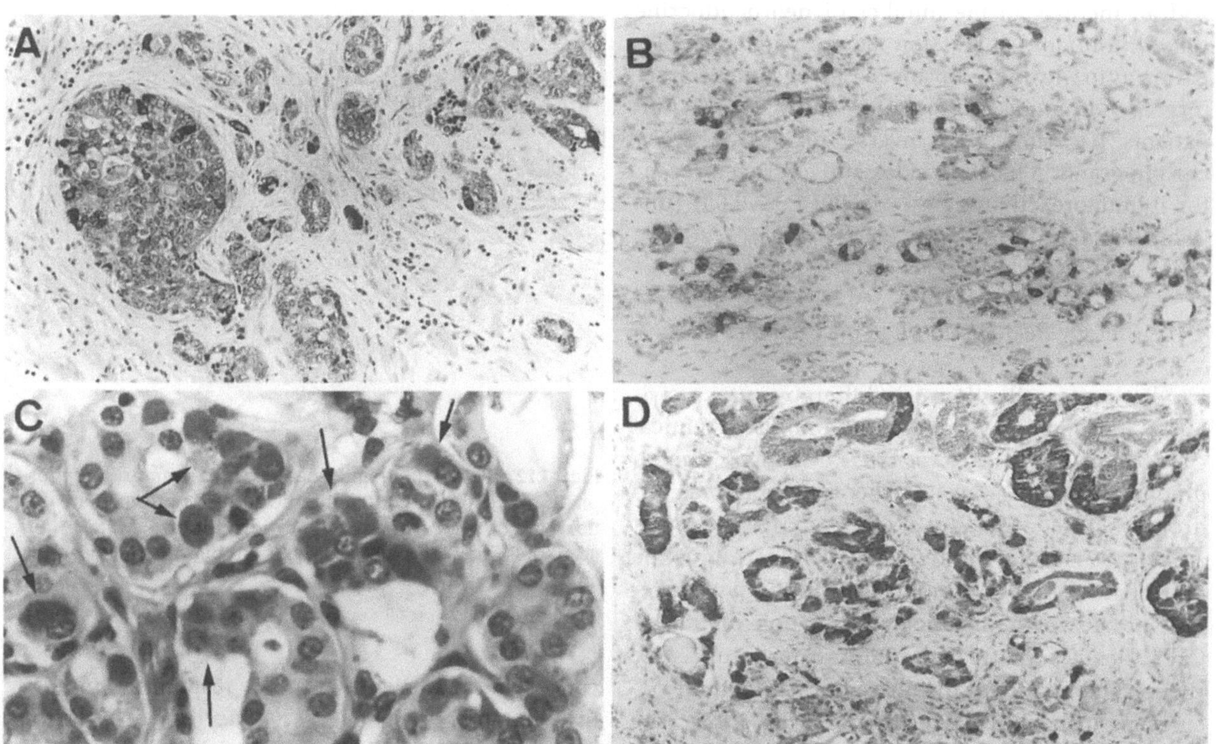

Fig. 4.11A–D. Neuroendocrine differentiation in CaP. **A** Single tumor cells, irregularly dispersed, are labeled with the neuroendocrine marker chromogranin A and **B** the amine serotonin (black cells) (×100). Sometimes, Paneth-like tumor cells (**C**) can be identified with coarse eosinophilic granules in their cytoplasm (*arrows*) (×400) that (**D**) stain bright red with Masson's trichrome (dark cells) (×200)

metastases (APRIKIAN et al. 1994a). The prognostic significance of this parameter, however, has been denied by other investigators (APRIKIAN et al. 1993; COHEN et al. 1994; BOSTWICK et al. 1994). We have confirmed the previously reported finding that the number of neuroendocrine cells increases with increasing Gleason score and progressing pathologic stage (ABRAHAMSSON et al. 1989; VAN DE VOORDE et al. 1995b). Examination of 213 untreated CaP patients also revealed a positive correlation between the chromogranin A labeling index and proliferation, assessed by mitotic figure count ($r = 0.4302$; $P \leq 0.0001$) and PCNA labeling index ($r = 0.2306$; $P \leq 0.01$) (unpublished data). Furthermore, the degree of neuroendocrine differentiation not only correlates well with the Gleason score and tumor volume but also can be considered an independent predictor of pathologic stage beyond, for example, the Gleason score (VAN DE VOORDE et al. 1995b). Finally, serum levels of NSE and chromogranin A are elevated in patients with an advanced stage of disease and those who become refractory to hormonal therapy (KADMON et al. 1991; TARLE et al. 1994). It has been shown that tumoral neuroendocrine cells most probably lack androgen receptors (BONKHOFF et al. 1993), and an increase in the number of neuroendocrine cells with tumor progression may provide an explanation as to why more advanced CaP becomes refractory to hormonal therapy. Our study of 113 CaP patients has shown an inverse relation between chromogranin A labeling index and androgen receptor immunoreactivity ($r = -0.199$; $P \leq 0.05$) (unpublished data).

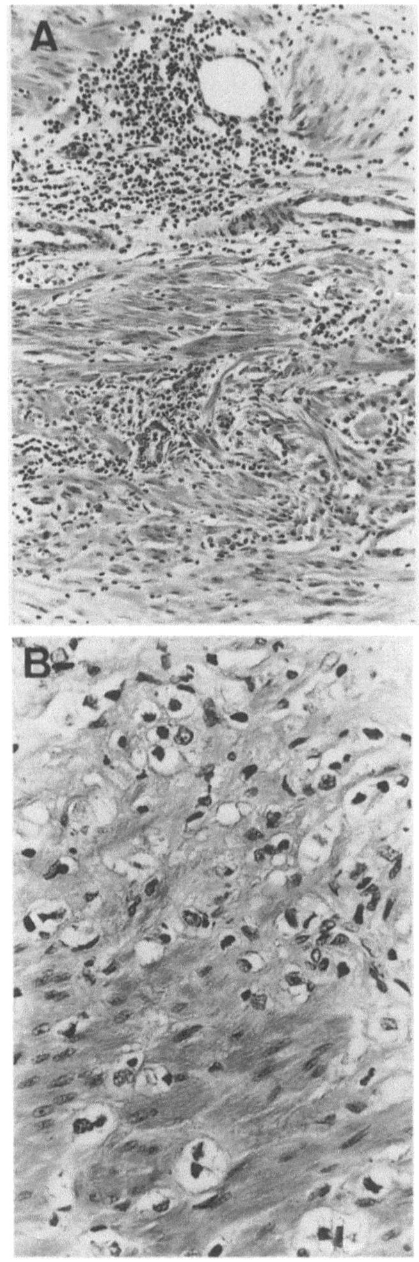

Fig. 4.12A,B. Morphologic changes in estramustine phosphate-treated CaP. **A** Altered tumor cells (*lower half*) are difficult to discern from lymphocytic infiltrates (*upper half*) (×100). **B** Detail of tumor cells with cytoplasmic vacuolization and nuclear pyknosis (×400)

4.4.5 Therapy-Related Morphologic Changes

Irradiation as well as hormonal therapy induce various morphologic and immunohistochemical changes in CaP (HELPAP 1985). Changes due to preoperative (neoadjuvant) therapy with total androgen blockade (ARMAS et al. 1994; MONTIRONI et al. 1994; SMITH and MURPHY 1994) and estramustine phosphate (VAN DE VOORDE et al. 1994b) may represent pitfalls in the histologic evaluation of treated CaP. Changes in treated tumors are cytoplasmic vacuolization, nuclear pyknosis, fibrosis, and the occurrence of lymphocytic infiltrates (Fig. 4.12). The altered morphology hampers recognition of cancerous tissue and influences histologic grading when using the Gleason system. It seems that a good response to therapy with more pronounced histologic changes paradoxically mimics a poorly differentiated cancer. In the presence of tumor response, immunohistochemistry will suggest a decreased secretion of PSA and PSAP, and a diminished proliferative activity.

In tumors treated with radiotherapy, the degree of fibrosis and nuclear changes are more evident. Polynuclear, bizarre tumor cells may be seen and sclerosis may be pronounced with serious difficulties in identifying malignant cells (BOSTWICK et al. 1982; HELPAP 1985).

4.5 Diagnosis of Prostatic Cancer

4.5.1 Needle-Core Biopsies

The ultrasound-guided needle-core biopsy provides a means to diagnose CaP in case of a palpable and/or ultrasonographically hypoechoic focal lesion (in the peripheral zone). Currently, urologists advocate six to eight systematic sextant biopsies of the prostate for patients with raised PSA without a clinically detectable nodule (see Chap. 7) to diagnose a T1c cancer.

Approximately one-half of needle-core biopsy samples performed for a suspicious focal lesion reveal CaP. In the remaining half benign prostatic tissue, (granulomatous) prostatitis, or, rarely, PIN are identified (EPSTEIN 1993). A small number of the negative biopsy samples with histologically benign prostatic glands are related to a so-called peripheral hyperplastic nodule (VAN DE VOORDE et al. 1995a).

Even limited adenocarcinoma can be detected on (systematic sextant) biopsies (EPSTEIN 1995), and can be readily graded according to the Gleason system (BOSTWICK 1994c). It has been shown that a minute focus of 3 mm or less of well-differentiated cancer on one needle biopsy out of six most likely corresponds to a clinically unimportant tumor of less than 0.5 cm^3 (MURPHY et al. 1994). Immunohistochemical staining for 34βE12 cytokeratin has been proven to be a useful tool in establishing the diagnosis of AAH versus well-differentiated CaP, and in confirming a small focus of cancer in needle biopsies (WOJNO and EPSTEIN 1995). However, one has to keep in mind that interpretation in the appropriate context is required. Negative staining of an entire suspicious focus can be taken as presumptive evidence when one is aware of the possible entrapment of benign glands. On the other hand, single acini may lack 34βE12 immunoreactivity in cases of AAH because of discontinuous staining around glands of this lesion.

4.5.2 Transurethral Resections

Transurethral resection of the prostate and simple subtotal prostatectomy or enucleation only remove the hyperplastic transition zone. Therefore, the most common lesions encountered in these specimens are BPH and related conditions such as AAH and basal cell hyperplasia (VAN DE VOORDE et al. 1994a). It is important that enough tissue, i.e., at least 60%, of the specimen is included for microscopic evaluation to detect a minute amount of cancer. The knowledge about differences in morphology of CaP according to the zone of origin influences the diagnostic interpretation, as shown in Table 4.5. Well-differentiated adenocarcinoma most often indicates a primary origin in the transition zone while the occurrence of even a few chips with poorly differentiated cancer corresponds to an advanced stage with poor prognosis.

4.5.3 Radical Prostatectomies

Radical prostatectomy specimens must be handled with care; the surface of the specimen has to be inked for evaluation of surgical margins and step-sectioned to include the whole tumor (EPSTEIN 1991; HALL et al. 1992). The report of the pathologist has to deal with histologic grade (GLEASON 1990), the pathologic stage (SCHRÖDER et al. 1992), the state of the surgical margins (EPSTEIN 1990), and estimation of the tumor volume (SCHMID and MCNEAL 1992).

Table 4.5. Interpretation of TURP specimens

No. of involved chips	Grade of CaP	
	Low grade (Gleason score ≤4)	High grade (Gleason score ≥7)
Few (<5%)	Most probably TZCa (T1a)	Probably extension of progressive (T3) PZCa
	PZCa very unlikely	TZCa unlikely
Many (>5%)	Probably TZCa (T1b)	Nearly always progressed (T3c–T4a)
	Extension of PZCa unlikely	(Inoperable) PZCa/TZCa

In approximately one-half of radical prostatectomies, although performed for clinically localized CaP, pathologic examination reveals non-organ-confined disease (Fair et al. 1993). *Capsular penetration* with extension of the tumor into extraprostatic tissue occurs in approximately 40% (Walsh et al. 1983) and may be related to prognosis (McNeal et al. 1990). It has been demonstrated that tumors with more extensive (established) capsular penetration have a higher risk of progression than those showing focal capsular penetration (Epstein et al. 1993b).

Surgical margins are considered to be positive in 30%–60% of specimens (Voges et al. 1992). Not all positive surgical margins are caused by capsular penetration; tumor may be transected due to capsular incision by the surgeon. Furthermore, positive surgical margins in the presence of only focal capsular penetration does not mean that recurrence is inevitable. Local recurrence occurs in about 10% of these patients. A total of 30%–40% of patients with focally positive margins progress at 5 years (Epstein et al. 1993c). The parameter that identified tumors with focal capsular penetration was the Gleason score. The 5-year progression rate in patients with focal capsular penetration increases with the increase in tumor grade. The potential for an artifactually positive margin in radical prostatectomy specimens is great, given the flimsy amount of periprostatic soft tissue surrounding the prostate, which may be easily disrupted either intraoperatively or postoperatively in the handling of the specimen (Epstein 1990).

Some 20% of radical prostatectomies demonstrate *invasion of seminal vesicles*, which is defined as invasion of the muscular wall. This phenomenon is associated with a poor prognosis, and may be influenced by the mechanism of seminal vesicle involvement (Ohori et al. 1993). In most cases, direct extension either along the ejaculatory complex and/or through the capsule into the seminal vesicles is encountered. A minority of patients are characterized by the finding of isolated deposits of cancer in the seminal vesicles, and show better progression-free survival rates.

4.6 Conclusions

Close interaction between the pathologist and the urologist is imperative in medical centers interested in the management of patients with prostatic carcinoma. The complexities of contemporary pathology of the prostate require the presence in such medical centers of a pathologist specifically interested in this area of urologic oncology. The evaluation of data from appropriate histologic studies of needle biopsy and prostatectomy specimens together with relevant biochemical and clinical information permits a reasonably accurate conclusion to be drawn as to the likelihood of a favorable treatment outcome. In view of the importance of CaP in Europe and North America, and the high potential for a favorable treatment outcome when treatment is given in a proper environment, it is strongly believed by the author that the management of CaP patients should be limited to specifically designated uro-oncology centers of excellence.

References

Abrahamsson P-A, di Sant'Agnese PA (1993) Neuroendocrine cells in the human prostate gland. J Androl 14:307–309

Abrahamsson P-A, Wadström LB, Alumets J, Falkmer S, Grimelius L (1986) Peptide-hormone- and serotonin-immunoreactive cells in normal and hyperplastic prostate glands. Pathol Res Pract 181:675–683

Abrahamsson P-A, Wadström LB, Alumets J, Falkmer S, Grimelius L (1987) Peptide-hormone- and serotonin-immunoreactive tumour cells in carcinoma of the prostate. Pathol Res Pract 182:298–307

Abrahamsson P-A, Falkmer S, Fäit K, Grimelius L (1989) The course of neuroendocrine differentiation in prostatic carcinomas. An immunohistochemical study testing chromogranin A as an "endocrine marker". Pathol Res Pract 185:373–380

Adlakha H, Bostwick DG (1994) Paneth cell-like change in prostatic adenocarcinoma represents neuroendocrine differentiation: report of 30 cases. Hum Pathol 25:135–139

Allsbrook WC, Simms WW (1992) Histochemistry of the prostate. Hum Pathol 23:297–305

Aprikian AG, Cordon-Cardo C, Fair WR, Reuter VE (1993) Characterization of neuroendocrine differentiation in human benign prostate and prostatic adenocarcinoma. Cancer 71:3952–3965

Aprikian AG, Cordon-Cardo C, Fair WR, Zhang Z-F, Bazinet M, Hamdy SM, Reuter VE (1994a) Neuroendocrine differentiation in metastatic prostate adenocarcinoma. J Urol 151:914–919

Aprikian AG, Sarkis AS, Fair WR, Zhang Z-F, Fuks Z, Cordon-Cardo C (1994b) Immunohistochemical determination of p53 protein nuclear accumulation in prostatic adenocarcinoma. J Urol 151:1276–1280

Armas OA, Aprikian AG, Melamed J et al. (1994) Clinical and pathobiological effects of neoadjuvant total androgen ablation therapy on clinically localized prostatic adenocarcinoma. Am J Surg Pathol 18:979–991

Aumüller H (1983) Morphologic and endocrine aspects of prostatic function. Prostate 4:195–214

Ayala AG, Ro JY, Babaian R, Troncosa P, Grignon DJ (1989) The prostatic capsule: does it exist? Its importance in the staging and treatment of prostatic carcinoma. Am J Surg Pathol 13:21–27

Benoit G, Jardin A, Gillot C (1993) Reflections and suggestions on the nomenclature of the prostate. Surg Radiol Anat 15:325–332

Berner A, Nesland JM, Waehre H, Silke J, Fossa SD (1993) Hormone resistant prostatic adenocarcinoma. An evaluation of prognostic factors in pre- and post-treatment specimens. Br J Cancer 68:380–384

Bonkhoff H, Remberger K (1993) Widespread distribution of nuclear androgen receptors in the basal cell layer of the normal and hyperplastic human prostate. Virchows Arch [A] 422:35–38

Bonkhoff H, Stein U, Remberger K (1993) Androgen receptor status in endocrine-paracrine cell types of the normal, hyperplastic, and neoplastic human prostate. Virchows Arch [A] 423:291–294

Bonkhoff H, Stein U, Remberger K (1994a) Multidirectional differentiation in the normal, hyperplastic, and neoplastic human prostate: simultaneous demonstration of cell-specific epithelial markers. Hum Pathol 25:42–46

Bonkhoff H, Stein U, Remberger K (1994b) The proliferative function of basal cells in the normal and hyperplastic human prostate. Prostate 24:114–118

Bookstein R, Allred D (1993) Recessive oncogenes. Cancer 71:1179–1186

Bookstein R, MacGrogan D, Hilsenbeck SG, Sharkey F, Allred DC (1993) p53 is mutated in a subset of advanced stage prostate cancers. Cancer Res 53:3369–3373

Bostwick DG (1994a) Prostate-specific antigen. Current role in diagnostic pathology of prostate cancer. Am J Clin Pathol 102 (Suppl 1):S31–S37

Bostwick DG (1994b) Grading prostate cancer. Am J Clin Pathol 102 (Suppl 1):S38–S56

Bostwick DG (1994c) Gleason grading of prostatic needle biopsies. Correlation with grade in 316 matched prostatectomies. Am J Surg Pathol 18:796–803

Bostwick DG, Egbert BM, Fajardo LF (1982) Radiation injury of the normal and neoplastic prostate. Am J Surg Pathol 6:541–551

Bostwick DG, Cooner WH, Denis L, Jones GW, Scardino PT, Murphy GP (1992a) The association of benign prostatic hyperplasia and cancer of the prostate. Cancer 70 (Suppl):291–301

Bostwick DG, Montironi R, Wagle R et al. (1992b) Current and proposed biologic markers in prostate cancer, J Cell Biochem Suppl 16H:65–67

Bostwick DG, Amin MB, Dundore P, Marsh W, Schultz DS (1993a) Architectural patterns of high-grade prostatic intraepithelial neoplasia. Hum Pathol 24:298–310

Bostwick DG, Graham SD, Napalkov P et al. (1993b) Staging of early prostate cancer: a proposed tumor volume-based prognostic index. Urology 41:403–411

Bostwick DG, Srigley J, Grignon D et al. (1993c) Atypical adenomatous hyperplasia of the prostate: morphologic criteria for its distinction from well-differentiated carcinoma. Hum Pathol 24:819–832

Bostwick DG, Dousa MK, Crawford BG, Wollan PC (1994) Neuroendocrine differentiation in prostatic intraepithelial neoplasia and adenocarcinoma. Am J Surg Pathol 18:1240–1246

Brinkman AO, Jenster G, Kuiper GGJM et al. (1992) The human androgen receptor: structure/function relationship in normal and pathological situations. J Steroid Biochem Mol Biol 41:361–368

Byar DP, Mostofi FK, VACURG (1972) Carcinoma of the prostate: prognostic evaluation of certain pathologic features in 208 radical prostatectomies examined by the step section technique. Cancer 30:5–13

Capella C, Usellini L, Buffa R, Frigerio B, Solcia E (1981) The endocrine component of prostatic carcinomas, mixed adenocarcinoma-carcinoid tumours and non-tumour prostate. Histochemical and ultrastructural identification of the endocrine cells. Histopathology 5:175–192

Casamento J, Abrahamsson P-A, Nakada SY, di Sant'Agnese PA, de Mesy Jensen KL, Cockett ATK (1992) Prognostic significance of neuroendocrine differentiation in prostatic carcinoma. J Urol 147:332A

Cher ML, Chew K, Rosenau W, Carroll PR (1995) Cellular proliferation in prostatic adenocarcinoma as assessed by bromodeoxyuridine uptake and Ki-67 and PCNA expression. Prostate 26:87–93

Chiarodo A (ed) (1991) National Cancer Institute roundtable on prostate cancer: future research directions. Meeting Report. Cancer Res 51:2498–2505

Chodak GW, Kranc DM, Puy LA, Tihada H, Johnson K, Chang C (1992) Nuclear localization of androgen receptor in heterogeneous samples of normal, hyperplastic and neoplastic human prostate. J Urol 147:798–803

Christensen WN, Partin AW, Walsh PC, Epstein JI (1990) Pathologic findings in clinical stage A2 prostate cancer. Relation of tumor volume, grade, and location to pathologic stage. Cancer 65:1021–1027

Christensen WN, Steinberg G, Walsh PC, Epstein JI (1991) Prostatic duct adenocarcinoma. Findings at radical prostatectomy. Cancer 67:2118–2124

Christopher ME, Seftel AD, Sorensen K, Resnick MI (1991) Small cell carcinoma of the genitourinary tract: an immunohistochemical, electron microscopic and clinicopathological study. J Urol 146:382–388

Cohen MK, Arber DA, Coffield KS, Keegan GT, McClintock J, Speights VO (1994) Neuroendocrine differentiation in prostatic adenocarcinoma and its relationship to tumor progression. Cancer 74:1899–1903

Cohen RJ, Glezerson G, Haffejee Z, Afrika D (1990) Prostatic carcinoma: histological and immunohistological factors affecting prognosis. Br J Urol 66:405–410

Cunha GR, Chung LWK, Shannon JM et al. (1980) Stromal-epithelial interactions in sex differentiation. Biol Reprod 22:19–42

Currin SM, Lee SE, Walther PJ (1988) Flow cytometric analysis of comedocarcinoma of the prostate: an uncommon histopathological variant of prostatic adenocarcinoma. J Urol 140:96–100

Dauge MC, Delmas V (1987) APUD type endocrine tumour of the prostate. Incidence and prognosis in association with adenocarcinoma. Prog Clin Biol Res 243:529–531

de la Torre M, Haggman M, Brandstedt S, Busch C (1993) Prostatic intraepithelial neoplasia and invasive carcinoma in total prostatectomy specimens: distribution, volume and DNA ploidy. Br J Urol 72:207–213

di Sant'Agnese PA (1992) Neuroendocrine differentiation in carcinoma of the prostate. Diagnostic, prognostic, and therapeutic implications. Cancer 70 (Suppl):254–268

di Sant'Agnese PA, Cockett ATK (1994) The prostatic endocrine-paracrine (neuroendocrine) regulatory system and neuroendocrine differentiation in prostatic carcinoma: a review and future directions in basic research. J Urol 152:1927–1931

di Sant'Agnese PA, de Mesy Jensen KL (1984) Endocrine-paracrine cells of the prostate and prostatic urethra: an ultrastructural study. Hum Pathol 15:1034–1041

di Sant'Agnese PA, de Mesy Jensen KL (1987) Neuroendocrine differentiation in prostatic adenocarcinoma. Hum Pathol 18:849–856

di Sant'Agnese PA, de Mesy Jensen KL, Churukian CJ, Agarwal MM (1985) Human prostatic endocrine-paracrine (APUD) cells. Distributional analysis with a comparison of serotonin and neuron-specific enolase immunoreactivity and silver stains. Arch Pathol Lab Med 109:607–612
Eggleston JC, Walsh PC (1985) Radical prostatectomy with preservation of sexual function: pathologic findings in the first 100 cases. J Urol 134:1146–1148
Elgamal AA, Van de Voorde W, Van Poppel H, Lauweryns J, Baert L (1994a) Immunohistochemical localization of prostate-specific markers within accessory male sex glands of Cowper, Littré and Morgagni. Urology 44:84–90
Elgamal AA, Van de Voorde W, Van Poppel H, Vandeursen H, Baert L, Lauweryns J (1994b) Exophytic papillary prostatic duct adenocarcinoma with endometrioid features, occurring in prostatic urethra after TURP. Urology 43:737–742
Epstein JI (1990) Evaluation of radical prostatectomy capsular margins of resection: the significance of margins designated as negative, closely approaching, and positive. Am J Surg Pathol 14:626–632
Epstein JI (1991) The evaluation of radical prostatectomy specimens. Therapeutic and prognostic implications. Pathol Annu 26:159–210
Epstein JI (1992) Differential diagnosis in pathology. Urologic disorders. Igaku-Shoin, New York, pp 108–109
Epstein JI (1993) Discrepancies between findings suspicious for prostate cancer at rectal examination and benign biopsy findings. Radiology 189:657–658
Epstein JI (1995) Diagnostic criteria of limited adenocarcinoma of the prostate on needle biopsy. Hum Pathol 26:223–229
Epstein JI, Lieberman PH (1985) Mucinous adenocarcinoma of the prostate gland. Am J Surg Pathol 9:299–308
Epstein JI, Carmichael M, Partin AW, Walsh PC (1993a) Is tumor volume an independent predictor of progression following radical prostatectomy? A multivariate analysis of 185 clinical stage B adenocarcinomas of the prostate with five years follow-up. J Urol 149:1478–1481
Epstein JI, Carmichael M, Pizov G et al. (1993b) Influence of capsular penetration on progression following radical prostatectomy: a study of 196 cases with long-term follow-up. J Urol 150:135–141
Epstein JI, Pizov G, Walsh PC (1993c) Correlation of pathologic findings with progression after radical retropubic prostatectomy. Cancer 71:3582–3593
Fair WR, Aprikian A, Sogani P, Reuter V, Whitmore WF (1993) The role of neoadjuvant hormonal manipulation in localized prostate cancer. Cancer 71 (Suppl):1031–1038
Gaudin PB, Epstein JI (1994) Adenosis of the prostate. Histologic features in transurethral resection specimens. Am J Surg Pathol 18:863–870
Gleason DF (1990) Histologic grading of prostatic carcinoma. In: Bostwick DG (ed) Pathology of the prostate. Churchill Livingstone, New York, pp 83–93
Gleason DF, Mellinger GT, VACURG (1974) Prediction of prognosis for prostatic carcinoma by combined histological grading and clinical staging. J Urol 111:58–64
Greene DR, Wheeler TM, Egawa S, Dunn JK, Scardino PT (1991) A comparison of the morphological features of cancer arising in the transition zone and in the peripheral zone of the prostate. J Urol 146:1069–1076
Greene DR, Fitzpatrick JM, Scardino PT (1995) Anatomy of the prostate and distribution of early prostate cancer. Semin Surg Oncol 11:9–22
Guerin D, Hasan N, Keen CE (1993) Signet ring cell differentiation in adenocarcinoma of the prostate: a study of five cases. Histopathology 22:367–371
Hall GS, Kramer CE, Epstein JI (1992) Evaluation of radical prostatectomy specimens. A comparative analysis of sampling methods. Am J Surg Pathol 16:315–324
Harper ME, Glynne-Jones E, Goddard L et al. (1992) Relationship of proliferating cell nuclear antigen (PCNA) in prostatic carcinomas to various clinical parameters. Prostate 20:243–253
Hedrick L, Epstein JI (1989) Use of keratin 903 as an adjunct in the diagnosis of prostate carcinoma. Am J Surg Pathol 13:389–396
Helpap B (1985) Treated prostatic carcinoma. Histological, immunohistochemical and cell kinetic studies. Appl Pathol 3:230–241
Hollstein M, Sidransky D, Vogelstein B, Harris C (1991) p53 mutations in human cancer. Science 253:49–53
Huggins C, Hodges CV (1941) Studies on prostatic cancer. The effect of castration, of estrogen and of androgen injection on serum phosphatases in metastatic carcinoma of the prostate. Cancer Res 1:293–297
Humphrey PA, Frazier HA, Vollmer RT, Paulson DF (1993) Stratification of pathologic features in radical prostatectomy specimens that are predictive of elevated initial postoperative serum prostate-specific antigen levels. Cancer 71:1821–1827
Isaacs JT, Coffey DS (1984) Adaptation versus selection as the mechanism responsible for relapse of prostate cancer to androgen ablation therapy as studied in the Dunning R-3327-H adenocarcinoma. Cancer Res 41:5070–5075
Ittmann M, Wieczorek R, Heller P, Dave A, Provet J, Krolewski J (1994) Alterations in the p53 and MDM-2 genes are infrequent in clinically localized, stage B prostate adenocarcinomas. Am J Pathol 145:287–293
Jones EC, Young RH (1994) The differential diagnosis of prostatic carcinoma. Its distinction from premalignant and pseudocarcinomatous lesions of the prostate gland. Am J Clin Pathol 101:48–64
Kadmon D, Thompson TC, Lynch GR, Scardino PT (1991) Elevated plasma chromogranin-A concentrations in prostatic carcinoma. J Urol 146:358–361
Kallakury BVS, Frigge J, Ross JS, Fisher HAG, Figge HL, Jennings TA (1994) Association of p53 immunoreactivity with high Gleason tumor grade in prostatic adenocarcinoma. Hum Pathol 25:92–97
Kellokumpu-Lehtinen P, Santti R, Pelliriemi LJ (1980) Correlation of early cytodifferentiation of the human prostate and Leydig cells. Anat Res 196:262–273
Klocker H, Culig Z, Hobisch A, Cato ACB, Bartsch G (1994) Androgen receptor alterations in prostatic carcinoma. Prostate 25:266–273
Lane DP (1994) The regulation of p53 function: Steiner Award Lecture. Int J Cancer 57:623–627
Larsen WJ (1993) Development of the urogenital system. In: Larsen WJ (ed) Human embryology. Churchill Livingstone, New York, pp 235–279
Lepor H, Gregerman M, Crosby R, Mostofi FK, Walsh PC (1985) Precise localization of the autonomic nerves from the pelvic plexus to the corpora cavernosa: a detailed anatomical study of the adult male pelvis. J Urol 133:207–212
Loda M, Fogt F, French FS, Posner M, Cukor B, Aretz HT, Alsaigh N (1994) Androgen receptor immunohistochemistry on paraffin-embedded tissue. Mod Pathol 7:388–391
Masai M, Sumiya H, Akimoto S, Yatani R, Chang C, Liao S, Shimazaki J (1990) Immunohistochemical study of androgen receptor in benign hyperplastic and cancerous human prostates. Prostate 17:293–300

Matzkin H, Soloway MS, Hardeman S (1991) Transitional cell carcinoma of the prostate. J Urol 146:1207–1212
McNeal JE (1980) Anatomy of the prostate: an historical survey of divergent views. Prostate 1:3–13
McNeal JE (1983) The prostate gland. Morphology and pathobiology. Monogr Urol 4:3–33
McNeal JE (1988a) Normal histology of the prostate. Am J Surg Pathol 12:619–633
McNeal JE (1988b) Significance of duct-acinar dysplasia in prostatic carcinogenesis. Prostate 13:91–102
McNeal JE (1992) Cancer volume and site of origin of adenocarcinoma in the prostate: relationship to local and distant spread. Hum Pathol 23:258–266
McNeal JE, Bostwick DG (1986) Intraductal dysplasia: a premalignant lesion of the prostate. Hum Pathol 17:64–71
McNeal JE, Bostwick DG, Kindrachuk RA, Redwine EA, Freiha ES, Stamey TA (1986) Patterns of progression in prostate cancer. Lancet 1:60–63
McNeal JE, Price HM, Redwine EA, Freiha FS, Stamey TA (1988a) Stage A versus stage B adenocarcinoma of the prostate: morphological comparison and histological significance. J Urol 139:61–65
McNeal JE, Redwine EA, Freiha FS, Stamey TA (1988b) Zonal distribution of prostatic adenocarcinoma. Correlation with histologic pattern and direction of spread. Am J Surg Pathol 12:897–906
McNeal JE, Villers AA, Redwine EA, Freiha FS, Stamey TA (1990) Capsular penetration in prostate cancer. Significance for natural history and treatment Am J Surg Pathol 14:240–247
McNeal JE, Alroy J, Villers A, Redwine EA, Freiha FS, Stamey TA (1991) Mucinous differentiation in prostatic adenocarcinoma. Hum Pathol 22:979–988
Montie JE, Wood DP Jr, Vanderburg Medendorp S, Levin HS, Pontes JE (1990) The significance and management of transitional cell carcinoma of the prostate. Semin Urol 8:262–268
Montironi R, Magi-Galluzzi C, Muzzonigro G, Prete E, Polito M, Fabris G (1994) Effects of combination endocrine treatment on normal prostate, prostatic intraepithelial neoplasia, and prostatic adenocarcinoma. J Clin Pathol 47:906–913
Mostofi FK, Price EB Jr (1973) Tumors of male genital system (Fascicle 8). Atlas of tumor pathology, 2nd series. Armed Forces Institute of Pathology, Washington DC, pp 236–338
Mostofi FK, Sesterhenn I, Sobin LH (1980) Histologic typing of prostate tumours. (International histological classification of tumours, no. 22). WHO, Geneva
Murphy GP, Busch C, Abrahamsson P-A et al. (1994) Histopathology of localized prostate cancer. Scand J Urol Nephrol Suppl 162:7–42
Myers RP (1991a) Anatomical variation of the superficial preprostatic veins with respect to radical retropublic prostatectomy. J Urol 145:992–993
Myers RP (1991b) Male urethral sphincteric anatomy and radical prostatectomy. Urol Clin North Am 18:211–227
Myers RP, Goellner JR, Cahill DR (1987) Prostate shape, external striated urethral sphincter and radical prostatectomy: the apical dissection. J Urol 138:543–550
Myers RB, Oelschlager D, Srivastave S, Grizzle WE (1994) Accumulation of the p53 protein occurs more frequently in metastatic than in localized prostatic adenocarcinomas. Prostate 25:243–248
Navone NM, Troncoso P, Pisters LL et al. (1993) p53 protein accumulation and gene mutation in the progression of human prostate carcinoma. J Natl Cancer Inst 85:1657–1669
Oesterling JE, Hauzeur CG, Farrow GM (1992) Small cell anaplastic carcinoma of the prostate: a clinical, pathological and immunohistological study of 27 patients. J Urol 147:804–807
Ohori M, Scardino PT, Lapin SL, Seale-Hawkins C, Link J, Wheeler TM (1993) The mechanisms and prognostic significance of seminal vesicle involvement by prostate cancer. Am J Surg Pathol 17:1252–1261
Pearse AGE (1969) The cytochemistry and ultrastructure of polypeptide hormone-producing cells of the APUD series and the embryologic, physiologic and pathologic implications of the concept. J Histochem Cytochem 17:303–313
Reese JH, Freiha FS, Gelb AB, Lum BL, Torti FM (1992) Transitional cell carcinoma of the prostate in patients undergoing radical cystoprostatectomy. J Urol 147:92–95
Reichlin S (1993) Neuroendocrine-immune interactions. N Engl J Med 329:1246–1253
Ro JY, Tetu B, Ayala AG, Ordonez NG (1987) Small cell carcinoma of the prostate. II. Immunohistochemical and electron microscopic studies of 18 cases. Cancer 59:977–982
Ro JY, Ayala AG, Wishnow KI, Ordonez NG (1988a) Prostatic duct adenocarcinoma with endometrioid features: immunohistochemical and electron microscopic study. Semin Diagn Pathol 5:301–311
Ro JY, Grignon DJ, Troncoso P, Ayala AG (1988b) Mucin in prostatic adenocarcinoma. Semin Diagn Pathol 5:273–283
Ro JY, Grignon DJ, Ayala AG, Fernandez PL, Ordonez NG, Wishnow KI (1990) Mucinous adenocarcinoma of the prostate: histochemical and immunohistochemical studies. Hum Pathol 21:593–600
Ruizeveld de Winter JA, Trapman J, Brinkmann AO et al. (1990) Androgen receptor heterogeneity in human prostatic carcinomas visualized by immunohistochemistry. J Pathol 161:329–332
Sadi MV, Barrack ER (1993) Image analysis of androgen receptor immunostaining in metastatic prostate cancer-heterogeneity as a predictor of response to hormonal therapy. Cancer 71:2574–2580
Sadi MV, Walsh PC, Barrack ER (1991) Immunohistochemical study of androgen receptors in metastatic prostate cancer. Comparison of receptor content and response to hormonal therapy. Cancer 67:3057–3064
Schmid H-P, McNeal JE (1992) An abbreviated standard procedure for accurate tumor volume estimation in prostate cancer. Am J Surg Pathol 16:184–191
Schröder FH, Hermanek P, Denis L et al. (1992) The TNM classification of prostate cancer. Prostate 4 (Suppl):129–138
Schröder F, Tribukait B, Böcking A et al. (1994) Clinical utility of cellular DNA measurements in prostate carcinoma. Scand J Urol Nephrol Suppl 162:51–64
Scott WW, Menon M, Walsh PC (1980) Hormonal therapy of prostatic cancer. Cancer 45 (Suppl):1929–1936
Siiteri PK, Wilson JD (1974) Testosterone formation and metabolism during male sexual differentiation in the human embryo. J Clin Endocrinol Metab 38:113–125
Smith DM, Murphy WM (1994) Histologic changes in prostate carcinomas treated with leuprolide (luteinizing hormone-releasing hormone effect). Distinction from poor tumor differentiation. Cancer 73:1472–1477
Sogani P, Israel A, Lieberman P et al. (1985) Gleason grading of prostatic cancer: a predictor of survival. Urology 25:223–227
Spires SE, Banks ER, Davey DD, Jennings CD, Wood DP, Cibull ML (1994) Proliferating cell nuclear antigen in pro-

static adenocarcinoma: correlation with established prognostic indicators. Urology 43:660–666

Stamey TA, Vang H, Hay AR, McNeal JE, Freiha FS, Redwine EA (1987) Prostate-specific antigen as a serum marker for adenocarcinoma of the prostate. N Engl J Med 317:909–916

Tarle M, Frkovic-Grazio S, Kraljic I, Kovacic K (1994) A more objective staging of advanced prostate cancer - routine recognition of malignant endocrine structures: the assessment of serum TPS, PSA, and NSE values. Prostate 24:143–148

Thomas DJ, Robinson M, King P et al. (1993) p53 expression and clinical outcome in prostate cancer. Br J Urol 72:778–781

Thompson SJ, Mellen K, Charlton RG, Marsh C, Robinson M, Neal DE (1992) p53 and Ki-67 immunoreactivity in human prostate cancer and benign hyperplasia. Br J Urol 69:609–613

Ullrich SJ, Anderson CW, Mercer WE et al. (1992) The p53 tumor suppressor protein, a modulator of cell proliferation. J Biol Chem 267:15259–15262

Van der Kwast TH, Schaller J, Ruizenveld de Winter JA, Van Vroonhoven CCJ, Mulder E, Boersma W, Trapman J (1991) Androgen receptors in endocrine therapy-resistant human prostate cancer. Int J Cancer 48:189–193

Van de Voorde WM, Baldewijns M, Lauweryns JM (1994a) Florid basal cell hyperplasia of the prostate. Histopathology 24:341–348

Van de Voorde WM, Elgamal AA, Van Poppel HP, Verbeken EK, Baert LV, Lauweryns JM (1994b) Morphologic and immunohistochemical changes in prostate cancer after preoperative hormonal therapy. A comparative study of radical prostatectomies. Cancer 74:3164–3175

Van de Voorde WM, Van Poppel HP, Haustermans K, Baert LV, Lauweryns JM (1994c) Mucin-secreting adenocarcinoma of the prostate with neuroendocrine differentiation and Paneth-like cells. Am J Surg Pathol 18:200–207

Van de Voorde WM, Oyen RH, Van Poppel HP, Wouters K, Baert LV, Lauweryns JM (1995a) Peripherally localized benign hyperplastic nodules of the prostate. Mod Pathol 8:46–50

Van de Voorde WM, Van Poppel HP, Verbeken EK, Oyen RH, Baert LV, Lauweryns JM (1995b) Morphologic and neuroendocrine features of adenocarcinoma arising in the transition zone and in the peripheral zone of the prostate. Mod Pathol 8:595–598

Van Poppel HP, Ameye F, Oyen R, Van de Voorde WM, Baert LV (1992) Radical prostatectomy for localized prostate cancer. Eur J Surg Oncol 18:456–462

Van Poppel HP, Ameye F, Oyen RH, Van de Voorde WM, Baert LV (1994) Accuracy of combined computerized tomography and fine needle aspiration cytology in lymph node staging of localized prostatic carcinoma. J Urol 151:1310–1314

Vesalainen S, Lipponen P, Talja M, Syrjänen K (1995) Mitotic activity and prognosis in prostatic adenocarcinoma. Prostate 26:80–86

Villers A, McNeal JE, Redwine EA, Freiha FS, Stamey TA (1989) The role of perineural space invasion in the local spread of prostatic adenocarcinoma. J Urol 142:763–768

Vogelstein B, Kinzler KW (1992) p53 function and dysfunction. Cell 70:523–526

Voges GE, McNeal JE, Redwine EA, Freiha FS, Stamey TA (1992) Morphological analysis of surgical margins with positive findings in prostatectomy for adenocarcinoma of the prostate. Cancer 65:520–526

Walsh PC, Lepor H, Eggleston JC (1983) Radical prostatectomy with preservation of sexual function: anatomical and pathological considerations. Prostate 4:473–485

Ware JL (1994) Prostate cancer progression. Implications of histopathology. Am J Pathol 145:983–993

Weinstein MH, Epstein JI (1993) Significance of high-grade prostatic intraepithelial neoplasia on needle biopsy. Hum Pathol 24:624–629

Wojno KJ, Epstein JI (1995) The utility of basal cell-specific anti-cytokeratin antibody (34βE12) in the diagnosis of prostate cancer. A review of 228 cases. Am J Surg Pathol 19:251–260

Wood DP Jr, Montie JE, Pontes JE, Vanderburg Medendorp S, Levin HS (1989) Transitional cell carcinoma of the prostate in cystoprostatectomy specimens removed for bladder cancer. J Urol 141:346–349

Xia T, Blackburn WR, Gardner WA (1990) Fetal prostate growth and development. Pediatr Pathol 10:527–537

5 Chromosome Abnormalities in Adenocarcinoma of the Prostate

P. Dal Cin and H. Van Den Berghe

CONTENTS

5.1 Introduction

Little is known about the genetic changes underlying the development and evolution of prostatic cancer. As in other tumors, however, identification of consistently occurring chromosome changes could allow for more orientated molecular studies at the sites of structural chromosome abnormalities. It is the purpose of this paper to review the chromosome changes which so far have been found in prostatic cancer.

5.2 Classical Cytogenetic Analysis and In Situ Hybridization

5.2.1 General Observations

The majority of adenocarcinomas of the prostate (approximately 75%) studied by classical cytogenetics has shown a normal diploid male karyotype, 46, XY (Sandberg 1992). Since prostatic tumors usually contain a mixture of neoplastic and nonneoplastic epithelial cells, stroma, and inflammatory cells, a high frequency of normal karyotypes could be explained by a lack of proliferation of karyotypically abnormal cells in vitro (Konig et al. 1993), even in the presence of growth factors (Peehl et al. 1988). In this respect, the introduction of in situ hybridization (ISH) techniques into the field of cancer cytogenetics has allowed more information to be gained from nondividing cells (Devilee et al. 1989). Evaluations of the ISH signals can be performed on isolated nuclei from fresh tumors as well as from paraffin-embedded or cryosection tissue preparations, thereby avoiding problems due to selection of cells during in vitro culture. In addition, ISH allows for the ascertainment of the origin of cells studied (neoplastic versus nonneoplastic cells) because tissue architecture is retained (Micale et al. 1993; Persons et al. 1994; Steilen et al. 1994).

5.2.2 Chromosome Abnormalities in Adenocarcinomas

5.2.2.1 Structural Changes

Structural changes of the long arm of chromosomes 7 and 10, with breakpoints at 7q22 and 10q24, have been identified in primary tumors (Atkin and Baker 1985; Brothman et al. 1990; Lundgren et al. 1988, 1992b; Arps et al. 1993) as well as in cell lines (Gibas et al. 1984; Iizumi et al. 1987; Konig et al. 1988, 1989).

As in other malignant solid tumors, structural abnormalities of chromosome 1 affecting both chromosome arms have been reported, without any obvious breakpoint clustering (Atkin and Baker 1985; Gibas et al. 1985; Pittman et al. 1987; Brothman et al. 1989, 1990; Lundgren et al. 1992b; Wullich et al. 1992; Arps et al. 1993). Band 1q12, however, seems to be an important breakpoint since a der(16)t(q12;q23) was found in two distinct adenocarcinomas (Wullich et al. 1992; Breitkreuz et al. 1993) and we recently found a del(1)(q12) in four cases (Qi et al. 1996), confirming a previous observation by Arps et al. (1993).

P. Dal Cin, PhD, Center for Human Genetics, University of Leuven, Herestraat 49, 3000 Leuven, Belgium
H. Van Den Berghe, PhD, Professor and Chairman, Department of Human Genetics and Head of Center for Human Genetics, University of Leuven, Herestraat 49, 3000 Leuven, Belgium

Double minute chromosomes indicating the presence of gene amplification have been observed in primary prostatic cancers (LIMON et al. 1989; BROTHMAN et al. 1990, 1991; LUNDGREN et al. 1992b; ARPS et al. 1993) as well as in prostatic cell lines (STONE et al. 1978; OHNUKI et al. 1980; BROTHMAN et al. 1989), but the nature of these amplified genes has not been elucidated. Rearrangements of 8p21, leading to loss of 8p21→pter, has been reported by several investigators (GIBAS et al. 1985; KONIG et al. 1989; LUNDGREN et al. 1992b).

5.2.2.2 Numerical Changes

Loss of the Y chromosome is the single most common numerical change found in prostatic tumors (ATKIN and BAKER 1985; BABU et al. 1990; BROTHMAN et al. 1990; LUNDGREN et al. 1992b; WULLICH et al. 1992; BREITKREUZ et al. 1993; ARPS et al. 1993). However, loss of this chromosome has been observed in a variety of other human neoplasms (MITELMAN 1994) and the significance of Y chromosome loss as a cancer-related abnormality is unclear.

Trisomy 7, as the sole abnormality and in conjunction with a missing Y, has been reported repeatedly (BABU et al. 1990; ARPS et al. 1993). The significance of trisomy 7 in neoplasia, however, is unclear as it has been found in nonneoplastic tissues as well (for review see JOHANSSON et al. 1993).

Few clinical-cytogenetic associations are known in solid tumors (FALOR and WARD 1976; TRENT et al. 1990; RYDHOLM et al. 1990). LUNDGREN and coworkers (1992a) showed that the presence of clonal chromosome changes in prostatic cancers was associated with a shorter survival time compared with those of patients with normal karyotypes.

5.3 In Situ Hybridization Results in Interphase Nuclei of Prostatic Cancers

In situ hybridization techniques using chromosome-specific α-satellite DNA probes for chromosomes 7,8,10,17,18,X,Y have been performed on human prostatic cancers by several groups on fresh isolated nuclei (JONES et al. 1994), touch imprinting preparations (TAKAHASHI et al. 1994; ZITZELSBERGER et al. 1994; JONES et al. 1994; BROWN et al. 1994), paraffin-embedded tissue sections and/or isolated nuclei (MACOSKA et al. 1993; MICALE et al. 1993; BREITKREUZ et al. 1993; ALCARAZ et al. 1994; BANDYK et al. 1994; VISAKORPI et al. 1994; ZITZELSBERGER et al. 1994; BROTHMAN et al. 1994).

Loss of chromosome 17 seems to be a relatively common event in prostatic tumors (JONES et al. 1994; BROWN et al. 1994; BROTHMAN et al. 1994), but it deserves further study.

In situ hybridization has confirmed the frequent loss of the Y chromosome; however, the significance of this is controversial as it seems to be a normal phenomenon in elderly men (UKCCG 1992). Some authors have found loss of the Y chromosome in carcinoma biopsies and not in benign prostatic tumors (VAN DEKKEN and ALERS 1993; MICALE et al. 1993). Gain of chromosome 8 has also been revealed by ISH analysis (MICALE et al. 1993; MACOSKA et al. 1993; BROWN et al. 1994; TAKAHASI et al. 1994).

The presence of trisomy 7 in nondividing prostatic cancer cells has been demonstrated by several investigators (JONES et al. 1994; BROWN et al. 1994; MICALE et al. 1993; ZITZELSBERGER et al. 1994). Recently, a significantly higher rate of trisomy 7 in advanced stages of prostatic tumors as well as bone marrow metastases has been reported (BANDYK et al. 1994), and has been associated with clinically aggressive prostatic cancer (TAKAHASHI et al. 1994; ALCARAZ et al. 1994). Trisomy 7 has been found in tumor parenchymal cells, but occasionally also in nonneoplastic tissues (ZITZELSBERGER et al. 1994).

5.4 Conclusions

The loss of chromosomal material of 7q, 8p, 10q, and 16q and structural changes of bands 7q22 and 10q24 seem to be the most common changes in adenocarcinomas of the prostate. These chromosome findings have also been confirmed by molecular investigations (for review see MACGROGAN et al. 1994; CHER et al. 1995). Band 1q12 seems to be an important breakpoint. Loss of the Y chromosome is the most frequent numerical change, but its significance remains to be clarified, as does that of trisomy 7.

References

Alcaraz A, Takahashi S, Brown JA et al. (1994) Aneuploidy and aneusomy of chromosome 7 detected by fluorescence in situ hybridization are markers of poor prognosis in prostate cancer. Cancer Res 54:3998–4002

Arps S, Rodewald A, Schmalenberger B, Carl P, Bressel M, Kastendieck H (1993) Cytogenetic survey of 32 cancers of the prostate. Cancer Genet Cytogenet 66:93–99

Atkin NB, Baker MC (1985) Chromosome studies of five cancers of the prostate. Hum Genet 70:359–364
Babu VR, Miles BJ, Cerny JC et al. (1990) Cytogenetic study of four cancers of the prostate. Cancer Genet Cytogenet 48:83–87
Bandyk MG, Zhao L, Troncoso P et al. (1994) Trisomy 7: a potential cytogenetic marker of human prostate cancer progression. Genes Chromosom Cancer 9:19–27
Breitkreuz T, Romanakis K, Lutz S, Seitz G et al. (1993) Genotypic characterization of prostatic carcinomas: a combined cytogenetic, flow cytometry, and in situ DNA hybridization study. Cancer Res 53:4035–4040
Brothman AR, Lesho LJ, Somers KD, Schellhammer PF, Ladaga LL, Merchant DJ (1989) Cytogenetic analysis of four primary prostatic cultures. Cancer Genet Cytogenet 37:241–248
Brothman AR, Peehl DM, Patel AM, McNeal JE (1990) Frequency and pattern of karyotypic abnormalities in human prostatic cancer. Cancer Res 50:3795–3803
Brothman AR, Peehl DM, Patel AM, MacDonald GR, McNeal JE, Ladaga LE, Schellhammer PF (1991) Cytogenetic evaluation of 20 cultured primary prostatic tumors. Cancer Genet Cytogenet 55:79–84
Brothman AR, Watson MJ, Zhu XL, Williams BJ, Rohr LR (1994) Evaluation of 20 archival prostate tumor specimens by fluorescence in situ hybridization (FISH) Cancer Genet Cytogenet 75:40–44
Brown JA, Alcaraz A, Takahashi S, Persons DL, Lieber MM, Jenkins RB (1994) Chromosomal aneusomies detected by fluorescent in situ hybridization analysis in clinically localized prostate carcinoma. J Urol 152:1157–1162
Cher ML, Ito T, Weidner N, Carroll PR, Jensen RH (1995) Mapping of regions of physical deletion on chromosome 16q in prostate cancer cells by fluorescence in situ hybridization (FISH). J Urol 153:249–254
Devilee P, Thierry RF, Keivits T et al. (1989) Detection of chromosome aneuploidy in interphase nuclei from human primary breast tumors using chromosome specific repetitive DNA probes. Cancer Res 48:5825–5830
Falor WH, Ward RM (1976) Cytogenetic analysis: a potential index for recurrence of early carcinoma of the bladder. J Urol 115:49
Gibas Z, Becher R, Kawinski E, Horoszewicz J, Sandberg AA (1984) A high-resolution study of chromosome changes in a human prostatic carcinoma cell line (LNCaP). Cancer Genet Cytogenet 11:399–404
Gibas Z, Pontes JE, Sandberg AA (1985) Chromosome rearrangements on a metastatic adenocarcinoma of the prostate. Cancer Genet Cytogenet 16:301–304
Iizumi T, Kyazaki T, Kanoh S, Kondo I, Koiso K (1987) Establishment of a new prostatic carcinoma cell line (TSU-PR1). J Urol 137:1304–1306
Johansson B, Heim S, Mandahl N, Mertens F, Mitelman F (1993) Trisomy 7 in nonneoplastic cells. Genes Chromosom Cancer 6:199–205
Jones E, Zhu XL, Rohr LR, Stephenson RA, Brothman AR (1994) Aneusomy of chromosomes 7 and 17 detected in FISH in prostate cancer and the effects of selection in vitro. Genes Chromosom Cancer 11:163–170
König JJ, Hagemeijer A, Smit b, Kamst E, Romijn JC, Schröder FH (1988) Cytogenetic characterization of an established xenografted prostatic cell line (PC-82). Cancer Genet Cytogenet 34:91–99
König JJ, Kamst E, Hagemeijer A, Romijn JC, Horoszewicz J, Schöder FH (1989) Cytogenetic characterization of several androgen responsive and unresponsive sublines of the hyman prostatic carcinoma cells line LNCap. Urol Res 17:79–86
König JJ, Teubel W, van Dongen JW, Hagemeijer A, Romijn JC, Schröder FH (1993) Tissue culture loss of aneuploid cells from carcinomas of the prostate. Genes Chromosom Cancer 8:22–27
Limon J, Lundgren R, Elfving P, Heim P, Kristoffersson U, Mandahl N, Mitelman F (1989) Double minutes in two primary adenocarcinomas of the prostate. Cancer Genet Cytogenet 39:191–194
Lundgren R, Kristofferson U, Heim S, Mandahl N, Mitelman F (1988) Multiple structural chromosome rearrangements, including del(7q) and del(10q), in an adenocarcinoma of the prostate. Cancer Genet Cytogenet 35:103–108
Lundgren R, Heim S, Mandahl N, Anderson H, Mitelman F (1992a) Chromosome abnormalities are associated with unfavorable outcome in prostatic cancer patients. J Urol 146:784–788
Lundgren R, Mandahl N, Heim S, Limon J, Henrikson H, Mitelman F (1992b) Cytogenetic analysis of 57 primary prostatic adenocarcinomas. Genes Chromosom Cancer 4:16–24
MacGrogan D, Levy A, Bostwick D, Wagner M, Wells D, Bookstein R (1994) Loss of chromosome arm 8p loci in prostate cancer: mapping by quantitative allelic imbalance. Genes Chromosom Cancer 10:151–159
Macoska JA, Micale MA, Sakr WA, Benson PD, Wolman SR (1993) Extensive genetic alterations in prostate cancer revealed by dual PCR and FISH analysis. Genes Chromosom Cancer 8:88–97
Micale MA, Sanford JS, Powell IJ, Sakr WA, Wolman SR (1993) Defining the extent and nature of cytogenetic events in prostatic adenocarcinoma: paraffin FISH vs. metaphase analysis. Cancer Genet Cytogenet 69:7–12
Mitelman F (1994) Catalog of chromosome aberrations in cancer, 5th edn. Wiley-Liss, New York
Ohnuki Y, Marnell MM, Babcock MS, Lechner JF, Kaighn ME (1980) Chromosomal analysis of human prostatic adenocarcinoma cell lines. Cancer Res 40:524–534
Peehl DM, Wong ST, Stamey TA (1988) Clonal growth characteristics of adult human prostatic epithelial cells. In Vitro Cell Dev Biol 24:530–536
Persons DL, Takai K, Gibney DJ, Ratzmann JA, Lieber MM, Jenkins R (1994) Comparison of fluorescence in situ hybridization with flow cytometry and static image analysis in ploidy analysis of paraffin-embedded prostate adenocarcinoma. Hum Pathol 25:678–683
Pittman S, Russell PJ, Jelbart ME, Wass J, Raghavan D (1987) Flow cytometric and karyotypic analysis of a primary small cell carcinoma of the prostate: a xenografted cell line. Cancer Genet Cytogenet 26:165–169
Qi H, Dal Cin P, Van de Voorde W et al. (1996) Del(1)(q12) in adenocarcinomas of the prostate. Cancer Genet Cytogenet (in press)
Rydholm A, Mandahl N, Heim S, Krreichbergs A, Willén H, Mitelman F (1990) Malignant fibrous histiocytomas with a 19p+ marker chromosome have increased relapse rate. Genes Chromosom Cancer 2:296
Sandberg AA (1992) Chromosomal abnormalities and related events in prostate cancer. Hum Pathol 23:368–380
Steilen H, Ketter R, Romanakis K et al. (1994) DNA aneuploidy in prostatic adenocarcinoma: a frequent event as shown by fluorescence in situ DNA hybridization. Hum Pathol 25:1306–1313
Stone KR, Mickey DD, Wunderli H, Mickey GH, Paulson DF (1978) Isolation of a human prostate carcinoma cell line (DU^U145) Int J Cancer 21:274–281

Takahashi S, Qian J, Brown JA, Alcaraz A, Bostwick DG, Lieber MM, Jenkins RB (1994) Potential markers of prostate cancer aggressiveness detected by fluorescence in situ hybridization in needle biopsies. Cancer Res 54:3574–3579

Trent JM, Meyskens FL, Salmon SE, Ryschon K, Leong SPL, Davis JR, McGee DL (1990) Relaton of cytogenetic abnormalities and clinical outcome in metastatic melanoma. N Engl J Med 322:1508

United Kingdom Cancer Cytogenetics Group (UKCCG)(1992) Loss of the Y chromosome from normal and neoplastic bone marrows. Genes Chromosom Cancer 5:83–88

Van Dekken H, Alers J (1993) Loss of chromosome Y in prostatic cancer cells, but not in stromal tissue. Cancer Genet Cytogenet 66:131–132

Visakorpi T, Hyytinen E, Kallioniemi A, Isola J, kallioniemi O-P (1994) Sensitive detection of chromosome copy number aberrations in prostate cancer by fluorescence in situ hybridization. Am J Pathol 145:624–630

Wullich B, Breitkreuz T, Zwergel T, Unteregger G, Seitz G, Zang KD (1992) Cytogenetic evidence of interatumoral focal heterogeneity in prostatic carcinomas. Urol Int 48:377–377

Zitzelsberger H, Szücs S, Weier H-U et al. (1994) Numerical abnormalities of chromosome 7 in human prostate cancer detected by fluorescence in situ hybridization (FISH) on paraffin-embedded tissue sections with centromere-specific DNA probes. J Pathol 172:325–335

6 Radioimmunoscintigraphy and Radioimmunotherapy in Cancer of the Prostate

D. Kahn and R.D. Williams

CONTENTS

6.1 Introduction

Despite the initial great promise, immunodiagnosis/therapy with monoclonal antibodies (MOABs) directed against human tumor-associated antigens has proven to be an elusive and less than "magic bullet." Nevertheless, currently highly specific techniques for isolating tumor antigens and developing designer-specific MOABs combined with improved imaging methods and innovative treatment strategies are stimulating renewed enthusiasm for immunodetection and immunotherapy of prostate cancer.

D. Kahn, MD, Associate Professor, Department of Radiology, The University of Iowa and Veterans Administration Medical Center, 200 Hawkins Drive, Iowa City, IA 52242-1089, USA
R.D. Williams, MD, Rubin H. Flocks Chair, Professor and Head, Department of Urology, 3 RCP, The University of Iowa, 200 Hawkins Drive, Iowa City, IA 52242-1089, USA

Most MOABs react to plasma membranes or cytoplasmic glycoproteins, glycolipids, or mucins. There are several investigative antibodies available for evaluating prostate cancer. The potential uses of MOABs in prostate cancer may be summarized as follows:

1. Diagnosis/progression
   a) Biomarkers in body fluids
   b) Pathologic tissue diagnosis
   c) Prognostic prediction
   d) Therapeutic response prediction
   e) Localization and staging by imaging
2. Treatment
   a) Native MOABs
   b) Conjugated with toxins or radioactive agents
   c) Autologous marrow cleansing
   d) Anti-idiotype vaccines

There are potential problems with using MOABs for the above purposes, including:

1. Development of human antimouse antibodies (HAMAs) against some murine MOABs
2. Low tumor specificity due to antigens common to multiple organs and tissue specificity not limited to neoplasia
3. Tumor antigen heterogeneity within the tumor
4. Insufficient MOAB access to tumor cells due to high tumor volume, poor vascularity, or tumor necrosis
5. MOAB-conjugate toxicity
6. Lack of MOAB-cytocidal activity.

The use of MOABs in the diagnosis or therapy of prostate cancer does, however, have specific advantages which include:

1. Abnormal cells can be targeted, thus sparing normal cells.
2. Diagnostic or therapeutic isotopes can be linked to MOABs.
3. Cancer of the prostate is radioresponsive.
4. Metastases are primarily small and highly accessible to MOAB delivery, and are thus ideal for beta-particle therapy.

5. Sufficient markers to indicate stage of disease and response to therapy are available.

6.2 Radioimmunoscintigraphy for the Detection of Prostate Cancer

The utilization of MOABs for prostate cancer tumor localization has held considerable interest due to the availability of prostatic acid phosphatase (PAP) and prostate-specific antigen (PSA) as potential antigen targets. The great hope is that MOAB imaging by radioimmunoscintigraphy (RIS) will improve the poor accuracy of conventional methods in detecting extraprostatic sites of cancer. Both computed tomography (CT) and magnetic resonance imaging (MRI), for example, are only able to detect nodes that are 1.0 cm or greater in size and are not capable of determining intranodal architecture. Imaging with MOABs has the potential of detecting finite numbers of tumor cells within lymph nodes or other tissues.

6.3 Radioimmunoconjugates

In the case of anti-cancer MOABs, a tumor-associated antigen (such as PSA) is commonly used to generate the antibody. To be used in RIS the antibody must first be radiolabeled. Each of the available radionuclides has certain advantages and disadvantages. Factors that influence the choice of radionuclide include the radiochemistry required for labeling, the integrity of the particular protein being labeled (particularly as measured by the immunoreactivity after the labeling procedure), the rate of clearance of the radioimmunoconjugate, the tumor site to be targeted within the body, and the biodistribution of the agent. Most whole anti-cancer antibodies used for RIS (including those used in patients with prostate cancer) are labeled with either ^{131}I (half-life 8 days) or ^{111}In (half-life 2.8 days). Protein labeling with ^{131}I is relatively simple using techniques such as the chloramine-T or iodogen methods. Another advantage of ^{131}I-labeled immunoconjugates is that the radioactivity which accumulates in the liver is usually relatively low, thus enhancing the target-to-noise (lesion-to-normal tissue) ratio. Liver lesions are therefore more readily detected with iodinated radioimmunoconjugates. The principal disadvantages of RIS with ^{131}I-labeled antibodies are the dehalogenation which occurs and the lower dose of ^{131}I that must be used for safety concerns (both of which degrade image quality). The latter problem can be overcome through the use of ^{123}I, but due to its shorter half-life (13 h) and much greater expense, its use is not practical on whole antibodies. Compared with iodinated antibodies, ^{111}In-labeled immunoconjugates offer the advantage of high-quality images (single-photon emission computerized tomography or SPECT) when between 3 and 6 mCi is administered, substantially more stable binding of the radioatom to the protein, and a physical half-life which is approximately equal to the biologic serum half-life of many murine whole MOABs. The main drawback of ^{111}In is that considerably more complex chemistry procedures are required for antibody labeling, and, unlike radioiodinated antibodies, a significantly higher fraction of the injected dose normally accumulates in the liver and bone marrow. This accumulation of activity degrades the lesion-to-background ratio such that tumor metastases in the bone and liver are often not detectable.

6.4 Imaging Technique

Radioimmunoconjugates are usually introduced into the body by intravenous injection. Patients are observed for a short period following injection in order to detect side-effects, such as an allergic response to the foreign protein. Since most radiolabeled whole antibodies normally have blood clearance half-times in excess of 24 h, imaging is typically delayed for at least 48 h following injection. In radiolabeled whole antibody fragments, such as Fab' or F(ab)2', the blood clearance times are considerably less than 24 h (even as short as 1–2 h). Imaging in patients receiving radiolabeled antibody fragments is thus often initiated by 4–6 h and completed by 18–24 h after injection. In either case, the principal reason for the delay between the time of injection and scanning is to permit the background activity in the blood and therefore in the body tissues to decline sufficiently that antibody preferentially attached to the target site (e.g., tumor) can be detected. With regard to most radioimmunoconjugates, the primary route of elimination of the radioactive atom is by urinary excretion.

After the appropriate delay for background elimination, imaging is carried out using conventional nuclear medicine gamma cameras. Initially a planar, whole-body set of images is obtained so as to evaluate the entire body for sites of disease. If no sites are seen on the whole-body scan, the patient will have multiplanar tomography performed of the region(s) of the body which is (are) most likely to have disease present. SPECT is more accurate than planar imaging when studying patients with cancer, and must be performed in all cases. Furthermore, when abnormal foci are detected with planar, whole-body imaging, SPECT, because of its three-dimensional display, can better define the precise location of an abnormality in the thorax or abdomen. Current gamma camera technology has advanced to the point that larger field-of-view multiheaded cameras, which can have their camera heads' orbits programmed to match a particular patient's body habitus, are considered state of the art.

6.4.1 Imaging Anti-prostate Cancer Radioimmunoconjugates in Humans

Twenty years ago KOHLER and MILSTEIN (1975) first reported producing a MOAB through the use of a hybridoma system. Until this new method of producing "pure" (monoclonal) murine antibodies became available, polyclonal antibodies had been used in clinical practice since about 1948, when PRESSMAN and KEIGHLEY (1948) reported investigations of the murine kidney in vivo. In the years that followed this work, a number of studies were performed using radioiodinated polyclonal antibodies directed against a variety of tissues, including the pioneering work of GOLDENBERG et al. (1978) and MACH et al. (1980) in the late 1970s. They demonstrated that radioimmunoconjugates directed against carcinoembryonic antigen could be successfully used to image primary and metastatic cancer and that their use in humans was generally safe.

6.4.2 Polyclonal Radioimmunoconjugates

The first report of RIS in patients with prostate cancer was published by GOLDENBERG et al. (1983), who later expanded their work in a larger group of patients with prostate cancer using the same polyclonal antibodies (GOLDENBERG and DELAND 1984). In these publications, anti-PAP IgG antibodies, which had been raised initially in rabbits and later in goats, were radioiodinated with ^{131}I. Primary prostate cancer lesions were successfully imaged with these radioimmunoconjugates, and the authors concluded that RIS with this agent was safe and reasonably effective. Importantly, bone lesions were not detected with this radioimmunoconjugate.

6.4.3 Monoclonal Radioimmunoconjugates: Anti-PSA and Anti-PAP Antibodies

Monoclonal antibodies of murine origin have also been investigated (Table 6.1). VIHKO et al. (1984) used ^{111}In- or ^{99m}Tc-labeled whole antibody or fragments directed against PAP. They injected varying doses of protein and radionuclide in four patients with prostate cancer. All sites of tumor, including the prostate, were visible with these immunoconjugates.

Table 6.1. Prostate cancer MOAB imaging

Reference	Antigen	MOAB	No. of patients	Scan results
GOLDENBERG et al. (1978)	PAP	Polyclonal	2	Primary tumor imaged; bone lesions not seen
VIHKO et al. (1984, 1987)	PAP	Monoclonal	4	Primary tumor and extraprostatic sites imaged
		Monoclonal	5	Periprostatic injection; 1/1 patients with positive LNs imaged; 4/4 true-negatives
DILLMAN et al. (1987)	PSA	PSA-399	4	55% of tumor sites imaged
	PAP	PAY-276	5	16% of tumor sites imaged
HALPERN et al. (1988)	PAP	PAY-276	10	15% of tumor metastases imaged with high dose
BABAIAN et al. (1987)	PAP	PAY-276	25	With high dose, bone sensitivity 75%; LN metastases not detected; HAMA incidence 50%
ABDEL-NABI et al. (1992)	PSMA (7E11-C5.3)	CYT-356	28	59% primary prostate cancer detected; 50% positive LNs imaged; scan correct in 93% with negative LNs
			40	55% of patients with bone metastases detected; HAMA incidence only 7%
BABAIAN et al. (1994)	PSMA	CYT-356	19	50% detection of positive LNs; HAMA not detected
KAHN et al. (1994, 1995)	PSMA	CYT-356	35	78% sensitivity and 77% specificity for prostate fossa

LN, lymph nodes; PSMA, prostate-specific membrane antigen

They also reported five patients who, prior to scheduled radical prostatectomy and lymphadenectomy, had 1.0 mg of ^{99m}Tc-labeled F(ab)2′ directed against PAP injected percutaneously into the periprostatic space (Vihko et al. 1987). Three sets of images were acquired in each patient over 24 h after injection. In one patient abnormal activity was detected in multiple lymph nodes including periaortic nodes. Histopathologic examination of multiple nodes in the obturator, iliac, and periaortic regions in this patient confirmed the positive scan. Histopathology also confirmed the negative scans in the four remaining patients. The authors concluded from their preliminary data that lymphoscintigraphy may accurately determine the extent of regional spread of prostate cancer prior to prostatectomy.

Dillman et al. (1987) studied four patients with an anti-PSA MOAB (^{111}In-labeled PSA-399) and five patients with an anti-PAP antibody (^{111}In-labeled PAY-276. With all doses administered, the fraction of tumor sites detected was 55% and 16% for the ^{111}In-labeled PSA-399 and the ^{111}In-labeled PAY-276, respectively. The results of this limited trial led the authors to conclude that antibodies directed against PSA appear more promising than those against PAP. This same group confirmed their experience with anti-PAP RIS in ten additional patients using ^{111}In-labeled PAY-276 (Halperne et al. 1988). Again, a low sensitivity (15%) for prostate cancer metastasis was demonstrated. In addition, some patients showed a decrease in white blood cell counts as a result of the antibody infusion, the mechanism for which is unknown.

Babaian et al. (1987), using the same anti-PAP MOAB (^{111}In-labeled PAY-276), studied a larger series of patients (n = 25) with escalating doses of unlabeled antibody and 1 mg of the radioimmunoconjugate. All patients had metastatic disease. They reported a high incidence of HAMA formation in 8 of 16 patients tested, but no other adverse reactions. Both lesion and patient sensitivity in the bone improved markedly in those cases that received the higher doses (20–80 mg) of unlabeled antibody (patient sensitivity increased from 40% to 100%, while lesion sensitivity increased from 23% to 75%). The enhanced lesion sensitivity in this report, compared with the series reported by Halpern et al. (1988), is possibly explained by the dose of unlabeled antibody. In many of Babaian's patients the dose was considerably higher than the dose used by Halpern. Importantly, however, lymph node metastases were not detected with this agent. Therefore, the authors concluded that while ^{111}In-labeled PAY-276 is reasonably sensitive for bone metastases (although less so than conventional bone scintigraphy), it is of little value in assessing the status of the lymph nodes and other soft tissues. Furthermore, the incidence of HAMA formation was too high for clinical use.

6.4.4 Monoclonal Antibody 7E11-C5.3

The murine monoclonal antibody 7E11-C5.3 is an IgG1 protein. It is produced from a hybridoma originating from the fusion of myeloma cells with spleen cells of mice immunized with the human prostate cancer cell line LNCaP and was originally reported by Horoszewicz et al. (1987). This antibody appears to recognize a prostate-specific membrane glycoprotein that is only expressed by prostatic epithelial cells (benign and malignant) and whose DNA coding sequence has significant homology to that of the human transferrin receptor (Israeli et al. 1993). The monoclonal antibody 7E11-C5.3 underwent site-specific conjugation with the linker-chelator glycyl-tyrosyl-(N, Σ-diethylene triamine penta-acetic acid)-lysine (GYK-DTPA) using the procedure developed by Rodwell et al. (1986). The resulting immunoconjugate, 7E11-C5.3 GYK-DTPA labeled with ^{111}In (^{111}In-CYT-356 or ^{111}In-capromab pendetide) has been investigated in numerous patients with prostate cancer prior to or following radical prostatectomy.

6.4.5 ^{111}In-Capromab Pendetide Studies in Patients with Prostate Cancer

A phase I/II trial using ^{111}In-capromab pendetide (CP) in patients with prostate cancer was reported by Abdel-Nabi et al. (1992). Two types of patients were scanned and formed the basis for their report: a group of men with no detectable metastatic disease prior to staging pelvic lymphadenectomy (n = 28) and a group of patients with known metastatic prostate cancer (n = 40). Pharmacokinetic evaluations were completed in nine men who received between 0.1 and 10 mg of protein. Mean ± SD serum half-life was 71.5 ± 25.3 h. There were no significant adverse effects. Serum HAMA measurements on 44 patients, 8 weeks after antibody infusion, revealed that only three (7%) had developed evidence of significant murine antibody development. Imaging results demonstrated that two of four surgically proven pelvic lymph node metastases were detected with the scan. The scan was correctly negative in 25 of 27 histologically confirmed negative lymph nodes. Sixteen of the 27 prostates (with confirmed cancer) were detected with the scan. In those patients with known metastatic disease, 38 of 40 had bony lesions previously documented by conventional radiographic modalities. The antibody scan detected these lesions in only 55% of the patients, and in only a minority of the patients were all bony lesions detected. Confirmatory biopsies of lesions, particularly those that were discordant with the scan, were not obtained. The scan was also positive in four of six patients with extraprostatic soft tissue lesions. Overall, ^{111}In-CP was safe, and was able to detect soft tissue lesions, but it seemed to have only modest sensitivity for bone lesions. Further antibody dose escalation beyond 0.5 mg did not improve scan accuracy.

Babaian et al. (1994) assessed the diagnostic accuracy of ^{111}In-CP for the detection of prostate cancer in the pelvic lymph nodes prior to bilateral pelvic lymph node dissection. They studied 19 patients with histologically confirmed prostate cancer clinically confined to the prostate, who underwent a single intravenous infusion of 5 mCi of ^{111}In-CP. Whole-body scanning and SPECT were performed twice between 48 and 120 h after administration. Mild and transient adverse reactions were seen in three patients. HAMA titers were not detected in any of the men. Scan results were compared with the histopathologic findings and the conventional radiographic appearance of the pelvic lymph nodes. Eight of the 19 patients had pathologic evidence of metastatic disease to the pelvic lymph nodes, with the scan detecting four (50%) of these cases. CT and MRI detected lymph node abnormalities in only one of the eight (12.5%) patients. The antibody scan was negative in 9 of 11 (82%) patients without prostate cancer metastatic to the pelvic nodes.

6.5 The University of Iowa/Iowa City VAMC Experience with ^{111}In-CP in Patients with Prostate Cancer

As part of the multicenter phase II and phase III trials, we have evaluated patients with suspected recurrent prostate cancer following bilateral pelvic lymph node dissection and radical prostatectomy with curative intent. Defined as "occult prostate cancer recurrence," subsequently all of the patients had residual or recurrent cancer as evidenced by a progressively elevated PSA (>0.4 ng/dl). The patient's physical examination and all other tests, such as bone scan, CT or MRI, and transrectal ultrasonography (TRUS) were negative for evidence of recurrent prostate cancer.

In the initial series, we and the Lahey Clinic Medical Center (Burlington, Mass.) studied 27 men with 5 mCi of ^{111}In-CP from 9 to 141 months (range) following radical prostatectomy (Kahn et al. 1994). Eight of these patients had at least one additional infusion at a later date. We did not detect a correlation between the serum PSA and the likelihood of exhibiting scan abnormalities. However, the initial pathologic stage of the tumor was related to the probability of an abnormal scan: those with disease confined to the prostate gland before radical prostatectomy were statistically less likely to have disease seen on scan compared to those with nonconfined disease (64% vs 94%). Based on scan findings from the initial infusion data, 22 of the 27 men had a positive scan in the prostatic fossa and/or extra-fossa sites (Figs. 6.1–6.3). In 11 of the 22 patients, some of the lesions were confirmed by CT or MRI or by fossa biopsy. Included in this group were men with a positive scan in the prostate fossa (biopsy confirmed, $n = 8$), mediastinum (radiographically confirmed, $n = 2$), abdominal lymph nodes (unconfirmed, $n = 5$), and lumbar spine (radiographically confirmed, $n = 1$). None of the men developed detectable HAMA titers during at least 8 weeks of follow-up. This preliminary data, like the data from the phase I/II trials described above, suggested that ^{111}In-CP imaging was able to detect prostatic fossa cancer recurrence and that extra-fossa sites of soft tissue metastases were also being imaged.

This initial trial provided some scan sensitivity data but little specificity data. Thus, a phase III trial was designed to confirm as accurately as possible (with either CT/MRI or biopsy) positive scan findings outside of the prostatic fossa, and (with TRUS) both positive and negative scans in the prostatic fossa.

In this trial, 0.5 mg of ^{111}In-CP was administered to 62 patients with occult prostate cancer recurrence as defined above. All prostatic fossa biopsies were performed within 8 weeks after the scan. We recently reported our preliminary results in these patients (Kahn et al. 1995). Thirty-five of the 36 patients entered completed the entire protocol. In the prostate fossa (based on biopsy results of this region), the sensitivity of the ^{111}In-CP scan was seven of nine

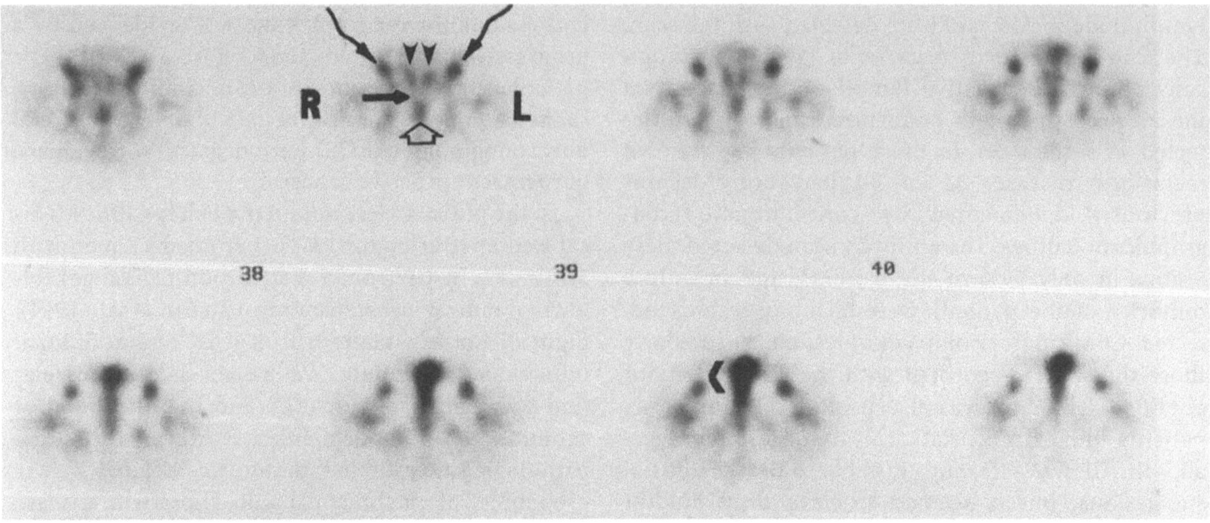

Fig. 6.1. Transaxial cuts of the pelvis from an ^{111}In-CP scan in a man who, following radical prostatectomy, had a rising PSA. Nonspecific uptake of ^{111}In-CP is seen in the marrow within the pubic bones (*arrowheads*), in the iliac vessels (*curved arrows*) and in the rectum (*open arrowhead*). The intense midline localization seen in the inferior cuts (*bottom row*) anteriorly and extending posteriorly represent activity in the bulb, crura and proximal corpus of the penis (*bracket*). No significant accumulation of the radiotracer is seen in the prostate fossa (*arrow*) inferior to the pubic marrow, superior to rectal activity. The patient had a negative TRUS-guided biopsy of the fossa, confirming the scan findings. The slices start in the *left upper corner* and progress to the *right lower corner*, moving superior to inferior. Gray scale depicts areas of increased activity as a darker shade of gray. R, right; L, left

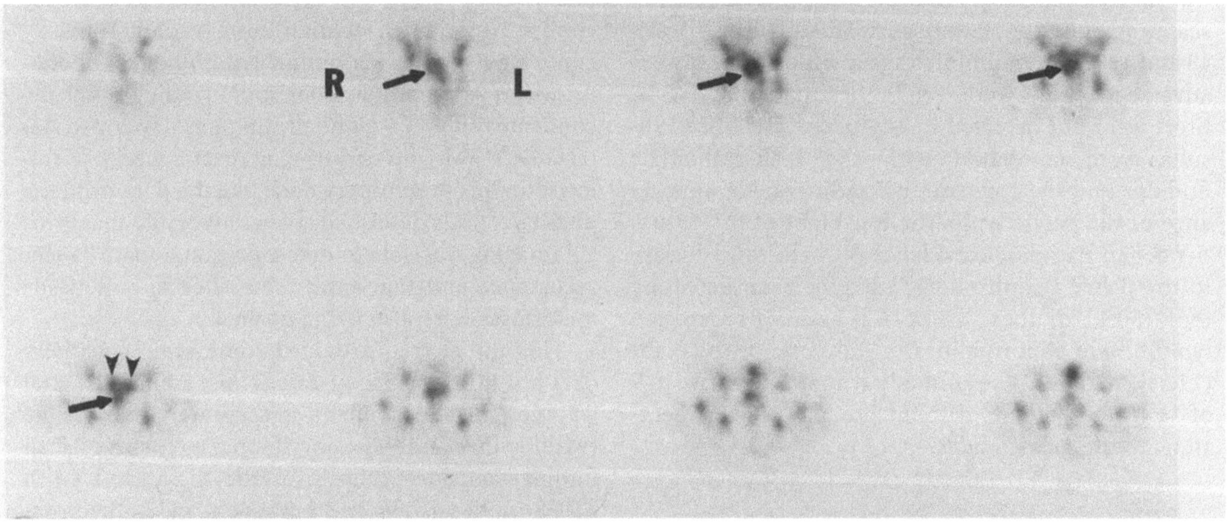

Fig. 6.2. Transaxial cuts of the pelvis from an ^{111}In-CP scan. This patient (not the patient shown in Fig. 6.1) was scanned following a radical prostatectomy when he demonstrated a rising PSA. An abnormal, intense focus of ^{111}In-CP uptake is seen in multiple cuts through the prostate fossa (*arrows*), posterior to the pubic bones (*arrowheads*). This lesion was biopsied and confirmed to be cancer. Image orientation is the same as in Fig. 6.1

(78%) and the specificity was 20 of 26 (77%). Sixteen of 36 (44%) patients had ^{111}In-CP scan positive areas detected outside of their prostate fossa. Twelve of 36 (33%) had no abnormalities detected on their scans. Follow-up continues in all the patients to determine whether: (a) scan-positive, prostate fossa biopsy-negative results were due to biopsy sampling error; (b) clinical outcome is related to scan findings (e.g., do patients with scan positivity limited to their prostate fossa respond to radiation therapy to the pelvis

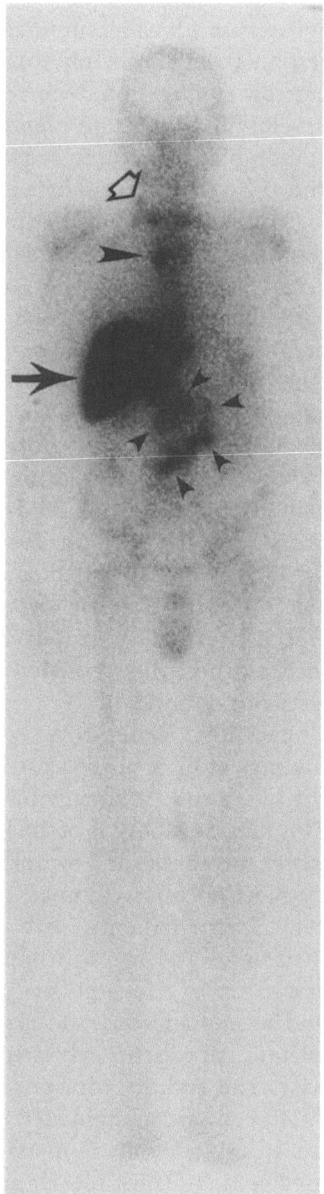

Fig. 6.3. Whole-body image of an ^{111}In-CP scan in a man with a rising PSA following radical prostatectomy. The usual pattern of nonspecific uptake is seen in the marrow, scrotum, liver (*arrow*) and within the blood pool. Multiple areas of abnormal ^{111}In-CP accumulation are seen in the abdomen (*small arrowheads*), the mediastinum (*large arrowhead*), and the right supraclavicular region (*open arrowhead*). CT scan of these regions did not demonstrate lymphadenopathy

whereas those with extra-fossa scan abnormalities do not); and (c) extraprostatic sites of disease can be confirmed with follow-up conventional imaging techniques or tissue confirmation. From our data it appears that, in patients treated with radical prostatectomy with curative intent, ^{111}In-CP is able to detect prostate fossa recurrences with reasonable accuracy. The scan was certainly superior to conventional techniques such as CT scanning, which has been shown to be relatively inaccurate (PLATT et al. 1987).

6.6 Potential Clinical Uses of RIS for Prostate Cancer

These studies indicate that RIS with ^{111}In-CP may be quite useful in several aspects of prostate cancer management. First, during initial staging of patients with prostate cancer, the scan can be utilized to define patients who have node-positive disease and are in need of biopsy confirmation prior to determining therapy, or those in whom node positivity is very unlikely and thus for whom curative radiation or surgical therapy should proceed. Second, in patients who have been treated for cure but demonstrate recurrence by serum PSA elevation, ^{111}In-CP scan can provide management direction such that if the scan shows activity confined to the prostate area further attempts at curative therapy directed at the pelvis may be beneficial. If, however, disseminated activity is noted beyond the pelvis, systemic therapy would be more appropriate. Third, ^{111}In-CP scan may be helpful in patients with known pelvic recurrence or systemic metastases to evaluate treatment results. This latter application has not been studied adequately and is thus more speculative than the two prior indications. Finally, as MOAB therapy is initiated (to be discussed subsequently) ^{111}In-CP may be used to determine candidate suitability and treatment response, particularly in patients with no clinical evidence of disease on conventional scans.

Radioimmunoscintigraphy, particularly with ^{111}In-CP, appears to have substantial promise for detecting extraprostatic or recurrent prostatic fossa sites of cancer of the prostate. However, further study is necessary to identify the precise sensitivity and specificity of the method so that absolute indications in management of prostate cancer can be determined.

6.7 Radioimmunotherapy of Prostate Cancer

Several therapeutic trials which were designed to treat patients with cancer using radiolabeled antibodies ("magic bullets") have been undertaken. Typically, the trials have been performed in patients with advanced stage neoplasms, usually those who had failed several prior antitumor therapies. Many of these patients were also suffering from adverse effects associated with these multiple therapies. With the exception of non-Hodgkin's lymphoma, where the response rates have been very impressive (Kaminski et al. 1993; Press et al. 1993), trials in patients with carcinomas have not shown significant rates of response. Few data, however, are available for radioimmunotherapy (RIT) of prostate cancer. It is likely that RIT of patients with large tumor burdens is destined to failure, probably as a result of inadequate levels of radiation being delivered to tumor sites. Thus, treatment efficacy might be improved if RIT, particularly in prostate cancer, was initiated in men with less advanced disease.

6.7.1 *Radioimmunoconjugates*

As in RIS, there are a variety of radionuclides which can and have been used in RIT. To date, the most commonly used radionuclides have included beta-emitting isotopes such as ^{131}I and ^{90}Y. These two in particular have offered the advantage of simpler chemistry for labeling. Many other radioatoms for therapy, including alpha-emitters, have been tested in animals and in early clinical trials in humans. Most trials which used ^{131}I- and ^{90}Y-labeled antibodies have shown that the dose-limiting organ is bone marrow. In part, the myelosuppressive effects of radiation have limited the therapeutic effectiveness of many of the radioimmunoconjugates that have been investigated. Ultimately, for RIT to be successful in carcinomas, it will be necessary to overcome two principal problems: tumor uptake of an inadequate fraction of the administered radioimmunoconjugate, and toxicity in the form of bone marrow suppression. Strategies designed to enhance uptake by tumor and to protect (or preserve for later autologous transplantation) the bone marrow are under intensive investigation.

6.7.2 *Anti-prostate Cancer RIT*

Meredith et al. (1994) reported a phase II trial of ^{131}I-CC49 in 15 men with metastatic disease who had failed conventional hormonal therapy. CC49 is a genetically engineered chimeric mouse/human antibody directed against the antigen TAG-72 (tumor-associated glycoprotein). After the appropriate preparation, subjects received 75 mCi/m^2 ^{131}I-CC49 i.v. Gamma camera imaging (with estimates of dosimetry) was performed. Standard radiographic and serum PSA measurements were used to assess response rates. The only toxicity was transient bone marrow suppression, with about half of the patients developing significant depressions of neutrophils and/or platelets (three required RBC transfusions, and two required prophylactic platelet transfusions for counts $<$25 000/m^3). No measurable antitumor responses were achieved using PSA or radiographic criteria. However, six of ten patients with pain had relief following infusion. Thirteen of 15 patients had tumor sites detected with ^{131}I-CC49, but consistently fewer sites of bone disease were seen when compared with bone scan findings. Estimates of whole-body radiation dose ranged from 84 to 145 cGy (mean = 114) with no detectable relationship between the whole-body dose and marrow suppression. Dose to individual bone lesions in four patients were calculated and ranged from 208 to 1083 cGy. The relatively low radiation doses (considerably below doses received from external beam therapy) probably provided an analgesic effect but were not tumoricidal.

Recently, Abdel-Nabi et al. (1995) published findings of their phase I preliminary work assessing the safety and maximally tolerated dose of ^{90}Y-KC4. This murine MOAB is of the IgG3 subclass and reacts with a membrane and cytoplasmic antigen expressed by most adenocarcinomas, including prostate cancer. Seven patients, five of whom had bone metastases and two of whom had a rising PSA, received up to 9 mCi/m^2 of the radiopharmaceutical and a simultaneous i.v. infusion of calcium disodium edetate. All patients exhibited mild hematologic toxicity. The authors concluded that this dose of ^{90}Y-KC4 can be administered without significant toxicities and that the maximally tolerated dose is greater than 9 mCi/m^2. Estimates of dosimetry and tumor responses rates to ^{90}Y-KC4 have yet to be defined but presumably will be included in future trials.

6.7.3 *^{90}Y-CP RIT in Patients with Prostate Cancer*

Preliminary results obtained from immunohistochemical staining studies of human prostate metastatic tissue samples have shown that staining of CYT-356 seems to be highest in androgen-independent lesions. Radioimmunoassay of LNCaP prostate cancer cells grown in androgen-stripped media has also demonstrated persistent 7E11-C5 production while the expression of PSA fell by 47%. A logical extension of this information is to predict that a therapeutic form of CYT-356 (e.g., beta-particle emitting ^{90}Y-labeled CYT-356) might preferentially target and destroy hormonally insensitive deposits of prostate cancer (Grob BM et al., unpublished). Because of the favorable targeting of prostate cancer with the diagnostic radioimmunoconjugate ^{111}In-CP described above, a phase I trial assessing the safety and maximally tolerated dose of ^{90}Y-CP in patients with prostate cancer metastatic to bone was started and is nearly completed (Maquire R, personal communication). The data have not been reported as yet but the labeled MOAB apparently can be given safely in possibly therapeutic doses. As expected, bone marrow toxicity is the dose-limiting factor. However, the results have been promising to the extent that a phase II trial will be undertaken. The phase II study will evaluate the antitumor response of ^{90}Y-CP in patients who, after radical prostatectomy, have evidence of recurrent or residual disease as indicated by a progressively elevated PSA and positive ^{111}In-CP scan. It is hoped that by choosing patients with a small tumor burden the ability of ^{90}Y-CP to affect scan-positive sites and serum PSA can be accurately determined.

6.8 Conclusion

Radioimmunodiagnostic scanning of human prostate cancer has been inaccurate using polyclonal and PAP monoclonal antibodies. The use of ^{111}In-CP (MOAB 7E11-C5.3) is promising for detection of tumorous pelvic lymph nodes and/or eliminating disseminated disease in the initial staging of newly diagnosed prostate cancer patients. In addition, patients with a rising PSA after radical prostatectomy can benefit from an ^{111}In-CP scan to detect prostate fossa recurrence and/or to exclude extrapelvic metastases. Further study is necessary to determine the absolute indications for prostate cancer RIS. Radioimmunotherapy with MOABs directed to prostate cancer antigens has not been adequately tested previously due to the lack of suitable agents. With the availability of ^{90}Y-CP appropriate trials have begun. Time alone will determine whether the renewed optimism regarding RIT for prostate cancer is realistic.

References

Abdel-Nabi H, Wright GL, Gulfo JV et al. (1992) Monoclonal antibodies and radioimmunoconjugates in the diagnosis and treatment of prostate cancer. Semin Urol 10:45–54

Abdel-Nabi H, Spaulding M, Farrel E, Derby L, Larmonica D (1995) Treatment of refractory prostate carcinoma with Y-90 KC4. J Nucl Med 36:215P

Babaian RJ, Murray JL, Lamki LM et al. (1987) Radioimmunological imaging of metastatic prostatic cancer with ^{111}indium-labeled monoclonal antibody PAY-276. J Urol 137:439–443

Babaian RJ, Sayer J, Podoloff DA, Steelhammer LC, Bhadkamkar VA, Gulfo JV (1994) Radioimmunoscintigraphy of pelvic lymph nodes with In-111-labeled monoclonal antibody CYT-356 J Urol 152:1952–1955

Dillman RO, Beauregard J, Ryan KP et al. (1987) Radioimmunodetection of cancer with the use of indium-111-labeled monoclonal antibodies. NCI Monogr 3:33–36

Goldenberg DM, DeLand FH (1984) Clinical studies of prostatic cancer imaging with radiolabeled antibodies against prostatic acid phosphatase. Urol Clin North Am 11:277–281

Goldenberg DM, DeLand F, Kim E et al. (1978) Use of radiolabeled antibodies to carcinoembryonic antigen for the detection and localization of diverse cancers by external photoscanning. N Engl J Med 298:1384–1386

Goldenberg DM, DeLand FH, Bennett SJ et al. (1983) Radioimmodetection of prostate cancer. In vivo use of radioactive antibodies against prostatic acid phosphatase for diagnosis and detection of prostatic cancer by nuclear imaging. JAMA 250:630–635

Halpern SE, Haindl W, Beauregard J et al. (1988) Scintigraphy with indium-labeled monoclonal antibodies: kinetics, biodistribution, and tumor detection. Radiology 168:529–536

Horoszewicz JS, Kawinski E, Murphy GP (1987) Monoclonal antibodies to a new antigenic marker in epithelial prostatic cells and serum of prostatic cancer patients. Anticancer Res 7:927–936

Israeli RS, Powel CT, Fair WR, Heston WDW (1993) Molecular cloning of a complementary DNA encoding a prostate-specific membrane antigen. Cancer Res 53:227–230

Kahn D, Williams RD, Seldin DW et al. (1994) Radioimmunoscintigraphy with ^{111}indium labeled CYT-356 for the detection of occult prostate cancer recurrence. J Urol 152:1490–1495

Kahn D, Miller S, Gerstbrein J, Maquire R, Williams RD (1995) Accuracy of In-111 capromab pendetide MAb scan for detecting prostate fossa tumor recurrence following radical prostatectomy. J Urol 153:519A

Kaminski MS, Zasadny KR, Francis IR et al. (1993) Radioimmunotherapy of B-cell lymphoma with I-131 anti-B1 (anti-CD20) antibody. N Engl J Med 329:459–465

Kohler G, Milstein C (1975) Continuous cultures of fused cells secreting antibody of predefined specificity. Nature 256:495–497

Mach JP, Carrel S, Forni M et al. (1980) Tumor localization of radiolabeled antibodies against carcinoembryonic antigen in patients with carcinoma. N Engl J Med 305:5–10

Meredith RF, Bueschen AJ, Khazaeli MB et al. (1994) Treatment of metastatic prostate cancer with radiolabeled antibody CC49. J Nucl Med 35:1017–1022

Platt JF, Bree RL, Schwab RE (1987) The accuracy of CT in the staging of carcinoma of the prostate. AJR 149:315–318

Press OW, Eary JF, Appelbaum FR et al. (1993) Radiolabeled-antibody therapy of B-cell lymphoma with autologous bone marrow support. N Engl J Med 329:1219–1224

Pressman D, Keighley G (1948) The zone of activity of antibodies as determined by the use of radioactive tracers: the zone of activity of nephrotoxic antikidney serum. J Immunol 59:141–146

Rodwell JD, Alvares VL, Lee C et al. (1986) Site-specific covalent modification of monoclonal antibodies: in vitro and in vivo evaluations. Proc Natl Acad Sci USA 83:2632–2636

Vihko P, Kontturi M, Lukkarinem O et al. (1984) Radioimaging of prostate and metastases of prostate carcinoma with Rc^{99m}-labeled prostatic acid phosphatase-specific antibodies and their Fab fragments. Am Clin Res 16:51–52

Vihko P, Kontturi M, Lukkarinen O et al. (1987) Immunoscintigraphic evaluation of lymph node involvement in prostate carcinoma. Prostate 11:51–57

7 Imaging Modalities in Diagnosis and Staging of Carcinoma of the Prostate

R.H. Oyen

CONTENTS

R.H. Oyen, MD, PhD, Professor, Department of Radiology, University Hospitals, Catholic University of Leuven, Herestraat 49, 3000 Leuven, Belgium

7.1 Introduction

7.1.1 Anatomy of the Prostate

The zonal description of the prostate by McNeal has led to a better understanding of the anatomy of this gland as visualized by transrectal ultrasonography (TRUS) and magnetic resonance imaging (MRI) and of the pathology involved. The applied anatomy has been discussed in Chap. 4.

7.1.2 Adenocarcinoma of the Prostate

Adenocarcinomas of acinar origin account for 95% of all prostatic carcinomas. Adenocarcinomas predominantly arise in the subcapsular area of the outer peripheral zone (PZ) of the gland (70%). Theoretically, cancers located in the PZ are more likely to be palpable at digital rectal examination (DRE). Approximately 30% of the adenocarcinomas arise in the transitional zone (TZ) of the prostate. The latter are not palpated at DRE; they are most frequently found incidentally during histologic examination of chips obtained at the time of transurethral resection (TURP), operative prostatectomy (enucleation), or random biopsies, or during histologic examination of whole-mount sections of a radical prostatectomy specimen. TZ cancers usually coexist with at least some degree of hyperplasia (i.e., lateral lobes). At transurethral or open adenomectomy, the hyperplastic TZ is partially or completely removed. Another important observation is that, because most adenocarcinomas originate in the PZ, the probability that men will develop a prostatic adenocarcinoma after the treatment remains as high as before. The central zone (CZ) is relatively resistant to both benign and malignant disease processes. The periurethral glands, which are exclusively found inside the confines of the proximal prostatic sphincter, are of limited importance. With pronounced benign hyperplasia of these tiny periurethral glands, however, a typical middle lobe narrows the bladder neck and subsequently causes outflow obstruction.

Other benign and malignant tumors of the prostate are uncommon. Their features at imaging are almost anecdotal, and therefore will only be briefly discussed at the end of this chapter.

7.1.3 Staging of Prostatic Adenocarcinoma

Accurate staging of adenocarcinoma of the prostate allows the treating physician to tailor therapy more exactly to the individual patient. There are a number of approaches to treating prostate cancer. These include radical prostatectomy, radiation therapy, hormonal chemotherapy, and in certain cases, a combination of these treatments. Treatment options depend on a number of factors, the most important being the extent of the malignancy. Patients with disease confined to the prostate are more amenable to radical prostatectomy or to curative radiotherapy. Continuous improvements in surgical technique and expertise have decreased morbidity and increased the popularity of radical prostatectomy in the past decade. Cryosurgery is a newer application that may be an appropriate treatment option for some cancers, but long-term evaluation is required to identify its true benefit in treating prostate cancer (Onik et al. 1993).

7.1.3.1 T Staging

Clinical staging using DRE may lead to understaging in up to 72% of cases (Catalona and Bigg 1990; Fair and Kadmon 1983). With advancing technology there has been a determined effort to develop a modality that accurately delineates the local extent of disease. Especially TRUS and MRI have been subject to several comparative studies correlating the T staging with these modalities and the pathologic staging (pT staging) obtained with whole-mount slices of radical prostatectomy specimens. Assurance of confinement of the disease to the prostate would make the morbidity of each treatment more acceptable to the man contemplating therapeutic options. Therefore, if imaging could be more accurate than clinical staging, it would have enormous potential in therapy planning.

7.1.3.2 N Staging

The presence or absence of lymph node metastases is an important prognostic factor. When considering treatment for localized disease, lymph node status should be determined with reasonable certainty. In general, a relationship exists between tumor (Gleason) grade, concentration of prostate specific antigen (PSA) in the serum, and lymph node status (Partin et al. 1993; Wolf et al. 1993a,b; Kleer et al. 1993).

It has been estimated that laparoscopic pelvic lymphadenectomy for the detection of lymph node metastases is indicated in patients with a PSA of 15 ng/ml or greater and a Gleason biopsy score of 7 or greater, or a PSA of 25 ng/ml or greater and a Gleason biopsy score of 5 or greater (Wolf et al. 1993b). A poorly differentiated carcinoma (Gleason combined score 8) with a PSA of 15 ng/ml may have a 20% risk of nodal disease. Data from a multicenter study confirm that any surgical pelvic lymphadenectomy is worthwhile only if the patients has a PSA of 10 ng/ml or greater or a Gleason biopsy score of 7 or greater (Narayan et al. 1994). Current series suggest that the incidence of lymph node metastases in a population of patients undergoing lymph node dissection before intended radical prostatectomy is approximately 10% (Petros and Catalona 1992; Bluestein et al. 1994). It has been estimated, however, that among candidates for radical prostatectomy only 2.5% would benefit from the use of preoperative imaging (Wolf et al. 1995). Therefore it may be desirable to limit any imaging modality to patients at high risk for lymph node metastases.

The only patients who benefit from imaging of pelvic lymph nodes are those in whom radical prostatectomy is aborted because the presence of lymph node metastases has been confirmed with fine-needle aspiration.

7.2 Transrectal Ultrasonography

7.2.1 Equipment and Techniques

A variety of transducers are now available for imaging the prostate in several spatial planes. A very convenient probe design is an endfiring, endviewing transducer which allows multiplanar imaging in oblique coronal and sagittal projections by simply tilting the transducer 90°. Other transducers allow biplanar imaging (axial and sagittal) by simply switching the direction of the crystals. Many of the latest electronic transrectal transducers enable color Doppler ultrasonography as well. Thus blood vessels that surround and supply the prostate are visualized.

Most ultrasonographers prefer the patient to be in

a left lateral decubitus position for transrectal scanning of the prostate. In this position both imaging and TRUS-guided biopsies can be performed without major discomfort for the patient.

Transrectal ultrasonography allows volume estimation of the prostate or parts of it (i.e., hyperplasia, tumor). The volume can be calculated according to the formula: $(W \times L \times H)/2$, where W is the width of the prostate on a transverse section, L is the distance between the bladder neck and the apex on a sagittal scan, and H is the anteroposterior diameter, measured perpendicular to the long axis of the prostate on a sagittal scan. This would give the best estimation of the prostate volume compared to planimetry, which is not routinely available on all ultrasound equipment. The elliptical volume measurement method (calculated with the formula: $8A^2/3\pi L$, where A is the area of the prostate on a transverse section and L is the transverse diameter of the prostate) allows a fast estimation of the volume of the gland, with a deviation range that is similar to that of other techniques. The underestimation of the volume of the prostate as measured by the elliptical volume method ranges between 10% and 20%.

7.2.2 Normal Anatomy of the Prostate

In men under the age of 30 years the zonal anatomy of the prostate as described by McNeal can be fully illustrated (OYEN 1994; OYEN et al. 1994a). In these young men, however, the paired TZ is hardly visible. The PZ and CZ are the major glandular zones that are displayed in young males.

With advancing age, in the majority of men the TZ gradually increases because of benign prostatic hyperplasia (BPH, lateral hyperplasia, lateral lobes). Hyperplasia can be diffuse and homogeneous, but in general the hyperplastic tissue appears to be multinodular. The nodules display a wide variety of echogenicity that ranges from hypoechoic to isoechoic and hyperechoic (Fig. 7.1). Purely stromal hyperplasia is usually hypoechoic, while pure glandular hyperplasia tends to be hyperechoic. Depending on the ratio of stromal to glandular hyperplasia, nodules with a mixed tissue composition display heterogeneous sonographic characteristics.

In the majority of men over 50 years of age with suspected or known prostatic cancer, the PZ and TZ can be differentiated by TRUS. The CZ, however, is difficult to recognize, but the ejaculatory duct complex provides an excellent landmark to evaluate this zone. Identification of this crossroads is important particularly for local T staging of prostate cancer (OYEN 1994).

The prostatic capsule cannot be seen entirely. The hypoechoic line at the posterior aspect of the prostate probably represents the capsule or a part of it.

The extraprostatic trapezoid area can be recognized at the apex of the gland on a midsagittal scan. In this area the prostatic capsule is thin or even

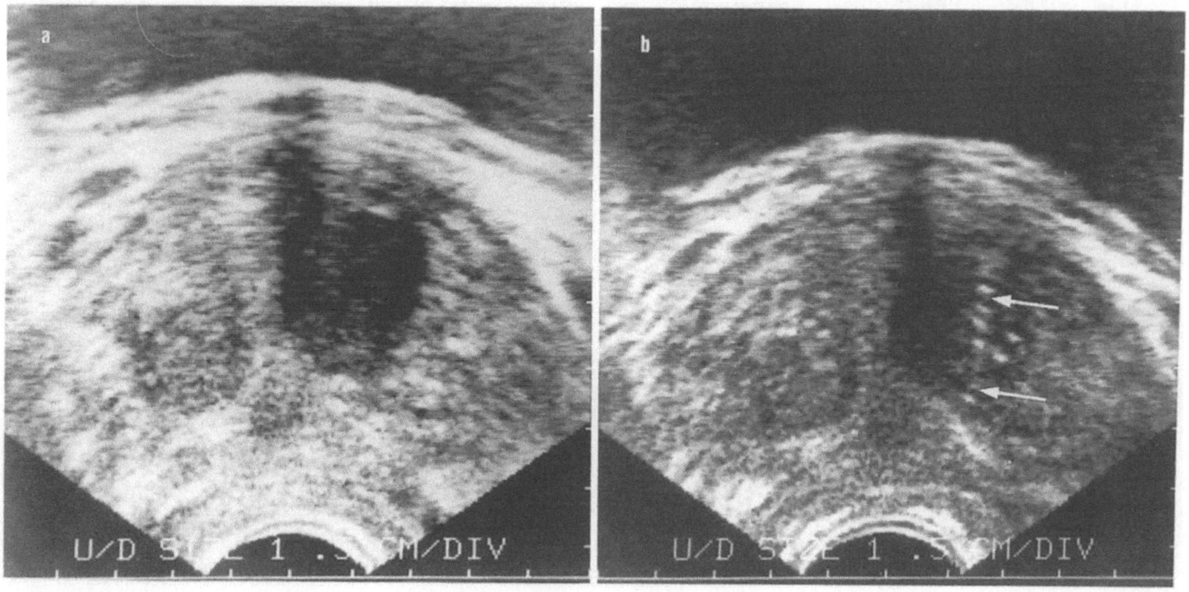

Fig. 7.1a,b. TRUS; transverse section of the prostate. Benign, multinodular hyperplasia of the TZ (**a**). Hypoechoic nodules are, in general, explained by stromal hyperplasia. They cannot be differentiated from prostatic carcinomas originating in the TZ. Because of the low prevalence of carcinoma in these hypoechoic nodules, systematic biopsy (*arrow*, needle path in **b**) is not warranted

completely absent. This area of weakness facilitates the spread of apical cancer beyond the confines of the gland. At the posterolateral surface of the prostate, on a transverse scan, the rounded section of the neurovascular bundle can be seen consistently. Of course, color Doppler imaging enables the visualization of branches of the neurovascular bundle penetrating the prostatic capsule. Again, areas of anatomic weakness are present, and in fact these are the routes of predilection along which prostatic cancer reaches the extraprostatic space.

7.2.3 Indications

The generally accepted indications for TRUS of the prostate in patients with known or suspected cancer are: (a) evaluation of the patient with an abnormal DRE; (b) evaluation of the patient with an abnormal laboratory test indicative of prostate cancer, including raised PSA or acid phosphatase or other evidence of metastatic disease; (c) guidance for directed biopsies; (d) staging of known prostatic cancer; (e) screening for prostate cancer; and (f) monitoring response following treatment for prostate cancer.

7.2.4 Echogenicity of Prostatic Adenocarcinoma

7.2.4.1 Hypoechoic Prostatic Adenocarcinoma

Most larger cancers, defined as prostatic cancers greater than 5 mm in diameter, and originating in the PZ, will be identified on TRUS as hypoechoic lesions (Shinohara et al. 1989; Rifkin et al. 1990) (Figs. 7.2, 7.3). Hypoechoic (or echopenic) cancers account for approximately 60% of all prostatic adenocarcinomas. Their hypoechogenicity is, at least partially, explained by the almost homogeneous cellular composition throughout the tumor. The appearance on TRUS is also correlated with the histologic grade and the degree of stromal fibrosis. Echopenic cancers are, in general, the better differentiated cancers with less fibrosis (Rifkin et al. 1989) and a nodular growth pattern (as opposed to an infiltrative growth pattern). In our experience, however, the histologic grade of the tumor does not influence its echogenicity: all tumors that we have diagnosed by TRUS and TRUS-guided transrectal needle core biopsy have appeared to be almost homogeneously hypoechoic regardless of the grade or Gleason score.

The infiltrative portion of a hypoechoic cancer may be completely isoechoic, i.e., indiscernible on TRUS. This behavior certainly explains why the vol-

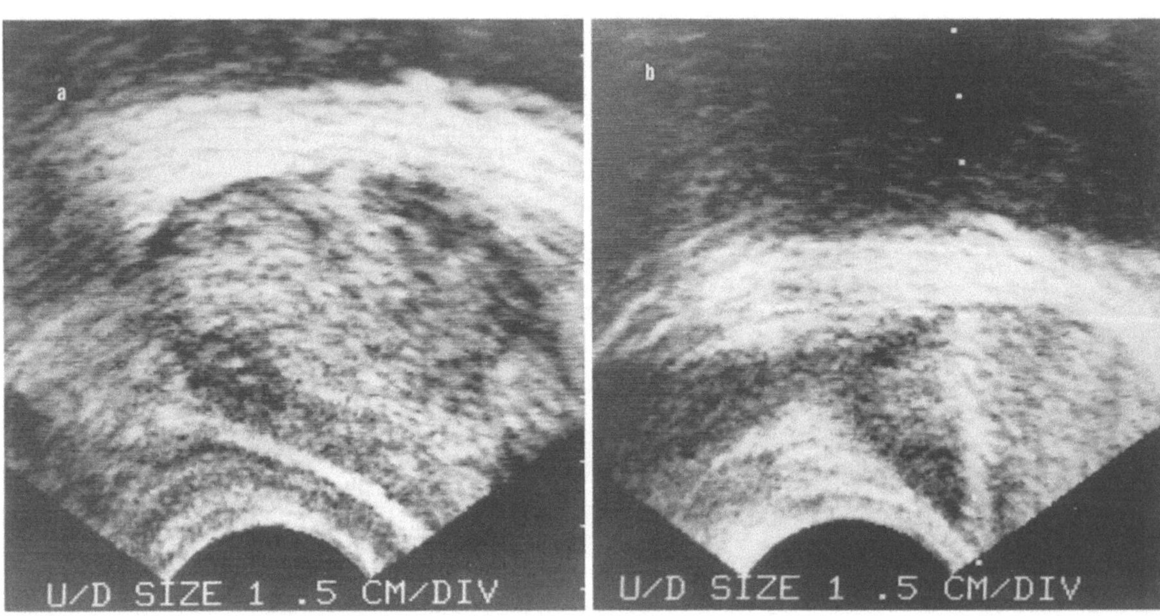

Fig. 7.2. TRUS; sagittal scans before (**a**) and during (**b**) TRUS-guided needle biopsy. A small hypoechoic lesion is present at the base of the left PZ (prostatic adenocarcinoma, Gleason score 5). TRUS-guided biopsy using a spring-driven automatic device enables representative biopsies to be obtained of virtually all focal lesions in any part of the gland

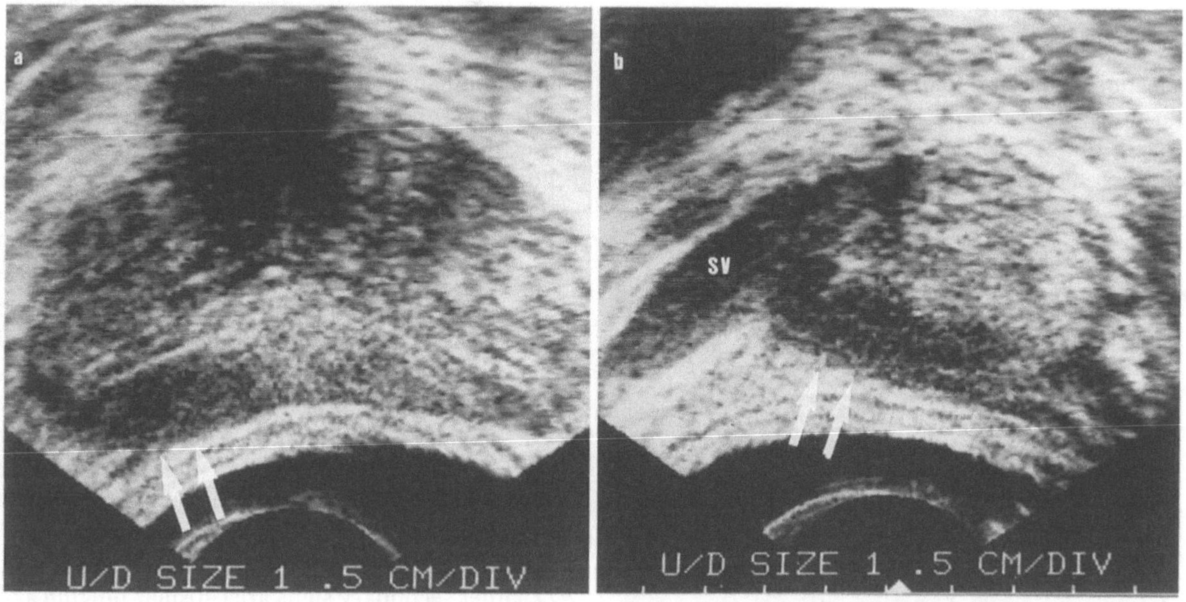

Fig. 7.3. TRUS; transverse (**a**) and sagittal (**b**) scans. A hypoechoic adenocarcinoma (Gleason score 7) is present in the PZ on the right side (*arrows*). It is difficult to predict whether the lesion is confined to the gland or not. The prostate capsule is not even definable on the contralateral side. The echogenicity of the tumor is the same as that of the seminal vesicle (*SV*). Since the tumor is small (less than 4 cm^3), the likelihood of seminal vesicle invasion is low

ume of prostatic cancers is generally underestimated on TRUS.

7.2.4.2 Hyperechoic Prostatic Adenocarcinoma

Hyperechoic tumors can be unusual ductal adenocarcinomas with central necrosis and dystrophic calcifications (Egawa et al. 1992). Another explanation for the heterogeneity and predominantly hyperechoic texture of some advanced cancers is that, while they spread, they incorporate preexisting brighter echoes from corpora amylacea or calculi (Fig. 7.4). Homogeneous hyperechoic carcinomas, thought, are not frequent and probably do not even exist at all (Fig. 7.5). Indeed, most if not all of these so-called hyperechoic cancers have a hypoechoic background with dispersed hyperechoic areas due to necrosis and (incorporated) calcifications (Fig. 7.4).

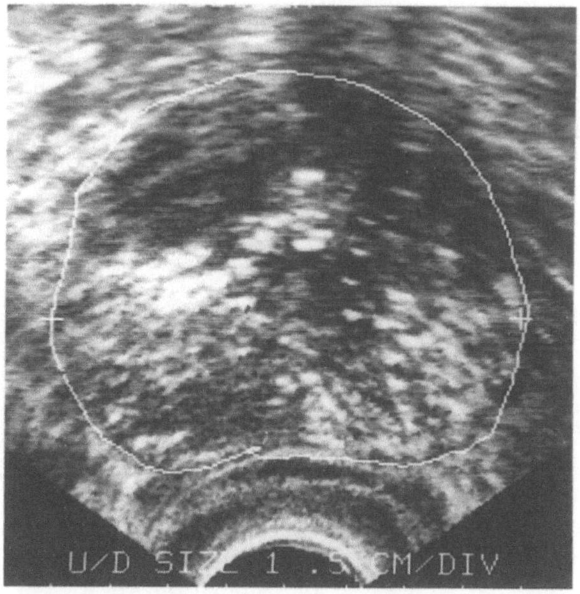

Fig. 7.4. TRUS; transverse scan. Diffusely heterogeneous aspect of the entire prostate. Note the hypoechoic background with dispersed coarse hyperechoic areas throughout the gland. All four of the quadrant biopsies revealed moderately differentiated adenocarcinoma (Gleason score 7)

7.2.4.3 Isoechoic Prostatic Adenocarcinoma

The other 40% of carcinomas are less visible or even not visible at all; these are termed isoechoic cancers. Theoretically, there reasons why so many prostatic carcinomas may be isoechoic. Firstly, the underlying echotexture at the site of the cancer may not be altered sufficiently to be distinguished from the uninvolved portions of the prostate (Fig. 7.6). This situation is not exclusive to subtle microscopic foci of cancer; rather, for the same reason even larger carcinomas may remain indiscernible. Similarly, cancers originating in the anterior extension of the PZ (i.e., in front of the hyperplastic TZ) may be isoechoic compared to the hypoechoic nonglandular fibromuscular stroma. Secondly, as already mentioned, the hyperplastic TZ displays heterogeneous sonographic characteristics with multiple nodules, some of them hypoechoic, and hence even large-volume cancers can remain indiscernible from the benign glandular or stromal tissue (Fig. 7.1). Moreover, subtle foci of cancer may originate from within these nodules, without focal alterations of the echogenicity.

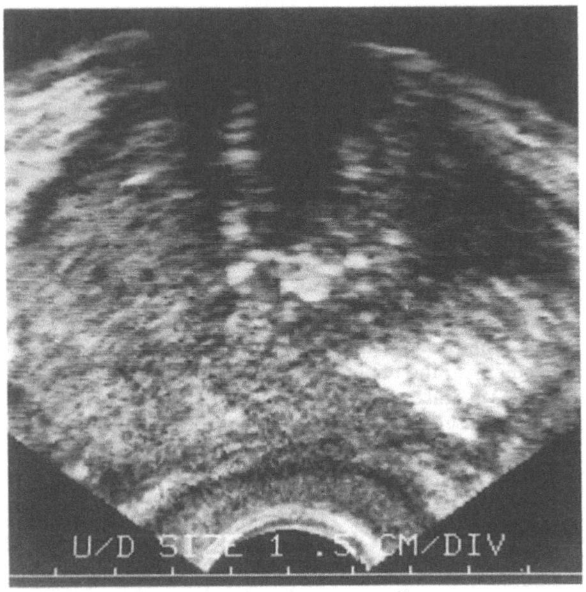

Fig. 7.5. TRUS; transverse view. Focal hyperechogenicity of the left PZ, felt as an induration at DRE. Fibrosis and chronic prostatitis were found in the biopsy cores

On histopathologic examination, isoechoic cancers (including those with subtle hyperechoic areas) more frequently display poor cellular differentiation and have a greater degree of stromal fibrosis. It can be seen grossly that they are larger and tend to blend into the background of hyperplasia. Again, considerable overlap among histologic types is seen (RIFKIN et al. 1989).

When an isoechoic cancer is present, it can be detected only when secondary signs of malignancy are appreciated. These include glandular asymmetry, which is most often obvious on transverse scans (Fig. 7.7). Other secondary signs are capsular bulging and areas of attenuation. Nevertheless, none of them is specific for malignant disease. It is therefore important to be aware of this pitfall and, if there is strong clinical suspicion of prostate cancer and a palpable nodule, to urge that a biopsy be performed even in the face of a negative TRUS examination.

Most isoechoic tumors are detected in biopsy specimens from a palpable nodule or by any set of (systematic) random biopsies. The sonographic false-negatives support the opinion of some that reliance on TRUS for screening is not appropriate.

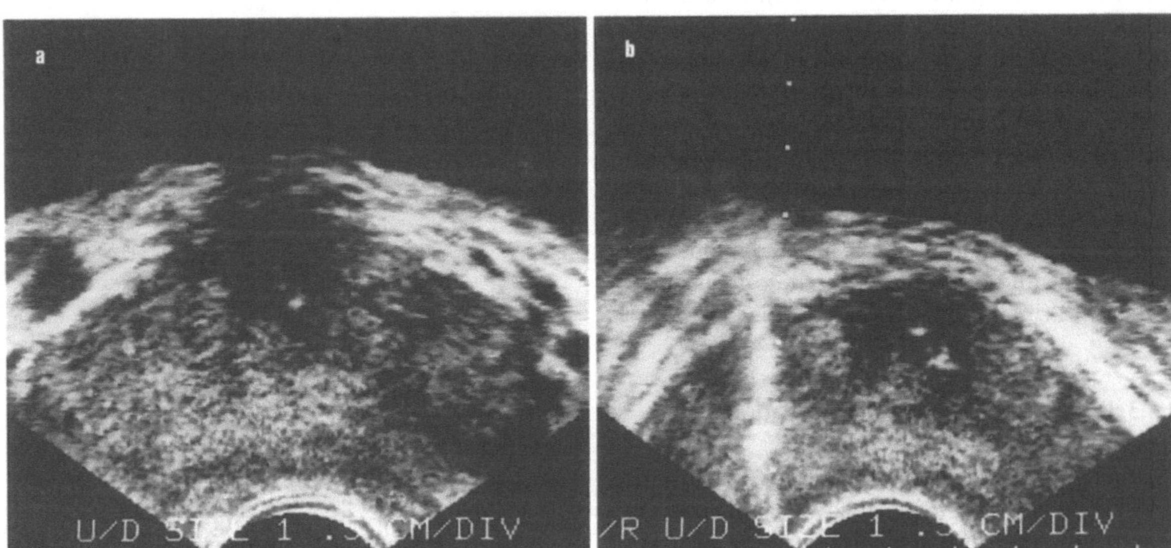

Fig. 7.6a,b. TRUS; transverse scans. Hypoechoic biopsy-proven prostatic adenocarcinoma (Gleason score 5) in the left PZ. One biopsy of the contralateral lobe (**b**) contained a 5-mm isoechoic focus of moderately well differentiated adenocarcinoma (Gleason score 5)

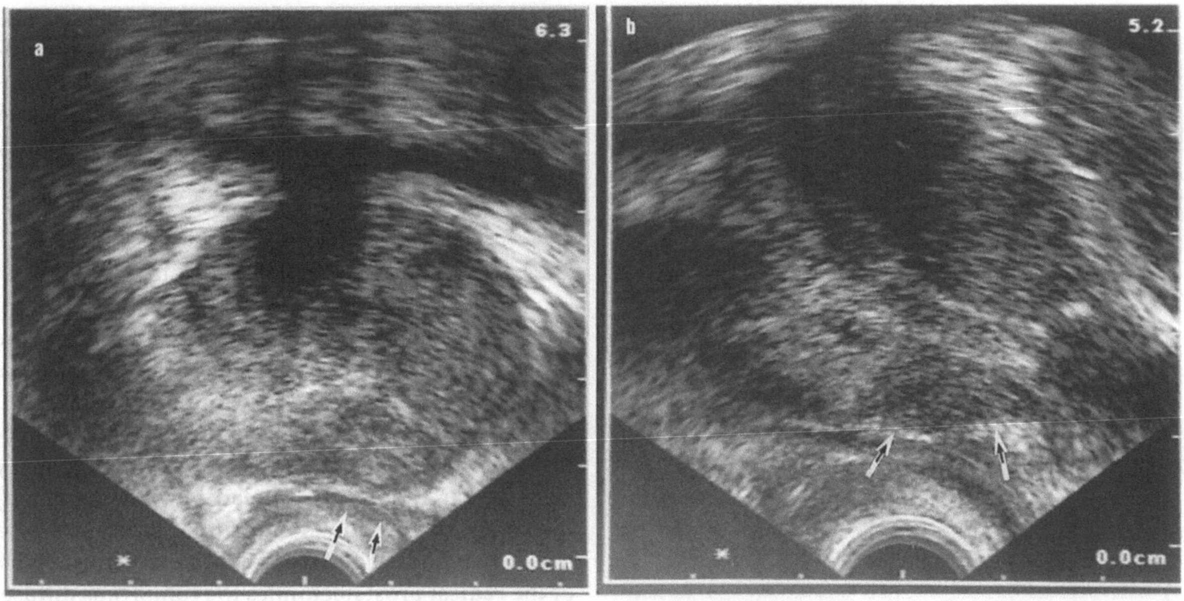

Fig. 7.7. TRUS; transverse (**a**) and sagittal (**b**) scans. Tumor is present in the PZ on the left side (*arrows*); there is bulging of the prostatic capsule, which shows some irregularity as well. This was correctly staged as a T3a lesion. Note that there are difficulties in assessing the size of the lesion, since it is isoechoic to the glandular tissue in the anterior and lateral aspects of the PZ

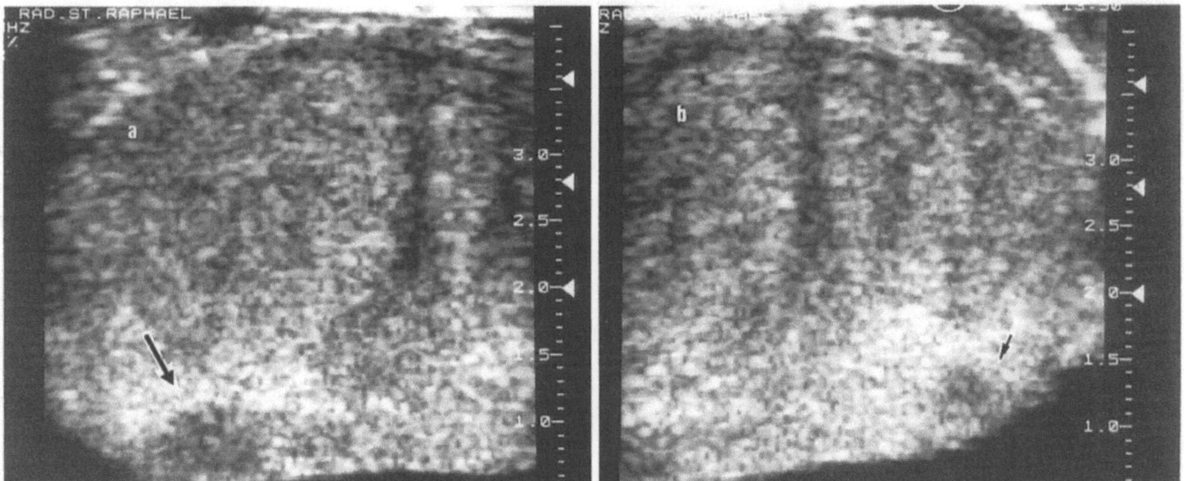

Fig. 7.8. Ultrasonography showing two subtle cancers in the PZ, originating in the subcapsular area. One has a diameter of approximately 8 mm (*large arrow*) and the other a diameter of approximately 3 mm (*small arrow*)

7.2.4.4 Multifocal Prostatic Adenocarcinoma

Often, prostate cancer is bilateral or, perhaps better, multifocal. The ultrasonographer may not appreciate the multiple foci when encountering a well-defined hypoechoic lesion (Fig. 7.8). This has been demonstrated in a multi-institutional trial in which TRUS was able to correctly identify only 59% of all lesions, and 72% of lesions larger than 1 cm (Rifkin et al. 1990). Similar figures have been found in our experience as well. In a large retrospective series of patients with just one biopsy-proven prostatic carcinoma and where the prostatectomy specimen was investigated with step-sectioned whole-mount slices, at least 71% had more than one focus of carcinoma. The tumors were bilateral in 61% of the cases. Some of those not seen were small lesions and represented secondary tumors in the gland with multiple foci. Multiple foci of cancer may be found either exclusively in the PZ (53.4% in our series), in both the PZ and the TZ (41.8%), or exclusively in the TZ (4.8%). In 39% of the cases, the tumor was bifocal; in 17.5% three different foci of cancer were present; in 9.7% four different foci were found. Cancers that originated in the TZ tended to be small and, in general, were well differentiated. PZ cancers, by contrast, were larger and were more often moderately differentiated or undifferentiated. This probably explains the variety in biologic behavior of carcinomas that originate in either the PZ or the TZ. Note that primary TZ cancers may show very aggressive behavior too.

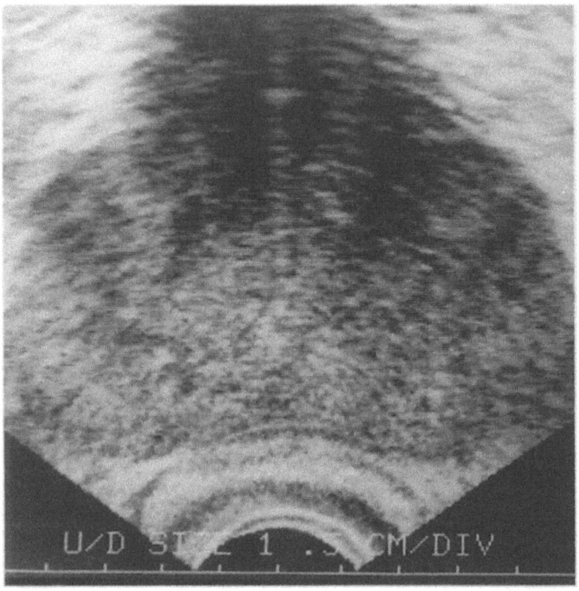

Fig. 7.9. TRUS; transverse scan. Heterogeneous, almost isoechoic gland in a patient with a PSA of 16 ng/ml and a firm gland on DRE. Systematic sextant biopsies showed tumor in all but one core (i.e., *center left*), Gleason score 5

7.2.4.5 Completely Isoechoic Prostate

If the gland is completely infiltrated by cancer, the prostate may become completely isoechoic and there may be no normal tissue for comparison (Fig. 7.9). The absence of the normal internal zonal architecture (and eventually the association with secondary signs of carcinoma, i.e., spread beyond the gland) then may be the only sonographic indication of a diffusely infiltrating carcinoma. In our series, in 5% of the radical prostatectomies the tumor was diffuse, so that the site of origin was completely obscured. It is obvious that DRE and the PSA will be abnormal, and that the gland may appear hypervascular on color Doppler ultrasonography.

7.2.4.6 Other Hypoechoic Lesions

Even in the hands of experienced ultrasonographers, only a limited number of hypoechoic areas in the PZ are positive for cancer upon histologic examination of the core biopsies. Thus, the positive predictive

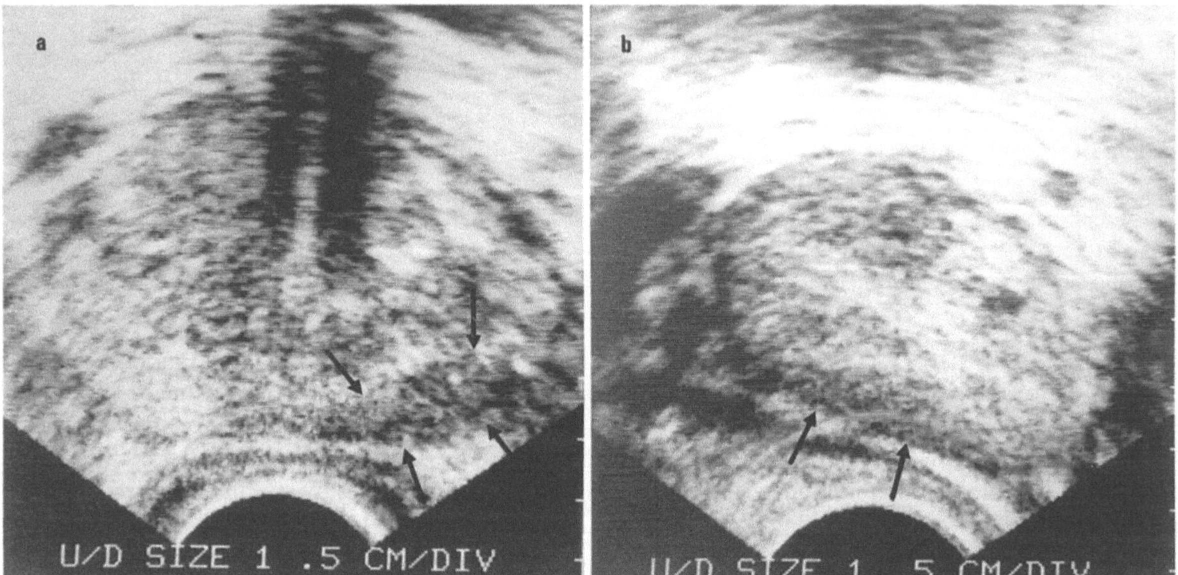

Fig. 7.10. TRUS; transverse (**a**) and sagittal (**b**) scans. A persistent hypoechoic area (*arrows*) is present in the PZ after an episode of subacute prostatitis and appropriate treatment. Biopsy yielded a well-differentiated adenocarcinoma, Gleason grade 2

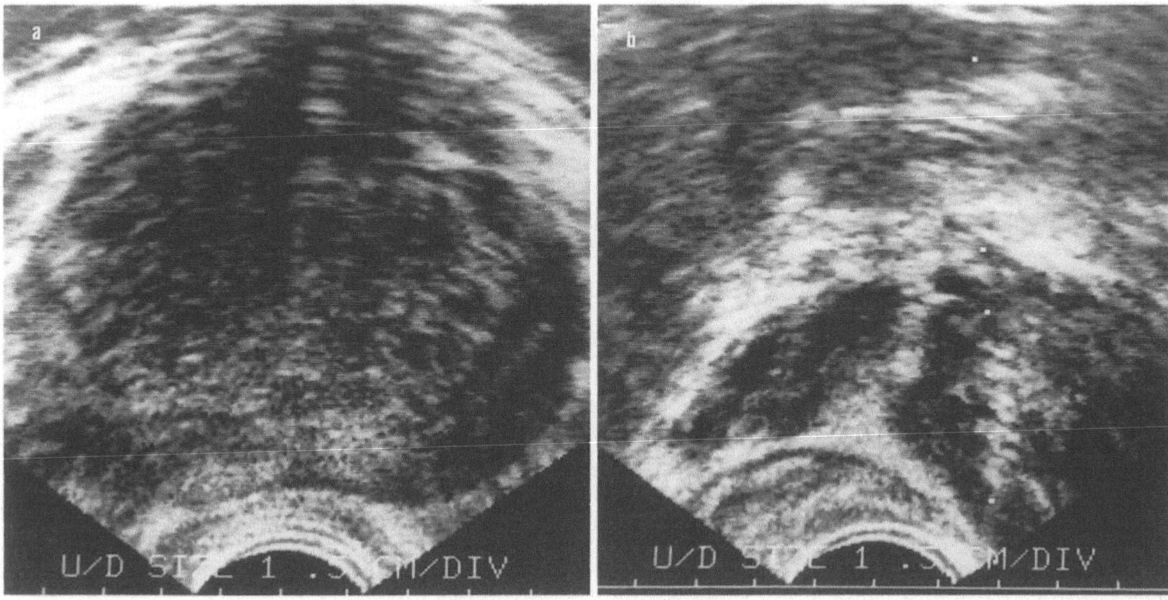

Fig. 7.11. TRUS; transverse (**a**) and sagittal (**b**) scans during needle biopsy. There is heterogeneous hypoechogenicity of the PZ in a male with a firm gland on DRE. The hypoechoic areas were explained as nonspecific prostatitis upon histologic examination of the needle biopsy cores

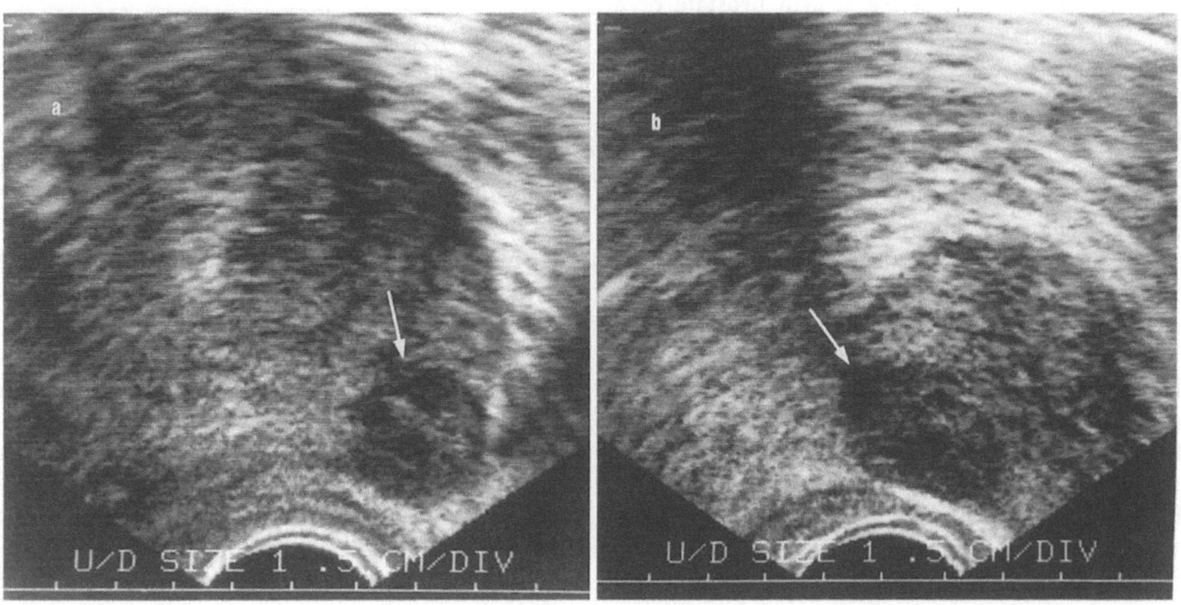

Fig. 7.12. TRUS; transverse (**a**) and sagittal (**b**) sections of the prostate. A hypoechoic nodule (*arrow*) is present in the left PZ, causing bulging of the prostatic capsule. There are some tiny cystic areas within the lesion. The lesion was soft on DRE. Although there is nothing specific about the diagnosis, the TRUS characteristics are suggestive of a benign hyperplastic nodule originating in the peripheral zone of the prostate

value of TRUS ranges from 16% to 40% only. Biopsies from noncancerous areas in the PZ usually show normal prostatic tissue, prostatitis (Figs. 7.10, 7.11), BPH, atrophy, prostatic intraepithelial neoplasia (PIN), infarction, and cyst. None of them can be differentiated based on gray-scale criteria only. The rare benign hyperplastic nodule originating in the PZ of the prostate can be recognized sonographically with somewhat greater confidence (Oyen et al. 1994b) (Fig. 7.12).

Equally disconcerting is the observation that (stromal) nodules of BPH in the TZ are normally hypoechoic, making it virtually impossible to diagnose prostate cancer in the TZ based on TRUS alone (Oyen 1994; Oyen et al. 1994a) (Fig. 7.1).

7.3 Differentiation of Benign from Malignant Lesions

7.3.1 TRUS and DRE and/or PSA

There have been many attempts to define parameters that would enable the differentiation of benign from malignant hypoechoic lesions in the PZ of the prostate. Combinations of a TRUS-hypoechoic lesion and DRE and/or serum PSA concentration (normal <4 ng/ml) or PSA-derived parameters (PSA index or PSA density, excessive PSA) have been proposed by several authors.

The positive predictive value of the combination of a palpable and hypoechoic lesion was 75% (in our series of more than 530 hypoechoic lesions), compared to 57% for TRUS as a single examination, and 65% for DRE. In this series, a firm prostate or a nodularity on DRE corresponding to the site of the hypoechogenicity on TRUS was considered an abnormality. If just these palpable hypoechoic lesions had had a TRUS-guided biopsy, 5% of the hypoechoic prostatic carcinomas that originated in the PZ of the prostate would not have had a confirmatory needle core biopsy at that time.

The serum PSA concentration is not a valid discriminator either. In the same series of patients with hypoechoic cancers originating in the PZ, 76 (of 306 cancers or 25% !) had a serum PSA concentration less than 4 ng/ml. Therefore, it seems reasonable to defend the strategy that a hypoechoic lesion in the PZ deserves a TRUS-guided biopsy, regardless of the serum PSA concentration. This is especially true when the nodule is palpable on DRE.

None of the PSA-related parameters, such as the PSA density or PSA index (i.e., the ratio of the serum PSA concentration over the volume of the prostate, expressed in no units) or excessive PSA (i.e., the difference between the serum PSA concentration and the predicted PSA concentration, where the predicted PSA concentration is calculated from the volume of the prostate multiplied by 0.12), have proven helpful in discriminating benign from malignant lesions (Lee F et al. 1992). The overlap between the values of these indices in patients with benign and patients with malignant hypoechoic lesions is too great to be of any use in clinical practice. This is similar to the experience of Brawer et al. (1993), who reported on the inability of the PSA index to enhance the predictive value of PSA in the diagnosis of prostatic carcinoma. It is likely that these parameters are imperfect because the epithelial-to-stroma ratio varies considerably from one prostate to the next and it is only the epithelium that produces the PSA. As a result, two prostates of similar size can produce markedly different amounts of PSA.

In conclusion, when one aims at a reduction of the number of negative biopsies, limitation of TRUS-guided biopsies to those echopenic nodules that are palpable on DRE seems to be an acceptable strategy. This is certainly true when both examinations, i.e., TRUS and DRE, are performed by different and experienced, well-skilled examiners. The number of biopsies of hypoechoic lesions is reduced by approximately 25%, while 5% of (small, i.e., less than 1 cm diameter) hypoechoic PZ cancers will not have a confirmative histologic diagnosis.

7.3.2 Color-Doppler Ultrasonography

The inability to make a specific diagnosis with conventional gray-scale TRUS has been a vexing problem. Color Doppler flow imaging has been proposed for the evaluation of prostate pathology to allow more elaborate and accurate differentiation of focal areas within the gland (Rifkin et al. 1993; Kelly et al. 1993). This technology displays the mean frequency shifts of flowing red blood cells within blood vessels as varying shades of color spectrum depending on the direction and speed of their flow. Unfortunately, the various blood flow speeds detected within the different types of tumor vessels may depend on a given instrument sensitivity. Both operator-independent and operator-dependent parameters such as gain, pulse repetition frequency, and wall filter settings may influence detection of these vessels and must be understood by the operator to optimize results.

Initial reports stressed the value of color Doppler in the diagnosis of prostate cancer. Owing to neovascularity, prostate cancer, either echopenic or isoechoic, has an increased flow within or at the periphery of the lesion as opposed to other focal processes that can affect the prostate (Fig. 7.13). Many other diseases, however, exhibit a diffusely or focally abnormal flow too. There is considerable overlap between carcinoma and acute prostatitis (Newman et al. 1995). It has now been accepted that in prostatitis, the flow is not significantly different from that in cancer (Fig. 7.14). Therefore, biopsies are still

Fig. 7.13. TRUS; sagittal scan (**a**) and sagittal color Doppler image (**b**). A focal hypervascular, hypoechoic malignant lesion is present in the subcapsular area. Although one would expect low compliance in the case of neovascularity, the resistive indices in this case are high (0.80). Color Doppler imaging could be used to detect isoechoic, hypervascular areas harboring cancer

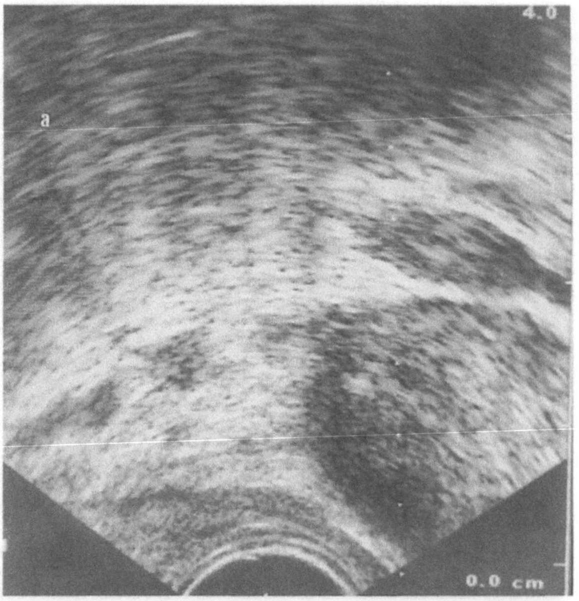

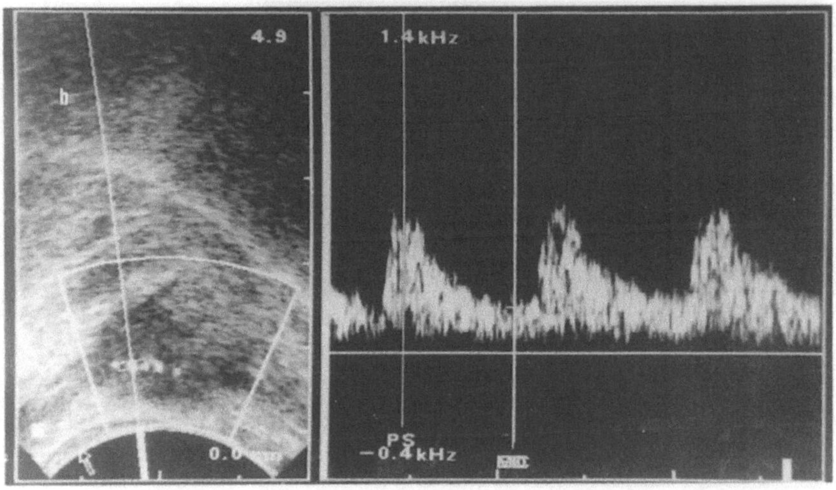

necessary to obtain a histologic diagnosis. The addition of objective, measurable flow-related criteria, such as the resistive index, does not provide a specific discriminator either: spectral wave form analysis of the area of potential concern shows no statistical difference in the mean resistive indices in any patients with focal hypoechoic lesions in the PZ (Rifkin et al. 1993) (Figs. 7.13, 7.14).

While there are still clinically significant cancers that are undetectable by TRUS, the use of color Doppler flow imaging has increased the ability to identify many subtle lesions. In Rikfin et al.'s series, 7% of prostate cancer patients had no obviously identifiable abnormality on gray-scale scanning but had distinctly abnormal flow on color Doppler (Rifkin et al. 1993). However, again, abnormal findings on color Doppler without abnormal findings on gray-scale scanning occurred in inflammatory foci (24%) and in 5% of other benign lesions. This has been confirmed by others as well (Kelly et al. 1993). Color Doppler imaging thus improves the positive predictive value of TRUS but appears to have little additional value over TRUS alone in the diagnosis of prostate cancer.

In conclusion, at present, focal increased PZ flow on color Doppler imaging is associated with a high likelihood of focal carcinoma or prostatitis on histologic examination. Many sites of neoplasm may be conspicuous on color Doppler yet manifest no definable gray-scale TRUS abnormality. However, color Doppler may improve biopsy yield by permitting determination of the appropriate site for biopsy in patients with elevated PSA levels and no focal grayscale abnormality. As color Doppler appears to have limited sensitivity for detection of all sites of

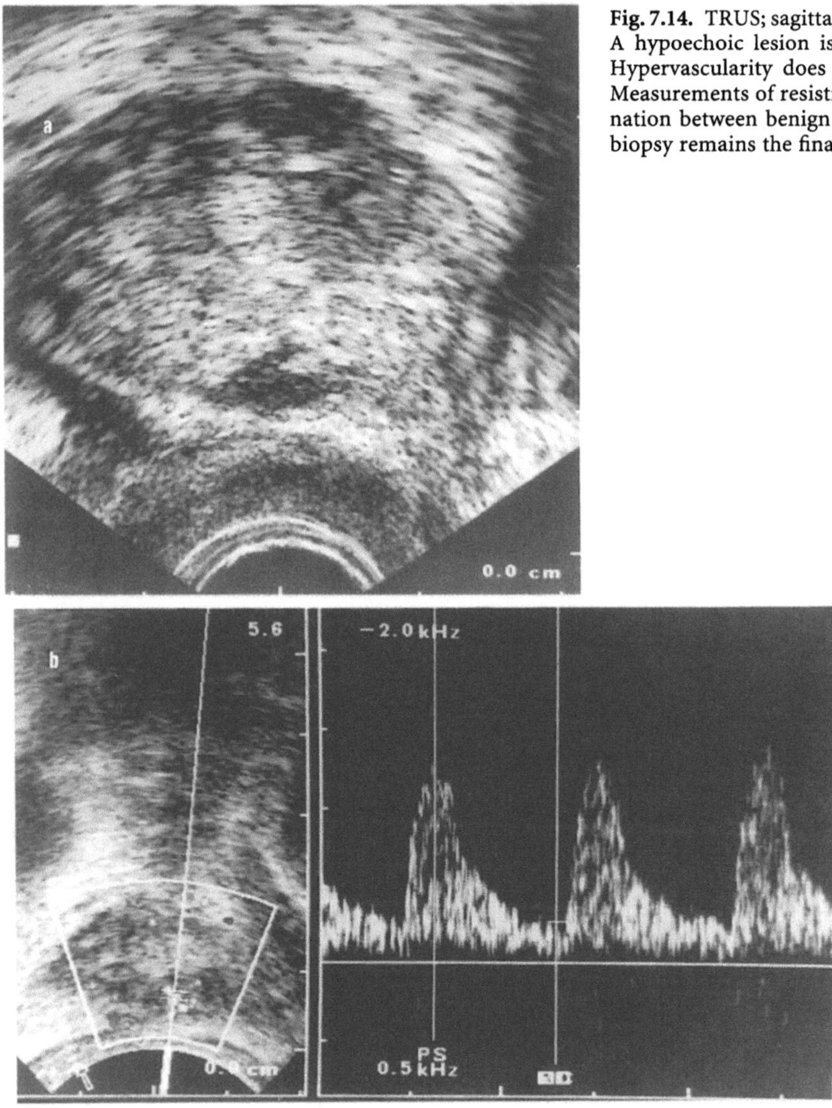

Fig. 7.14. TRUS; sagittal view (**a**) and color Doppler image (**b**). A hypoechoic lesion is located at the base of the prostate. Hypervascularity does not necessarily indicate malignancy. Measurements of resistive indices are not helpful in discrimination between benign and malignant lesions. TRUS-guided biopsy remains the final discriminator

involvement by prostate cancer in any given patient, however, negative findings on both color Doppler and gray-scale TRUS should not preclude the performance of random or systematic prostate biopsies.

7.3.3 Image Processing

With image processing, tissue characterization in the prostate is performed to assess the probability of malignancy. The gray-scale characteristics of a newly found lesion are compared by the computer with the set of tissue characteristics obtained from other previously histologically proven lesion patterns. A sensitivity of 80.6% and a specificity of 77.1% have been achieved in a retrospective study (Huynen et al. 1994). In a prospective study, the results were 80.0% and 88.2% respectively; the prospective predictive value for cancer was 85.7% (Huynen et al. 1994).

A disadvantage is that the technique is limited to one particular type of sonographic gray-scale equipment and that extrapolation of the results to other machines is not readily possible. A large set of biopsy-proven hypoechoic lesions is necessary for gray-scale equipment to provide enough reference parameters to the computer to make it a useful tool in practice. In an individual case, image-processed lesion differentiation does not exclude malignancy. This technique obviates the need for any kind of repeat examination, and probably ultimately TRUS-guided biopsy, in about 15% of the patients.

7.3.4 Sonoelasticity

With sonoelasticity tissue is vibrated with a low-frequency source and tissue motion is detected and displayed as a color image superimosed on the conventional gray-scale ultrasound image. The theory of sonoelasticity imaging is based on the postulate that low-frequency vibrations are easily conducted through soft tissue and muscle; discrete stiff tumors, however, create a detectable disturbance in vibration pattern. Early investigations demonstrated a clear correlation between vibration image deficits and areas of palpable stiffness (Lee F Jr et al. 1991b). A recent in vitro study of impalpable areas of prostate cancer concluded that sonoelasticity imaging was more sensitive for tumor detection and more accurate for assessment of tumor location than was conventional TRUS (Rubens et al. 1995). Sensitivity and specificity with sonoelasticity imaging were 85% and 84%, respectively, and 30% and 100% with ultrasound when compared with pathologic findings. In this particular study, 64% of pathologically confirmed tumors detected on sonoelasticity imaging were completely isoechoic on conventional US images. Large-scale studies are required to judge whether this technique deserves a place in the diagnostic algorithm of diffuse or focal prostatic lesions.

7.3.5 TRUS-Guided Biopsies

7.3.5.1 Biopsy Techniques

The role of TRUS in the diagnosis of prostate cancer by imaging alone remains controversial. In general, when TRUS is performed, identification of an abnormal lesion or an area of asymmetry warrants further evaluation. As described above, the addition of color Doppler imaging does not allow reliable lesion discrimination. It has become clear, however, that adding TRUS-guided biopsy procedures to the diagnostic examination adds a significant dimension to prostate ultrasonography.

The current most popular biopsy technique is with the use of a transrectal approach. Needle guidance systems are available for the probes with guides that clamp onto the side of the probe and place electronic guide lines showing the needle path on the monitor (Figs. 7.2, 7.6, 7.11). A common needle device for transrectal prostate biopsies is the automatic spring-driven biopsy gun. This device allows precise needle localization and performs a core type of biopsy with minimal manipulation and with remarkable safety due to the speed at which the biopsy is performed. Usually an 18 gauge needle is used with a slot of approximately 17 mm in length.

TRUS guidance for transrectal biopsy is a safe and relatively painless procedure for the patient and is more accurate than digitally guided biopsy, even for palpable lesions (Rifkin et al. 1991). It can be performed without significant complications on an outpatient basis with little or no prior preparation. The use of a cleansing enema is sometimes recommended but is not mandatory. It has become standard practice to administer a rapidly absorbed antibiotic just prior to the biopsy. One of the newer broad-spectrum antibiotics (such as fluoroquinolone) will almost completely eliminate the risk of major complications associated with prostate biopsies. If biopsy is performed, continued treatment with the antibiotic for a period of a few days has also been suggested.

Risks of the biopsy include bleeding and sepsis. Neither is a significant risk if one of the automatic biopsy devices, usually supplied with 18-gauge needles or smaller, is used and antibiotics are administered. Urosepsis occurs in far less than 1% of cases, and although about 25% of men develop bleeding (hematuria, hematochezia, or hematospermia), it is rarely clinically important. Prostatitis has been described as a complication in 2% of cases (Billebaud et al. 1990). The risk of complication from biopsy does not increase significantly in men who are using low-dose salicylates prophylactically, although stronger anticoagulants do represent a relative contraindication.

Controversy still exists over whether TRUS guidance is necessary to biopsy palpable prostatic nodules. When a palpable abnormality is not discovered sonographically, it should be biopsied with conventional digital techniques. Conversely, when a digitally guided biopsy is negative in a suspicious gland, repeat biopsy with TRUS guidance may yield cancer in up to 30% of cases.

7.3.5.2 Biopsy Results

7.3.5.2.1 Focal lesions. Positive biopsy rates range from a low of 20% in small hypoechoic masses to a high of 65% in all suspected masses in different series of patients. DRE remains the most valuable single examination in the diagnosis of prostate cancer. TRUS increases the sensitivity of DRE if both are positive. When there is a discrepancy between the two examinations, the biopsy yield is low. When both are positive, a high cancer yield is obtained, TRUS having additional value in directing the biopsy needle to the suspicious site (Shapiro et al. 1994). If sonographic abnormalities are correlated with tumor size, DRE, and PSA, it has been shown that normal PSA and DRE can obviate the need for biopsy, particularly when lesions are 1 cm or smaller. When lesions are detected which are 1 cm or larger, and biopsy is performed, up to 70% of these lesions may represent cancer. The majority of tumors less than 3 cm^3 in volume show no tumor spread beyond the capsule.

Spencer suggested guidelines for biopsy in men with normal PSA and suspected of having prostate cancer (Spencer et al. 1993). Predictors of malignancy on ultrasonography of the PZ in men with normal PSA levels include (a) the size of the lesion, (b) the degree and focality of hypoechogenicity, and (c) correspondence with the site of DRE abnormality. The size of the lesion and the degree of the hypoechogenicity are unfortunately subjective criteria and are therefore felt to be of limited value in clinical practice.

7.3.5.2.2 Systematic and Random Biopsies. Several authors (Hodge et al. 1989a; Billebaud et al. 1990; Vallancien et al. 1991b) realized that six systematic, spatially oriented biopsies into each sextant of the prostate under TRUS guidance might provide more valuable histologic information than is acquired when biopsy sites are limited to either hypoechoic areas or the estimated area of palpable abnormalities. It is indeed impossible to histologically examine whole prostate at 3-mm intervals in men not known to have prostate cancer without finding a 40% incidence of invasive prostate cancer (Franks 1954; Stamey et al. 1993b). Six biopsy cores are sufficient to sample a prostate of moderate volume ($\leq$ 40 ml). When the prostate volume is larger, additional anteriorly oriented biopsies are indicated to sample the anterior part of the TZ and the anterior extension of the PZ. Many carcinomas arise within this area and remain undetected with a standard set of sextant biopsy samples.

In our experience, systematic biopsies result in a 13.6% increase in overall cancer detection. The positive predictive value of a set of random biopsies in patients without focal lesions on TRUS is only 0.7% when the serum PSA concentration is less than the predicted PSA concentration. The positive predictive value increases to 23.6% when the serum PSA concentration exceeds the predicted PSA concentration [predicted PSA concentration = volume (v) of the prostate $\times 0.12$, or: ePSA = sPSA − ($V \times 0.12$)]. Finally, the predictive value is 52% when the serum PSA concentration exceeds the predicted PSA concentration by at least 2 ng/ml and the prostate is abnormal on DRE (firm or nodular). If the radical prostatectomy specimens of these men are carefully investigated, it becomes obvious that most of the cancers originate in the hyperplastic TZ. These include subtle (insignificant ?) microscopic foci and large-volume cancers.

It has also been estimated by other investigators that 25% of all PZ or CZ prostate cancers treated by radical prostatectomy can be detected only by systematic, spatially separated biopsies, a figure that does not include TZ cancers (Stamey 1995). Assuming that half of the TZ cancers may be considered clinically significant, probably one-third of all prostate cancers can only be detected by systematic, spatially separated biopsies under TRUS guidance (Stamey 1995). Large (isoechoic) TZ cancers may explain the 10% incidence of men who present with metastatic prostate cancer and a normal rectal examination, much of the discrepancy between focal cancer on biopsy and large cancers in radical prostatectomy specimens, and why some men have very high PSA levels and organ-confined cancer at prostatectomy (Stamey et al. 1993a).

It is stated that systematic biopsies detect many significant isoechoic tumors that would have been missed by directed biopsies, and provide invaluable information about the distribution and Gleason grade of the cancer. However, there is also a probability of detecting a clinically insignificant cancer. Clinically insignificant cancers have been defined as those less than 0.5 cm^3 in volume (Stamey and McNeal 1992). The chance of detecting these small cancers theoretically increases when multiple biopsies are taken.

Measurement of the extent of cancer within the tissue core has been emphasized as providing important information on volume (Hodge et al. 1989a). Based on these findings it is justified to repeat biopsies in patients in whom 3 mm or less of cancer is identified in only one of the multiple biopsy cores. When such a small focus of adenocarcinoma is detected on biopsies it is difficult to determine whether the biopsy has traversed a clinically insignificant volume or whether the biopsy has sampled only a small area of a large, and significant tumor. Greater than 3 mm of cancer on repeat biopsy appears to support the latter possibility. Patients with no cancer or only another tiny focus of cancer on repeat biopsies may be managed conservatively. This conservative management consists of repeat PSA concentration measurements and DRE every 6–12 months, and repeat TRUS and biopsies at 12–24 months. That this conservative approach is warranted is not only supported by the cystoprostatectomy study, which suggests that cancers less than 0.5 ml are unlikely to achieve clinical significance in a patients' lifetime (Stamey and McNeal 1992), but also by recent data indicating that small-volume clinical cancers require 3–4 years to double in volume at least when measured by PSA (Schmid et al. 1992).

Such an approach employing systematic biopsies combined with rebiopsy if a single biopsy contains 3 mm or less of cancer results in a reduction in the number of radical prostatectomy specimens with less than 0.5 cm³ of cancer. In patients with minimal cancer, these repeat biopsies are more reliable predictors of substantial cancer volume than patient age, tumor grade on biopsy, DRE, or PSA concentration. This procedure could be applied at a hypoechoic or digitally suspicious area, if the inital biopsy contains 3 mm or less of cancer in only one of the (multiple) cores (Terris et al. 1992a).

Isolated high-grade PIN on needle biopsy of the prostate is a strong predictor of malignancy on repeat evaluation. The cancer will be found on the same side of the prostate in approximately two-thirds of cases. Directing the repeat biopsy only towards the site of PIN on initial biopsy will miss the cancer in about 35% of cases. Repeat biopsy for PIN should include systematic biopsies of both sides of the prostate (Shepard et al. 1995).

In conclusion, it is true that any set of multiple biopsies has the potential to detect an insignificant prostate cancer. The real question that arises is whether this early diagnosis is useful for the patient, since presently there is no certainty of any therapeutic benefit in terms of quantity and quality of life (Terris et al. 1992a,b; Vallancien et al. 1991a). Nevertheless, it has gradually become evident that PSA-detected, impalpable cancer is rarely insignificant and it adds further emphasis that patients diagnosed by PSA elevation have, for the most part, significant cancer that should be treated aggressively.

7.3.5.2.3 Biopsies of the Contralateral Lobe. Many ultrasonographers routinely perform random biopsies of the contralateral lobe in patients with a prostatic nodule (Fig. 7.6). Because approximately 60% of patients have bilateral carcinoma, it is obvious that, when performing biopsies of the opposite lobe in patients with a unilateral TRUS or DRE abnormality, the rate of positive biopsies will be higher. The incidence of contralateral cancer in patients with a tumor digitally localized to one prostatic lobe ranges between 14% and 50% (Carter et al. 1989; Daniels et al. 1992; Dyke et al. 1990; Hodge et al. 1989a,b; Lee F Jr et al. 1991a). In general, these patients tend to have higher serum PSA concentrations and a larger tumor volume than those with negative contralateral biopsies. These findings further demonstrate that contralateral negative biopsies in patients with unilaterally palpable disease predict low-volume, localized tumor and a negligible likelihood of surgical margin compromise when using a contralateral nerve-sparing approach. Bilaterally positive biopsies, however, suggest a larger tumor volume with a greater likelihood of adverse pathologic findings and recurrence (Daniels et al. 1992).

7.4 Staging of Prostatic Adenocarcinoma by Transrectal Ultrasonography

Radical prostatectomy is the most frequently utilized therapy for localized prostatic carcinoma. Surgical cure depends on the complete extirpation of tumor, defined as negative surgical margins at radical prostatectomy. Extraprostatic tumor in the form of positive surgical margins, seminal vesicle involvement, or lymph node metastases is a poor prognostic sign. Unfortunately, at present, the incidence of positive surgical margins remains high, with reported values ranging from 35% to 50%, even in those patients with no seminal vesicle involvement. The main causes of positive surgical margins are large tumor volume, cancer with extracapsular extension, or inadvertent dissection into the gland leaving residual tumor. These patients are then classified as stage pT3, and are at high risk for tumor progression, with 47% and 60% progression rates at 5 and 10 years after surgery, respectively.

7.4.1 T Staging

7.4.1.1 Size of the Carcinoma

The intraprostatic volume of prostatic carcinoma is a strong predictor of extraprostatic extension and prognosis (Stamey et al. 1988, 1993b). Suspicious for non-capsule-confined cancer is a lesion greater than 1.5 cm (>3 cm³) (Lee F et al. 1989). Almost all tumors of this size have a high Gleason score and a high probability of extracapsular tumor extension. DRE is known to be a poor predictor of cancer volume whereas TRUS imaging has correlated well with cancer volume. Step section planimetry correlates with the volume of hypoechoic PZ cancers with a coefficient of 0.93 (TERRIS et al. 1995). This technique is not available on all machines, and it is relatively time consuming. In general, however, there is a wide range of error that prevents general application of the technique (TERRIS et al. 1992b; SHINOHARA et al. 1989; MCSHERRY et al. 1991). Sonographic studies have shown that TRUS tends to underestimate the size and volume of individual lesions, making size a less accurate factor in determining the significance of a lesion. This is particularly problematic due to the irregular shape of many prostate cancers and the isoechoic appearance when they infiltrate into BPH (Fig. 7.7). Underestimation of the tumor volume by up to 40% has been reported. If has been proposed that an average TRUS tumor dimension be calculated based on the formula: $[(W + H + L)/3]$ where W is the width of the lesions measured on transverse images, and L the length and H the height on longitudinal sections (LEE F et al. 1989). This is indeed an easy and reproducible method, which, however, suffers from the disadvantages of every TRUS-based method of volume measurement.

As already stated, measurement of the extent of cancer within the tissue core can provide important volume information (see Sect. 7.3.5.2.2 for details).

Recently, incorporation of all available preoperative information has been proposed to produce an algorithm for estimating tumor volume. Serum PSA concentration, volume of the PZ and/or CZ hypoechoic lesions as measured by step-section planimetry, and the amount of cancer in the six systematic biopsies have been proposed to estimate the cancer volume (TERRIS et al. 1995). These algorithms correctly predicted 97% of cancer 1.0 cm^3 or greater in volume and 99% of cancers greater than 12 cm^3 in volume. However, since the cure rate with radical prostatectomy falls rapidly between 4 and 12 cm^3, it is felt that there is a need to predict these intermediate volume ranges with greater accuracy than is now possible (STAMEY 1995).

7.4.1.2 The Prostatic Capsule

TRUS is known to be highly operator dependent; it is widely used for cancer staging, with results which are highly variable. SCARDINO et al. (1989) reported an 86% staging accuracy rate but ANDREOLE et al. (1989) found understaging in 62% of their patients. Some investigators have found sensitivities for local extension into the capsule (or seminal vesicles) as high as 90%. Others have found less accuracy in the ability of TRUS to define local invasion, with sensitivities ranging between 40% and 60%. More importantly, specificities for invasion have ranged from 46% to 90%. As expected, these figures have depended on the patient mix in a given study. It is accepted that capsule-confined cancer is overdiagnosed in 9.1% of cases and missed in 31.3% (HAMPER et al. 1991). Correlation of radiologic and pathologic findings revealed that TRUS correctly staged 66% of patients with advanced disease and only 46% of those with localized disease. In patients with advanced disease correctly staged by TRUS, there was agreement between the site of periprostatic invasion detected by TRUS and that identified by pathologic examination in 71% of patients (RIFKIN et al. 1990).

The use of three-dimensional TRUS has also been proposed in the local staging of prostate cancer. In a study of 30 patients, a sensitivity of 83%, a specificity of 93%, and a positive predictive value of 96% have been reported for the detection of extracapsular extension. For the evaluation of seminal vesicle involvement, the results were 87%, 100%, and 100%, respectively (STRASSER et al. 1995).

A positive TRUS-diagnosis of extracapsular tumor spread correlates moderately well with the depth of penetration demonstrated at final pathologic examination of the radical prostatectomy specimen. Large tumors can be easily seen to extend outside of the capsule due to the loss of symmetry and capsule irregularity (Figs. 7.15–7.18). Anatomically, however, the prostate does not contain a true capsule but a fibromuscular band. This creates a dilemma for the pathologist and urologist in determining the exact significance of the depth of invasion outside this band and into the periprostatic tissues. It has been shown that in patients with benign disease, the histologic capsule is frequently absent and correlates poorly with the consistent TRUS findings of a regular, well-defined sonographically visible capsule. Therefore it would be better to replace the term capsule as a tumor-staging landmark with more realistic terminology. Carcinoma may be described as intra- or extraprostatic, or confined or unconfined with respect to the gland. This is further substantiated by the observation that in malignant prostates, there is no correlation between morphologically unconfined cancers and an irregular or absent ultrasound capsule when corresponding areas are compared. This disparity must contribute to an underestimation of tumor extent with TRUS (YOUNG et al. 1993).

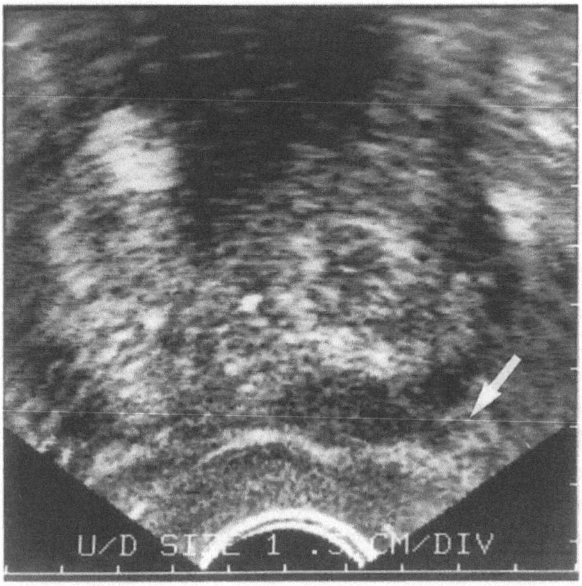

Fig. 7.15. TRUS; transverse scan showing hypoechoic adenocarcinoma in the left posterior PZ. The tumor is isoechoic to and therefore indiscernible from the neurovascular bundle (*arrow*). TRUS-guided needle biopsy of this structure might be indicated for staging, if appropriate

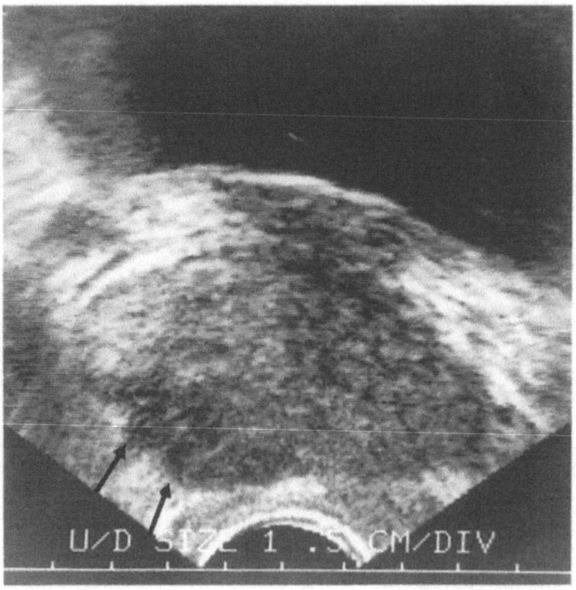

Fig. 7.16. TRUS; oblique scan. A rather small (less than 2 ml), poorly differentiated adenocarcinoma (Gleason score 9) with capsular transgression (*arrow*) is observed in a patient presenting with symptoms related to bone metastases

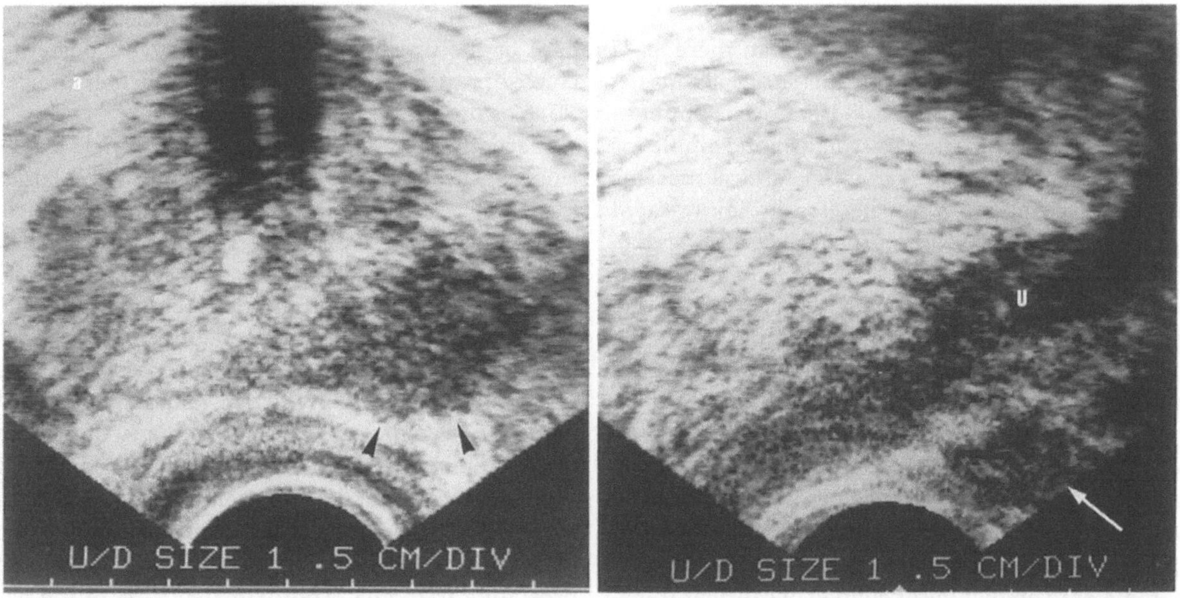

Fig. 7.17. TRUS; transverse (**a**) and sagittal (**b**) scans. Adenocarcinoma in the PZ on the left side. In this case there is really no doubt that there is capsular transgression (*arrowheads*). The tumor is indistinguishable from the membranous urethra (*U*). In these cases, TRUS-guided needle biopsies of the apex and of the external sphincter can be helpful for pretherapeutic staging. Note that there is tumor (*arrow*) in the trapezoid area. The spread of the cancer occurs preferentially along the inner surface of the prostatic capsule. This case illsutrates that if one were to measure the amount of tumor in a biopsy core perpendicular to the prostate capsule, the size of the tumor would clearly be underestimated

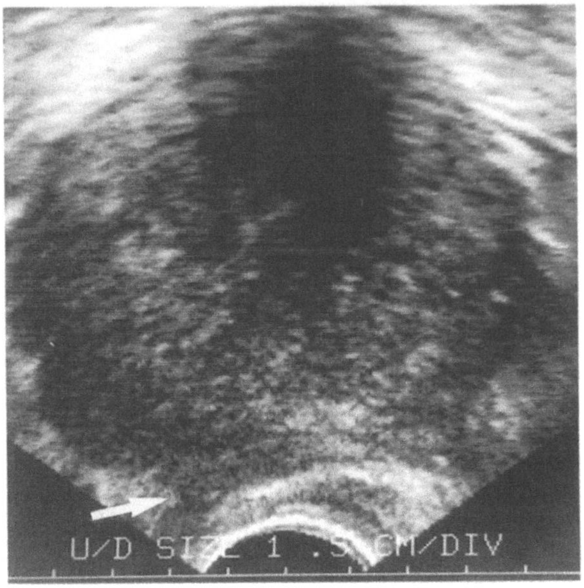

Fig. 7.18. TRUS; transverse scan. A large hypoechoic tumor (Gleason score 7) is present in the PZ on the right side, infiltrating the TZ and with capsular transgression (*arrow*) towards the serosal surface of the rectum

Nevertheless, capsular transgression is not necessarily indicative of positive surgical margins. This means that even if one proves that there is a (microcopic) transgression of the surgical capsule, surgery still may be curative. Moreover it is doubtful whether microcopic transgression is unfavorable for the patient's prognosis: even if the surgical marigns are positive, this does not necessarily imply rapid tumor progression or poor prognosis (HERING et al. 1990; EPSTEIN et al. 1993).

Intraglandular perineural invasion correlates well with capsular penetration, which along with large tumor volume represents a risk for positive surgical margins and seminal vesicle involvement. In our series, two-thirds of the patients with perineural, invasion demonstrated transgression of the prostatic capsule. Thus, it seems important for the pathologist to mention whether there is perineural invasion in the biopsy core sample or not, since this is a useful parameter to predict the likelihood of capsular transgression. Together with other features (e.g., volume, grade, PSA concentration). This may influence further diagnostic and/or therapeutic management. Evidence of perineural invasion in prostatic needle biopsy samples might warrant staging biopsies of areas of potential involvement (such as the neurovascular bundle) or endorectal coil MRI.

While early results suggested great accuracy of TRUS, more rigorous and scientific studies including correlation with the pathology specimen have shown that MRI is a more accurate tool (RIFKIN et al. 1990).

7.4.1.3 The Seminal Vesicles

There are several ways in which a prostatic cancer can spread to the seminal vesicles (WHEELER 1989). The tumor can reach the seminal vesicles by direct extension via the ejaculatory ducts. Direct invasion of the vesicles either from the base of the prostate or from the periprostatic area is another common possibility. Finally, isolated areas of cancer in the seminal vesicles may occur without any evidence of extracapsular disease, presumably due to hematogenous tumor spread.

Whatever the mode of tumor spread may be, prostatic cancers invading seminal vesicles tend to be isoechoic with those vesicles and hence remain indiscernible on TRUS (Fig. 7.3). Alterations in the echogenicity of the seminal vesicles are not specific either. The sensitivity of TRUS in detecting seminal vesicle invasion was determined by RIFKIN et al. (1990) to be 22%, while the specificity was 88%. OHORI et al. (1993) add to hypoechoic lesions at the base of the prostate, adhesion signs and posterior convexity of the seminal vesicles as further indications of seminal vesicle invasion.

Recently, it was stated that seminal vesicle extension can be identified sonographically by enlargement of the seminal vesicle, seminal vesicle asymmetry, and loss of the seminal vesicle beak (CUMMINGS et al. 1994). If one chooses a total seminal vesicle volume of 15 cm^3 as a cutoff value, the specificity and sensitivity of predicting extracapsular spread of cancer is 84% and 38%, respectively. The positive and negative predictive values are 54% and 72% (CUMMINGS et al. 1994). Asymmetry of the size of the seminal vesicles is generally well shown. If asymmetry is defined as one seminal vesicle having twice the volume of the other, it seems that this can be used as a marker of extracapsular extension of prostatic carcinoma. Approximately 44% of the patients with non-organ-confined disease were found by CUMMINGS et al. (1994) to have asymmetry of the seminal vesicles, as opposed to 12.9% of patients with confined tumors; specificity, sensitivity, and positive and negative predictive values were 87%, 44%, 63%, and 75%, respectively. The ability to detect non-organ-confined disease is improved by combining seminal vesicle volume and asymmetry determinations. CUMMINGS et al. (1994) reported that 69% of men with extracapsular disease had either a total seminal vesicle volume of 15 cm^3 or greater and asymmetry, as opposed to 22.6% of those with confined cancers. The specificity and sensitivity of this finding were 77% and 69%, respectively; positive and negative predictive values were 58% and 82%, respectively. This means that only 18% of men with a total seminal vesicle volume of less than 15 cm^3 with symmetric seminal vesicles will have non-organ-confined prostatic carcinoma (CUMMINGS et al. 1994).

In a personal review of more than 200 radical prostatectomy specimens, it has become obvious that tumor spread to the seminal vesicles is directly related to the volume of the cancer. Eighty percent of patients with a tumor volume greater than 4 cm^3 had invasion of the seminal vesicles, as opposed to none of the patients with a tumor volume of less 3 cm^3 Two patients with a tumor volume between 3 and 4 cm^3 had seminal vesicle invasion. In conclusion, 82% of men with a tumor volume greater than 3 cm^3 had invasion of the seminal vesicles. It is worthwhile to add that in the subgroup of patients with a tumor volume of greater than 4 cm^3 and invasion of the seminal vesicles, 80% had positive surgical margins as well. For this reason in spite of its well-known limitations it is reasonable to try to determine the volume of the cancer. Systematic biopsies of the seminal vesicles are indicated for large-volume cancers (>3 cm^3) (VALLANCIEN et al. 1991a). A valuable alternative to avoid staging biopsies of the seminal vesicles is MRI, especially when an endorectal surface coil and/or phased array coils are applied. Perhaps this is the only true indication for MRI in the local staging of prostatic cancer. False-positives are to be expected in cases of hemorrhage in the seminal vesicles (from previous TRUS-guided biopsies of the prostate), atrophy and fibrosis of the seminal vesicles, and amyloidosis.

7.4.2 Color Doppler Ultrasonography

The suggestion has been made by several investigators that tumor vascularization correlates well with its potential for rapid growth and distant metastases. Moreover, in recent microvessel density studies of prostatic carcinoma, BRAWER et al. (1994) supported this concept of neovascularity as a prerequisite for tumor progression. These investigators have also observed a high degree of correlation with the disease stage, which may provide important prognostic information. Therefore, color Doppler-detected neovascularity that ultimately would correlate well with a biologically more aggressive cancer would enable identification of a clinically important subgroup of patients.

7.4.3 TRUS-Guided Staging Biopsies

The comprehensive description of the zonal anatomy, which is now generally accepted, has identified the likely sites of cancer within the gland and provides further understanding of the way in which prostatic tumors spread. It is well known that the primary sites of tumor escape are different for PZ and TZ cancers. PZ cancers escape through the capsule, apex, neurovascular bundle, seminal vesicles, and anterior fibromuscular stroma. TZ cancers escape only through the apex and the anterior fibromuscular stroma (LEE F et al. 1991). Furthermore, PZ cancers show more highly aggressive behavior of both histologic and biologic nature (see Chap. 4).

TRUS can be used to direct biopsies to suggestive and potentially involved areas, including the prostate capsule, the neurovascular bundles and their penetrating fascicles (Figs. 7.15, 7.16), the seminal vesicles, the invaginated extraprostatic space, the trapezoid area (Fig. 7.17), and adjacent lymph nodes (TERRIS et al. 1993). Strategic biopsies of these areas allow for accurate tumor mapping and staging relying on the knowledge of the modes of internal spread and escape of cancer (LEE F et al. 1991). Such biopsies can be performed on an outpatient basis and do not increase the morbidity of the TRUS-guided biopsy technique. Color Doppler imaging may be helpful in targeting these areas of potential. Staging biopsies are useful if the specimen demonstrates cancer. A negative specimen (i.e., one not infiltrated by tumor), however, does not ensure that the cancer has not spread beyond the gland. If a small specimen has been obtained, it may not be representative of the entire pathologic process.

The technique of staging biopsies has been well investigated for the evaluation of tumor spread to the seminal vesicles. It has been shown that biopsy of the seminal vesicles improves the preoperative staging before radical prostatectomy (VALLANCIEN et al. 1991a; TERRIS et al. 1993). It has been generally agreed that negative biopsies are a good predictor of the absence of lymph node metastases.

7.5 Magnetic Resonance Imaging

7.5.1 Equipment and Techniques

A number of MRI approaches should be considered before performing the examination. High-resolution MRI of the prostate is best performed with 1.5-T scanners allowing for the acquisition of thin-section images (3–5 mm). Usually, conventional spin-echo (SE) techniques with multiparameter, multiplanar imaging are recommended. The pulse sequence parameters obtained are T1- and T2-weighted. Standard T2-weighted images are now being replaced by T2-weighted fast SE sequences which shorten the examination time and improve the image resolution.

Three kinds of coil are employed: body coils, external surface coils, and endorectal coils. Body coils evaluate the prostate as well as the pelvis and lymph nodes. If an endorectal coil is combined with external coils placed on the anterior pelvis, as part of a multicoil array, high-resolution images of the entire pelvis, including bladder and plevic lymph nodes, can be obtained (RIFKIN 1990). When an endorectal coil is used, supplementary body coil imaging of the abdomen and pelvis is required to evaluate lymph node status.

7.5.2 Normal Anatomy of the Prostate

Each zone of the prostate has a characteristic signal intensity on T1- and T2-weighted images (OYEN et al. 1994a; OYEN 1994). There are no significant differences in the internal architecture of the gland on T1-weighted sequences. T2-weighted SE images define the intrinsic tissues of the prostate and involvement of these areas by a variety of disease processes. The anterior fibromuscular stroma is a low-signal-intensity nonglandular zone that covers the anterior surface of the prostate and forms its anterior boundary. The many fluid-containing glands in the PZ are responsible for its high signal intensity on T2-weighted images (Fig. 7.19). The TZ has a lower signal intensity than the PZ on T2-weighted images, and is similar in intensity to the CZ (Fig. 7.19). The CZ and TZ together are often termed the "the central gland." Even when the TZ is involved by BPH, it usually has a lower signal intensity than the PZ on T2-weighted images. With BPH the TZ enlarges and produces either a homogeneous low signal or, more often and as the hyperplasia progresses, a heterogeneous mixture of low- and high-signal areas on T2-weighted sequences (ALLEN et al. 1989) (Figs. 7.20, 7.21). High-signal areas are due to cystic involution of areas of hyperplasia. Low-signal areas are explained by predominant stromal hyperplasia. As the BPH progresses, the PZ becomes gradually compressed (Fig. 7.20).

It is doubtful that the thin band of low signal intensity surrounding the prostate on T2-weighted images obtained with endorectal coil imaging really represents the prostatic capsule.

On T1-weighted images, the seminal vesicles are of low to intermediate signal intensity within the tubules, while the walls are of low signal intensity. On T2-weighted images the seminal vesicles are of very high and bright intensity.

On T1-weighted images, the periprostatic fat appears with high signal intensity, while the neurovascular bundles located in the retroprostatic fat at 5 and 7 o'clock are of low signal intensity and contrast against the fat.

Axial images, whatever technique is ultimately used, are most suitable to identify tumor, neurovascular bundle involvement, and laterally originating disease and/or tumor extension. Asymmetry of the anatomy due to pathology is often best identified on the transverse views.

Coronal images allow the best evaluation of the apex of the prostate. Subtle seminal vesicle infiltration may be well seen in this orientation.

Sagittal images are frequently used to localize and view the apex and base of the gland. Subtle seminal vesicle invasion may also be identified.

7.5.3 Prostatic Adenocarcinoma

7.5.3.1 Adenocarcinoma of the Peripheral Zone

Prostate cancer is usually isointense to normal prostate on T1-weighted images, which are most useful for determining the extraprostatic extent of the cancer. When cancer is present in the PZ, it replaces the normal fluid-filled acini with solid malignant tissue. Therefore, the normal high-signal areas on T2-weighted images are replaced by low-signal-intensity tumor (RIFKIN 1990; SCHIEBLER et al. 1993) (Figs. 7.19, 7.21–7.23). Focal hypointensity is, however, not specific for prostatic cancer as chronic inflammation, purely stromal BPH, and prostatic infarcts may have exactly the same signal intensity (LOVETT et al. 1992). Rarely, the lesion is of high signal intensity, as with the rare mucin-producing adenocarcinoma.

It should be remembered that, although MRI is highly sensitive in demarcating disease, low signal

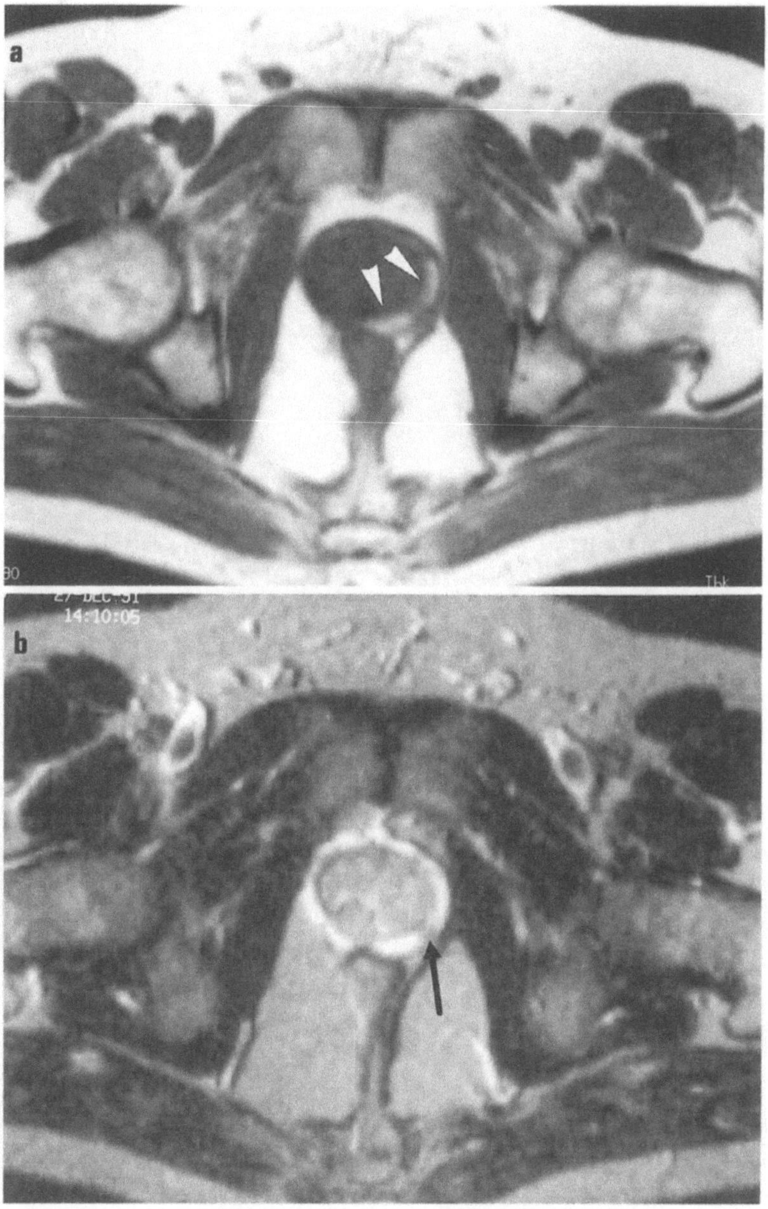

Fig. 7.19. MRI; axial T1-weighted (**a**) and T2-weighted (**b**) images. A hyperintense left PZ is seen (*arrowheads*) due to hemorrhage of a previous TRUS-guided biopsy (10 days earlier). The carcinoma in the PZ is well visible on the T2-weighted image (*arrow*). Artifacts caused by hemorrhage can mask the tumor and can lead to either under- or overestimation of the local T stage of the prostatic carcinoma. It is suggested that an interval of at least 3 weeks be allowed after the biopsy before considering MRI for local staging

foci are relatively non-specific and may also be seen in cases of chronic inflammation. This in fact limits the usefulness of MRI in the absence of biopsy-proven cancer.

7.5.3.2 Adenocarcinoma of the Transitional Zone

Transitional zone (and CZ) carcinomas are difficult to recognize because the intrinsic signal intensity of the central gland is low and thus, theoretically, identical to most tumors (Fig. 7.22). A problem affecting MRI is those tumors involving the central gland, the signal of which is usually a composite of high and low intensities. Even large low-signal prostate cancers may be difficult or impossible to detect when they occur in a low-signal central gland. Therefore, care must be taken in using MRI as a diagnostic modality for prostate cancer: a positive result is not

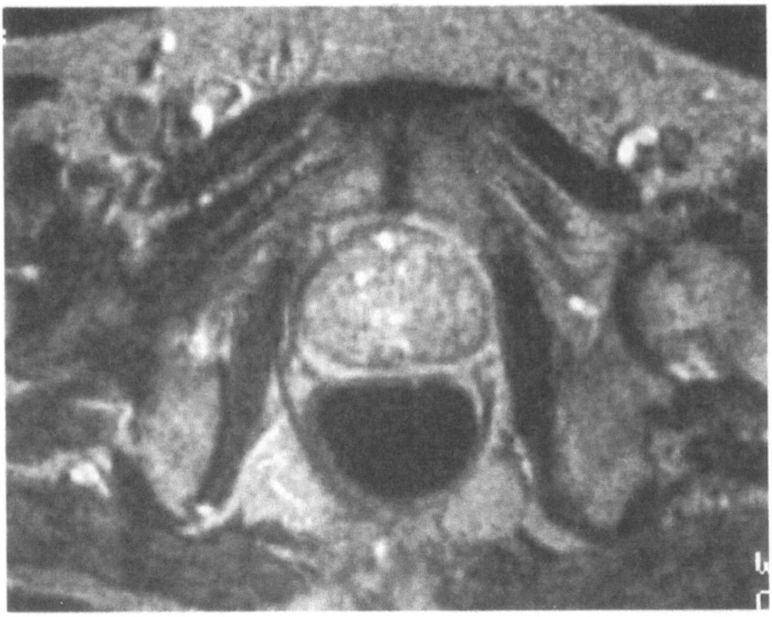

Fig. 7.20. MRI; T2-weighted image. There is pronounced hyperplasia of the TZ with heterogeneous signal characteristics. The hyperintense outer PZ is compressed by the hyperplastic inner prostate: just a thin rim of PZ is visible. In such cases MRI diagnosis of prostatic carcinoma is difficult or even impossible

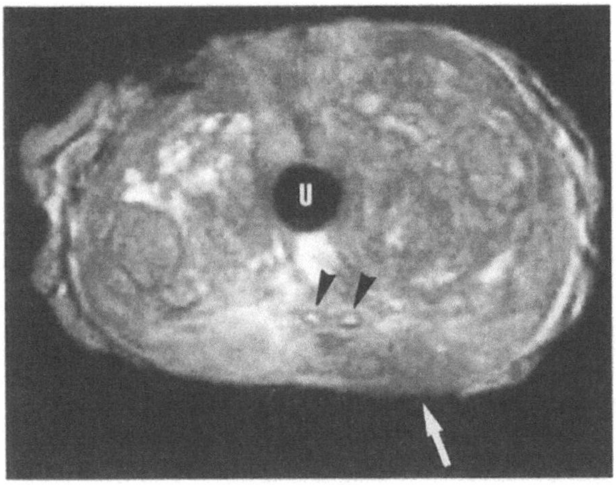

Fig. 7.21. MRI; T2-weighted image of a radical prostatectomy specimen. Note the heterogeneous aspect of the multinodular benign hyperplasia of the transitional zone on either side of the urethra (*U*). Hypointense adenocarcinoma is present in the PZ on the left side (*arrow*), posterolateral to the hyperintense ejaculatory ducts (*arrowheads*). Some of the nodular parts of the cancer have sharp margins; the lateral infiltrative part of the cancer has blurred margins

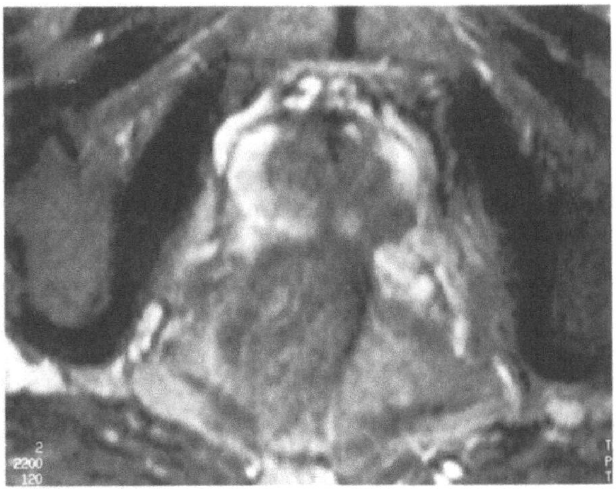

Fig. 7.22. MRI; T2-weighted image. Large tumor in the left PZ, clearly extending beyond the confines of the gland (T3a). Such "macroscopic" transcapsular penetration can be visualized with TRUS as well, and is obvious on DRE. Microscopic transcapsular spread cannot be detected with MRI, TRUS, or DRE. Note that the tumor is isointense compared to the hyperplastic TZ. It is clear that a tumor that originates in the TZ will not be distinguished on MRI

conclusive, nor does a negative result exclude the diagnosis.

7.5.3.3 Contrast-Enhanced MRI

Regions of BPH and cancer enhance the signal to a similar degree following intravenous injection of gadolinium, though BPH enhancement is more heterogeneous than cancer enhancement. No advantages in detecting prostate cancer, in differentiating cancer from BPH or normal prostatic tissue, or in assessing extraprostatic spread of cancer are observed for routine contrast-enhanced studies as compared to T2-weighted (fast) SE imaging (Sommer et al. 1993).

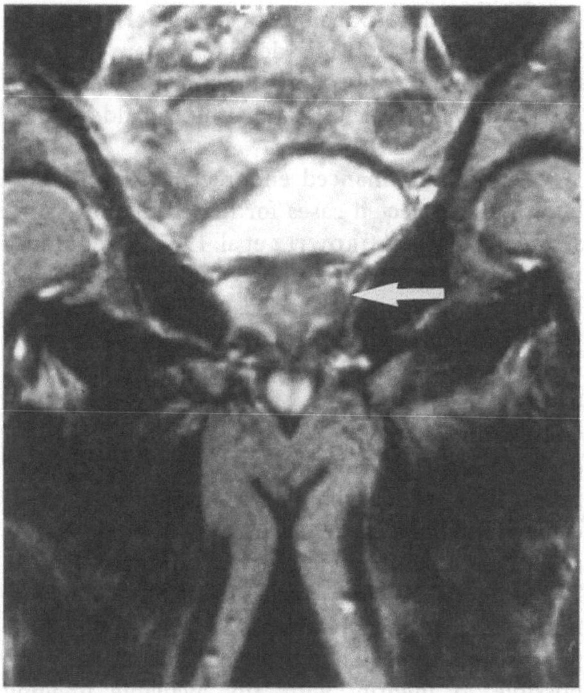

Fig. 7.23. MRI; T2-weighted coronal image. Prostatic adenocarcinoma in the left PZ (*arrow*) is confined to the prostate (T2) and is indiscernible from the hyperplastic TZ. At radical prostatecomy, there was microscopic transgression of the prostatic capsule (pT3a)

7.6 Staging of Prostatic Adenocarcinoma by Magnetic Resonance Imaging

7.6.1 T Staging

Currently, most radiologists consider MRI the method of choice for determining whether prostatic carcinoma is confined to the gland or has spread beyond it. Its advantages over other techniques are its multiplanar capabilities, the high soft tissue contrast, and the absence of ionizing radiation.

7.6.1.1 The Prostate Capsule

Prostatic cancer that penetrates through the capsule into the periprostatic tissues interrupts or obliterates the hypoechoic rim, whereas an intact rim indicates that the tumor is probably confined to the gland (Figs. 7.22, 7.23). Tumor in the periprostatic fat is optimally demonstrated on T1-weighted images. Multiplanar images are often required to obtain the best accuracy. Obliteration of the high-tubular-intensity venous plexus is a reliable sign of macroscopic extracapsular tumor spread.

Biopsy-related changes may account for some discrepancies. Postbiopsy hemorrhage may produce high or low signal artifact depending on the age of the hematoma (Fig. 7.19). This may lead to overestimation of the extent of disease if it is not recognized as biopsy related (Schnall et al. 1991). With experience, however, one can recognize biopsy sites on T1-weighted images by identifying the high signal intensity of the blood and correlating this information with corresponding T2-weighted images to differentiate low signal intensity secondary to blood from that due to tumor (Oyen et al. 1994a; White et al. 1995). Nevertheless, this does raise the question of whether it might be justifiable to perform prebiopsy MRI of the prostate when the suspicion of prostatic cancer is high. If this is not the case, and if artifacts from biopsy are absolutely to be avoided, a delay of 4–6 weeks between the biopsy and MRI is necessary. Postbiopsy changes persist as long as 4 1/2 months (Rubens et al. 1995; White et al. 1995). Less than 21 days after biopsy, there is a tendency to overestimate tumor presence and extracapsular extension. After 21 days, tumor presence is underestimated but the positive predictive value for extracapsular extension has improved (Rubens et al. 1995; White et al. 1995).

The accuracy of MRI in differentiating stage T2 (B) from stage T3 (C) disease has been well studied. A PZ defect 1 cm or greater with an ill-defined border and of low signal proved 100% sensitive for extracapsular spread of prostatic carcinoma. MRI is found to have 54% specificity with a high degree of interobserver agreement. Data from the multi-institutional trial of Rifkin et al. comparing the accuracy of various methods of staging have imputed an accuracy of 70% to body MRI (Rifkin et al. 1990). However, surface coil imaging appears to have taken staging to a new level of accuracy, with results nearing 90% (Schnall et al. 1991). Periprostatic extension is readily detectable, and the overall accuracy of separating confined from unconfined cancer is approximately 90%, excluding microscopic extension, which cannot be recognized (Schnall et al. 1991). Tumors involving the prostatic apex and those not within the high-signal-intensity PZ remain somewhat of a problem.

The accuracy in staging advanced disease in general is better than that in staging localized disease (74% vs 64%; Chelsky et al. 1993). The accuracy in staging advanced disease is significantly affected by the diagnostic criterion used for defining extraprostatic extension. Irregular capsular bulge as a criterion for extraprostatic extension is an indirect finding and appears to be suggestive rather than diagnostic of capsular penetration (Chelsky et al. 1993; Schnall et al. 1991). If an irregular capsule is not used as a criterion for stage T3 disease, the specificity of endorectal surface coil MRI for determining stage T3 disease is significantly improved (96% vs 78%) but the sensitivity is decreased (38% vs 58%) (Chelsky et al. 1993). The overall staging accuracy is 68%, with a 74% accuracy in staging advanced disease and a 91% accuracy for depiction of seminal vesicle involvement (Chelsky et al. 1993).

7.6.1.2 The Seminal Vesicles

The high soft tissue contrast of MRI is extremely helpful in assessing the spread of prostate cancer, particularly to the seminal vesicles. Normally, seminal vesicle images show high signal from the fluid in the tubules on T2-weighted sequences, whereas the walls of the tubules show low signal. Invasion of the seminal vesicles is denoted by unilateral or bilateral low-signal T2-weighted images, which may or may not be associated with enlargement of the structure (Fig. 7.24).

The accuracy in identifying seminal vesicle involvement is 91%, with a sensitivity of 63% and a specificity of 97% (Chelsky et al. 1993). This is significantly better than the sensitivity and specificity for TRUS (22% and 88%, respectively) and body coil MRI (28% and 88%, respectively) Rifkin et al. 1990). Failure to recognize microscopic extracapsular spread is again responsible for the majority of staging inaccuracies. MRI is definitely more sensitive than TRUS in the detection of tumor involvement of the seminal vesicles and the bladder base (Chadwick et al. 1991).

Gadolinium-enhanced endorectal coil MRI may be useful in selected cases for the evaluation of the seminal vesicles (Mirowitz et al. 1993). Gadolinium may be required to differentiate between postbiopsy hemorrhage, amyloidosis, and prostate cancer. The last-mentioned will increase in signal intensity, while the former two will have similar signal intensities as before.

In conclusion, MRI of the prostate with an endorectal surface coil appears to be the most accurate method of identifying advanced disease, especially seminal vesicle involvement. It is, however, less accurate in identifying and staging localized disease. This is almost certainly due to the fact that in a large number of clinically localized cases, there is microscopic extension of disease that is virtually impossible to identify with any available imaging modality.

7.6.2 N Staging

The value of MRI in assessing the nodal involvement (N staging) in men with prostate cancer has been the subject of several studies. Metastatic and reactive enlarged lymph nodes cannot be differentiated on the basis of their signal intensities. For practical pur-

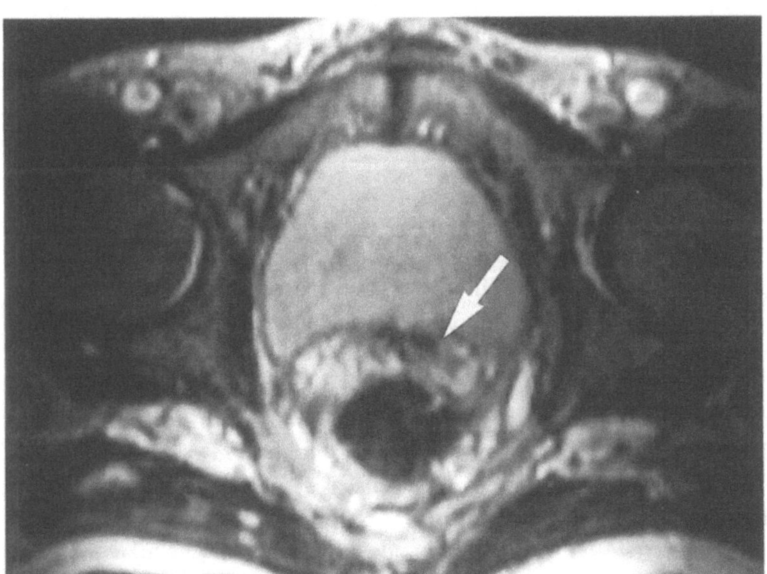

Fig. 7.24. MRI; axial T2-weighted image. Hypointense area in the base of the left seminal vesicle (*arrow*) indicative of spread of cancer into these structures

poses, clusters of nodes larger than 1 cm in diameter are considered pathologic (Fig. 7.25). Recently, a sensitivity of 25% and a specificity of 97% have been reported (Wolf et al. 1995).

Thin-slice (1.2 mm) multiplanar reconstruction has recently been described as a valuable technique to select patients with enlarged metastatic lymph nodes (Barentsz et al. 1995). In this particular study, to determine longitudinal and minimal axial size, multiplanar reconstruction was performed in planes parallel and perpendicular to the long axis of the nodes. 3D MP-RAGE evaluation of nodal metastases resulted in high accuracy (91%), sensitivity (77%), specificity (99%), and positive predictive value (97%). This 3D technique facilitated successful multiple angulated MR-guided biopsy.

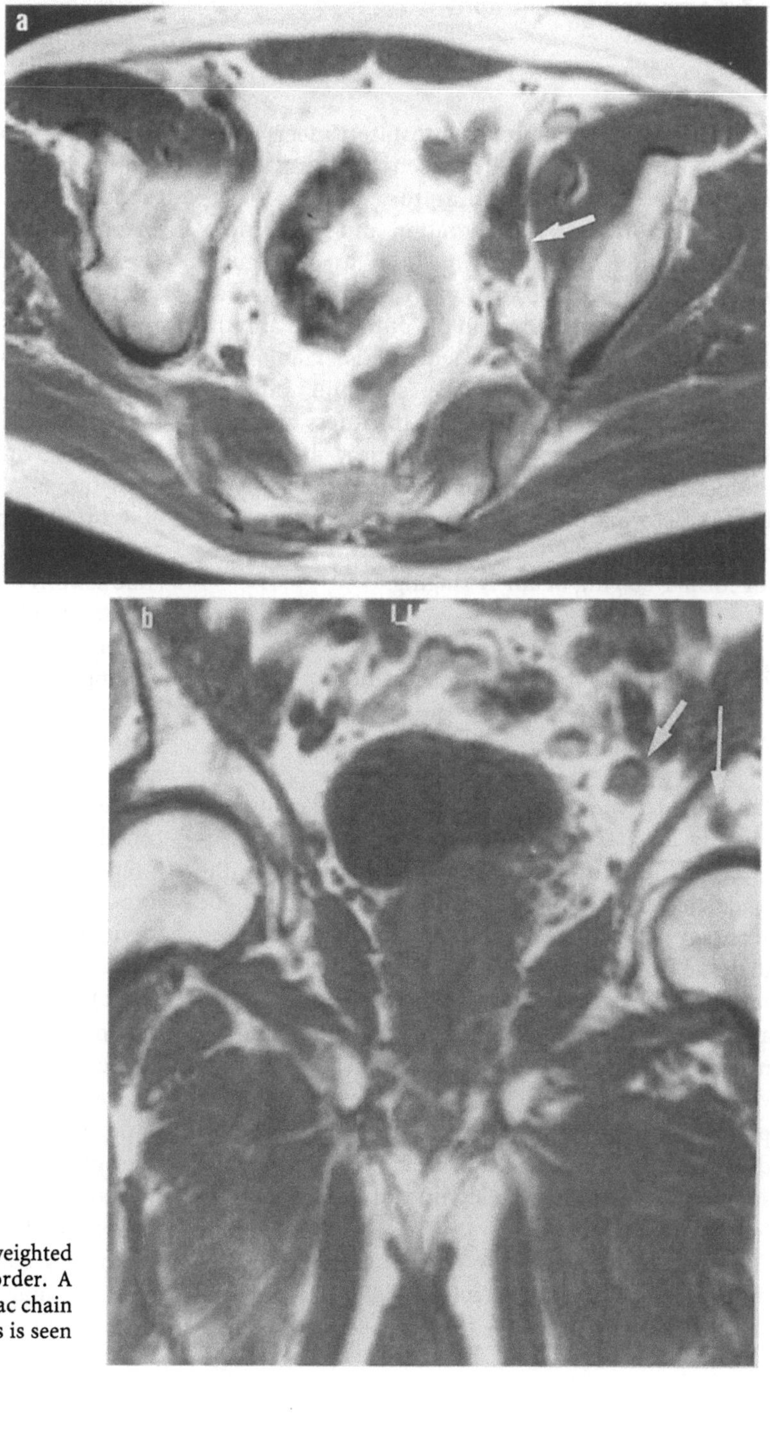

Fig. 7.25. MRI; axial (**a**) and coronal (**b**) T1-weighted images. Enlarged prostate with irregular border. A large lymph node is present in the external iliac chain on the left side (*thick arrow*). Bone metastasis is seen in the left acetabulum (*thin arrow*)

7.6.3 Bone Metastases

Magnetic resonance imaging is an excellent complementary technique when bone scan findings are equivocal. MRI appears to be quite sensitive and probably more specific for metastasis in certain locations of the spine (GOSFIELD et al. 1993; TURNER et al. 1993; OYEN 1994) (Fig. 7.25).

7.7 Computed Tomography

7.7.1 Techniques

Patients with biopsy-proven prostate cancer and a need to be evaluated for the presence of lymph node disease are scanned according to a routine procedure. After oral bowel preparation and intravenous administration of contrast medium to distinguish vascular and intestinal strutures from lymph nodes, scans are performed between the public arch and the aortic bifurcation. The scanned area is extended up to the diaphragm whenever suspect lymph nodes are found in the pelvic area. The slice thickness is usually 8–10 mm and the table incrementation is 10 mm in the pelvis and 15 mm in the abdomen (OYEN et al. 1994a). Reformatting of the raw data in spatial planes other than the axial is not considered useful, either for local T staging or for N staging.

7.7.2 Staging of Prostatic Adenocarcinoma

7.7.2.1 T Staging

Computed tomography has very limited ability to identify local extension of cancer. CT cannot accurately identify focal disease within the prostate, the ejaculatory ducts, or the neurovascular bundles. The accuracy of CT in these conditions has been reported to range from 35% to 55% (PLATT et al. 1987). On the rare occasion when intraprostatic carcinoma is seen as a low-density focus, it is likely that hemorrhage or necrosis within the tumor is responsible. Seminal vesicle size is found to be a poor predictor of pathologic involvement when compared with tumor differentiation (LARNER et al. 1993). Invasion of the seminal vesicles must be significant before it is detectable on CT.

A variety of symmetric abnormalities are commonly seen on postprostatectomy pelvic CT. Seminal vesicle-like soft tissue in the rectovesical space is commonly demonstrated. These structures should not be confused with local tumor recurrence (SUMMERS et al. 1993).

7.7.2.2 N Staging

The role of CT (and MRI) with or without fine-needle aspiration in the assessment of pelvic lymph nodes in patients with prostate cancer is now under discussion.

Imaging is superior to no imaging only when the pretest probability of pelvic lymph node metastases is high. The most important parameter is the sensitivity of cross-sectional imaging for lymphadenopathy. When the sensitivity is 36%, the probability of lymph node metastases required for imaging to be beneficial is 32% (WOLF et al. 1995). The reported data indicate that patients with a PSA of 20–25 ng/ml or greater and a Gleason score of 7 or greater have a 50% likelihood of lymph node metastases (PARTIN et al. 1993; WOLF et al. 1993a). The high-risk groups in these series comprise 5%–10% of the patients undergoing surgery and included 20%–50% of those with pelvic lymph node metastases. In another series 43% of patients with a PSA of 20 ng/ml or greater and a primary Gleason grade of 4 or 5 had lymph node metastases (BLUESTEIN et al. 1994).

For the aforementioned reasons, and due to the use of biochemical and histologic parameters, CT is no longer considered such a useful diagnostic tool as in the past. Furthermore, CT cannot differentiate lymph nodes enlarged by tumor involvement from those enlarged by benign processes, nor can it identify normal-sized lymph nodes that have been infiltrated by a tumor. Nevertheless, it has been shown in a recent study that the CT accuracy increases when fine-needle aspiration biopsies (FNAB) are applied to virtually all visible and asymmetric lymph nodes in patients with prostatic carcinoma (OYEN et al. 1994c). The proposed staging procedure by CT scan in combination with FNAB has proven to be a highly efficient method. Percutaneous needle aspiration can be used to confirm a CT-positive or suspicious lymph node, if such confirmation is required for further therapy planning (Fig. 7.26). Positive cytology for metastasis will confirm the imaging diagnosis, thus preventing the possibility of patients not receiving potentially curative therapy on the basis of a false-positive diagnostic imaging study. Surgical or laparoscopic staging procedures can still be consid-

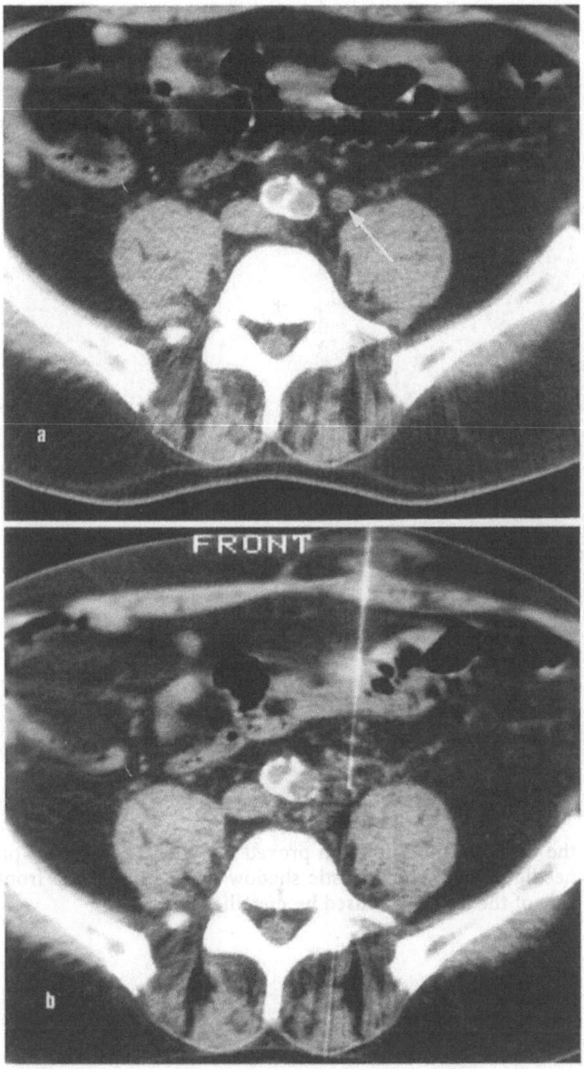

Fig. 7.26a,b. CT. **a** Rounded lymph node (*arrow*) of 1 cm diameter on the left side of the aortic bifurcation. **b** Transperitoneal FNAB confirms the presence of metastasis of a prostatic carcinoma. The infiltration of the fat indicates some retroperitoneal hemorrhage

ered in those patients with equivocal CT and FNAB staging results or in those with unfavorable prognostic indicators such as advanced clinical stage, high PSA, and tumor aneuploidy.

In conclusion, most authors now agree that there is no real justification for routine use of CT in patients with preoperative PSA of less than 20–25 ng/ml. This suggests that significant cost savings can be realized by abandoning the practice of routine CT scanning for lymph node metastases in all patients with newly diagnosed prostate cancer.

7.8 Imaging Prostatic Adenocarcinoma After Treatment

Hypoechoic lesions in the PZ or the TZ should be biopsied after transurethral resection (TUR) before expectant management of stage T1 prostate cancer is considered. The sensitivity of TRUS for tumors confined to the TZ is very low (Fig. 7.27). TRUS-directed systematic biopsies in clinical stage T1 prostate cancer reveal cancer in 28% of the cases, and in 47% with more anteriorly directed biopsies (TERRIS et al. 1992c).

Transrectal ultrasonography is useful in the follow-up of patients with prostate cancer who are receiving hormone therapy. In general, the volume of the prostate decreases after 12 months and the echo structure changes in two-thirds of the patients. The gland becomes isoechoic in the majority of the patients and the tumor is completely obscured. Therefore, a set of biopsies may be required if residual cancer in the prostate has to be excluded.

Knowledge of the baseline anatomy depicted on TRUS after radical prostatectomy may be useful in the selection of patients for TRUS-guided biopsy when the PSA is elevated (WASSERMAN et al. 1992a,b). Tumor relapse usually appears as a

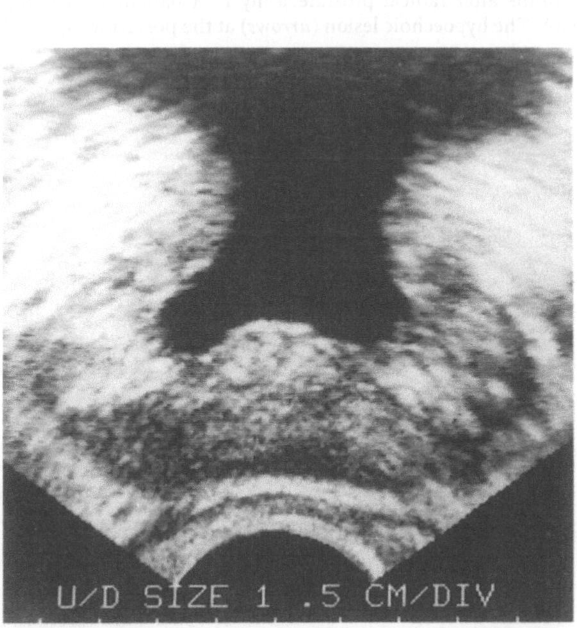

Fig. 7.27. TRUS; transverse scan after TUR. The hypoechoic area in the PZ proved to be prostatic adenocarcinoma on needle biopsy (Gleason score 6). Theorectically, because most cancers originate in the PZ, the chance of a male developing a cancer after TUR is nearly as high as in males who do not undergo TUR

hypoechoic nodule in or around the vesico-urethral junction (Fig. 7.28). Again, hypoechogenicity is not specific to cancer and subtle microscopic recurrencies cannot be detected (Fig. 7.29).

Percutaneous transperineal TRUS-directed interstitial radiotherapy is an attractive and elegant technique for the administration of high-dose local radiotherapy to the prostate. The complications

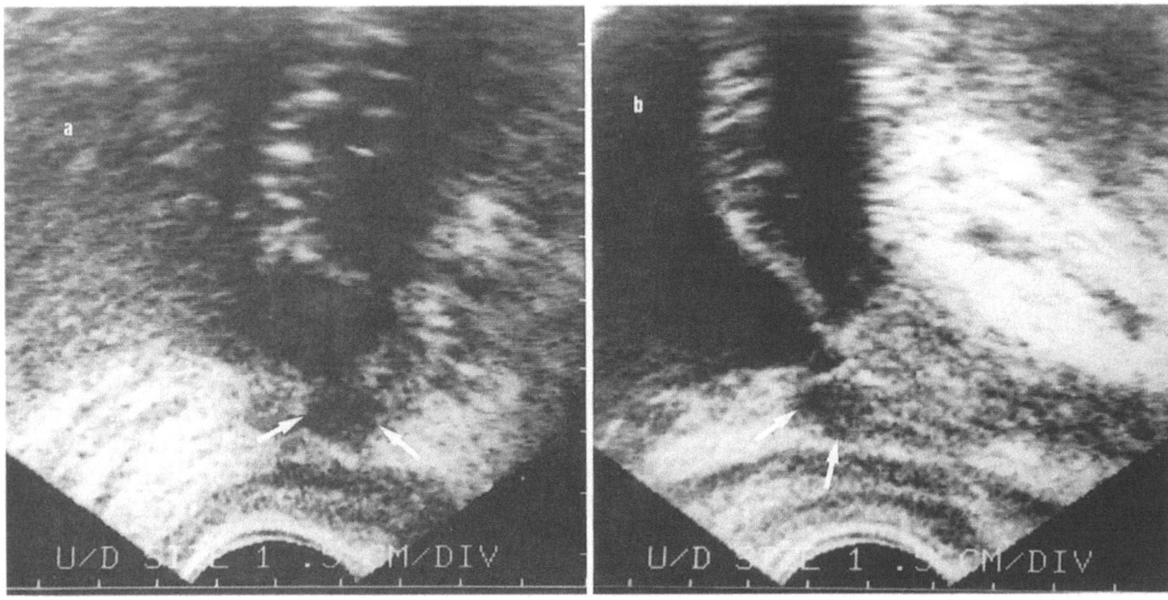

Fig. 7.28. TRUS; transverse (**a**) and sagittal scans (**b**) 12 months after radical prostatectomy in a patient with rising PSA. The hypoechoic lesion (*arrows*) at the posterior aspect of the vesicourethral junction proved to be local recurrence on needle biopsy. The acoustic shadow originating at the front side of the lesion is caused by metallic clips

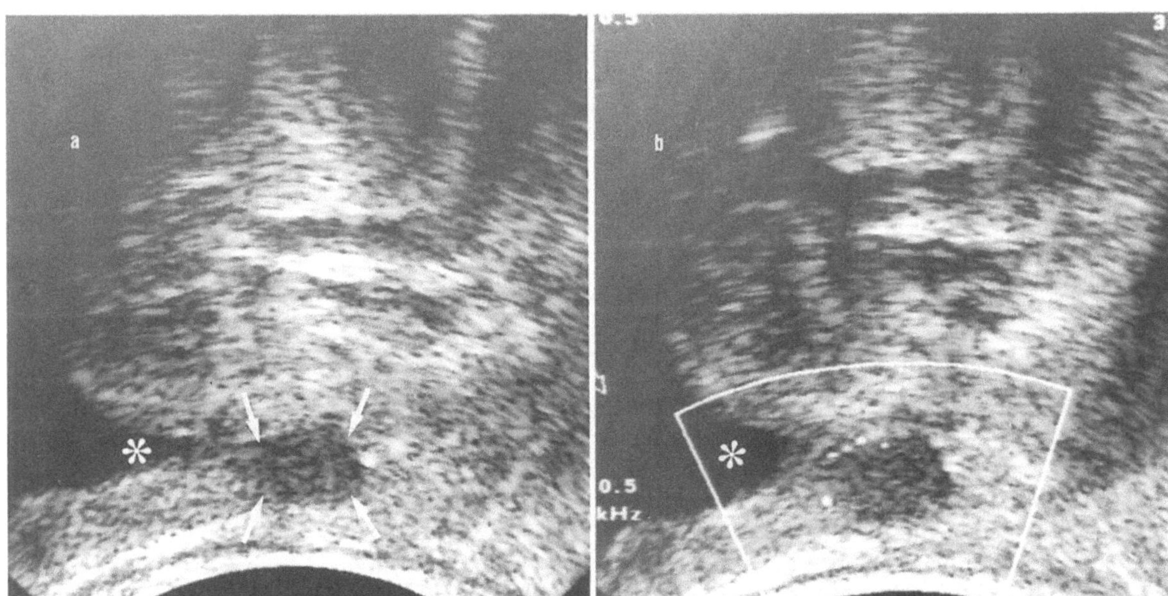

Fig. 7.29. TRUS; sagittal view (**a**) 14 months after radical prostatectomy. The hypoechoic nodule (*arrows*) at the vesicourethral junction proved to be granulomatous prostatitis on TRUS-guided needle biopsy. There is a marked resemblance to the malignant lesion (i.e., prostatic carcinoma) in Fig. 7.28. Color Doppler imaging (**b**) is not helpful in lesion discrimination. *Asterisk*, bladder neck

of seed implantation are those associated with radiation and the technique of implantation. Brachytherapy, however, has not provided impressive local control of disease or prolonged survival.

Transrectal ultrasonography is thought to be particularly valuable for monitoring the response of prostate cancer to radiotherapy. Dramatic changes in the echo pattern of the prostate and of the seminal vesicles may be expected following radiotherapy, and these may be difficult to evaluate. Similar limitations apply to MRI of the prostate after radiotherapy. Therefore, based on imaging (i.e., TRUS or MRI) it may be impossible to differentiate between radiation fibrosis, residual tumor, and tumor relapse. Biopsies targeted at focal (hypoechoic) lesions, or a set of random biopsies, may be required to obtain an objective mapping of the histologic status of the prostate.

7.9 Conclusions on the Imaging of Prostatic Adenocarcinoma

It has been generally accepted that imaging can and should be used for both the diagnosis and staging of prostate cancer. In the process of making a diagnosis, TRUS is the most – and perhaps the only – appropriate imaging tool. Its sensitivity can be further increased by systematically applying color Doppler ultrasonography; its specificity, however, is not increased by adding this technique.

Magnetic resonance imaging is the most useful tool for evaluation of potential local extension of prostate cancer, especially to the seminal vesicles. Like TRUS, however, MRI has its limitations, particularly in the evaluation of microscopic disease.

Given the limits of resolution inherent to any imaging technique, it is not possible to resolve pathologic processes at the microscopic level, and minute extracapsular disease seems destined to remain unrecognizable using imaging techniques for the foreseeable future. Some recent reports, however, suggest that minimal extracapsular extension of prostatic carcinoma may not adversely affect the surgical cure rate (Hering et al. 1990; Epstein et al. 1993). If this is true, the radiologist's failure to detect small foci of malignant cells beyond the prostatic capsule may prove to be less clinically important. Imaging modalities such as TRUS and MRI are, however, of major importance in identifying tumor extension beyond the capsule.

Routine use of cross-sectional pelvic imaging before radical prostatectomy, solely for the purpose of detecting pelvic lymph node metastases, is not justified at this time. However, it may remain useful and cost-effective in a limited number of patients with high PSA values and appropriate histologic parameters (high Gleason grade or sum). Thus, it is presumed that patients at increased risk of pelvic lymph node metastases from prostate cancer, in whom radical prostatectomy would be considered only in the absence of nodal involvement, are most likely to benefit from cross-sectional pelvic imaging and subsequent fine-needle aspiration cytology when lymphadenopathy is found (Amis 1994; Wolf et al. 1995).

7.10 Other Malignancies Originating in the Prostate

Carcinomas other than adenocarcinoma of acinar origin are uncommon, and description of their imaging characteristics is anecdotal and incomplete.

7.10.1 Small Cell Carcinoma

Undifferentiated small cell (oat cell) carcinoma is a rare prostatic neoplasm that merely coexists with a low-grade adenocarcinoma. Ectopic ACTH production and Cushing's syndrome have been reported. From time to time apparently primary prostatic carcinoid tumors are reported. Because these neoplasms stain positive for PSA and prostate acid phosphatase (PAP), they are regarded as primary prostatic carcinomas.

7.10.2 Adenoid Cystic Carcinoma

Adenoid cystic carcinomas, which arise from ectopic seromucinous glands in the prostate, exhibit large anechoic areas on TRUS and are hyperintense on T2-weighted MR images.

7.10.3 Transitional Cell Carcinoma

Transitional cell carcinoma originating in the distal prostatic ducts was first recognized only 25 years ago. Some patients present with bladder outlet obstruction. Therefore the diagnosis is usually obtained at transurethral resection or through systematic random biopsies of the prostate, including the TZ.

Histologically, prostatic transitional cell carcinoma shows predominant central involvement of distal prostatic ducts, which are dilated and commonly filled with the neoplastic proliferation. Not uncommonly, the tumor cells in the center of the dilated ducts show necrosis, resulting in a comedo pattern. Retrograde spread into distal prostatic ducts is variable; stromal invasion of the prostate is frequent. Tumor cells may spread along the basement membrane to involve the urethra and the bladder, obscuring the primary site of origin. The associated finding of transitional cell hyperplasia with atypia (carcinoma in situ) within prostatic ducts establishes the prostate as the primary site. Bony metastases are frequently osteolytic, and hormonal therapy is ineffective.

7.10.4 Prostatic Ductal Adenocarcinoma

Prostatic ductal adenocarcinoma (previously called "endometrial" carcinoma) is a papillary adenocarcinoma of the prostate that originates in the distal prostatic ducts and is a histologic variant of ductal carcinoma and not of müllerian origin, as initially proposed. The expanded ducts in prostatic ductal adenocarcinoma are filled with a papillary proliferation, in contrast to the solid or comedo patterns of prostatic transitional cell carcinoma (Oyen 1994).

7.10.5 Malignant Mesenchymal Tumors

Malignant mesenchymal tumors of the prostate are extremely rare. They account for less than 1% of primary prostatic neoplasms (Tannenbaum 1975). Most of these tumors occur before the age of 50, and a third are seen in children. Rhabdomyosarcoma is the most common prostatic malignancy of childhood; there is a second peak after 50 years. In the pediatric age group rhabdomyosarcomas originate more commonly in the bladder. When there is extensive growth with involvement of both organs, the site of origin may be inapparent.

Leiomyosarcoma occurs in older males. This neoplasm has a typical prolonged course, with multiple recurrences (Smith and Dehner 1972). Leiomyosarcomas of the prostate tend to present with large masses with central hemorrhage or necrosis similar to gastrointestinal leiomyosarcomas.

Other soft tissue sarcomas have also been described in the prostate. These include malignant schwannoma and malignant fibrous histiocytoma (Bain et al. 1985).

7.10.6 Metastases to the Prostate

Metastatic disease to the prostate from a distant primary tumor is uncommon and is usually diagnosed late in the course of the disease. Leukemic infiltration, melanoma, and lung carcinoma are the most common metastases. Although the prostate is rarely involved by lymphoma, the diagnosis must be considered because of its amenability to treatment when a large prostatic mass is palpated in a young male. Non-Hodgkin's lymphoma is more likely to affect the prostate than is Hodgkin's disease.

References

Allen KS, Kressel HY, Arger PH, Pollack HM (1989) Age-related changes of the prostate: evaluation by MR imaging. Am J Roentgenol 152:77–81
Amis ES (1994) Role of CT and CT-guided nodal biopsy in staging of prostate cancer. Radiology 190:309–314
Andreole GL, Coplen DE, Mikkelson DJ, Catalona WJ (1989) Sonographic and pathological staging of patients with clinically localized prostate cancer. J Urol 142:1259–1263
Bain GO, Danyluk JM, Shnikata TK, Jewell LD, Manickavel V (1985) Malignant fibrous histiocytoma of the prostate gland. Urology 26:89–91
Barentsz JO, Jager G, Oosterhof G, Wites F, Ruijs SHJ (1995) The value of MR imaging using a three dimensional sequence in lymph node staging of urinary bladder carcinoma and prostate cancer. Eur Radiol 5 (Suppl):228
Billebaud T, Sibert A, Dauge MC et al. (1990) Intérêt des biopsies systématiques multiples échoguidés dans le diagnostic précoce du cancer de prostate. Ann Urol 24:524–529
Bluestein DL, Bostwick DG, Bergstralh EJ, Oesterling JE (1994) Eliminating the need for bilateral pelvic lymphadenectomy in select patients with prostate cancer. J Urol 151:1315–1319
Brawer MK, Aramburu EAG, Chen GL et al. (1993) The inability of prostate specific antigen index to enhance the predictive value of prostate specific antigen in the diagnosis of prostatic carcinoma. J Urol 150:369–373
Brawer MK, Deering RE, Brown M, Preston SD, Bigler SA (1994) Predictors of pathologic stage in prostatic carcinoma: the role of neovascularity. Cancer 73:678–687
Carter HB, Hamper UM, Sheth S et al. (1989) Evaluation of transrectal ultrasound in the early detection of prostate cancer. J Urol 142:1008–1010
Catalona WJ, Bigg SW (1990) Nerve-sparing radical prostatectomy: evaluation of results after 250 patients. J Urol 143:538–543
Chadwick DJ, Cobby M, Goddard P, Gingell JC (1991) Comparison of transrectal ultrasound and magnetic resonance imaging in the staging of prostate cancer. Br J Urol 67:616–621
Chelsky MJ, Schnall MD, Seidmon EJ, Pollack HM (1993) Use of endorectal coil magnetic resonance imaging for local staging of prostate cancer. J Urol 150(2):391–395

Cummings JM, Bouillier JA, Sankari BR, Parra RO (1994) Seminal vesicle volume as a sonographic predictor of prostatic cancer stage. Urology 44:206–210
Daniels GF, McNeal JE, Stamey TA (1992) Predictive value of contralateral biopsies in unilaterally palpable prostate cancer. J Urol 147:870–874
Dyke CH, Toi A, Sweet JM (1990) Value of random US-guided transrectal prostate biopsy. Radiology 176:345–349
Egawa S, Wheeler TM, Greene DR, Scardino PT (1992) Unusual hyperechoic appearance of prostate cancer on transrectal ultrasonography. Br J Urol 69:169–174
Epstein JI, Carmichael MJ, Pizov G, Walsh P (1993) Influence of capsular penetration on progression following radical prostatectomy: a study of 196 cases with long-term followup. J Urol 150:135–141
Fair WR, Kadmon D (1983) Carcinoma of the prostate – diagnosis and staging, current status and future prospects. World J Urol 1:3
Franks LM (1954) Latent carcinoma of the prostate. J Pathol 68:603–616
Gosfield E, Alavi A, Kneeland B (1993) Comparison of radionuclide bone scans and magnetic resonance imaging in detecting spinal metastases. J Nucl Med 34:2191–2198
Hamper UM, Sheth S, Walsh PC, Holtz PM, Epstein JI (1991) Capsular transgression of prostatic carcinoma: evaluation with transrectal US with pathologic correlation. Radiology 178:791–795
Hering F, Rist M, Roth J et al. (1990) Does microinvasion of the capsule and/or micrometastases in regional lymph nodes influence disease-free survival after radical prostatectomy? Br J Urol 66:177–181
Hodge KK, McNeal JE, Terris MK, Stamey TA (1989a) Random systematic versus directed ultrasound guided transrectal core biopsies of the prostate. J Urol 142:71–74
Hodge KK, McNeal JE, Stamey TA (1989b) Ultrasound guided transrectal core biopsies of the palpable abnormal prostate. J Urol 142:66–70
Huynen AL, Giesen RJB, De La Rosette MCH, Aarnink RG, Debruyne FMJ, Wijkstra H (1994) Analysis of ultrasonographic prostate images for the detection of prostatic carcinoma: the automated urologic diagnostic expert sytem. Ultrasound Med Biol 20:1–10
Kelly IMG, Lees WR, Rickards D (1993) Prostate cancer and the role of color Doppler US. Radiology 189:153–156
Kleer E, Larson-Keller JJ, Zincke H, Oesterling JE (1993) Ability of preoperative serum prostate-specific antigen value to predict pathologic stage and DNA ploidy. Influence of clinical stage and tumor grade. Urology 41:207–216
Larner J, Gay S, Grizos W, Fortier G, Malcom R (1993) Significance of CT-scan-detected seminal vesicle enlargement in prostate cancer: a pilot study. Urology 41:259–261
Lee F, Torp-Pedersen ST, Littrup JL et al. (1989) Hypoechoic lesions of the prostate: clinical relevance of tumor size, digital rectal examination, and prostate specific antigen. Radiology 170:29–32
Lee F, Siders DB, Torp-Pedersen ST et al. (1991) Prostate cancer: transrectal ultrasound and pathology comparison. A preliminary study of outer gland (peripheral and central zones) and inner gland (transition zone) cancer. Cancer 67:1132–1142
Lee F, Littrup PJ, Loft-Christensen L et al. (1992) Predicted prostate specific antigen results using transrectal ultrasound gland volume. Cancer 70:211–220
Lee F Jr, Bronson JP, Lee F et al. (1991a) Nonpalpable cancer of the prostate: assessment with transrectal US. Radiology 178:197–199
Lee F Jr, Bronson JP, Lerner RM, Parker KJ, Huang SR, Rach DJ (1991b) Sonoelasticity imaging: results in vitro tissue specimens. Radiology 181:237–239
Lovett KL, Rifkin MD, McCue PA, Choi H (1992) MR imaging characteristics of noncancerous lesions of the prostate. J Magn Reson Imaging 2:35–39
McSherry SA, Levey F, Schiebler ML, Keefe B, Dent GA, Mohler JL (1991) Preoperative prediction of pathological tumor volume and stage in clinically localized prostate cancer: comparison of digital rectal examination, transrectal ultrasonography and magnetic resonance imaging. J Urol 146:85–89
Mirowitz SA, Brown JJ, Heiken JP (1993) Evaluation of the prostate and prostatic carcinoma with gadolinium-enhanced endorectal coil MR imaging. Radiology 186:153–157
Narayan P, Fournier G, Viswanathan G et al. (1994) Utility of preoperative serum prostate specific antigen concentration and biopsy Gleason score in predicting risk of pelvic lymph node metastases in prostate cancer. Urology 44:519–523
Newman JS, Bree RL, Rubin JM (1995) Prostate cancer: diagnosis with color Doppler sonography with histologic correlation with each biopsy site. Radiology 195:86–90
Ohori M, Shinohara K, Wheeler TM et al. (1993) Ultrasonic detection of non-palpable seminal vesicle invasion: a clinicopathological study. Br J Urol 72:799–808
Onik GM, Cohen JK, Reyes GD, Rubinsky B, Chang Z, Baust J (1993) Transrectal ultrasound guided percutaneous radical cryosurgical ablation of the prostate. Cancer 72:1291–1299
Oyen RH (1994) Contemporary imaging of the prostate. In: Petrovich Z, Baert L (eds) Benign prostatic hyperplasia: innovations in management. Springer, Berlin Heidelberg New York, pp 77–139
Oyen RH, Baert AL, Bockisch A (1994a) Prostata, Samenblasen und Samenwege. In: Lüning M, Felix R (eds) Komplexe bildgebende Diagnostik – Becken. Thieme Stuttgart, p 114–139
Oyen RH, Van de Voorde WA, Van Poppel HP et al. (1994b) Benign prostatic nodules in the peripheral zone of the prostate. Radiology 189:707–711
Oyen RH, Van Poppel HP, Ameye FE, Van de Voorde WA, Baert AL, Baert LV (1994c) Lymph node staging of localized prostatic carcinoma with CT and CT-guided fine needle aspiration biopsy: prospective study of 285 patients. Radiology 190:315–321
Partin AW, Yoo J, Carter HB, Pearson JD, Chan DW, Epstein JI, Walsh PC (1993) The use of prostate specific antigen, clinical stage, and Gleason score to predict pathological stage in men with localized prostate cancer. J Urol 150:110–114
Petros JA, Catalona WJ (1992) Lower incidence of unsuspected lymph node metastases in 521 consecutive patients with clinically localized prostate cancer. J Urol 147:1574–1575
Platt JF, Bree RL, Schwab RE (1987) The accuracy of CT in the staging of carcinoma of the prostate. AJR 149:315–321
Rifkin MD (1990) MR imaging of the prostate. Crit Rev Diagn Imaging 31:223–262
Rifkin MD, Alextientseucci T (1991) Ultrasound-guided prostate biopsy: superior accuracy compared to digital guided biopsy of palpable masses. Radiology 179:41–42
Rifkin MD, McGlyn ET, Choi H (1989) Echogenicity of prostate cancer correlated with histologic grade and stromal fibrosis: endorectal US studies. Radiology 170:549–552
Rifkin MD, Zerhouni EA, Gatsonis CA et al. (1990) Comparison of MR imaging and ultrasonography in staging early

prostate cancer: results of a multiinstitutional cooperative trial. N Engl J Med 323:621–626

Rifkin MD, Alexander AA, Pisarchick J, Matteucci T (1991) Palpable masses in the prostate: superior accuracy of US-guided biopsy compared with accuracy of digitally guided biopsy. Radiology 179:41–42

Rifkin MD, Sudakoff GS, Alexander AA (1993) Color Doppler imaging of the prostate: techniques, results and potential applications. Radiology 186:509–513

Rubens DJ, Hadley MA, Alam SK, Gao L, Mayer RD, Parker KJ (1995) Sonoelasticity imaging of prostate cancer: in vitro results. Radiology 195:379–383

Scardino PT, Shinohara K, Wheeler TM, Carter SS (1989) Staging of prostate cancer. Value of ultrasonography. Urol Clin North Am 16:713

Schiebler ML, Schnall MD, Pollack HM et al. (1993) Current role of MR imaging in staging of adenocarcinoma of the prostate. Radiology 189:339–352

Schmid HP, McNeal JE, Stamey TA (1992) Observations on the doubling time of prostate cancer as measured by serial PSA in untreated patients with prostate cancer. N Engl J Med

Schnall MD, Imai Y, Tomaszewski J, Pollack HM, Lenkinski RE, Kressel HY (1991) Prostate cancer: local staging with endorectal surface coil MR imaging. Radiology 178:797–802

Shapiro A, Lebensart PD, Pode D, Bloom RA (1994) The clinical utility of transrectal ultrasound and digital rectal examination in the diagnosis of prostate cancer. Br J Radiol 67:668–671

Shepard D, Keetch DW, Stahl D, Huphrey PA (1995) Rebiopsy strategy in men with isolated prostatic intraepithelial neoplasia on prostate needle biopsy. AUA 153 (suppl):420A

Shinohara K, Wheeler TM, Scardino PT (1989) The appearance of prostate cancer on transrectal ultrasonography: correlation of imaging and pathological examinations. J Urol 142:76–82

Smith BH, Dehner LP (1972) Sarcoma of the prostate gland. Am J Clin Pathol 58:43–50

Sommer FG, Nghiem HV, Herfens R, McNeal JE (1993) Gadolinium-enhanced MRI of the abnormal prostate. Magn Reson Imaging 11:941–947

Spencer JA, Alexander AA, Gomella L, Matteucci T, Goldberg BB (1993) Clinical and US findings in prostate cancer: patients with normal prostate specific antigen levels. Radiology 189:389–393

Stamey TA (1995) Making the most out of six systematic sextant biopsies. Urology 45:2–12

Stamey TA, McNeal JE (1992) Adenocarcinoma of the prostate. In: Walsh PC, Retik AB, Stamey TA, Vaughan ED Jr (eds) Campbell's urology, 6th edn. Saunders, Philadelphia, pp 1159–1160

Stamey TA, McNeal JE, Freiha FS, Redwine E (1988) Morphometric and clinical studies on 68 consecutive radical prostatectomies. J Urol 139:1235–1241

Stamey TA, Dietrick DD, Issa MM (1993a) Large, organ confined, impalpable transition zone cancer: association with metastatic levels of prostate specific antigen. J Urol 149:510–515

Stamey TA, Freiha FS, McNeal JE, Redwine EA, Whittemore AS, Schmid HP (1993b) Localized prostate cancer. Relationship of tumor volume of clinical significance for treatment of prostate cancer. Cancer 71:933–938

Strasser H, Janetschek G, Rissigl A, Helweg H, Bartsch G (1995) Three-dimensional transrectal sonography: staging of prostate cancer. Eur Radiol 5 (Suppl):227

Summers RM, Korobkin M, Quint LE, Ellis JH, Grossman HB, Sandler HM, Mandell SH (1993) Pelvic CT findings after radical prostatectomy. J Comput Assist Tomogr 17:767–771

Trannenbaum M (1975) Sarcomas of the prostate gland. Urology 5:810–824

Terris MK, McNeal JE, Stamey TA (1992a) Detection of clinically significant prostate cancer by transrectal ultrasound-guided systematic biopsies. J Urol 148:829–832

Terris MK, McNeal JE, Stamey TA (1992b) Estimation of prostate cancer volume by transrectal ultrasound imaging. J Urol 147:855–857

Terris MK, McNeal JE, Stamey TA (1992c) Transrectal ultrasound imaging and ultrasound guided prostate biopsies of residual carcinoma in clinical stage A carcinoma of the prostate. J Urol 147:864–869

Terris MK, McNeal JE, Freiha FS, Stamey TA (1993) Efficacy of transrectal ultrasound guided seminal vesicle biopsies in the detection of seminal vesicle invasion by prostate cancer. J Urol 149:1035–1039

Terris MK, Haney DJ, Johnstone IM, McNeal JE, Stamey TA (1995) Prediction of prostate cancer volume using prostate-specific antigen levels, transrectal ultrasound, and systematic sextant biopsies. Urology 45:75–80

Turner JW, Hawes DR, Williams RD (1993) Magnetic resonance imaging for detection of prostatic cancer to bone. J Urol 149:1482–1484

Vallancien G, Prapotnich D, Veillon B, Brisset JM, Andre-Bougaran J (1991a) Seminal vesicle biopsies in the preoperative staging of prostatic cancer. Eur Urol 19:196–200

Vallancien G, Prapotnich D, Veillon B et al. (1991b) Systematic prostatic biopsies in 100 men with no suspicion of cancer at digital rectal examination. J Urol 146:1308–1312

Van de Voorde WM, Van Poppel HP, Verbeken EK, Oyen RH, Baert LV, Lauweryns JM (1995) Morphologic and neuroendocrine features of adenocarcinoma arising in the transition zone and in the peripheral zone of the prostate. Mod Pathol 8:591–598

Wasserman NF, Kapoor DA, Hildebrandt WC et al. (1992a) Transrectal US in evaluation of patients after radical prostatectomy. I. Normal postoperative anatomy. Radiology 185:361–366

Wasserman NF, Kapoor DA, Hildebrandt WC et al. (1992b) Transrectal US in evaluation of patients after radical prostatectomy. II. Transrectal US and biopsy findings in the presence of residual and early recurrent prostatic cancer. Radiology 185:367–372

Wheeler TM (1989) Anatomic considerations in carcinoma of the prostate. Urol Clin North Am 16:623–634

White S, Hricak H, Forstner R et al. (1995) Prostate cancer: effect of postbiopsy hemorrhage on interpretation of MR images. Radiology 195:385–390

Wolf JS Jr, Shinohara K, Carroll PR, Narayan P (1993a) Combined role of transrectal ultrasonography, Gleason score, and prostate-specific antigen in predicting organ-confined prostate cancer. Urology 42:131–137

Wolf JS Jr, Shinohara K, Kerlikowske KM, Narayan P, Stoller ML, Carroll PR (1993b) Selection of patients for laparoscopic pelvic lymphadenectomy: a decision analysis. Urology 42:680–687

Wolf JS Jr, Cher M, Dall'era M, Presti JC, Hricak H, Carroll PR (1995) The use and accuracy of cross-sectional imaging and fine needle aspiration cytology for detection of pelvic lymph node metastases before radical prostatectomy. J Urol 153:993–999

Young MPA, Jones DR, Griffiths GJ, Peeling WB, Roberts EE, Parkinson MC (1993) Prostatic "capsule": a comparative study of histological and ultrasonic appearances. Eur Urol 24:479–482

8 Conservative Management of Carcinoma of the Prostate

B.J. Norlén

CONTENTS

8.1 Introduction

Conservative management of carcinoma of the prostate is based on the assumption that the natural course of the disease, i.e., the course of the disease if no treatment were to be given, is extremely slow or is not influenced by the treatments available. Autopsy studies (Franks and Durh 1956; Sakr et al. 1993) indicate a high prevalence of so-called latent prostatic carcinomas in men above the age of 50. It is well known that most of these men will succumb to other diseases and will die with their prostatic carcinoma rather than from it. In the Western world there is an increase in the incidence of prostatic carcinomas and this increase in incidence is mainly due to the detection of localized disease. Especially in countries where case finding or screening programs have been launched, this increase in incidence is dramatic. Information on the natural history of prostatic cancer before the era of hormone therapy is available from a few studies (Nesbit et al. 1946; Barnes and Ninan 1972; Whitmore 1973). In his paper in *Cancer*, Whitmore wrote: "In the face of the variable and unpredictable natural history of prostatic cancer the end results of uncontrolled treatment regimens are subject to varying interpretations. It is morally and ethically impossible in the present era to obtain data regarding the natural history of the disease which might resolve some of the existing questions regarding therapy but, as in the remarkably analogous problem of female breast cancer, controlled clinical trials would answer some of the legitimate therapeutic questions." Unfortunately, 22 years later there is still only one published randomized controlled study with a primary untreated control arm (Graversen et al. 1990), but randomized controlled studies are in progress both in Scandinavia (Norlén 1994) and in the United States (Prorok 1994).

B.J. Norlén, MD, PhD, Associate Professor and Head, Department of Urology, University Hospital, 75185 Uppsala, Sweden

8.2 The VACURG Study

The VACURG study, carried out from 1967 to 1975 (Graversen et al. 1990), compared initial radical prostatectomy with initial placebo treatment. In 1994, Madsen presented a 20-year follow-up of this study comprising 111 evaluable patients out of 142. There was no difference in survival between the two groups. Due to the limited number of patients in this study the statistical efficacy is low and the study has also been criticized for a relatively high dropout of patients. In addition there is a high proportion of well-differentiated tumors, which might explain the few lethal events due to prostatic cancer.

8.3 Scandinavian Studies

In 1985 Larsson and Norlén, in a supplement of the *Scandinavian Journal of Urology and Nephrology*, published an abstract on a 5-year follow-up of patients with localized prostatic carcinoma initially referred to expectant management. The patients were collected from a university hospital setting and selected from all patients referred to the institution from January 1976 to September 1979. The material consisted of 31 patients, 15 with low-grade, 14 with medium-grade, and two with high-grade carcinoma. Of the 15 patients with well differentiated tumors, seven did not show any progression, five showed local progression, and three developed distant metastasis. After a follow-up of 6.5 years all these patients were in remission. Of the 16 patients with medium- or high-grade carcinoma, three showed local progression and the remaining 13 developed distant metastasis. The average time from diagnosis to progression was 3.1 years. The conclusion of this study was that younger patients with well differentiated tumors should be considered for aggressive therapy, as should those with lower tumor grades.

In a register study published by Adami et al. (1986), an annual excess death rate of about 8% was found in patients with prostatic carcinoma when compared to the general population, even after an observation period of more than 10 years. The conclusion from this study was that low long-term relative survival rates contradicted the concept that biologically inactive (latent) tumors constitute a significant proportion of the prostatic cancers diagnosed in clinical practice.

Improvements in the surgical techniques for radical retropubic prostatectomy by Walsh et al. (1983), the randomized study by Paulson et al. (1982) suggesting superior survival for patients subjected to radical prostatectomy than those subjected to irradiation, and the above-cited studies turned many Swedish urologists away from a conservative attitude to localized prostatic cancer towards a more aggressive therapeutic approach.

8.3.1 Two Prospective Cohort Studies from Sweden

8.3.1.1 The Örebro Study

In a series of articles Johansson et al. have published the most frequently cited studies on watchful waiting for early-stage prostatic cancer (Johansson et al. 1989; Johansson 1994). During the 7-year period beginning from 1977, 654 new patients with prostatic cancer were diagnosed in the Örebro area, where there is only one hospital and the population is very stable. Of the 306 localized cases, 223 were left without primary treatment and constituted the cohort from which the natural course of the disease was studied. Thus, 83 patients were excluded from the study and this is one of the main criticisms of it. During the first 2 years, only patients with well differentiated tumors (grade 1) were included in the untreated group. During the following 5 years, patients with moderately or poorly differentiated tumors were randomized to receive either local irradiation or no treatment. There was a high incidence of well differentiated tumors in this study population. The number of patients with grade 1 tumors was 148 (66%) compared to 66 (30%) with moderately differentiated tumors and nine (4%) with poorly differentiated tumors. In most series there have been few poorly differentiated tumors, but generally there has been a better balance between well and moderately differentiated carcinomas. In the Örebro study the mean age was 72 years and after a mean observation period of 12.5 years 77 (35%) patients showed progression of their disease. In 28 (13%) patients metastatic disease was identified. During the observation period, 66% of these patients died but only 10% from their prostatic cancer. The calculated survival rate without signs of progression was 55% at 10 years. The observed survival rate after 10 years was 42% and the cancer-specific survival rate was 85%. The cancer-specific survival curve was very similar to the relative survival curve, indicating an appropriate estimation of the cause of death. During the mean follow-up period of 12.5 years, 30 (13%) of the 223 study patients were subjected to transurethral resection of the prostate due to infravesical obstruction. Four patients (2%) were treated with percutaneous nephropyelostomy due to upper tract obstruction and an additional six (3%) patients suffered severe gross hematuria necessitating hospital admission. In a multivariate analysis tumor grade was a more important prognostic factor predicting tumor progression and death, as compared with stage of disease or age at diagnosis.

A subset of 58 (26%) patients below the age of 70 years and in the retrospective analysis who were considered good candidates for radical prostatectomy were analyzed. These patients showed a better survival rate than the cohort as a whole, with a corrected 5-year survival rate of 98% and a corrected 10-year survival rate of 88%. The rate of tumor progression was 60% higher in this subgroup than in the total cohort, whereas the risk of dying of prostatic cancer did not differ significantly. Unfortunately, the distribution of well differentiated versus moderately well differentiated tumors in this subgroup of 58 patients was not reported. Nor do we have any information concerning the clinical stage of these patients.

The conclusions from Johansson's study were that after 12.5 years the mortality from prostatic cancer for patients with localized disease was 10%–15%, the corrected survival was 85%, and very few additional years could be gained with aggressive curatively intended treatment.

8.3.1.2 The Stockholm Study

The Stockholm study comprised 122 patients with well or moderately well differentiated tumors collected between 1978 and 1982 (ADOLFSSON et al. 1992). The background population in this study was not reported and no N-staging was done either in this study or in the Örebro study. The mean age of the patients was 68 years, and treatment was instituted upon local progression or distant spread. After a mean observation period of 91 months, 45 of patients had received some treatment. In most cases this treatment was hormonal, but in 15% of patients curatively intended treatment was given. In this study, as in the Örebro study, there was a high intercurrent mortality (38%) but only 7% of the patients succumbed to their prostatic cancer. Thus, the rates for tumor progression and mortality were very similar for the two studies. A subgroup analysis of 61 patients younger than 70 years at diagnosis revealed that after an observation period of 86 months nine (15%) patients had distant metastasis and four (7%) had died from their prostatic cancer. Another four patients had succumbed to intercurrent diseases.

8.3.2 The Oslo Study

WAALER and STENWIG in 1993 reported their experience with 94 patients with T0–T2NxN0 prostatic cancer evaluated for progression within 2–7 years and for cancer-specific mortality within 4–9 years. The patients received no anticancer treatment. A significant difference was found according to the initial T-category both in tumor progression rates and in the incidence of cancer-related death. The investigators also found a significant difference in progression rates and cancer-related deaths according to histologic grade. No difference could be demonstrated according to patient age. These authors found nine (10%) deaths due to prostatic cancer among the 94 patients during an observation period of 4–9 years. In contrast to the findings of JOHANSSON and ADOLFSSON, there was an increased risk of death with increasing T-category. WAALER and STENWIG found a 5-year corrected survival rate of 100% for T0 focal, 93% for T0 diffuse, and 70% for T1–T2 tumors. These statistically significant findings contrast with the corresponding survival rates found by JOHANSSON et al. (96%, 94%, and 92.4%, respectively).

8.3.3 The Gothenburg Study

In a report from Gothenburg by AUS et al. (1994), a completely different technique was used to study prostatic cancer. This paper was read at the SIU meeting in Sydney 1994 and is accepted for publication in the *Journal of Urology*. The study was made possible by the registration of all new cancers in Sweden in the Swedish National Cancer Register. All 535 patients with prostatic carcinoma in the community of Gothenburg who died during the years 1988–1990 were identified. A retrospective analysis was then performed, all records were reviewed, and tumor stage was classified according to UICC 1992 and tumor grade according to MOSTOFI (1991). In patients with stage M0 at diagnosis (n = 301) the overall cancer-specific mortality was 50% and for those who survived more than 10 years an even higher mortality due to prostatic cancer of 63% was found. The most important conclusion from this study was that there is a progressive mortality in prostatic cancer stage M0 when follow-up is longer than 10 years in patients who have received noncurative treatment. This study has been criticized mainly by biostatisticians considering the disease-specific mortality to be excessive from a methodological point of view. One criticism is that Kaplan Meier curves cannot be used in a study starting from a point where all patients have died and then estimating survival backwards. Another criticism is that the incidence of prostatic carcinoma is not stable during the period of observation and according to the statisticians this may introduce a systematic over-evaluation of the risk of dying from prostatic carcinoma. However, this study might indicate a completely different view on the risk of dying from prostatic carcinoma after a longer period of observation, and further statistical analysis and additional studies are needed to resolve this extremely important issue.

8.4 American Studies

8.4.1 Pooled Analysis of Six Nonrandomized Studies

Chodak et al. (1994) published in the *New England Journal of Medicine* (1994) a pooled analysis on 828 patients with localized cancer of the prostate. In this analysis the following studies were included: the two Swedish cohorts (Johansson et al. 1989; Adolfsson et al. 1992), two cohorts from the United States (Whitmore et al. 1991; Jones 1992), one from Israel (Moskovitz et al. 1987), and one from the United Kingdom (Goodman et al. 1988). The 10-year disease-specific survival was 87% for the 492 patients with well differentiated tumors and 87% for the 265 patients with moderately differentiated tumors but significantly lower, 34%, for the 63 patients with poorly differentiated tumors. The corresponding 10-year metastasis-free survival rate was 81%, 58%, and 26% for tumor grades 1, 2, and 3, respectively. The observed survival for the prostatic cancer patients did not differ significantly from the expected survival of the matched group of the general population in Sweden and the United States. It must be stressed, however, that at 10 years following diagnosis 42% of the patients with moderately well differentiated tumors revealed metastasis. This might indicate a decreased survival after a longer period of observation. For the time being, and in the absence of randomized studies, this pooled analysis has probably provided the most reliable results concerning deferred treatment for patients with early localized prostatic cancer.

8.4.2 The Memorial Sloan Kettering Study

In the Memorial Sloan Kettering study, included in the above pooled analysis, Whitmore et al. (1991) reported their experience with 75 retrospectively reviewed patients receiving no therapy for at least 1 year after diagnosis. In this series, 21% of B1, 46% of B2, and 22% of B3 tumors developed recognized distant metastases. The actuarial survival at 15 years was 67%, 39%, and 63% for patients with B1, B2, and B3 lesions, respectively. The study emphasized the importance of efforts to prospectively identify patients with localized prostatic cancer in whom the evolution of the tumor, response to palliative therapy, and competing mortality might obviate the need for putatively curative therapy.

8.4.3 The Howard University College Study

The Howard University College study, reported by Jones (1992), was also included in the above-mentioned pooled analysis. In this study 233 patients with localized stage A and B cancer were observed prospectively and conservatively for a total period of 22 years. All patients were managed conservatively until signs or symptoms of disease progression were noted. Of the 233 study patients, 44 (19%) were treated with iodine-125 irradiation implantation and pelvic lymphadenectomy. The overall survival of these patients managed with watchful waiting did not differ statistically from the United States life-table survival probability for men of similar ages. The conclusion of this study was that, because of the favorable results in this expectant management of patients, it appears prudent that all patients with localized prostatic cancer should have this management option as well as radical surgery or external irradiation.

8.4.4 The Mayo Clinic Study

In a very early study from the Mayo Clinic (Hanash et al. 1972) the fate of 195 patients with histologically proved, conservatively treated carcinomas of the prostate was analyzed. It was found that age at diagnosis and histologic tumor grade were the most important factors for tumor progression and death from prostatic carcinoma.

8.5 British Studies

8.5.1 The George Study

One of the early and most cited studies on conservative therapy for localized prostatic cancer was published in the *Lancet* by George (1988). He compiled the complete records of 120 out of 152 patients without metastasis at diagnosis. The mean age in this cohort was 75 years. Local tumor increased to palpable dimensions in 100 (84%) of these patients but metastasis developed in only 13 (11%), the mean time to bone scan conversion being 36 months. Twenty-three (19%) patients were withdrawn from the study and treated because of concern about increasing tumor size, and in one of these patients metastasis developed. Five patients (4%) died of prostatic cancer but there were 48 (40%) additional non-cancer-related deaths. The 5- and 7-year actuarial survival rates were 80% and 75%, respectively. The conclusion from this study was that the likelihood that prostatic cancer will cause death within 7 years is indicated primarily by the scintigraphic findings at diagnosis. Thus, patients with metastatic disease have a high cancer mortality whereas patients without metastasis have an extremely high intercurrent mortality. It should be noted, however, that the mean age of patients in this series was quite high, i.e., 75 years, with a range from 62 to 90 years.

8.5.2 The Edinburgh Study

RANA et al. (1993) reported a study of 614 men with newly diagnosed prostatic carcinoma. Of these, 107 (17%) had early disease at presentation and their management was based on regular surveillance and deferred treatment until disease progression or development of symptoms. Of these 107 patients, four (4%) developed local failure, 11 (10%) bone metastases, and only three (3%) died of cancer with a median survival of 6.3 years. During this observation period, 34 (32%) died of intercurrent disease with a median survival of 2.6 years. The observed 12-year survival for the entire group of 614 patients was similar to the expected survival for an age-matched population in Scotland. Thus, the British studies revealed findings similar to those of the two Swedish studies from Örebro and Stockholm.

8.6 Japanese Study

EGAWA et al. (1993) presented the clinical outcome of 107 patients with localized prostatic cancer. Of these 107, 52 (49%) patients did not receive any antitumor treatment until cancer progression. Fifty-five (51%) received immediate endocrine therapy after diagnosis. Overall, 22 (20%) patients out of the 107 died of prostatic cancer while 45 (42%) died of other causes. During a mean observation period of 37 months, 25% of patients experienced progression of the disease. The cancer-specific survival rate for the 107 patients was 78% at 5 years and 71% at 10 years. The presence of poorly differentiated tumor was the strongest predictor of tumor progression and cancer death. In spite of the low incidence of prostatic cancer in Asia, prostatic cancer survival and mortality do not seem to differ significantly among races, once the disease has become clinically manifest.

8.7 Incidental Carcinoma of the Prostate

Several studies have been published on this subject (BEYNON et al. 1983; EPSTEIN et al. 1986; BLUTE et al. 1986; GOODMAN et al. 1988; LOWE and LISTROM 1988). To summarize these studies, it seems evident that the risk of progression for tumors with a small volume (less than 5% cancer volume in the surgical specimen = T0A) can be calculated at 5% at 5 years, 15%–20% at 10 years, and 25%–35% at 15 years. Following a long observation period some of these patients will succumb to their tumor. If the tumor volume is large (T1B), however, the risk of tumor progression and death from prostatic cancer is considerably higher.

8.8 Discussion

All published studies on the natural history of localized prostatic cancer have been subjected to criticism. The main criticism has been patient selection favoring well differentiated tumors, which are known to have a low tendency for progression. Another criticism has been the presence of a high proportion of elderly men with a high risk of intercurrent mortality soon after diagnosis. Some of the studies have been population based (JOHANSSON et al. 1989; WAALER et al. 1993) but at least in the Örebro study there was a selection favoring patients with well differentiated tumors. In spite of these problems, comparison between the different patient subpopulations with different histologic grades with respect to tumor progression and death from prostatic cancer should be possible.

Further difficulties in comparing different studies are the varying diagnostic techniques and the different staging systems. For example, we know that with fine needle aspiration biopsy there is a higher frequency of well differentiated tumors than with core biopsies (WAISMAN et al. 1991). During the period of inclusion of patients in the different studies, several classification systems have been used and also the classifications have been changed, e.g., for incidental carcinomas. In surgically treated patients the pathologic stage is often used and the tumor grading is based on whole mount step-sectioned material.

The tumors included in the different studies with long observation periods and thus recruited many years previously probably differ in many respects from the tumors referred to the urologist today. Nowadays a substantial number of patients are referred and diagnosed due to elevated prostate-specific antigen (PSA) values.

In series reporting the results of curatively intended treatment most patients have been subjected to lymph node staging. Subsequently those with positive lymph nodes have been excluded from further analysis; on the other hand, in most observation studies lymph node staging generally has not been performed. Most authors consider a lymph node staging unethical in patients in whom no curative treatment is planned.

Another extremely difficult problem in this kind of study is retrospective evaluation of the cause of death. There are no generally accepted criteria in prostatic cancer patients for evaluating which factors are responsible for death, which are contributory, and which are irrelevant. It can also be discussed whether, for example, cardiovascular death in patients on estrogen treatment is a death due to the cancer or to intercurrent disease.

8.9 Conclusion

Most patients with localized prostate cancer exhibit low mortality rates from their disease, especially if the tumor is of small volume and well differentiated. Patients with poorly differentiated tumors have a very poor prognosis. Within an observation period of 10 years, 10%–20% of well and moderately well differentiated tumors will lead to the death of their host. Many researchers, however, have major concern over what happens to their cancer patients with observation periods beyond 10 years. Furthermore, the series so far available for analysis do not include PSA-detected tumors or tumors found by screening. There is an urgent need for randomized studies comparing radical curative treatment with deferred treatment in patients with expected survival exceeding 10 years. It is also of utmost importance that patients' quality of life is evaluated in these prospective studies. Such studies are underway, both in Scandinavia and in the United States.

References

Adami HO, Norlén BJ, Malker B, Meirik O (1986) Long-term survival in prostatic carcinoma, with special reference to age as a prognostic factor. Scand J Urol Nephrol 20:107–112

Adolfsson J, Carstensen J (1991) Natural course of clinically localized prostatic carcinoma in men less than 70 years old. J Urol 146:96–98

Adolfsson J, Carstensen J, Löwhagen T (1992) Deferred treatment in clinically localized prostatic carcinoma. Br J Urol 69:183–187

Aus G, Hugosson J, Norlén L (1994) Prostate cancer: long-term survival after noncurative therapy. Abstract 158, Société Internationale d'Urologie, 23rd Congress, Sept 18–22, 1994, Sydney

Barnes RW, Ninan CA (1972) Carcinoma of the prostate: biopsy and conservative therapy. J Urol 108:897–900

Beynon LL, Bussuttil A, Newsam JE, Chisholm GD (1983) Incidental carcinoma of the prostate: selection for deferred treatment. Br J Urol 55:733–736

Blute ML, Zinke H, Farrow GM (1986) Long-term follow-up of young patients with stage A adenocarcinoma of the prostate. J Urol 136:840–843

Chodak GW, Thistedt RA, Gerber GS et al. (1994) Results of conservative management of clinically localized prostate cancer. N Engl J Med 330:242–248

Egawa S, Go M, Kuwao S, Shoji K, Uchida T, Koshiba K (1993) Long-term impact of conservative management on localized prostate cancer. Urology 42:520–526

Epstein JI, Paull G, Eggleston JC, Walsh PC (1986) Prognosis of untreated stage A1 prostatic carcinoma: a study of 94 cases with extended follow-up. J Urol 136:837–839

Franks IM, Durh MB (1956) Latency and progression in tumours: the natural history of prostatic cancer. Lancet 17:1037–1039

George NJR (1988) Natural history of localised prostatic cancer managed by conservative therapy alone. Lancet 1:494–497

Goodman CM, Busuttil A, Chisholm GD (1988) Age and size and grade of tumour predict prognosis in incidentally diagnosed carcinoma of the prostate. Br J Urol 62:576–580

Graversen PH, Corle DK, Nielsen KT, Madsen PO, Casser TC (1990) Radical prostatectomy versus expectant primary treatment in stage I and II prostatic cancer. A fifteen-year follow-up. Urology 36:493–498

Hanash KA, Utz DC, Cooke EN, Taylor WF, Titus JL (1972) Carcinoma of the prostate: a 15 year follow-up. J Urol 107:450–453

Johansson J-E (1994) Expectant management of early stage prostatic cancer: Swedish experience. J Urol 1252:1753–1756

Johansson J-E, Adami H-O, Andersson S-O, Bergström R, Krusemo UB, Kraaz W (1989) Natural history of localised prostatic cancer. A population based study in 223 untreated patients. Lancet 1:799–803

Johansson J-E, Adami H-O, Andersson S-O, Bergström R, Holmberg L, Krusemo UB (1992) High 10-year survival rate in patients with early untreated prostatic cancer. JAMA 167:191–196

Jones GW (1992) Prospective conservative management of localized prostate cancer. Cancer 70 (Suppl):307–310

Larsson A, Norlén BJ (1985) Five-year follow-up of patients with localized prostatic carcinoma initially referred for expectant treatment. Scand J Urol 19 (Suppl 93):30

Lowe BA, Listrom MD (1988) Incidental carcinoma of the prostate: an analsis of the predictors of tumor progression. J Urol 140:1340–1344

Madsen PO (1994) Prospective, randomized study of radical prostatectomy vs delayed treatment in early carcinoma of the prostate, a 20-year follow-up. Abstract 622, Société

Internationale d'Urologie, 23rd Congress, Sept 18–22, 1994, Sydney
Moskovitz B, Nitecki A, Levin D (1987) Cancer of the prostate: is there a need for aggressive treatment? Urol Int 42:49–52
Mostofi FK, Sesterhenn I, Sobin LH (1991) International histological classification of tumors of prostate. World Health Organisation, Geneva.
Nesbit RM, Plumb RT, Arbor A (1946) Prostatic carcinoma. Surgery 20:263–272
Norlén BJ (1994) Swedish randomized trial of radical prostatectomy versus watchful waiting. Can J Oncol 4 (Suppl 1):38–42
Paulson DF, Lin GH, Hinshaw W, Stephani S. The Uro-Oncology Research Group (1982) Radical surgery versus radiotherapy for adenocarcinoma of the prostate. J Urol 128:502–504
Prorok P (1994) The National Cancer Institute multi-screening trial. Can J Oncol 4 (Suppl 1):98–101
Rana A, Chisholm GD, Christodoulou S, McIntyre, Elton RA (1993) Audit and its impact in the management of early prostatic cancer. Br J Urol 71:721–727
Sakr WA, Haas GP, Cassin BF, Pontes JE, Crissman JD (1993) The frequency of carcinoma and intraepithelial neoplasia of the prostate in young male patients. J Urol 150:379–385
Waaler G, Stenwig AE (1993) Prognosis of localised prostatic cancer managed by "watch and wait" policy. Br J Urol 72:214–219
Waisman J, Adolfsson J, Löwhagen T, Skoog L (1991) Comparison of transrectal prostate digital aspiration and ultrasound-guided core biopsies in 99 men. Urology 37:301–307
Walsh PC, Lepor H, Eggleston JC (1993) Radical prostatectomy with preservation of sexual function: anatomical and pathological considerations. Prostate 4:473–485
Whitmore WF (1973) The natural history of prostatic cancer. Cancer 32:1104–1112
Whitmore WF Jr, Warner JA, Thompson IM (1991) Expectant management of localized prostatic cancer. Cancer 67:1091–1096

9 Surgical Treatment of Carcinoma of the Prostate

H. Van Poppel, D. De Ridder, H. Goethuys, A.A. Elgamal, and L. Baert

CONTENTS

9.1 Introduction

Prostate cancer is nowadays, after lung cancer, the second most common cause of cancer-related death in men (Boring et al. 1994). The risk of developing a clinically significant prostate cancer is about 10%, and approximately 25% of men with prostate cancer die of the disease (Cupp and Oesterling 1993). As a matter of fact, prostate cancer has become a major health problem. The debate on the usefulness (and the method) of screening for prostate cancer continues, but the management policy is also still the subject of debate.

Although it has been suggested that early prostate cancer can be followed without treatment (Johansson et al. 1992), patients with clinically localized prostate cancer are at substantial risk of dying from prostate cancer (Lerner et al. 1991). Therefore, aggressive therapy is usually advocated in patients with a life expectancy of 10 or more years (Chodak et al. 1994). Radical surgery is one of the curative treatments that is performed by many, although expert urologists, oncologists, and radiation oncologists in various parts of the world would prefer nonsurgical therapy if they themselves were to have a localized prostate cancer (Moore et al. 1988).

Attempts to compare the efficacy of surgery and radiotherapy have not been very successful because of differences in patient selection, clinical and surgical staging, and assessment of treatment failure. Moreover, owing to recent advances in detection and follow-up modalities, much of the existing literature is outdated. Therefore, decision-making about treatment by the clinician is dictated much more by the patient's general health, the clinical tumor stage, the pathologic grade, and quality of life factors, than by information about the established value of various treatments gained from the literature (Catalona 1994).

9.2 History

Radical prostatectomy, the oldest mode of treatment of prostate cancer with curative intent, was already applied at the beginning of this century. The first

H. Van Poppel, MD, PhD, Professor, Department of Urology, St. Pieter's Hospital, Catholic University of Leuven, Brusselsestraat 69, 3000 Leuven, Belgium
D. De Ridder, MD, Consultant Urologist, Department of Urology, St. Pieter's Hospital, Catholic University of Leuven, Brusselsestraat 69, 3000 Leuven, Belgium
H. Goethuys, MD, Senior Resident, Department of Urology, St. Pieter's Hospital, Catholic University of Leuven, Brusselsestraat 69, 3000 Leuven, Belgium
A.A. Elgamal, MD, Consultant Urologist and Research Fellow, Department of Urology, St. Pieter's Hospital, Catholic University of Leuven, Brusselsestraat 69, 3000 Leuven, Belgium
L. Baert, MD, PhD, Professor and Chairman, Department of Urology, St. Pieter's Hospital, Catholic University of Leuven Brusselsestraat 69, 3000 Leuven, Belgium and Clinical Professor, Department of Urology and Radiation Oncology, University of Southern California, 1441 Eastlake Avenue, Los Angeles, CA 90033, USA

well-described radical prostatectomy, defined as resection of the prostate, the seminal vesicles, Denonvilliers' fascia, and the bladder neck, was performed by H. Young, assisted by W. Halsted, in 1904 at Johns Hopkins University, Baltimore (YOUNG 1905). He used a perineal approach and published the technique and treatment results, insisting on the ease of the operation and on the importance of wide excision in order to achieve tumor control (YOUNG 1945). Among 184 cases, followed up for 5–27 years, he noted a cure rate of 55% and a mortality of 6.5%. TURNER and BELT (1957) reported on the same technique applied in 225 cases with a 5-year survival rate of 70%. Although these results were obviously excellent with respect to tumor control, the technical difficulty of the perineal approach precluded it from gaining overwhelming popularity.

In 1948 Millin, for the first time, used the retropubic approach for adenomectomy and for radical prostatectomy (MEMMELAAR and MILLIN 1949). In 1954 the retrograde technique of radical retropubic prostatectomy was described in detail (CHUTE 1954) and a few years later CAMPBELL (1959) described the antegrade procedure. Nevertheless, radical prostatectomy remained unpopular because of its morbidity. The high amounts of blood loss and the frequency of urinary incontinence and erectile impotence were considered too high a price to pay for cure of a disease that has a very protracted, non-life-threatening course in many cases. Therefore in the 1960s and 1970s, localized prostate cancer in Europe was mainly treated with irradiation although it was well recognized that radiotherapy only eradicates the radiation-sensitive cell populations and, when not administered cautiously, may result in severe complications (VAN POPPEL et al. 1987).

In 1979 Walsh described the anatomy of the dorsal venous complex and the technical aspects necessary to control Santorini's plexus (REINER and WALSH 1979), thereby reducing dramatically the blood loss during radical retropubic prostatectomy. Anatomic dissection at the level of the urethral sphincter allowed improvement of urinary continence rates. A few years later further anatomic work led to the recognition of the neurovascular bundles, responsible for erection, that could be spared under certain conditions, avoiding erectile impotence (WALSH and DONKER 1982).

At the present time most experts consider radical prostatectomy to be the treatment of choice to achieve local eradication of early prostate cancer. Indeed, the anatomic approach to radical prostatectomy has reduced the mortality to less than 1% and significant incontinence to less than 2%, while potency often can be preserved.

9.3 Indications for Radical Prostatectomy

In men with localized prostate cancer and a life expectancy of 10 years or more, the goal of management is to eradicate the disease. Watchful waiting can be advocated in patients with a shorter life expectancy with low-stage and low-grade tumor but is not acceptable in younger men at higher risk of tumor progression (CHODAK et al. 1994). Primary hormonal treatment may be given in patients with clinically localized prostate cancer when they are not suitable candidates for more aggressive treatment. In fact there is no age limit for radical prostatectomy in an individual patient. It has been shown in a group of patients between 70 and 79 years of age that those who underwent radical prostatectomy did not frequently die of intercurrent disease and had acceptable morbidity. Therefore, men should not be denied radical prostatectomy on the grounds of age alone (CORRAL and BAHNSON 1994).

Radical prostatectomy offers the best chance to eradicate clinically organ-confined cancer, i.e., T1 and T2 tumors (TNM classification, SCHRÖDER et al. 1992a), but with increasing experience a lot of centers are now performing surgery also for locally advanced (T3) tumors, and some have proposed combined treatment for patients with any localized stage with pelvic lymph node involvement (N1–2).

9.3.1 Stage T1 Prostate Cancer

T1 tumors are clinically inapparent cancers that are not palpable at digital rectal examination nor visible by imaging. At the age of 50 years, approximately one man out of three has incidental prostatic carcinoma detected on an autopsy, while only one out of ten of these men is at risk of developing a clinically significant carcinoma. Therefore it is questionable whether every case of prostate cancer found incidentally on transurethral resection or needle biopsy warrants aggressive treatment.

9.3.1.1 Stage T1a and T1b

Stage T1a prostate cancer is a cancer that is an incidental histologic finding in 5% or less of tissue samples, while T1b is diagnosed when more than 5%

of the tissue resected by transurethral resection or adenomectomy contains cancer. Although the risk of progression of untreated T1a prostate cancer after 5 years is only 5%, it has been clearly demonstrated that with longer follow-up (10–13 years) these cancers can progress in about 50% of these patients (LOWE and LISTROM 1988b). Therefore, although older T1a cancer patients often will not need aggressive treatment, in younger patients who are expected to survive 15 years or more the chance of progression is real, especially when high-grade tumor is present (BLUTE et al. 1986; EPSTEIN et al. 1986).

About half of the patients with T1b tumors can be expected to show disease progression after 5 years (LOWE and LISTROM 1988a) and therefore aggressive treatment is more often warranted. This makes the distinction between T1a and T1b tumors a relevant problem. A repeat transurethral resection of the prostate (TURP) upstages only 10% of patient from a T1a to a T1b tumor, although 85% may have a residual cancer (LOWE and BARRY 1990). Moreover a repeat TURP can render a radical prostatectomy more difficult because of the small amount of tissue left within the capsule, hindering proper recognition of the apex on the one hand, and causing periprostatic fibrosis on the other (VAN POPPEL et al. 1992b). Although a nerve-sparing radical prostatectomy should be curative for virtually all patients with T1 tumors while ensuring good continence, a prior repeat TURP can be responsible for higher incontinence rates and make preservation of the neurovascular bundles more difficult.

Therefore, in our medical center, when a T1a disease is diagnosed on TURP or adenomectomy, a new evaluation is done after 3 months. This evaluation includes: physical examination, prostate specific antigen (PSA) and transrectal ultrasonography (TRUS). Often the expansion of a formerly compressed peripheral zone makes the sonographic evaluation easier. Small hypoechoic lesions can then be recognized and selectively biopsied. When no suspect foci are seen, six ultrasound-guided needle biopsies are taken. In this situation if one or more biopsies are positive for carcinoma, the tumor is considered to be T1b.

As for a poorly differentiated T1a, T1b patients are offered a radical prostatectomy when they have a life expectancy of 10 years or more. When no cancer is found on biopsy, patients are routinely followed once a year with digital rectal examination, PSA, and TRUS. In some cases, when after the TURP nearly no residual prostate is palpable and the ultrasonographically measured weight is below 10 g, we are inclined to propose radiotherapy as a definitive treatment.

9.3.1.2 Stage T1c

The clinically inapparent tumor (not palpable and not visible) that is identified by needle biopsy (e.g., because of an elevated PSA) is becoming increasingly common. TRUS-guided needle biopsies in individual patients do not provide adequate information for differentiating between clinically insignificant and life-threatening prostate cancer (CUPP et al. 1995). Recent reports stress the fact that PSA-detected tumors are frequently significant tumors and should not be left untreated (EPSTEIN et al. 1994b; REITER et al. 1995; ELGAMAL et al. 1995; DOUGLAS et al. 1995). The presence or absence of the tumor on TRUS is irrelevant to the final outcome (FERGUSON et al. 1995).

It has been shown that 84% of T1c cancers are significant tumors either by volume or by grade (EPSTEIN et al. 1994a). Among our patients, 15% of radical prostatectomies were done for PSA-detected cancers. Only 14% of the latter were considered insignificant tumors (≤0.2 cc and Gleason score ≤4). Of the T1c patients treated, 25% had pT3a cancer and 48% had large tumors (mean 3.34 ± 3.9 cc).

Inability to palpate T1c tumors or to visualize them on imaging studies is sometimes due to small tumor size but is more often the consequence of location of the tumor in the heterogeneously echogenic transition zone or in the anterior commissure of the prostate. Transition zone cancers differ from those originating in the peripheral zone. The latter usually have a higher grade and more prostatic intraepithelial neoplasia (PIN) (GREENE et al. 1991). Analysis of the actuarial rate of treatment failure after radical prostatectomy in these patients clearly showed that transition zone cancers are inherently less aggressive than peripheral zone cancers (OHORI et al. 1995). Nevertheless, it remains impossible to recognize those cancers that might only be followed, without the need for immediate therapy. A relatively low PSA or, better, a PSA density between 0.1 and 0.15, with less than 3 mm of low-grade cancer in one core is considered a favorable preoperative finding. The above parameters retrospectively enabled us to identify correctly 60% of insignificant tumors (EPSTEIN et al. 1994b). It might be reasonable to follow some patients whose tumors are very likely insignificant. However, in general a radical prostatectomy should be advocated for T1c tumors, keeping in mind that significant tumors will be found in the majority of these patients.

Finally, men with a persistently elevated serum PSA value after an initial negative prostate biopsy should undergo at least one repeated biopsy including transition zone sampling. This is in order to exclude adequately the presence of detectable prostate cancer (KEETCH et al. 1994). We do not agree that radical prostatectomy should be performed without pathologic proof of malignancy. We accept that there is a subset of men with benign prostatic hyperplasia (BPH) who have very high PSA levels (STAMEY 1995). They should undergo open adenomectomy in order to facilitate a correct diagnosis.

9.3.2 Stage T2 Prostate Cancer

When the tumor involves half of a lobe or less and is confined to the prostate (=T2a), progression can be expected in most patients who are long-term survivors. The median time to progression of untreated T2 disease is reported to be 6–10 years (GRAVERSON et al. 1990). T2a patients with a 10-year life expectancy should be offered radical prostatectomy since after 5 years 35%–55% will have disease progression if not treated.

Among patients with T2b–c cancer, still confined to the prostate but involving more than half of a lobe or both lobes, progression will occur in more than 70% within 5 years. The prognosis is excellent after radical prostatectomy if the tumor is confined to the prostate on pathologic examination (GIBBONS 1988). In high-grade tumors capsular penetration will often occur and the expected incidence of local control will be much lower.

A watchful waiting policy has been proposed for T2 tumors on the grounds that patients are at higher risk of dying from causes unrelated to cancer (JOHANSSON and ANDERSSON 1991). It is important to note that only a few of the patients described by these authors had high-grade tumors. If one proposes watchful waiting for low-grade T2 cancer, one should bear in mind that the preoperative assessment of the tumor grade by needle biopsy is frequently unreliable (EPSTEIN and STEINBERG 1990). On the other hand it has been clearly shown that most poorly differentiated tumors extend outside of the prostate. Those high-grade tumors which are confined to the prostate have an excellent prognosis (OHORI et al. 1994a).

9.3.3 Stage T3 Prostate Cancer

Locally extensive prostate cancer is seen in about 40% of all clinically diagnosed tumors and its management remains controversial (SCHRÖDER et al. 1992b). T3a cancer is defined as having unilateral and T3b bilateral extracapsular extension while in T3c the seminal vesicles are also invaded.

In extracapsular tumors, radical prostatectomy will often not succeed in achieving complete tumor excision. The patients may have higher morbidity and are expected to have a substantial local recurrence rate; most will finally progress systemically. Therefore, it has been questioned whether the T3 prostate cancer patient should be a candidate for radical prostatectomy.

The main problem is the clinical staging of the prostate cancer. Not only will clinical T2 tumors (cT2) frequently prove to be pathologic T3 (pT3) but also 20% of clinical T3 patients in fact have pT2 tumors (BOSCH et al. 1987). Patients with T3 tumors have a much worse outcome than those with pT2, and about 50% of them will develop metastases within 5 years. It is, however, apparent that only a radical prostatectomy can recognize those few patients who can be cured by surgery for a cT3pT2 cancer (VAN DEN OUDEN et al. 1994).

Some authors have tried to recognize prior to treatment which tumors will prove to be pT3. Digital examination is disappointing for this purpose (VARENHORST et al. 1993). PSA and Gleason score are useful but only when they are either very low or very high. However, when PSA, Gleason score, and clinical stage are combined, this indeed predicts well the pathologic stage (PARTIN et al. 1993a).

Transrectal ultrasonography is better than digital rectal examination in evaluating the tumor volume. Tumor volume has been shown to correlate well with the presence of extracapsular disease once it exceeds 3.0 cc (STAMEY et al. 1988). It is apparent that extraprostatic tumor spread through the neurovascular bundles can be preoperatively recognized but it has been shown that TRUS frequently underestimates the tumor extent (SHINOHARA et al. 1989). Finally, TRUS can be used to assist in staging biopsies from the seminal vesicles, from the trapezoid area, and from the neurovascular bundles when tumor invasion of these structures is suspected (RAVERY et al. 1994). As has been shown by others, we found that TRUS-guided biopsies of the seminal vesicles are highly accurate (TERRIS et al. 1993). Also the number of positive sextant biopsies appeared to be an important prognostic indicator of the pT classification. Patients with four or more positive sextant biopsies had a greater likelihood of pT3 disease (PELLER et al. 1995). In experienced hands, the presence and precise location of microscopic extracapsular extension can be determined preoperatively with reasonable accuracy using TRUS combined with digital rectal examination (OHORI et al. 1994b).

Body coil magnetic resonance imaging (MRI) appears to offer no or little advantage over TRUS for T3 cancer staging. The role of endorectal surface coil MRI has not been fully established (SCHNALL et al. 1991).

Stage T3 tumors represent a spectrum of disease ranging from a well-differentiated pathologic T3 with focal extracapsular extension to a poorly differentiated bulky clinical T3 (WOLF and MONTIE 1994). The TNM classification (SCHRÖDER et al. 1992a) with three subclassifications for T3 adenocarcinoma is not always useful to distinguish prognostic substages, e.g., because PSA levels are not included in this staging (CORN et al. 1995). Moreover the same TNM system as is applied for clinical staging has to be applied for pathologic staging. The assessment of pathologic extracapsular extension can be obvious in many cases. There are differences in the importance of extracapsular extension for a given pT category of a tumor with positive surgical margins at the level of the apex or the anterior commissure, where the prostate capsule is absent. Should the invasion of the seminal vesicle, in continuity with the tumor, or metastatic spread in the seminal vesicle and invasion of the perivesicular fat represent the same stage pT3c? Is focal capsular penetration expected to have the same outcome as extensive capsular penetration and will specimen-confined and margin-positive T3 cancer have the same failure rates?

These considerations explain why published reports on treatment outcomes in patients with cT3 and pT3 are difficult to interpret. One therefore has to develop different prognostic categories based on the pathologic findings (EPSTEIN et al. 1993a), distinguishing focal and more extensive capsular penetration, Gleason score lower or higher than 7, and the presence of negative or positive surgical margins. Based on the different combinations of these factors, different progression rates were observed at 5 years. We feel that pre- and postoperative PSA should also be included when deciding on one or another adjuvant treatment modality such as hormonal manipulation or radiation therapy. Indeed, the indication for adjuvant treatment after radical prostatectomy for a pT3 prostate cancer with or without positive margins remains controversial. Hopefully, ongoing phase III prospective randomized trials on the administration of early postoperative radiotherapy in pT3 prostate cancer not only will show that the local recurrence rate is reduced (as expected) but also will demonstrate in which patients overall and cancer-related survival can be improved. Additionally, it is expected that a group of patients will be identified in whom adjuvant therapy is not beneficial at all or can be delayed with comparable result.

Although the best indication for radical prostatectomy is T1 and T2 cancer, we are not convinced that the preoperatively diagnosed pT3 prostate cancer should never be considered for radical prostatectomy. It seems that a subgroup of patients with locally extensive prostate cancer will have long-term benefit from radical prostatectomy. Wide resection of the neurovascular bundles can result in specimen-confined, margin-negative radical prostatectomy, the definitive outcome of which will be better with respect to both cancer-related progression and survival (SMITH et al. 1995). It is of importance to note that, even when progression does occur in these patients, it will be systemic progression: the local problems related to invasion of the bladder and the rectum will not occur, thus giving the patient a real advantage in terms of a better quality of life.

It is obvious that embarking on radical prostatectomy for T3 cancer necessitates sufficient surgical expertise in order to keep the morbidity acceptable. It has been acknowledged that increased overall surgical experience has contributed to the decreased operative morbidity from radical prostatectomy for clinical T3 cancer (BLUTE et al. 1995).

9.3.4 Nodal Disease

The indication for radical prostatectomy in all previously described T stages assumes the pathologically proven absence of nodal involvement. Lymph node-positive disease will be followed by systemic progression. Indeed, all patients with significant N^+ disease will ultimately fail if followed for a sufficient period.

The prevalence of nodal disease has decreased dramatically over the past several years, possibly due to earlier detection of prostate cancer. Only a few years ago all patient with histologically proven prostatic adenocarcinoma underwent bone scan and pelvic CT scan in order to rule out skeletal and nodal involvement. At that time we investigated the accuracy of combined computerized tomography and fine-needle aspiration cytology in detecting lymph node involvement. False-negative staging results were found in only 10 out of 285 patients scheduled for radical prostatectomy (Van Poppel et al. 1994). Most of these patients had high Gleason scores and pathologically proven extracapsular extension. These results enabled us to omit peroperative frozen sections of the lymph nodes before continuing with the radical prostatectomy.

Presently, with a significantly lower incidence of pelvic node involvement (Petros and Catalona 1992), urologists have tried to identify those patients for whom pelvic lymph node involvement is very uncommon. This would imply that preoperative staging by CT could be omitted, with important economic repercussions in terms of health care costs (Optenberg and Thompson 1990). Also, pelvic lymph node dissection could become superfluous, allowing, for instance, for radical perineal prostatectomy without lymph node staging. There is no doubt that patients with stage T1, T2, or T3a tumors and with high-grade disease should have their lymph nodes evaluated when the expected risk of nodal involvement exceeds 30% (Partin et al. 1994). The relationship between the tumor grade, clinical stage, and PSA and the lymph node status has been clearly demonstrated (Bosch et al. 1987; Partin et al. 1993a; Wolf et al. 1993). Patients with a Gleason score less than 7 and a PSA below 20 ng/ml have a low risk of nodal metastases. In patients with well-differentiated tumors and a PSA below 10, this risk is extremely low and lymph node assessment by any means becomes a useless excercise (Van Poppel et al. 1994). Preoperative lymph node assessment by CT scan and staging lymphadenectomy in these patients is superfluous and could only be advocated in patients treated in clinical studies (Bishoff et al. 1995).

In patients who are at risk of having lymph node invasion we believe CT scan is mandatory and, in experienced hands and combined with fine-needle aspiration cytology (FNAC), it is a very reliable diagnostic study. The CT scan should be performed after oral and intravenous contrast medium administration, to distinguish vascular and intestinal structures from lymph nodes. A CT slice thickness of 8 mm and a table incrementation of 10 mm is recommended. In an unselected group of 285 radical prostatectomy candidates, metastatic pelvic lymph nodes were suspected in 43 patients (17%). Of these 43 patients, 35 had pathologically confirmed N^+ on FNAC and were offered hormonal therapy only (Van Poppel et al. 1994). Our excellent results with CT and FNAC have not been confirmed by other authors who continue to rely only on lymph node dissection performed either during open surgery or by laparoscopy.

Most urologists are reluctant to perform radical prostatectomy for clinical N^+ disease or will cancel radical prostatectomy when frozen section shows lymph node invasion. On the other hand, many urologists face the situation where they have performed radical prostatectomy in patients who, after definitive pathologic examination, are found to have microscopic lymph node disease. The incidence of tumor progression is lower in patients with fewer involved lymph nodes and in those with microscopic disease only. Therefore a subclassification to the N stage was proposed, distinguishing a stage pN1.1 (=a single microscopic focus) and pN1.2 (=macroscopically detectable unilateral invasion of one node) (Rutishauser and Hering 1988). These authors found no significant difference in disease-free survival between pN0 and pN1.1, and others have also found no survival difference between the two groups (Prout et al. 1980; Gervasi et al. 1989).

The situation is, of course, different when lymphadenopathy is recognized with nodal stages $\geq$ pN1.1. Some suthors have felt that the presence of abnormal lymph nodes is no reason not to perform radical prostatectomy, claiming instead that it should be performed in conjunction with immediate hormonal treatment. Myers et al. (1992), in a retrospective study of a large number of patients with diploid cancer, showed that those treated by radical prostatectomy and early endocrine treatment did significantly better than a similar group who had no early hormonal therapy, mainly with respect to disease-free survival (Myers et al. 1992). A more recent analysis concluded that for patients with N^+ disease, radical prostatectomy and radiotherapy, when combined with orchiectomy, produce a similar outcome. The question remains as to whether N^+ patients need any local treatment at all. Those who are in favor of radical prostatectomy will cite the prevention of local complications although it is clear that local control may be obtained by hormonal treatment associated with transurethral resection. In any case, a surgical approach to patients with minimal nodal disease can only be proposed when the available surgical expertise is such that a low incidence of complications can be anticipated.

In conclusion, patients with a preoperative diagnosis of N^+ disease are not good candidates for radical prostatectomy. Mostly they will have significant ≥pN2 disease and will be treated by hormonal manipulation. As an exception, we have performed radical prostatectomy in patients with urinary retention and very large prostates that would need open adenomectomy in order to resolve their micturition disturbances. This was followed by early hormone therapy. In patients who prove to be pN+ after radical prostatectomy one should advocate adjuvant hormonal treatment although no randomized study has to date shown any advantage of early versus delayed treatment in these patients.

9.4 Surgical Aspects of Radical Prostatectomy

Although radical prostatectomy was originally performed through the perineum, the retropubic operation has become a more popular procedure. The retropubic approach has, to a large extent, replaced the perineal operation for three reasons:

1. It is possible to evaluate the lymph nodes during the same procedure. Nowadays surgical lymph node staging can be reliably done by CT scan and fine-needle aspiration cytology (Van Poppel et al. 1994) or can be omitted in the presence of well-differentiated tumors with low PSA (Danella et al. 1993). When lymph node dissection is considered necessary, the open retropubic approach can be replaced by laparoscopic or pelvioscopic surgery that enables an equally reliable lymph node assessment (Parra et al. 1992; Mazeman et al. 1992; Parra et al. 1994; Levy and Resnick 1994).
2. The nervi erigentes could be better spared during retropubic prostatectomy.
3. It is presumed that perineal radical prostatectomy results in less radical surgery, with a higher incidence of positive margins. However, whether this is the case remains controversial and some recent reports have attempted to demonstrate at least equivalence between the two techniques (Harris et al. 1995). The techniques have been applied in different medical centers, and some may use both the perineal and the retropubic approach. Important prospective studies comparing the operative techniques in respect of complication rate and tumor control rates are not yet available.

9.4.1 General Remarks on Retropubic and Perineal Prostatectomy

Both types of radical prostatectomy can be performed under general or under spinal or epidural anesthesia. Most anesthesiologists feel more comfortable with general anesthesia. In our institute, we offer the patient the advantage of an epidural anesthesia, which remains in place for the first 48 h, in combination with a general anesthesia for the surgery itself. This continuous epidural anesthesia can then be used "on demand" by the patient, while it does not hinder postoperative recovery or lower limb mobility.

All patients are required to undergo complete bowel preparation the day before operation (anticipating problems when the rectum is entered) and are put on a low molecular weight subcutaneous anticoagulant.

When lymphadenectomy is performed by open surgery or percutaneously, in one step or as a first-stage procedure, it is not considered a therapeutic procedure but a staging procedure only. Usually a modified iliac-obturator lymphadenectomy is performed, removing the lymph nodes lying underneath the iliac vein in the obturator fossa, starting with Cloquet's ganglion and extending to the bifurcation of the iliac artery. Care is taken not to damage the lymphatics that drain the lower limbs, avoiding postoperative lymphedema. Additionally, we secure the lymphatics with metal clips, avoiding lymphorrhea and lymphocele. The obturator nerve is preserved to avoid problems with adduction of the thigh (Brendler et al. 1980).

The removed lymphatic tissue can be sent for frozen section or for conventional processing and pathologic examination. One should avoid postponing the radical prostatectomy itself (scheduled as a second surgical time) for longer than 2 or 3 days since adhesions occurring after the lymph node dissection can make the dissection of the endopelvic fascia more difficult.

9.4.2 Radical Retropubic Prostatectomy

Anatomic radical retropubic prostatectomy was developed and described in detail by Walsh (Walsh et al. 1983).

The patient lies in a supine position, with an indwelling bladder catheter, and an incision is made between the symphysis and the pubis. The retrograde procedure is the most commonly performed. The endopelvic fascia is bilaterally incised. The puboprostatic ligaments are divided and the dorsal venous complex (both the superficial and the deep part of the plexus of Santorini) is ligated and transected. Then the urethra is identified at the prostatic apex and is divided sharply, avoiding excessive traction on the urethra that could result in impaired continence recovery. The apical dissection is the most critical part of the procedure: resecting a part of the striated muscle or mobilizing the urethral stump out of the pelvic floor can cause incontinence while a too cautious resection may result in positive margins, due to apical extension of the tumor or to inadvertent intracapsular dissection.

The neurovascular bundles lie just adjacent to the posterolateral aspect of the urethra and the urologist has to decide at this time whether the neurovascular bundles should be divided together with the urethra or swept off from the apex and preserved. Once the urethra is divided, the rectourethralis muscle is transected, allowing development of the dissection plane between the rectal wall and Denonvilliers' fascia. The dissection of the lateral prostatic wall, where the neurovascular bundles penetrate the prostate, is done either with wide resection of the bundles or very close to the prostate when a nerve-sparing procedure is justified. The dissection is continued cranially towards the prostate base. From now on the surgeon can either continue in a retrograde fashion by dissecting the seminal vesicles and the vasa deferentia, or first transect the prostatovesical junction and remove the seminal vesicles in an antegrade way. When the bladder is incised at the level of the prostatovesical junction care must be taken not to damage the ureteral orifices. The bladder neck is reconstructed and the mucosa is everted before making the urethrovesical anastomosis with four sutures on a Foley catheter, which is cautiously taped to the skin in order to avoid accidental withdrawal.

In cases of difficult apical dissection some authors have advocated an antegrade approach, starting the radical prostatectomy at the bladder neck and dividing the urethra as the last step (Petros and Catalona 1991). Other groups have modified some steps of this procedure. Different ways of controlling the dorsal venous complex have been proposed (Myers 1989; Goldwasser and Zincke 1989; Bressel 1990; Hrebinko and O'Donnell 1993; Wise and Fialk 1993). Measures to simplify the vesicourethral anastomosis have been described (Hanash 1992; Maggio et al. 1992; Bell 1993; Klein 1993), as have alternative approaches for apical dissection (Miller and Larson 1994), for bladder neck reconstruction (Steiner et al. 1993; Breul and Hartung 1994), and for nerve sparing (Ruckle and Zincke 1995).

The problem in evaluating the results of nerve-sparing procedures is a relative paucity of prospective studies with objective assessment of potency status before and after surgery. Before anatomic radical perineal prostatectomy was performed, recovery of potency was reported in just 8% of patients (Finkle and Williams 1985) whereas with the nerve-sparing technique 60%–80% of preoperatively potent patients regain erectile capacity (Eggleston and Walsh 1985). The best results have been shown to be obtained in younger patients with a lower stage of disease where a bilateral nerve-sparing procedure is performed (Catalona and Dresner 1985; Walsh 1987; Catalona and Bigg 1990; Leandri et al. 1992; Zimmern and Leach 1995). Systematic biopsies of the contralateral side can help to identify a unilateral nerve-sparing side without risk of positive margins in T2 cancers (Huland et al. 1994).

There is no agreement on whether a nerve-sparing technique will improve continence because of the more meticulous dissection at the prostatic apex. Although some authors have found no relation between preservation or wide excision of the neurovascular bundle and continence status (Steiner et al. 1991), others have concluded that a non-nerve-sparing technique is more likely to induce partial urethral denervation, resulting in a higher postoperative incontinence rate (O'Donnell and Finan 1992).

Another matter of discussion is the value of bladder neck preservation for improving urinary continence after radical retropubic prostatectomy. We have used this technique since 1990 in more than 150 patients. It consists in careful dissection between the bladder and prostate in order to preserve the bladder neck fibers. Also the intraprostatic urothelium can be dissected out and preserved. When necessary the neo-bladder neck can be narrowed by two or three semicircular muscular sutures, followed by eversion of the urethral mucosa upon the continent bladder neck. We are convinced that bladder neck preservation has several advantages: first, damage to the ureteral orifice is very unlikely; second, anastomotic strictures are avoided; and third, the time required to regain continence is reduced. Other groups have published their results with this technique (Gomez et al. 1993) while recent reports have addressed the same question (MARCUCCI 1994; PERETSMAN et al. 1994; BASLER et al. 1994; LICHT et al. 1994; KLEIN and LICHT 1995), all confirming that the bladder neck-sparing modification is safe and provides excellent continence rates and a low incidence of anastomotic strictures without compromising tumor control.

Bladder neck preservation cannot be performed in all patients: it is an unsafe procedure when the tumor is located at the prostate base and it can be very difficult when a large adenoma has elongated the bladder neck fibers. Similar problems are present after transurethral resection or adenomectomy, or in the presence of a median lobe, where opening of the bladder neck cannot be avoided.

After the surgery, recovery is usually very quick and patients are mobilized on the first postoperative day. We prefer to withdraw the suction drains after 2–5 days, when lymphorrhea stops and the patients are sufficiently mobilized. We withdraw the indwelling catheter on the 15th postoperative day. We do not perform a contrast study as others have recommended (PARIVAR et al. 1994). These studies are done in order to show any extravasation, but we believe that this has no clinical implications.

Early hospital discharge is possible after radical retropubic prostatectomy but most patients prefer to stay in hospital for the duration of indwelling catheterization. Those who leave the hospital early do so after a few days and return for 1 or 2 days at the time of catheter withdrawal. This can result in a significant hospital cost saving without increasing morbidity (LICHT and KLEIN 1994).

9.4.3 Radical Perineal Prostatectomy

Historically prostate cancer was first operated on via a perineal approach, although retropubic prostatectomy has now gained widespread acceptance. Recently, however, urologists have expressed renewed interest in radical perineal prostatectomy. The perineal approach has some disadvantages: simultaneous lymph node assessment is not possible and exposure and complete removal of the seminal vesicles are more difficult. Furthermore it was originally thought that preservation of potency was not possible with the perineal approach. It has been demonstrated, however, that by application of similar principles as are adopted in preserving the neurovascular bundles in retropubic prostatectomy, impotence can be avoided. The fascia containing the neurovascular bundles can be identified through a perineal incision, though the problem of sparing potency remains in patients with a small pelvic outlet or a big prostate (WELDON and TAVEL 1988).

Still, the perineal approach offers other advantages that include good urethral exposure, enabling easy anastomosis between bladder and urethra, and reduced blood loss. Indeed, the dissection is performed from behind the prostate, below the dorsal venous complex, which can cause severe hemorrhage using the retropubic technique (SCHRÖDER and BELT 1975; DOUBLET et al. 1994).

The patient is placed in an exaggerated lithotomy position. The perineal skin incision is made between the ischial tuberosities and a blunt dissection leads to the exposure of the ischiorectal fossa bilaterally. The central tendon is divided and a Lowsley retractor is used to pull the prostate into the incision. The rectourethralis muscle is then divided and the posterior surfaces of the prostate and seminal vesicles are separated from the rectum. The urethra is identified and transected followed by insertion of the straight Lowsley retractor. Then the anterior surface of the prostate is exposed and dissected beneath the puboprostatic ligament and more anteriorly located veins towards the bladder neck. The latter is incised and the prostate resected from the trigone. Now the neurovascular bundles can be identified and separated from the gland or resected when nerve sparing is not attempted. Finally, the seminal vesicles and vasa deferentia are removed en bloc with the prostate, the bladder neck is narrowed, and the vesicourethral anastomosis is performed. One suction drain is inserted before closing, and it can generally be removed after 2 or 3 days. The bladder draining Foley catheter is usually withdrawn after 10–14 days, while early ambulation can start on the first or second postoperative day.

Potency-sparing radical perineal prostatectomy is feasible but necessitates a vertical incision on the lateral reflection of the clinical posterior layer of Denonvilliers' fascia over the apex of the prostate (WELDON and TAVEL 1988). Inappropriate recognition of the fascial layers can result in intracapsular dissection or tumor transection in locally advanced tumors, giving rise to positive surgical margins.

9.5 Results of Radical Prostatectomy

The treatment outcome in patients with localized prostate cancer depends not only on the treatment itself but also (indeed, above all) on the inherent tumor biology (GLEASON 1988).

While there is agreement that small prostate cancers can be cured by radical prostatectomy, the role of surgery in locally advanced disease is still controversial. Unfortunately, clinical discrimination between locally confined and locally extensive (possibly disseminated) disease is not obvious. In any case, however, radical prostatectomy has become a standard treatment for prostate cancer with a low morbidity and nearly no mortality.

The treatment results of radical prostatectomy for prostate cancer are difficult to define. The prostate cancer population has changed over the years and now patients with early stages of prostate cancer more frequently constitute the radical prostatectomy population. Also staging modalities have improved during the past several years and PSA has become a reliable parameter for the detection of early treatment failure. On the other hand, early prostate cancer will often need a very long follow-up that is not yet obtained in PSA-monitored patients after surgery. Therefore reports on survival rates after radical prostatectomy are still used to assess the value of radical prostatectomy in the treatment of localized prostate cancer.

9.5.1 Survival Rates

An attempt has been made, looking at older and more recent literature, to compare crude survival and clinical disease-free survival rates in all stages of prostate cancer following radical prostatectomy. Considerable differences in treatment results have been noted in different series (VAN POPPEL and BAERT 1994). The 10-year survival rates after radical prostatectomy for stage T1a disease have recently been reported to be 73%, and the 15-year crude survival rate was nearly 60%. For T1b tumors the same authors showed similar 10-year survival rates and a 15-year survival of 45% (ZINCKE et al. 1991).

For T2 tumors reported 15-year crude survival rates are about 50% (WALSH and JEWETT 1986) and 15-year disease-free survival rates, 60% (GIBBONS 1988). No randomized studies on treatment outcomes in T2 prostate cancer are yet available but the survival of these patients after radical prostatectomy is believed to be comparable to the expected survival of an age-matched control group (GIBBONS et al. 1989). The disease-specific survival, differentiating death from cancer or intercurrent disease with or without tumor activity, was reported to be about 93%, as compared to 84% for deferred treatment and 75% for radiotherapy (ADOLFSSON et al. 1993).

VAN POPPEL and BAERT (1994) compared the crude survival rates cited in a number of older and more recent reports with respect to locally advanced prostate cancer (T3). The problem in comparing results in T3 patients is the fact that some patients will have received early or delayed hormonal treatment while others will not.

The largest reported study in T3 prostate cancer patients treated with radical prostatectomy in combination with hormonal treatment showed 5-, 10-, and 15-year survival rates of 91%, 68%, and 46%, respectively (CHENG et al. 1993). It has also been shown that adjuvant hormonal treatment only delays tumor progression and has no impact on overall survival or cancer-related death rate (ZINCKE et al. 1986; MYERS et al. 1992; CHENG et al. 1993).

On the other hand it is noteworthy that locally advanced prostate cancer is not per se an incurable disease. Radical prostatectomy can cure some patients with pT3 tumors when tumors are specimen confined and of low grade with a low PSA level (FROHMÜLLER and WIRTH 1993; VAN DEN OUDEN et al. 1994).

9.5.2 PSA Relapse Rate

More recent publications have not focused only on the survival data but also on PSA relapse after radical prostatectomy in order to evaluate overall treatment efficacy in controlling the disease process. PSA relapse-free survival data for patients with T1 and T2 prostate cancer have been summarized in a recently published report (VAN POPPEL and BAERT 1994). The 5-year risk of PSA recurrence after radical prostatectomy for T1 and T2 tumors was about 20% (MORTON et al. 1991; ZINCKE et al. 1991; STEIN et al. 1992; FRAZIER et al. 1993). A recent publication on 925 patients evaluated for PSA relapse 5 years after radical prostatectomy for clinical T1 and T2 tumors showed 78% of patients to be without PSA or clinical recurrence. For T1c patients this figure was 97%, for T2 it was 74%, and for pT2, 91%. Again, the Gleason score was the most important factor with respect to PSA-free survival (CATALONA and SMITH 1994).

Among pT3 or margin-positive patients, PSA elevation has been reported to occur within 5 years in 45%–75% of those treated by radical prostatectomy (EPSTEIN et al. 1993a; FRAZIER et al. 1993; PARTIN et al. 1993b; ROBINOW et al. 1993). This variation in the

PSA outcome is likely due to differences in patient selection and in prognostic factors of which the most relevant are tumor volume and Gleason score (CHENG et al. 1993).

A recent report on PSA follow-up after radical prostatectomy alone for prostate cancer with extracapsular extension suggested that clinical T3 cancer can be managed successfully by surgery alone in those patients without a high PSA level and/or poor tumor differentiation (VAN DEN OUDEN et al. 1994).

9.5.3 Radical Prostatectomy and Adjuvant Treatment

Results of a multivariate analysis of clinical and pathologic factors that could predict PSA failure after radical prostatectomy were recently presented, showing that in T3 patients with a Gleason score below 8 and uninvolved seminal vesicles, the margin status (negative or positive) and the extent of extracapsular extension (focal or established) were the two most relevant prognostic factors (D'AMICO et al. 1995). It was advocated that all of the different risk factors predicting tumor progression be taken into consideration when deciding on the need for adjuvant treatment (EPSTEIN et al. 1993a).

The combination of radical prostatectomy with early adjuvant hormonal treatment was recently studied in a group of more than 5000 clinical T3 patients. It was shown that radical prostatectomy with adjuvant hormonal treatment provides excellent control of the primary tumor (BLUTE et al. 1995) without improving survival (MORGAN et al. 1993).

The combined surgical and radiation therapeutic approach for locally advanced tumors is still under investigation. It is noteworthy that some authors advocate radical prostatectomy and radiotherapy without hormonal manipulation in patients with nodal involvement; indeed, a survival rate equivalent to that in age- and race-matched controls has been found, with excellent control of extensive primary T3 tumors (FREEMAN et al. 1994). For pathologic stage T3N0 the same group has reported a survival advantage over historical controls with a 45-Gy radiation dose given postoperatively. This was done primarily in patients with well and moderately well differentiated tumors without seminal vesicle involvement, and no major or clinically important complications were reported (PETROVICH et al. 1991; FREEMAN et al. 1993; YAMADA et al. 1994). These results were similar to the previous reports where investigators were using higher radiation doses and witnessed a higher morbidity.

Recently, the benefit of postoperative radiotherapy has been evaluated and some authors have reported that adjuvant radiotherapy might exacerbate or cause incontinence (KANE et al. 1995) and therefore radiotherapy should only be considered in patients with positive margins (JONSSON et al. 1995). On the other hand it could well be that only patients with initially undetectable postoperative PSA levels will benefit from postoperative radiotherapy (MCCARTHY et al. 1994).

9.5.4 Conclusions

Radical prostatectomy should be reserved for prostate cancer patients who have a high probability of cure and who will live long enough (≥10 years) to benefit from this treatment. Radical prostatectomy cures the majority of men with organ-confined disease or with well to moderately well differentiated tumors that have penetrated the prostate capsule to the extent where it is possible to obtain clear surgical margins (WALSH et al. 1994).

The role for radical prostatectomy in margin-positive disease and in poorly differentiated extracapsular tumors remains controversial. Furthermore, the use of combination treatments with hormonal manipulation and/or radiotherapy as neoadjuvant or adjuvant therapy is still under investigation. Well-designed prospective randomized studies will be of help in defining the role of these therapeutic approaches (BOLLA et al. 1994).

9.6 The European Experience with Radical Prostatectomy

Radical prostatectomy has become the standard treatment for locally confined prostate cancer in certain parts of Europe. The treatment modalities used in the management of prostate cancer are different in different European countries. In Scandinavia, for example, watchful waiting is popular. Within Scandinavia, the Danish physicians are the most conservative, while the most active intervention strategies are recorded in Finland (HEGGESTAD et al. 1993). In the United Kingdom, radical prostatectomy is rather unpopular and many urologists will treat prostate cancer patients with radical radiotherapy (MOORE et al. 1988). In Norway only about 5% of patients with localized prostate cancer receive radical prostatectomy (Tveter and Otnes 1994).

No data are available on how many prostatectomies are currently performed in different European centers. Some of these centers have, however, published their experience with radical prostatectomy. These publications mainly address staging, surgical complications, the degree of continence, potency, and other important quality of life parameters. Only very few European reports have discussed the oncological results of radical prostatectomy (Bressel 1990; Frohmüller et al. 1991; Rossignol et al. 1992; Van Poppel et al. 1992b; Frohmüller and Wirth 1993; Schröder and van den Ouden 1993; van den Ouden et al. 1994; Frohmüller and Theiss 1995). Long-term follow-up data (≥10 years) have been reported by a few authors, with survival rates comparable to those seen in American studies (Bressel 1990; Frohmüller and Theiss 1995). Of particular interest is a paper on radical prostatectomy as monotherapy for T3 prostate cancer, showing that cure can be obtained for those T3 cancer patients who present with favorable prognostic factors and concluding that only patients with poorly differentiated tumors, a PSA level above 20 ng/ml, and lymph node involvement should not be considered for radical surgery (van den Ouden et al. 1994).

We started performing radical prostatectomies in 1986, whereas formerly all patients with N0M0 prostate cancer were treated with radiotherapy. Since 1993, more than 100 radical prostatectomies have been performed per year in our institute. We have analyzed the early results of 310 radical prostatectomies performed prior to 1995.

The clinical and pathologic staging of these patients is given in Table 9.1. Of the 310 patients treated, 205 (66%) underwent a non-nerve-sparing procedure, while 63 (20%) had a bilateral and 28 (9%) a unilateral nerve-sparing operation. With a mean follow-up of 18 months, 25 patients presented PSA progression only, 15 had local recurrence, and seven had metastatic disease.

Of the 25 patients with PSA progression, four had cT1, 14cT2, and seven cT3-4 disease, and 11 (44%) had a Gleason score of ≥7 in the needle biopsy. Following surgery, nine patients had pT2, eight pT3a–b, six pT3c, and two pT4, and 20 (80%) had a Gleason score of ≥7 (Table 9.2).

Eight (5.3%) of the 150 pT2 patients and 15 (12.7%) of the 118 pT3-4 patients showed PSA progression.

Table 9.1. Clinical (cT) and pathologic (pT) stage in 310 radical prostatectomy patients treated at the Catholic University of Leuven

cT	No.	%	pT	No.	%
cT1b	20	7			
cT1c	31	11			
cT2a	102	39	pT2a	46	17
cT2b	36	13	pT2b	29	11
cT2c	24	9	pT2c	75	28
cT3a	44	16	pT3a	63	24
cT3b	8	3	pT3b	23	9
cT3c	4	1	pT3c	20	7
CT4a	3	1	pT4	12	4

Table 9.2. Clinical (CS) and pathologic stage (PS) and Gleason score in 25 patients with PSA recurrence

CS	No.	%	PS	No.	%
cT1	4	16			
cT2	14	56	pT2	9	36
cT3-4	7	28	pT3a–b	8	32
	25	100	pT3c	6	24
			pT4	2	8
				25	100

Gleason score (needle biopsy) ≥7: 11/25 (44%)
Gleason score (surgical specimen) ≥7: 20/25 (80%)

Local recurrence developed in 15 patients and 12 had a Gleason score of ≥7. Seven patients developed metastatic disease and all of them had poorly differentiated tumors. These results confirm that the final Gleason score is the most relevant prognostic factor predicting tumor progression. It is more important than pathologic stage in predicting early PSA or local or systemic tumor progression (Zincke et al. 1994).

The impact of margin-positive disease was not analyzed since patients were randomized into an EORTC protocol for immediate adjuvant radiotherapy versus no early adjuvant treatment (Bolla et al. 1994).

9.7 Neoadjuvant Hormonal Treatment

Local recurrence after radical prostatectomy is likely to occur when the resection of the tumor is incomplete, leaving a microscopic or macroscopic amount of neoplastic tissue behind in the pelvis. The presence of positive surgical margins, either because of extracapsular tumor extension or because of intracapsular dissection, is known to unfavorably influence the treatment outcome (EPSTEIN et al. 1993b; VAN DEN OUDEN et al. 1993; CATALONA and SMITH 1994; D'AMICO et al. 1995; SMITH et al. 1995). Wide excision of the neurovascular bundles is one measure that can result in a specimen-confined radical prostatectomy (PARTIN et al. 1993b) despite tumor extension beyond the prostatic capsule. Overemphasis on preservation of potency may result in a suboptimal procedure leaving some patients with persistent local disease (ROSEN et al. 1992).

In any case, positive surgical margins are a common problem in radical prostatectomy patients - not only in those with extracapsular extension but also in those with clinically locally confined tumors. To improve the results of surgery by reducing the number of positive margins, temporary androgen deprivation was proposed as a neoadjuvant treatment prior to radical prostatectomy. Impressive results have been published by some authors (MONFETTE et al. 1989), renewing the interest in hormonal manipulation before surgery (FAIR 1991). Over the past few years many investigators have used this approach. All have reported considerable downsizing of the prostate volume and a decrease in serum PSA levels after preoperative hormonal treatment. Some of these investigators have also claimed downstaging (from T3 to pT2 or from T2 to pT0) and downgrading TÊTU et al. 1991; FLAMM et al. 1991; FAIR et al. 1993; SCHULMAN and SASSINE 1993; VILLAVICENCIO et al. 1994; SOLOWAY et al. 1994), though others could not confirm these interesting findings (KENNEDY et al. 1992; VAN POPPEL et al. 1992b; MCFARLANE et al. 1993; OESTERLING et al. 1993). Additional benefits of hormonal treatment, such as a decrease in blood loss, facilitation of the surgical procedure, and improved continence, have been reported in some studies (SCHULMAN and SASSINE 1993), while others have found no difference in these parameters in patients with and patients without preoperative hormonal treatment (VAN POPPEL et al. 1992a, 1995; DE RIDDER et al. 1994).

An ideal neoadjuvant treatment will be nontoxic and well tolerated by patients, decrease the tumor volume within a reasonable interval, and inhibit the metastatic potential of the tumor cells. Recently, it was suggested that neoadjuvant androgen deprivation therapy could result in a significantly decreased incidence of micrometastatic disease. This could mean that a significantly higher number of patients might be rendered tumor free and potentially cured by the use of neoadjuvant therapy (FAIR et al. 1995b). These interesting results will need further confirmation.

Most investigators have used maximal androgen blockade. Some of them have used LHRH agonists alone (KENNEDY et al. 1992; AUS et al. 1994), cyproterone acetate (GOLDENBERG et al. 1995), estramustine phosphate (VAN POPPEL et al. 1995), or a pure antiandrogen alone (VAN POPPEL et al. 1992b; VAN DE VOORDE et al. 1994). The effects of all of the various hormonal manipulations as determined by pathologic examination are comparable and have been extensively described (TÊTU et al. 1991; HELLSTRÖM et al. 1993; VAN DE VOORDE et al. 1994). Benign parts of the prostate present atrophy and squamous metaplasia and the tumor itself shows cytoplasmic vacuolation, nuclear pyknosis, fibrosis, and lymphocytic infiltration. Some authors have reported a also significant decrease in the prevalence and extent of high-grade prostatic intraepithelial neoplasia (PIN), considered a precursor of prostate cancer (TÊTU et al. 1991; FERGUSON et al. 1994; VAN DE VOORDE et al. 1994; CIVANTOS et al. 1995). Neoadjuvant administration of a pure antiandrogen in monotherapy has given rise to much less impressive morphologic and immunohistochemical changes (VAN DE VOORDE et al. 1994).

There is no agreement on the duration of neoadjuvant therapy. Most investigators administer this therapy for 3 months. This means that surgery must be postponed for this period, potentially causing patients psychological distress on the one hand and leaving the question of insensitive tumor clone progression (GODET et al. 1992). Therefore, the duration of preoperative hormonal treatment should be kept as short as possible. This is why, in our study, we used estramustine phosphate: with this agent the decrease in prostate and tumor volume is most pronounced in the first 4 weeks of treatment. Prostate involution continues at a much lower rate after this period (VAN POPPEL et al. 1995). Other groups have used neoadjuvant hormonal treatment for a longer period (MONFETTE et al. 1989). Some investigators have shown that the efficacy of endocrine treatment is even higher when used for 6 months (SOLOMON et al. 1993). Recently, it was reported that maximal biochemical and pathologic downstaging requires 8 months of neoadjuvant hormonal therapy, during which time there should be no risk of tumor progression of androgen-independent clones as shown by PCNA and Ki-67 studies (SULLIVAN et al. 1994; GLEAVE et al. 1995).

Downsizing of the prostate gland by hormonal therapy is a widely recognized phenomenon (TÊTU et al. 1991; KENNEDY et al. 1992; MCFARLANE et al. 1993), while the downstaging effect of this therapy remains controversial. Digital rectal examination is frequently unable to correctly stage prostate cancer before, and even less so after hormonal therapy. So the clinical impression of downstaging is questionable (GODET et al. 1992). Also TRUS is not well suited to evaluate the tumor extent, since the hormonal treatment renders the peripheral zone less echogenic, making tumor volume appreciation difficult or impossible (VAN POPPEL et al. 1992a,b).

The PSA decrease which almost always occurs in neoadjuvantly treated patients cannot be considered a good measure of effective downstaging. Serum PSA has indeed been shown to be a completely unreliable tumor marker after hormonal deprivation (OESTERLING et al. 1993; AUS et al. 1994). The early drop in PSA after neoadjuvant hormonal treatment is due to decreased androgen-related PSA synthesis and not to decreased tumor volume. The further slower reduction in PSA after the first sharp decrease is probably related to a decrease in tumor volume. For this reason neoadjuvant treatment could be prolonged until the nadir in PSA has been reached (GLEAVE et al. 1995).

The outcome of surgery seems to be related to the PSA "response." It was shown by SCHULMAN and SASSINE (1993) that when PSA became undetectable after hormonal treatment, most patients had pT2 and some, pT3 tumors. By contrast, all patients in whom the PSA level remained above 4 ng/ml had pT3T4 cancers; these patients should probably not be considered for radical prostatectomy.

The assessment of the influence of neoadjuvant hormonal treatment on tumor grade is also problematic. The assignment of a certain grade after hormonal deprivation is difficult because involutional changes are hard to distinguish from malignancy (MURPHY et al. 1991; VAN POPPEL et al. 1992b; VAN DE VOORDE et al. 1994). Moreover, sampling errors with pretherapeutic prostate needle biopsies are inevitable (EPSTEIN and STEINBERG 1990). At the present time, we believe that in an individual patient, the presence or absence of downgrading by hormonal treatment cannot be accurately assessed.

Whether downstaging can be obtained by hormonal treatment is also a matter of controversy. Although some authors have stated that androgen ablation therapy prior to radical prostatectomy induces tumor necrosis and selective perineural kill (LEE et al. 1993), it is very unlikely that a tumor extending through the prostatic capsule can be transformed into organ-confined disease (a T3 tumor becoming pT2); unfortunately, this issue cannot be resolved with certitude, given the well-known inherent staging errors that attend all techniques, including digital rectal examination, TRUS, and MRI. As to the possibility of achieving complete tumor regression (pT0) with hormonal treatment, this, too, appears highly unlikely. While several authors have reported anecdotal cases in which no tumor was found after neoadjuvant treatment (TÊTU et al. 1991; SCHULMAN and SASSINE 1993; VILLAVICENCIO et al. 1994; GOLDENBERG et al. 1995), it should be noted that the changes induced by hormonal treatment represent pitfalls in the diagnosis of residual carcinoma; thus there is a chance of confusing pyknotic nuclei and the lymphocytic infiltration which is often present (VAN DE VOORDE et al. 1994; CIVANTOS et al. 1995). Many authors are in fact convinced that downstaging cannot be obtained by androgen deprivation prior to radical prostatectomy (GODET et al. 1992; OESTERLING et al. 1993; NARAYAN et al. 1994; VOGES et al. 1994). Only prospective randomized studies will give an insight into what actually happens with prostate cancer treated by neoadjuvant hormonal therapy and radical prostatectomy.

The results of some such randomized phase III studies have recently been published (DE RIDDER et al. 1994; VAN POPPEL et al. 1995) or reported at international meetings (FAIR et al. 1995a; GOLDENBERG et al. 1995; PEDERSEN et al. 1995; SOLOWAY et al. 1995), and may be summarized as follows: For clinical T2 tumors there seems to be a significant reduction in the incidence of positive surgical margins. This effect was not confirmed for clinical T3 tumors (VAN POPPEL et al. 1995). It should, however, be noted that the interpretation of margin-positive disease after hormonal therapy is difficult. After androgen deprivation, residual foci of atrophic glands can be difficult to identify, raising concerns that low positive margin rates may result from failure to identify cancer cells at the margins (GLEAVE et al. 1995).

Positive surgical margins have been shown to be a good predictor of local relapse (ANSCHER and PROSNITZ 1991) and of PSA failure (D'AMICO et al. 1995). On the other hand, not all patients with margin-positive disease will show tumor progression. Different outcomes have been noted in patients with focal or extensive positive margins (EPSTEIN et al. 1993a) and in patients with apical or posterolateral positive margins (FESSEHA et al. 1995; WELDON et al. 1995). Moreover there could be a problem of false-positive surgical margins caused by artifacts due to improper handling and processing of the specimens

(Epstein et al. 1993b). For this reason the indication for adjuvant treatment based on the finding of margin positivity alone is still a topic of debate.

It is unclear why neoadjuvant hormonal treatment seems not to be beneficial in T3 prostate cancer (Oesterling et al. 1993; Van Poppel et al. 1995). It is possible that the hormonal treatment has not been given long enough or that it is not an efficient treatment in more advanced tumors that are often poorly differentiated and relatively hormone insensitive. It has also been suggested that hormonal treatment could give the urologist a false impression that the tumor has been clinically downstaged and therefore a less extensive resection might be performed, resulting in margin-positive disease (Walsh 1993).

In conclusion, the role of neoadjuvant therapy before radical prostatectomy for locally confined prostate cancer as well as for locally advanced prostate cancer remains to be defined. The decrease in margin positivity obtained in T2 tumors does not per se mean that the likelihood of surgical cure is improved or that the time to progression or cancer-related survival will be prolonged (Graham et al. 1995). Longer follow-up data from the ongoing randomized studies have to be awaited.

9.8 Conclusion

Although the discussion on conservative management or aggressive intervention, and on surgery or irradiation for localized prostate cancer will continue, radical prostatectomy has become a frequently performed, efficient, and safe treatment modality.

Detection of cancers by reference to PSA levels is becoming increasingly important, and such tumors should not be considered insignificant. In T1 tumors that deserve treatment, nerve-sparing radical prostatectomy can be offered. In T2a cancers, which are often understaged, a contralateral nerve-sparing procedure can be proposed. In T2b and T2c cancer a nerve-sparing attempt will often result in positive surgical margins and give rise to a local failure. Some well or moderately well differentiated T3 cancers with a low PSA can be cured by radical prostatectomy, possibly followed by adjuvant treatment. This adjuvant treatment could consist in combination treatment with hormones and radiotherapy, which might be beneficial in pT3 patients. Specimen-confined pT3 tumors are expected to have a better outcome than margin-positive ones.

Neoadjuvant hormonal manipulation before radical prostatectomy reduces the frequency of positive margins in T2 cancer but its role in cure of the disease and in the treatment of T3 tumors is still under investigation.

Radical prostatectomy, like most cancer surgery, is a one-chance treatment and should therefore be performed by experienced urologists who can achieve a good balance between extensive local resection and avoidance of surgical complications.

Acknowledgement. Special thanks are due to Mrs. Agnes Goethuys for her motivation and help in the outline, wordprocessing, and typing of the paper.

References

Adolfsson J, Steineck G, Whitmore WF (1993) Recent results of management of palpable clinically localized prostate cancer. Cancer 72:310–322

Anscher MS, Prosnitz LR (1991) Multivariate analysis of factors predicting local relapse after radical prostatectomy – possible indications for postoperative radiotherapy. Int J Radiat Oncol Biol Phys 21:941–947

Aus G, Brandstedt S, Haggman M, Pedersen K, de la Torre M, Hugosson J (1994) Effects of 3 months neoadjuvant hormonal treatment with a GnRH analogue prior to radical retropubic prostatectomy on PSA and tumor volume in prostate cancer. Eur Urol 26:22–28

Basler J, Figenshau R, Bullock A, McCarthy J, Arcangeli C (1994) Does bladder neck sparing radical prostatectomy improve continence or compromise margins of resection (abstract)? J Urol 151 (Suppl):255A

Bell DG (1993) A simple technique to facilitate vesicourethral anastomosis following radical prostatectomy. Br J Urol 72:124–125

Bishoff JT, Clair SR, Reyes A, Gomella L, Thompson IM, Butzin CA, Harris MJ (1995) Pelvic lymphadenectomy can be omitted in selected patients with carcinoma of the prostate: development of a system of patient selection. Urology 45:270–274

Blute ML, Zincke H, Farrow GM (1986) Longterm follow-up of young patients with stage A adenocarcinoma of the prostate. J Urol 136:840–844

Blute ML, Lerner SE, Berstralh EJ, Eickholt JT, Zincke H (1995) Extended experience with radical prostatectomy for clinical stage T3 prostate cancer: outcome and contemporary morbidity (abstract). J Urol 153 (Suppl):313A

Bolla M, Gonzalez D, Van Tienhoven G et al. (1994) External irradiation and adjuvant hormonal treatment, and postoperative irradiation in prostatic carcinoma revisited. Rationale, trial design, eligibility criteria, statistical considerations. Contrib Oncol 47:111–123

Boring CC, Squires TS, Tong T, Montgomery S (1994) Cancer statistics 1994. CA Cancer J Clin 44:7–26

Bosch RJHL, Kurth KH, Schröder FH (1987) Surgical treatment of locally advanced (T3) prostatic carcinoma – early results. J Urol 138:816–822

Brendler CB, Cleeve LK, Anderson EE (1980) Staging lymphadenectomy for carcinoma of the prostate: risk versus benefit. J Urol 124:849–851

Bressel M (1990) Radical prostatectomy - indication, surgical technique, results. Akt Urol 21:115–120
Breul J, Hartung R (1994) Reconstruction of the bladder neck after radical retropubic prostatectomy using a tubular bladder flap. Urologe [A] 33:20–23
Campbell EW (1959) Total prostatectomy with preliminary ligation of the vascular pedicles. J Urol 81:464–467
Catalona WJ (1994) Management of cancer of the prostate. N Engl J Med 331:996–1004
Catalona WJ, Bigg SW (1990) Nerve sparing radical prostatectomy: evaluation of results after 250 patients. J Urol 143:538–544
Catalona WJ, Dresner SM (1985) Nerve sparing radical prostatectomy: extraprostatic tumor extension and preservation of erectile function. J Urol 134:1149–1152
Catalona WJ, Smith DS (1994) 5 year tumor recurrence rates after anatomical radical retropubic prostatectomy for prostate cancer. J Urol 152:1837–1842
Cheng WS, Frydenberg M, Bergstralh EJ, Larson-Keller JJ, Zincke H (1993) Radical prostatectomy for pathologic stage C prostate cancer: influence of pathologic variables and adjuvant treatment on disease outcome. Urology 42:283–295
Chodak GW, Thisted RA, Gerber GS et al. (1994) Results of conservative management of clinically localized prostate cancer. N Engl J Med 330:242–248
Chute R (1954) Radical retropubic prostatectomy for cancer. J Urol 71:347–372
Civantos F, Marcial MA, Banks ER et al. (1995) Pathology of androgen deprivation therapy in prostate carcinoma. A comparative study of 173 patients. Cancer 75:1634–1641
Corn BW, Hanks GE, Lee WR, Schultheiss T (1995) Do the current subclassifications of stage T3 adenocarcinoma of the prostate have clinical relevance? Urology 45:484–490
Corral DA, Bahnson RR (1994) Survival of men with clinically localized prostate cancer detected in the eighth decade of life. J Urol 151:1326–1329
Cupp MR, Oesterling JE (1993) Prostate specific antigen, digital rectal examination and transrectal ultrasonography: their roles in diagnosing early prostate cancer. Mayo Clin Proc 68:297–306
Cupp MR, Bostwick DG, Myers RP, Oesterling JE (1995) The volume of prostate cancer in the biopsy specimen cannot reliably predict the quantity of cancer in the radical prostatectomy specimen on an individual basis. J Urol 153:1543–1548
D'Amico AV, Whittington R, Malkowicz SB, Schnall M, Tomaszewski JE, Schultz D, Wein A (1995) A multivariate analysis of clinical and pathological factors which predict for PSA failure after radical prostatectomy for prostate cancer (abstract). J Urol 153 (Suppl):430A
Danella JF, deKernion JB, Smith RB, Steckel J (1993) The contemporary incidence of lymph node metastases in prostate cancer: implications for laparoscopic lymph node dissection. J Urol 149:1488–1491
De Ridder D, Elgamal A, Werbrouck P et al. (1994) Hormone therapy before radical prostatectomy. Effects on surgical methods and resection margins. Acta Urol Belg 62:61–65
Doublet JD, Lagrange L, Ciofu C, Thibault P, Gattegno B (1994) Radical prostatectomy: comparison of the perineal and retropubic route (40 patients): preliminary results. Prog Urol 4:33–39
Douglas TH, Sesterhenn IA, Moul JW, McLeod DG (1995) The significance of PSA-detected non-palpable adenocarcinoma of the prostate (stage T1c) (abstract). J Urol 153 (Suppl):251A
Eggleston JC, Walsh PC (1985) Radical prostatectomy with preservation of sexual function: pathological findings in the first 100 cases. J Urol 134:1146–1148
Elgamal AA, Van de Voorde WM, Van Poppel HP, Lauweryns JM, Baert LV (1995) Selective zonal distribution of tumor volume versus grade in T1c prostate cancer. J Urol 153 (Suppl):484A (Abstr. no 1024)
Epstein JI, Steinberg GD (1990) The significance of low-grade prostate cancer on needle biopsy. A radical prostatectomy study of tumor grade, volume and stage of the biopsied and multifocal tumor. Cancer 66:1927–1932
Epstein JI, Paull G, Eggleston JC, Walsh PC (1986) Prognosis of untreated stage A1 prostate carcinoma: a study of 94 cases with extended follow-up. J Urol 136:837–839
Epstein JI, Carmichael MJ, Pizov G, Walsh PC (1993a) Influence of capsular penetration on progression following radical prostatectomy: a study of 196 cases with long-term follow-up. J Urol 150:135–141
Epstein JI, Pizov G, Walsh PC (1993b) Correlation of pathologic findings with progression after radical retropubic prostatectomy. Cancer 71:3582–3593
Epstein JI, Walsh PC, Brendler CB (1994a) Radical prostatectomy for impalpable prostate cancer: the Johns Hopkins experience with tumors found on transurethral resection (stages T1a and T1b) and on needle biopsy (stage T1c). J Urol 152:1721–1729
Epstein JI, Walsh PC, Carmichael M, Brendler CB (1994b) Pathologic and clinical findings to predict the tumor extent of non-palpable (stage T1c) prostate cancer. JAMA 271:368–374
Fair WR (1991) Why not neo-adjuvant therapy for prostatic carcinoma? Prog Clin Biol Res 370:305–312
Fair WR, Aprikian A, Sogani P, Reuter V, Whitmore WF (1993) The role of neoadjuvant hormonal manipulation in localized prostatic cancer. Cancer 71 (Suppl):1031–1038
Fair WR, Wang Y, Cohen D et al. (1995a) Neoadjuvant androgen deprivation therapy in patients with clinically localized prostate cancer. Effect on positive margins and postoperative PSA (abstract). J Urol 153 (Suppl):313A
Fair WR, Israeli RS, Wang Y, Nawabi MD, Edwards T, Heston WDW (1995b) Neoadjuvant androgen deprivation therapy prior to radical prostatectomy results in a significantly decreased incidence of residual micrometastatic disease as detected by nested RT-PCR with PSM primers. J Urol 153 (Suppl):391A (Abstr. no 652)
Ferguson J, Zincke H, Ellison E, Bergstralh E, Bostwick DG (1994) Decrease of prostatic intraepithelial neoplasia following androgen deprivation therapy in patients with stage T3 carcinoma treated by radical prostatectomy. Urology 44:91–95
Ferguson JK, Bostwick DG, Suman V, Zincke H, Oesterling JE (1995) PSA detected prostate cancer: pathological characteristics of ultrasound visible versus ultrasound invisible tumors. Eur Urol 27:8–12
Fesseha T, Pontes JE, Montie JM, Haas GP, Powell I, Crignon D, Sakr W (1995) Prognostic significance of a positive apical margin in radical prostatectomy specimens (abstract). J Urol 153 (Suppl):430A
Finkle AL, Williams RD (1985) Sexual potency before and after radical prostatectomy. West J Med 143:475–479
Flamm J, Fischer M, Hoeltl W, Pfluger H, Tumschi W (1991) Complete androgen deprivation prior to radical prostatectomy in patients with stage T3 cancer of the prostate. Eur Urol 19:192–195
Frazier HA, Robertson JE, Humphrey PA, Paulson DF (1993) Is prostate specific antigen of clinical importance in evalu-

ating outcome after radical prostatectomy? J Urol 149:516–518

Freeman JA, Lieskovsky G, Cook DW, Petrovich Z, Chen SC, Groshen S, Skinner DG (1993) Radical retropubic prostatectomy and postoperative adjuvant radiation for pathologial stage C (pCN0). Prostate cancer from 1976 to 1989: intermediate findings. J Urol 149:1029–1034

Freeman JA, Cook DW, Lieskovsky G et al. (1994) Adjuvant radiation, chemotherapy, and androgen deprivation therapy for pathologic stage D1 adenocarcinoma of the prostate. Urology 44:719–725

Frohmüller HG, Theiss M (1995) Long-term results of radical prostatectomy. 15 year follow-up of 100 patients. Eur Urol 27 (Suppl 2):41–44

Frohmüller HG, Wirth MP (1993) Radical prostatectomy for carcinoma of the prostate: long-term results. Recent Results Cancer Res 126:43–49

Frohumüller HG, Wirth MP, Manseck A, Theiss M (1991) Selection criteria for radical prostatectomy with reference to long-term results. Urologe [A] 30:394–400

Gervasi LA, Mata J, Easley JD, Wilbanks JH, Seale Hawkins C, Carlton CE, Scardino PT (1989) Prognostic significance of lymph nodal metastases in prostate cancer. J Urol 142:332–336

Gibbons RP (1988) Total prostatectomy for clinically localized prostatic cancer: long term surgical results and current morbidity. NCI Monogr 7:123–126

Gibbons RP, Correa RJ, Brannen GE, Weissman RM (1989) Total prostatectomy for clinically localised prostatic cancer: long-term results. J Urol 141:564–566

Gleason DF (1988) Histologic grade, clinical stage and patient age in prostate cancer. NCI Monogr 7:15–18

Gleave ME, Goldenberg SL, Jones EC, Bruchovsky N, Sullivan LD (1995) Maximal biochemical and pathological downstaging requires 8 months of neoadjuvant hormonal therapy prior to radical prostatectomy (abstract). J Urol 153 (Suppl):392A

Godet DA, Knönagel H, Hauri D (1992) Endocrine treatment prior to radical retropubic prostatectomy in patients with T3 prostate cancer: a retrospective study of 22 patients. Urol Int 49:141–145

Goldenberg SL, Klotz LH, Jewett MAS et al. (1995) Randomized controlled study of neoadjuvant reversible androgen withdrawal therapy with cyproterone acetate in the surgical management of localized prostate cancer (abstract). J Urol 153 (Suppl):254A

Goldwasser B, Zincke H (1989) Modified Deschamps needle for securing dorsal vein complex and urethra during radical retropubic prostatectomy. Urology 33:324

Gomez CA, Soloway MS, Civantos F, Hachiya T (1993) Bladder neck preservation and its impact on positive surgical margins during radical prostatectomy. Urology 42:689–693

Graham SD, Keane TE, Petros JA, Sanders WH (1995) Perioperative hormonal therapy in locally advanced adenocarcinoma of the prostate. Cancer 75:1969–1971

Graverson PH, Nielsson KT, Gasser TC, Corle DK, Madsen PO (1990) Radical prostatectomy versus expectant primary treatment in stages I and II prostatic cancer. A 15 year follow-up. Urology 36:493–498

Greene DR, Wheeler TM, Egawa S, Dunn JK, Scardino PT (1991) A comparison of the morphological features of cancer arising in the transition zone and in the peripheral zone of the prostate. J Urol 146:1069–1076

Hanash KA (1992) Balloon pull-out or push-in technique for vesicourethral anastomosis. Urology 40:243–244

Harris M, Schow D, Renfer L, Rozanski T, Thompson I (1995) Morbidity and cancer control with radical perineal prostatectomy (abstract). J Urol 153 (Suppl):501A

Heggestad T, Jonsson PM, Danneskiold B, Leisti S (1993) Prostate cancer in Scandinavia. Variations in practice and attitude to radical treatment. Nord Med 108:104–106

Hellström M, Häggman M, Brändstedt S et al. (1993) Histopathological changes in androgen-deprived localised prostatic cancer. Eur Urol 24:461–465

Hrebinko RL, O'Donnell WF (1993) Control of the deep dorsal venous complex in radical retropubic prostatectomy. J Urol 149:799–801

Huland H, Hübner D, Henke RP (1994) Systematic biopsies and digital rectal examination to identify the nerve-sparing side for radical prostatectomy without risk of positive margin in patients with clinical stage T2, No prostatic carcinoma. Urology 44:211–214

Johansson JE, Andersson SO (1991) Deferred treatment in localized prostatic cancer. Acta Oncol 30:221–223

Johansson JE, Adami HO, Anderssson SO, Bergström R, Holmberg L, Krusemo UB (1992) High 10-years survival rate in patients with early, untreated prostatic cancer. JAMA 267:2191–2196

Jonsson E, Gibbons RP, Correa RJ, Weissman RM, Hafermann MD, Dail DH (1995) Postoperative radiotherapy for patients with clinically localized prostate cancer found to have pathologic stage C tumors (abstract). J Urol 153 (Suppl):501A

Kane JC, Narayan PA, Presti JC Jr (1995) Effect of adjuvant radiation therapy on urodynamic parameters of patients after radical retropubic prostatectomy (abstract). J Urol 153 (Suppl):384A

Keetch DW, Catalona WJ, Smith DS (1994) Serial prostatic biopsies in men with persistently elevated serum prostate specific antigen values. J Urol 151:1571–1574

Kennedy TJ, Sonneland AM, Marlett MM, Troup RH (1992) Luteinizing hormone-releasing hormone downstaging of clinical stage C prostate cancer. J Urol 147:891–893

Klein EA (1993) Modified apical dissection for early continence after radical prostatectomy. Prostate 22:217–223

Klein EA, Licht MR (1995) The impact of bladder neck preservation during radical prostatectomy on continence and cancer control (abstract). J Urol 153 (Suppl):383A

Leandri P, Rossignol G, Gautier JR, Ramon J (1992) Radical retropubic prostatectomy: morbidity and quality of life. Experience with 620 consecutive cases. J Urol 147:883–887

Lee F, Siders DB, Newby JE, Hugh TA, Solomon MH (1993) The role of transrectal ultrasound-guided staging biopsy and androgen ablation therapy prior to radical prostatectomy. Clin Invest Med 16:458–470

Lerner SP, Seale-Hawkins C, Carlton CE, Scardino PT (1991) The risk of dying of prostate cancer in patients with clinically localized disease. J Urol 146:1040–1045

Levy DA, Resnick MI (1994) Laparoscopic pelvic lymphadenectomy and radical perineal prostatectomy: viable alternative to radical retropubic prostatectomy. J Urol 151:905–908

Licht MR, Klein EA (1994) Early hospital discharge after radical retropubic prostatectomy: impact on cost and complication rate. Urology 44:700–704

Licht MR, Klein EA, Tuason L, Levin H (1994) Impact of bladder neck preservation during radical prostatectomy on continence and cancer control. Urology 44:883–887

Lowe BA, Barry JM (1990) The predictive accuracy of staging transurethral resection of the prostate in the management of stage A cancer of the prostate: a comparative evaluation. J Urol 143:1142–1144

Lowe BA, Listrom MB (1988a) Incidental carcinoma of the prostate: an analysis of the predictors of progression. J Urol 140:1340–1344

Lowe BA, Listrom MB (1988b) Management of stage A prostate cancer with a high probability of progression. J Urol 140:1345–1347

Maggio MI, Costabile RA, Foley JP (1992) Endoscopically controlled placement of urethrovesical anastomotic sutures after radical retropubic prostatectomy. J Urol 147:903–904

Marcucci PA, Fuselier HA, Bardot SF (1994) Optimal continence with bladder neck sparing radical prostatectomy (abstract). J Urol 151 (Suppl):254A

Mazeman A, Wurtz A, Gilliot P, Biserte J (1992) Extraperitoneal pelvioscopy in lymph node staging of bladder and prostatic cancer. J Urol 147:366–370

McCarthy JF, Catalona WJ, Hudson MA (1994) Effect of radiation therapy on detectable serum PSA levels following radical prostatectomy: early versus delayed treatment. J Urol 151:1575–1578

McFarlane MT, Abi-Aad A, Stein A, Danella J, Belldegrun A, deKernion JB (1993) Neoadjuvant hormonal deprivation in patients with locally advanced prostate cancer. J Urol 150:132–134

Memmelaar J, Millin T (1949) Total prostatovesiculectomy; retropubic approach. J Urol 62:340–348

Miller JI, Larson TR (1994) Simplified technique for improving exposure of the apical prostate during radical retropubic prostatectomy. Urology 44:117–118

Monfette G, Dupont A, Labrie F (1989) Temporary combination therapy with flutamide and tryptex as adjuvant to radical prostatectomy for the treatment of early stage prostate cancer. In: Labrie F (ed) Diagnosis and choice of therapy. Elsevier, New York, pp 41–51

Moore MJ, O'Sullivan B, Tannock IF (1988) How expert physicians would wish to be treated if they had genito-urinary cancer. J Clin Oncol 6:1736–1745

Morgan WR, Bergstralh EJ, Zincke H (1993) Long-term evaluation of radical prostatectomy as treatment for clinical stage C (T3) prostate cancer. Urology 41:113–120

Morton RA, Steiner MS, Walsh PC (1991) Cancer control following anatomical radical prostatectomy: an interim report. J Urol 145:1197–1200

Murphy WM, Soloway MS, Barrows GH (1991) Pathologic changes associated with androgen deprivation therapy for prostate cancer. Cancer 68:821–828

Myers RP (1989) Improving the exposure of the prostate in radical retropubic prostatectomy: longitudinal bunching of the deep venous plexus. J Urol 142:1282–1283

Myers RP, Larson-Keller JJ, Bergstralh EJ, Zincke H, Oesterling JE, Lieber MM (1992) Hormonal treatment at time of radical retropubic prostatectomy for stage D1 prostate cancer: results of long-term follow-up. J Urol 147:910–915

Narayan P, Lowe BA, Carroll PR, Thompson IM (1994) Neoadjuvant hormonal therapy and radical prostatectomy for clinical stage C carcinoma of the prostate. Br J Urol 73:544–548

O'Donnell PD, Finan BF (1992) Continence following nerve-sparing radical retropubic prostatectomy. J Urol 142:1227–1229

Oesterling JE, Andrews PE, Suman VJ, Zincke H, Myers RP (1993) Preoperative androgen deprivation therapy: artificial lowering of serum PSA without downstaging the tumor. J Urol 149:779–782

Ohori M, Goad JR, Wheeler TM, Eastham JA, Thompson TC, Scardino PT (1994a) Can radical prostatectomy alter the progression of poorly differentiated prostate cancer? J Urol 152:1843–1849

Ohori M, Egawa S, Shinohara K, Wheeler TM, Scardino PT (1994b) Detection of microscopic extracapsular extension prior to radical prostatectomy for clinically localized prostate cancer. J Urol 74:72–79

Ohori M, Dunn JK, Wheeler TM, Goto Y, Scardino PT (1995) Is there really a difference between peripheral zone and transition zone prostate cancer (abstract)? J Urol 153 (Suppl):517A

Optenberg SA, Thompson IM (1990) Economics of screening for carcinoma of the prostate. Urol Clin North Am 17:719–739

Parivar F, Fournier GR, Narayan P (1994) Urethral anastomotic healing after radical retropubic prostatectomy: impact on positive urethral margin. Urology 44:705–709

Parra RO, Andrus C, Boullier J (1992) Staging laparoscopic pelvic lymph node dissection: comparison of results with open pelvic lymphadenectomy. J Urol 147:875–878

Parra RO, Boullier JA, Rauscher JA, Cummings JM (1994) The value of laparoscopic lymphadenectomy in conjunction with radical perineal or retropubic prostatectomy. J Urol 151:1599–1602

Partin AW, Yoo J, Carter HB, Pearson JD, Chan DW, Epstein JI, Walsh PC (1993a) The use of PSA, clinical stage, and Gleason score to predict pathological stage in men with localized prostate cancer. J Urol 150:110–114

Partin AW, Borland RN, Epstein JI, Brendler CB (1993b) Influence of wide excision of the neurovascular bundle(s) on the prognosis in men with clinically localized prostate cancer with established capsular penetration. J Urol 150:142–148

Partin AW, Lee BR, Carmichael M, Walsh PC, Epstein JI (1994) Radical prostatectomy for high grade disease: a reevaluation 1994. J Urol 151:1583–1586

Pedersen KV, Lundberg S, Hugosson J, Aus G, Schelin S, Schain M, Ahlgren G, Abrahamsson PA (1995) Neoadjuvant hormonal treatment with triptorelin versus no treatment prior to radical prostatectomy: a prospective randomized multicenter study (abstract). J Urol 153 (Suppl):391A

Peller PA, Young DC, Marmaduke DP, Marsh WL, Badalament RA (1995) Sextant prostate biopsies. A histopathologic correlation with radical prostatectomy specimens. Cancer 75:530–538

Peretsman SJ, Seay TM, Wood DP (1994) Bladder neck biopsies during radical prostatectomy: incidence and implications of benign and malignant prostate tissue (abstract). J Urol 151 (Suppl):255A

Petros JA, Catalona WJ (1991) Antegrade approach to radical retropubic prostatectomy in patients with difficult apical dissection. J Urol 145:994–997

Petros JA, Catalona WJ (1992) Lower incidence of unsuspected lymph node metastases in 521 consecutive patients with clinically localized prostate cancer. J Urol 147:1574–1575

Petrovich Z, Lieskovsky G, Langholz B, Luxton G, Jozsef G, Skinner DG (1991) Radiotherapy following radical prostatectomy in patients with adenocarcinoma of the prostate. Int J Radiat Oncol Biol Phys 21:949–954

Prout GR, Heaney JA, Griffin PP, Daly JJ, Shipley WU (1980) Nodal involvement as a prognostic indicator in patients with prostatic carcinoma. J Urol 124:226–229

Ravery V, Boccon-Gibod LA, Dauge-Geffroy MC et al. (1994) Systematic biopsies accurately predict extracapsular extension of prostate cancer and persistent/recurrent PSA after radical prostatectomy. Urology 44:371–376

Reiner WG, Walsh PC (1979) An anatomical approach to the surgical management of the dorsal vein and Santorini's plexus during radical retropubic surgery. J Urol 121:198–203

Reiter RE, Wheeler T, Carlton CE, Scardino PT, Miles BJ (1995) Radical perineal versus retropubic prostatectomy in clinical T1c prostate cancer: a pathologic comparison (abstract). J Urol 153 (Suppl):501A

Robinow JS, Schild SE, Tomera KM, Wolfe JT, Buskirk SJ (1993) Postoperative prostate specific antigen levels in pathologic stage C adenocarcinoma of the prostate in patients treated with radical prostatectomy alone (abstract). Int J Radiat Oncol Biol Phys 27 (Suppl):228

Rosen MA, Goldstone L, Lapin S, Wheeler T, Scardino PT (1992) Frequency and location of extracapsular extension and positive surgical margins in radical prostatectomy specimens. J Urol 148:331–337

Rossignol G, Leandri P, Ramon J, Gautier JR (1992) Radical prostatectomy in the management of stage A carcinoma of the prostate. Eur Urol 21:269–273

Ruckle HC, Zincke H (1995) Potency-sparing radical retropubic prostatectomy: a simplified anatomical approach. J Urol 153:1875–1877

Rutishauser G, Hering F (1988) Lymph node staging in potentially curable prostatic carcinoma. Prog Clin Biol Res 269:227–236

Schnall MD, Imai Y, Tomaszewski J, Pollack HM, Lenkiski RE, Kressel HY (1991) Prostate cancer: local staging with endorectal surface coil magnetic resonance imaging. Radiology 178:797–802

Schröder FH, Belt E (1975) Carcinoma of the prostate: a study of 213 patients with stage C tumor treated by total perineal prostatectomy. J Urol 114:257–260

Schröder FH, van den Ouden D (1993) Rationale and results of radical surgery for prostatic cancer. Forum Trends Exp Clin Med 3:252–263

Schröder FH, Hermanek P, Denis L, Fair W, Gospodarowicz M, Pavone-Macaluso M (1992a) The TNM classification of prostate carcinoma. Prostate 4 (Suppl):129–138

Schröder FH, van den Ouden D, Davidson P (1992b) The limits of surgery in the cure of prostatic carcinoma. Eur Urol Update Series 1:18–23

Schulman CC, Sassine AM (1993) Neoadjuvant hormonal deprivation before radical prostatectomy. Eur Urol 24:450–455

Shinohara K, Scardino PT, Carter SSC, Wheeler TM (1989) Pathologic basis of the sonographic appearance of the normal and malignant prostate. Urol Clin North Am 16:675–691

Smith RC, Brendler CB, Partin AW (1995) Extended follow-up of the influence of wide excision of the neurovascular bundle(s) on prognosis in men with clinically localized prostate cancer (abstract). J Urol 153 (Suppl):392A

Solomon MH, McHugh TA, Dorr RP, Lee F, Siders DB (1993) Hormone ablation therapy as neoadjuvant treatment to radical prostatectomy. Clin Invest Med 16:532–538

Soloway MS, Hachiya T, Civantos F, Murphy WM, Gomez CC, Ruiz HE (1994) Androgen deprivation prior to radical prostatectomy for T2b and T3 prostatic cancer. Urology 43 (Suppl):52–56

Soloway MS, Sharifi R, Wood D, Wajsman Z, McLeod D, Puras A (1995) Randomized comparison of radical prostatectomy alone or preceded by androgen deprivation for cT2b prostate cancer (abstract). J Urol 153 (Suppl): 391a

Stamey TA (1995) Making the most out of six systematic sextant biopsies. Urology 45:2–11

Stamey TA, McNeal JE, Freiha FS, Redwine E (1988) Morphometric and clinical studies on 68 consecutive radical prostatectomies. J Urol 139:1235–1241

Stein A, deKernion JB, Smith RB, Dorey F, Patel H (1992) Prostate specific antigen levels after radical prostatectomy in patients with organ confined and locally extensive prostate carcinoma. J Urol 147:942–946

Steiner MS, Morton RA, Walsh PC (1991) Impact of anatomical radical prostatectomy on urinary incontinence. J Urol 145:512–515

Steiner MS, Burnett AL, Brooks JD, Brendler CB, Stutzman RE, Carter HB (1993) Tubularized neourethra following radical retropubic prostatectomy. J Urol 150:407–409

Sullivan L, Gleave M, Goldenberg L, Bruchovsky N, Jones EC (1994) Long-term neoadjuvant hormonal therapy prior to radical prostatectomy in localized prostate cancer (abstract). J Urol 151 (Suppl):435A

Terris MK, McNeal J, Freiha FS, Stamey TA (1993) Efficacy of transrectal ultrasound-guided seminal vesicle biopsies in the detection of seminal vesicle invasion by prostate cancer. J Urol 149:1035–1039

Têtu B, Srigley JR, Boivin JC, Dupont A, Monfette G, Pinault S, Labrie F (1991) Effect of combination endocrine therapy (LHRH agonist and Flutamide) on normal prostate and prostatic adenocarcinoma. Am J Surg Pathol 15:110–120

Turner R, Belt E (1957) A study of 229 consecutive cases of total perineal prostatectomy for cancer of the prostate. J Urol 77:62–77

Tveter KJ, Otnes B (1994) Radical treatment of localized prostatic cancer. Tidsskr Nor Laegeforen 114:162–165

van den Ouden D, Bentvelsen FM, Boeve ER, Schröder FH (1993) Positive margins after radical prostatectomy: correlation with local recurrence and distant progression. Br J Urol 72:489–494

van den Ouden D, Davidson PJT, Hop W, Schröder FH (1994) Radical prostatectomy as monotherapy for locally advanced (stage T3) prostate cancer. J Urol 151:646–651

Van de Voorde WM, Elgamal AA, Van Poppel HP, Verbeken EK, Baert LV, Lauweryns JM (1994) Morphological and immunohistochemical changes in prostate cancer after preoperative hormonal therapy. A comparative study of radical prostatectomies. Cancer 74:3164–3175

Van Poppel H, Baert L (1994) Clinical results of radical prostatectomy. Contrib Oncol 47:57–72

Van Poppel H, Van Uytsel L, Claes H, Baert L, van der Schueren E (1987) Late complications of multiple fraction radiotherapy for prostate cancer. In: Verhandlungsbericht der Deutschen Gesellschaft für Urologie. Springer, Berlin Heidelberg New York, pp 253–254

Van Poppel H, Ameye F, Oyen R, Van de Voorde W, Baert L (1992a) Neoadjuvant hormonotherapy does not facilitate radical prostatectomy. Acta Urol Belg 60:73–82

Van Poppel H, Ameye F, Oyen R, Van de Voorde W, Baert L (1992b) Radical prostatectomy for localized prostate cancer. Eur J Surg Oncol 18:456–462

Van Poppel H, Ameye F, Oyen R, Van de Voorde W, Baert L (1994) Accuracy of combined computerized tomography and fine needle aspiration cytology in lymph node staging of localized prostatic carcinoma. J Urol 151:1310–1340

Van Poppel H, De Ridder D, Elgamal AA et al. (1995) Neoadjuvant hormonal therapy before radical prostatectomy decreases the number of positive surgical margins in stage T2 prostate cancer. Interim results of a prospective randomized trial. J Urol 154:429–434

Varenhorst E, Berglund K, Lofman O, Pedersen K (1993) Interobserver variation in assessment of the prostate by digital rectal examination. Br J Urol 72:173–176

Villavicencio H, Laguna P, Ponce de Leon J (1994) Clinical impact of neoadjuvant treatment to radical prostatectomy in locally advanced prostatic cancer. Acta Urol Esp 18 (Suppl):404–408

Voges GE, Mottrie AM, Stöckle M, Müller SC (1994) Hormone therapy prior to radical prostatectomy in patients with clinical stage C prostate cancer. Prostate (Suppl)5P:4–8

Walsh PC (1987) Radical prostatectomy, preservation of sexual function, cancer control: the controversy. Urol Clin North Am 14:663–673

Walsh PC (1993) Editorial comment. J Urol 150:269

Walsh PC, Donker PJ (1982) Impotence following radical prostatectomy: insight into etiology and prevention. J Urol 128:492–497

Walsh PC, Jewett HJ (1986) Radical surgery for prostate cancer. Canceer 45:1906–1910

Walsh PC, Lepor H, Eggleston JC (1983) Radical prostatectomy with preservation of sexual function: anatomical and pathological considerations. Prostate 4:473–485

Walsh PC, Partin AW, Epstein JI (1994) Cancer control and quality of life following anatomical radical retropubic prostatectomy. Results at 10 years. J Urol 152:1831–1836

Weldon VE, Tavel FR (1988) Potency-sparing radical perineal prostatectomy: anatomy, surgical technique and initial results. J Urol 140:559–562

Weldon VE, Tavel FR, Neuwirth H, Cohen R (1995) Patterns of positive specimen margins and detectable PSA after radical perineal prostatectomy. J Urol 153:1565–1569

Wise HM, Fialk GS (1993) Instrument for ligation of dorsal vein complex in radical prostatectomy. Urology 41:476

Wolf JS, Shinohara K, Carroll PR, Narayan P (1993) Combined role of transrectal ultrasonography, Gleason score and PSA in predicting organ confined prostate cancer. Urology 42:131–137

Wolf MC, Montie JE (1994) Locally advanced cancer of the prostate: diagnosis and management. Current Opin Urol 4:261–265

Yamada AH, Lieskovsky G, Petrovich Z, Chen SC, Groshen S, Skinner DG (1994) Result of radical prostatectomy and adjuvant therapy in the management of locally advanced, clinical stage TC, prostate cancer. Am J Clin Oncol 17:277–285

Young H (1905) Radical perineal prostatectomy. Johns Hopkins Hosp Bull 16:315–321

Young HH (1945) The cure of cancer of the prostate by radical perineal prostatectomy (prostato-seminal vesiculectomy): history, literature and statistics of Young's operation. J Urol 53:188–256

Zimmern PE, Leach GE (1995) Nerve-sparing radical retropubic prostatectomy for localized prostate cancer. The pros and cons. Cancer 75:1944–1948

Zincke H, Utz DC, Taylor WF (1986) Bilateral pelvic lymhadenectomy and radical prostatectomy for clinical stage C prostatic cancer: role of adjuvant treatment for residual cancer and in disease progression. J Urol 135:1199–1205

Zincke H, Blute ML, Fallen MJ, Farrow GM (1991) Radical prostatectomy for stage A adenocarcinoma of the prostate: staging errors and their implications for treatment recommendations and disease outcome. J Urol 146:1053–1058

Zincke H, Oesterling JE, Blute ML, Bergstralh EJ, Myers RP, Barrett DM (1994) Long-term (15 years) results after radical prostatectomy for clinically localized (stage T2c or lower) prostate cancer. J Urol 152:1850–1857

10 Patterns of Failure in Surgically Treated Patients

H. Van Poppel, A.A. Elgamal, H. Goethuys, D. De Ridder, W.M. Van de Voorde, R.H. Oyen, and L. Baert

CONTENTS

10.1 Introduction

Radical prostatectomy is considered the treatment of choice for achieving local eradication of organ-confined prostate cancer. Nevertheless, many patients develop recurrent disease, either local or systemic, indicating that even when the disease has been locally eradicated, cure may not be obtained. In fact, "recurrent disease" is an incorrect term because most malignant disease after radical prostatectomy is not a relapse of malignancy but rather the progression of persistent disease that was already present at surgery. Therefore it is better to discuss failure of treatment rather than tumor recurrence after treatment.

Treatment failure on the basis of persistent disease can be diagnosed as local, systemic, or both local and systemic disease. With the use of prostate specific antigen (PSA) after radical prostatectomy another type of failure has been recognized, namely biochemical progression. PSA relapse-free survival is being widely used in studies assessing tumor control by surgery. On the other hand, increase in PSA after radical prostatectomy has created a new therapeutic dilemma in oncologic urology: there is still no consensus on how and when to treat positive margins, asymptomatic local recurrence, or metastatic disease after radical prostatectomy; consequently the treatment options for PSA relapse only, without evidence of local or systemic recurrence, are even more controversial.

10.2 Local Failure

The incidence of local "recurrence" after radical prostatectomy is difficult to estimate. Detection of local recurrence by digital rectal examination requires a long follow-up but early suspicion of local failure is raised by the use of PSA. In older series local failure rates, determined by digital rectal examination only, were estimated to be between 40% and 80%, while recent series report an incidence of local failure of 10%–30% (Zietman et al. 1993). Probably much of this difference is due to a longer postoperative follow-up in the older series. Nowadays, however, the use of PSA in the postoperative period has dramatically changed the follow-up strategy. Increase in PSA will force the urologist to look for local recurrence that is not yet clinically obvious. It is therefore very likely that a higher incidence of

H. Van Poppel, MD, PhD, Professor, Department of Urology, St. Pieter's Hospital, Catholic University of Leuven, Brusselsestraat 69, 3000 Leuven, Belgium
A.A. Elgamal, MD, Consultant Urologist and Research Fellow, Department of Urology, St. Pieter's Hospital, Catholic University of Leuven, Brusselsestraat 69, 3000 Leuven, Belgium
H. Goethuys, MD, Senior Resident, Department of Urology, St. Pieter's Hospital, Catholic University of Leuven, Brusselsestraat 69, 3000 Leuven, Belgium
D. De Ridder, MD, Consultant Urologist, Department of Urology, St. Pieter's Hospital, Catholic University of Leuven, Brusselsestraat 69, 3000 Leuven, Belgium
W.M. Van de Voorde, MD, PhD, Professor, Department of Pathology, University Hospitals (K.U. Leuven), Minderbroedersstraat 12, 3000 Leuven, Belgium
R.H. Oyen, MD, PhD, Professor, Department of Radiology, University Hospitals, Catholic University of Leuven, Herestraat 49, 3000 Leuven, Belgium
L. Baert, MD, PhD, Professor and Chairman, Department of Urology, St. Pieter's Hospital, Catholic University of Leuven, Brusselsestraat 69, 3000 Leuven, Belgium and Clinical Professor, Department of Urology and Radiation Oncology, University of Southern California, 1441 Eastlake Avenue, Los Angeles, CA 90033, USA

recurrence will be reported in the future as compared to former reports.

When a radical prostatectomy is performed, the surgical margins surrounding the prostate are only a few millimeters away from the gland. Indeed in the pelvis, the prostate is very closely surrounded by important structures, such as the rectum, the trigone, and the bony pelvis, that limit the extent of resection in healthy tissue. For this reason it was suggested that this operation be termed total rather than radical prostatectomy (EGGLESTON and WALSH 1985).

Local failure after radical prostatectomy with curative intent for clinically localized prostate cancer means that a certain number of cancer cells are (still) present in the pelvis after radical prostatectomy. Therefore, two kinds of local failure should be distinguished; the first should be called immediate local failure, relying on the presence of positive surgical margins, and the second, later local failure, this form of failure being present when a recurrent tumor is suspected because of an increase in PSA or because it can be palpated, visualized on an imaging study, or demonstrated on biopsy. All of these circumstances indicate that complete eradication of tumor has not been achieved by the surgery.

10.2.1 Margin-Positive Disease or Immediate Local Failure

Immediate local failure is identified by pathologic examination of the radical prostatectomy specimen showing a microscopic amount of residual tumor. This is illustrated by the presence of a positive surgical margin, where malignant glandular structures reach the border of resection. This identification process is facilitated by inking of the specimen after its removal.

10.2.1.1 Incidence

The increased popularity of radical prostatectomy for locally confined prostate cancer has dramatically increased the number of radical prostatectomies performed. Histologic examination of the resected specimen has become a routine practice and has increased the awareness of the presence of tumor invasion of the periprostatic tissue.

Positive surgical margins are often found in locally confined prostate tumors and are very common in locally advanced cancer. The incidence of positive resection margins differs widely between series, ranging from 10% to 69% (EGGLESTON and WALSH 1985; JONES 1990; STAMEY et al. 1990; ROSEN et al. 1992; ACKERMAN et al. 1993; EPSTEIN et al. 1993d). This wide range is most likely due to major differences in surgical indications for prostatectomy (T1/T2/T3), the use of different surgical techniques for prostatectomy (nerve sparing, non-nerve sparing, perineal, or retropubic), differences in pathologic stages (with or without capsular penetration), and different histologic preparation and evaluation of surgical specimens.

For prostate cancer clinically extending outside the capsule (cT3), more than 50% of radical prostatectomies performed by an expert urologist will end up with positive margins (MOUL and PAULSON 1991). In patients with cT2 organ-confined tumors this incidence is more than 30%, and for cT1 tumors it is ca. 20%. The incidence of positive margins is also related to the occurrence of seminal vesicle invasion and histologic grade of tumor (ROSEN et al. 1992; VAN DEN OUDEN et al. 1993). Our own pathology data on 213 radical prostatectomies showed positive margins in 22% of pT2 patients (25/114), 48% of pT3a–b patients (31/64), and 80% of pT3c–pT4a patients (28/35), all of these rates being comparable to data from the literature (Table 10.1).

The most frequent sites of margin-positive disease are the prostate apex (MCNEAL et al. 1990) and the posterolateral and lateral aspects of the gland, with a reported incidence varying between 15% and 60% (STAMEY et al. 1990; ROSEN et al. 1992; ACKERMAN et al. 1993; EPSTEIN et al. 1993d). Less often the bladder neck or the prostate base show positive resection margins, the reported incidence being below 15% (STAMEY et al. 1990; ROSEN et al. 1992; EPSTEIN et al. 1993d; BASLER et al. 1994). In nearly half of the patients positive margins are multifocal (FENDLER and PERRIN 1994).

Table 10.1. Pathologic outcome in 213 radical prostatectomy patients with regard to surgical margins

Pathologic stage	No.	Margin pos.		Margin neg.	
		No.	%	No.	%
pT2	114	25	22	89	78
pT3a–b	64	31	48	33	52
pT3c–pT4a	35	28	80	7	20
Total	213	84	39.4	129	60.6

10.2.1.2 Diagnosis

The assessment of the histopathologic evidence of margin-positive disease is not without controversy. It is widely recognized that the processing of the radical prostatectomy specimen is very important to the proper evaluation of the resection margins. The specimen should be fixed in formalin and coated with ink. The prostate should then be transversely sliced from the urethral margin to the bladder neck at 3- to 4-mm intervals. The tissue blocks can be further divided into halves or quarters but they should remain properly oriented. Whole mount specimen sections, which will, of course, better display the topography, are not really superior to sections mounted on standard-sized glass slides (COHEN et al. 1994). Particular care should be taken in the investigation of the apical margin since the apex is often invaded by the tumor and is not covered by the capsule. Correct processing by making separate radial slides of the amputated apex (AYALA et al. 1989) is necessary to properly recognize apical margin positivity and to avoid reporting positive margins in every patient with apical tumor extension. It is possible that the touch preparation cytologic examination of specimens will open up new opportunities in the assessment of margin-positive disease (PEARLE et al. 1994).

The pathologist will often have problems with the interpretation of surgical margins, especially in differentiating between margins that are negative, equivocal or focally positive. When the neoplastic glands are surrounded by an intact rim of prostate capsule or periprostatic tissue, the margin is undoubtedly negative. When, however, malignancy reaches the inked margin this can be due to the presence of artifacts. The periprostatic tissue is easily disruptable because of the desmoplastic reaction surrounding the prostate at the level of the tumor. Therefore, even when the surgical resection is done in healthy tissue, neoplastic cells may reach the margin because the healthy surrounding tissue is removed from the tumor during surgery or specimen handling (VAN POPPEL et al. 1992). Sometimes the urethral margin is made falsely positive because, after transection of the urethra, the urethral edge may retract in the prostatic apex.

All these considerations show that a positive surgical margin does not per se equal locally persistent tumor (EPSTEIN 1990). Close cooperation between an experienced pathologist and the urologist in examining the slides is the only guarantee of reducing the incidence of false-positive margins and thus avoiding overtreatment of patients who do not need any adjuvant therapy.

10.2.1.3 Significance

The finding of tumor at the resection margin after radical prostatectomy has been shown to be a predictor of local relapse (ANSCHER and PROSNITZ 1991; EPSTEIN et al. 1993a) and of PSA failure (CATALONA and SMITH 1994; D'AMICO et al. 1995). However, not all patients with positive margins will show tumor progression: some patients never have tumor progression. This may be due to misinterpretation of margin positivity (EPSTEIN et al. 1993d). As pointed out above, just because the margin is positive, this does not mean that cancer has been left behind (EPSTEIN 1990).

The degree of margin invasion in patients with capsular penetration can be classified as negative, equivocal, focal, extensive, or macroscopic. Resection margins are diagnosed as being negative when any amount of nonneoplastic tissue separates the inked surface of the prostate from the tumor. Equivocal margins are diagnosed when the surface of the prostate has a disrupted appearance and the tumor reaches the inked edge of the gland. Focal positive margins are present when tumor is found at the inked transected exterior surface but the involved sites are limited, being present in only one or two areas. Cases with extensive positive margins are those with multiple positive margins present at different sites of the prostate (EPSTEIN et al. 1993d).

It is important to distinguish between these different categories of margin status. Indeed, the amount of persistent tumor has been shown to be related to outcome and therefore different adjuvant treatment strategies may be warranted (EPSTEIN et al. 1993c,d; WALSH et al. 1994).

The significance of margin positivity also depends on its location. Positive margins at the lateral, basal, or posterolateral aspect and at the level of the prostate apex have been shown to have different outcomes. Although posterior and posterolateral positive margins obviously are related to tumor progression, positive margins at only the apex do not influence the time to progression (VAN DEN OUDEN et al. 1993; WELDON et al. 1995). In patients with a positive apical margin only, PSA relapse was shown to occur in less than 10% by FESSEHA et al. (1995). It is possible that this reflects the problem with the recognition of the apical margin.

In our experience positive margins also occur at the level of the anterior commissure and the anterior fibromuscular stroma, mainly in T1c tumors and in large transition zone cancers (ELGAMAL et al. 1995a). This kind of margin positivity has not been reported in the literature and its clinical significance is still uncertain.

Finally, recognition of the cause of margin positivity is also important. It is obvious that the outcome of a tumor with extracapsular extension (pT3) and a positive margin because of the local extent will be different from the outcome of a pT2 tumor that was intracapsularly transected by inadvertent opening of the prostate capsule during dissection of the posterior wall, e.g., in a nerve-sparing attempt (ROSEN et al. 1992).

Although a positive margin following radical prostatectomy should be considered as an independent risk factor for recurrence, its prognostic impact is strongly related to other poor prognostic factors such as seminal vesicle involvement, lymph node invasion, high Gleason score, and extracapsular extension (CATALONA 1993; EPSTEIN et al. 1993c). A multivariate analysis of clinical and pathologic factors which predict PSA failure after radical prostatectomy showed that in T3 cases with a Gleason score below 8 and without seminal vesicle involvement, the margin status is the strongest predictor of tumor progression, followed by the extent of capsular penetration (D'AMICO et al. 1995). Others have shown the influence of Gleason score and margin status on tumor progression. In patients with extensive extracapsular extension, who obviously bear a higher risk of progression than those with focal extracapsular extension, three groups of tumors have been identified (EPSTEIN et al. 1993c) with increasing risk of progression:

1. Negative margins and low tumor grade: excellent prognosis
2. Positive margins or high tumor grade: approximately 50% will progress
3. Positive margins and high tumor grade: ca. 75% will show progression.

10.2.1.4 Etiology and Prevention

Surgical margins may be positive in a radical prostatectomy specimen because of factors inherently related to the tumor (e.g., tumor stage, size, prostate architecture) but positive margins can also be due to surgery-related factors (e.g., nerve-sparing procedures, perineal or retropubic approach, and bladder neck-sparing operations).

10.2.1.4.1 Tumor-Related Factors. The most important tumor-related factor responsible for a positive surgical margin is the local tumor extent. It is well known that clinical T1 and T2 tumors will often prove to be pT3. When the extracapsular penetration is extensive, margin positivity is virtually certain.

Tumor volume is also predictive of positive margins (VOGES et al. 1992). We noted in our patients that even in transition zone cancers, often T1c tumors, careful pathologic examination showed positive margins, not at the posterolateral or lateral side but at the level of the apex or the anterior fibromuscular stroma (ELGAMAL et al. 1995a). In a total group of 213 radical prostatectomies we found 49 transition zone cancers, defined as having the index tumor located in the transition zone and having a Gleason score of ≤6. Five of these 49 tumors (10%) had a positive margin at the apex only. Their mean tumor volume was 7.8 cc (range 1.4–29.2 cc). Five other tumors (10%) had a positive margin anteriorly. The tumor volume ranged from 0.9 to 9.8 cc (mean 4.1 cc). The urologist has to be aware of the possibility of this type of positive margin in these patients, who often have T1c tumors.

It has recently been reported that neoadjuvant therapy for clinical T3 tumors may increase the number of positive surgical margins (whereas for clinical T2 tumors it decreases the number) (VAN POPPEL et al. 1995). This suggests that the clinically apparent regression of tumor induced by the hormonal treatment misdirects the surgeon from performing appropriate wider resection, resulting in positive margins (WALSH, 1993). Also when small glands are neoadjuvantly treated with hormones before radical prostatectomy, shrinkage of the gland could, instead of making surgery easier, render it more difficult (VAN POPPEL et al. 1992).

The performance of radical prostatectomy can be difficult in patients with very small prostates following very thorough transurethral resection that leaves behind only a small amount of tissue in the peripheral zone. This makes proper recognition of the apex difficult, which can result in laceration of the anterior commissure of the gland (RAMON et al. 1994).

Finally, the specific architecture of the prostate apex can be responsible for a risk of positive margin, when not correctly assessed during the operation. Indeed, benign prostatic hypertrophy can develop an anterior commissure and dissection of the apex is then more easy (MYERS et al. 1987). When an anterior notch is present, by virtue of the absence of glandular hypertrophy at the anterior apex, transection of the urethra at the level of the notch can cause a portion of the posterior apical prostate to be left behind. When the apex is invaded, as is very often the case, this will frequently lead to a positive resection margin (VAN POPPEL et al. 1992).

10.2.1.4.2 Surgery-Related Factors. Theoretically organ-confined tumors should never have positive margins because experienced surgeons should not make incisions into the prostate. Nevertheless, positive margins occur in pT2 tumors (MCMEAL et al. 1990). This is obviously due to inadvertent intracapsular dissection during a nerve-sparing attempt, which becomes a cancer-sparing operation. It has been shown that excision of the neurovascular bundles allows a significant reduction in the positive margin rate (ROSEN et al. 1992). Other authors, however, have found no difference in margin positivity in nerve-sparing versus non-nerve-sparing operations (JONES 1990; WAHLE et al. 1990; KILLEEN et al. 1991; VAN DEN OUDEN et al. 1993).

The problem of margin positivity caused by neurovascular bundle preservation is mainly related to the pathologic stage of the tumor. When a pT2 tumor is operated on in a non-nerve-sparing way, positive margins are not likely to occur. When a pT3 tumor is subjected to a similar treatment, positive margins will often occur. Therefore the discussion continues on how the cT2pT3 tumor can be recognized preoperatively or intraoperatively in order not to overemphasize the need for nerve preservation in these patients.

Some authors have proposed three prostate needle biopsies on the contralateral side of the T2 tumor (HULAND et al. 1994) or a tangential biopsy to identify perineural invasion on the ipsilateral side (BASTACKY et al. 1993). This is important in order to reduce the risk of positive margins with unilateral nerve preservation. On the other hand, men who undergo nerve-sparing radical retropublic prostatectomy will be at a higher risk for positive surgical margins. It is not clear whether a non-nerve-sparing radical prostatectomy confers a survival advantage (ZIMMERN and LEACH 1995). Recently, the follow-up in radical prostatectomy patients after wide resection of the neurovascular bundle(s) was updated. Initially, no survival benefit was found (PARTIN et al. 1993b). The 30-month follow-up, however, showed that wide excision of the bundles, in order to achieve negative surgical margins, does confer a sustained survival advantage (SMITH et al. 1995).

We currently propose nerve-sparing radical prostatectomy only in patients with T1 and T2a tumors. However, in T1 tumors one should be particularly careful: First, care must be exercised in the apical dissection, since nonpalpable transition zone cancers can often extend into the apex, and nerve preservation can result in a positive resection margin. Second, the control of the dorsal venous complex should be carried out cautiously in order to avoid margin positivity at the level of the anterior fibromuscular stroma. After section of the puboprostatic ligaments, the transection of Santorini's plexus is performed caudally and control of bleeding is done by transfixion sutures. For a small, clinically and ultrasonographically obvious intracapsular T2a tumor a bilateral nerve-sparing procedure may be performed. In larger T2a tumors only the contralateral bundle is preserved in order to reduce the probability of non-specimen-confined pT3 tumors.

It remains controversial whether retropubic or perineal prostatectomy carries more risk of positive margins. There could be an advantage in performing perineal prostatectomy to reduce the probability of positive apical margins (WELDON et al. 1995). However, other authors have not identified superiority of one over the other approach in reducing the incidence of positive margins (FRAZIER et al. 1992).

Preservation of the bladder neck in order to improve time to continence and avoid anastomotic strictures and ureteral damage during radical retropubic prostatectomy has been shown not to compromise the surgical margins (BASLER et al. 1994; LICHT et al. 1994). Among our radical prostatectomy patients, 150 underwent a bladder neck-sparing procedure. None of these patients had positive margins at the bladder base without having positive margins at another site. We believe that the bladder neck can be preserved during radical retropubic prostatectomy without increased risk of margin-positive disease.

10.2.1.5 Treatment Options

There is still no definite consensus on what should be done when surgical margins after radical prostatectomy are found to be positive. Indeed, just because the margins are positive, it does not necessarily mean that cancer is left behind. In patients with positive margins the pattern of failure has not been clearly identified (WALSH and EPSTEIN 1993).

When adjuvant treatment for positive margins is considered, one can choose between radiotherapy and hormonal treatment. Radiotherapy decreases the frequency of local recurrence (EISBRUCH et al. 1994); however, no impact on survival has been identified (LEE and HANKS 1995; COETZEE and PAULSON 1995), and randomized studies are required to demonstrate whether such a benefit accrues (BOLLA et al. 1994). Although our own experience with early adjuvant radiotherapy has been excellent with respect to the low incidence of complications, one should weigh the probable benefit of irradiation against possible complications such as incontinence, bladder neck contracture, and impotence. These issues are discussed in detail in Chaps. 11 and 20.

Hormonal treatment has not yet been shown to improve survival in patients with extracapsular extension or margin-positive disease (CHENG et al. 1993). At the present time no rationale exists for routine use of adjuvant hormonal treatment in patients with positive margins (BEYER et al. 1993).

10.2.2 PSA Failure and Local Recurrence

Locally persistent disease after radical prostatectomy is almost always microscopic and cannot be palpated or visualized on an imaging study in the immediate postoperative period. Therefore local "recurrence" will always be detected some time after the surgery, unless a macroscopic positive margin has been identified, reflecting an unacceptable inexperience in preoperative staging.

The use of PSA has dramatically changed the follow-up policy for detection of a locally persistent tumor. It is apparent that the sooner a local recurrence is detected, the better should be the outcome of an adjuvant local treatment.

Local recurrence, as reported in the literature, is usually detected within 5 years of surgery (MORTON et al. 1991). When local recurrence occurs later than 7 years after radical prostatectomy it is nearly always seen together with systemic progression (CATALONA et al. 1988).

In patients operated on for T1 and T2 prostate cancer the 10-year incidence of an isolated elevation of PSA was 23%, the incidence of systemic recurrence was 7%, and the incidence of local recurrence was 4% (WALSH et al. 1994). It is very likely that all patients with PSA relapse will ultimately progress and that many of them will do so not by local but by systemic recurrence.

10.2.2.1 Etiology

The etiology of local recurrence is nearly the same as that described for positive margins, including tumor- and surgery-related factors. It is presumed that when a true positive surgical margin is left untreated, with time it will become a clinically detectable recurrent tumor.

The predictors of local relapse after radical prostatectomy have been investigated by univariate and multivariate analysis. High Gleason score, seminal vesicle involvement, and positive margins were found by ANSCHER and PROSNITZ (1991) to be the most powerful predictors of local recurrence.

Another possible cause of local recurrence might be considered. Cytologic examination of the seminal and prostatic fluid that is expressed through the urethra during surgical manipulation for radical prostatectomy shows the obvious presence of malignant cells in patients with locally advanced tumors. It has been suggested that malignant cells shed during radical prostatectomy and seed the surgical bed and can be responsible for some instances of local tumor recurrence (ABI AAD et al. 1993; KASSABIAN et al. 1993). Although this mechanism of tumor relapse is difficult to prove, surgeons should keep it in mind in order to minimize the probability of seeding from this source.

10.2.2.2 Diagnosis

The most readily available tool to evaluate a patient for local recurrence is digital rectal examination (DRE). Local recurrence can be manifested by an induration or a nodularity in the prostatic fossa. DRE is, however, an unreliable early indicator of recurrent local cancer following surgery (LIGHTNER et al. 1990): Many transrectally palpable irregularities can be noted after surgery, making it difficult to distinguish recurrent cancer from benign scar tissue; furthermore, tumor will often be detected while the DRE remains unremarkable (WASSERMAN et al. 1992; FOSTER et al. 1993). Nevertheless, DRE is an important examination for the detection of gross tumor recurrence in the prostatic fossa and most clinicians continue to perform DRE in the serial assessment of postprostatectomy patients.

Transrectal ultrasonography (TRUS) has been used in the evaluation of patients with an elevated PSA after surgery. The sonographic visualization of a mass in the prostate bed or loss of integrity of the retroanastomotic fat plane has been shown to correlate strongly with recurrent or residual tumor (SALOMON et al. 1993). Indeed, some investigators have been able to detect recurrent lesions of less than 0.1 g, corresponding to an increase in PSA of 0.2–0.5 ng/ml (SANDERS et al. 1995). Nevertheless, TRUS after radical prostatectomy has a low sensitivity and specificity. Mature scar tissue is hypocellular and rich in collagen, having few acoustic interfaces, and thus appears on TRUS as a hypoechoic lesion in relation to the surrounding fat. This can make it very hard to distinguish such scar tissue from recurrent tumor (WASSERMAN et al. 1992), even though it has been clearly shown that more than 50% of proven recurrences are not hypoechoic but isoechoic (ABI AAD et al. 1992). Other investigators have found the appearance of the vesicourethral anastomosis after radical prostatectomy in patients with recurrence to be indistinguishable from that in patients without recurrent tumor (KAPOOR et al. 1993).

Whatever its limitations, TRUS can be a useful method to sequentially monitor the region of the urethrovesical anastomosis. Different features of the "neoanatomy" after radical prostatectomy have been described in postprostatectomy patients who are free of disease recurrence, such as anastomotic rings and anterior tissue nodules. Because of the distinct variations in the neoanatomy of different patients it is recommended that postoperative TRUS be performed early to establish a baseline image for each individual case. When the patient subsequently has an increase in PSA, TRUS-guided biopsy can be more accurately directed to suspicious areas, detected by comparison with the baseline study (GOLDENBERG et al. 1992). This follow-up policy for detection of early recurrence needs further confirmation.

In conclusion, TRUS has only a limited value as a screening tool for early recurrence after surgery. However, when recurrence is suspected, TRUS is useful in guiding biopsies of the vesicourethral anastomosis to obtain histologic confirmation of the tumor.

Other imaging techniques have also been used for early detection of local failure, though without success. Pelvic computed tomographic (CT) findings have been described. Local recurrence is very difficult to recognize on CT. Seminal vesicle-like soft tissue structures are routinely visualized and a horizontal bar of soft tissue is commonly demonstrated in the retrovesical space. These structures should not be confused with local tumor recurrence (SUMMERS et al. 1993). We do not expect that CT scan will ever be superior to TRUS in its ability to diagnose local recurrence. By contrast, rectal coil magnetic resonance imaging could perhaps become helpful (see Chap. 7 for more details).

Measurement of PSA has become an excellent tool for identification of tumor recurrence (BENTVELSEN et al. 1993). In theory, no circulating PSA should be present after radical prostatectomy when all prostatic tissue, benign and malignant, has been removed. The half-life of serum PSA is 2.2–3.2 days (STAMEY et al. 1987). This relatively long biological half-life requires a period of several weeks for the complete elimination of PSA from the serum after curative radical prostatectomy. Determination of serum PSA less than 1 month after radical prostatectomy is thus of limited value for the detection or exclusion of residual malignant disease (VAN STRAALEN et al. 1994). On the other hand, it has been suggested that the half-life of PSA elimination after radical prostatectomy could provide additional prognostic information for predicting outcome in patients who have undergone potentially curable radical prostatectomy (SEMJONOW et al. 1993).

The available assays display limited precision in the determination of very low PSA levels. Therefore a real zero reading is not possible at this time. The biologic detection limit is the lowest level of PSA measurable by the assay for which a high degree of confidence exists that PSA actually is present in the test serum (TAKAYAMA et al. 1993a). Recently, ultrasensitive PSA assays have been developed that can detect recurrent cancer up to 9–12 months earlier than the conventional assays (STAMEY et al. 1993; TAKAYAMA et al. 1993b; PRESTIGIACOMO and STAMEY 1994). The clinical value of even lower detection levels of PSA remains uncertain (FERGUSON and OESTERLING 1994).

Production of PSA is not limited to cells within the prostate. By means of immunohistochemistry we have identified prostate-specific markers in the accessory sex glands of Cowper, Littré, and Morgagni (ELGAMAL et al. 1994). The urinary PSA levels measured after radical prostatectomy indeed originate from the urethra (TAKAYAMA et al. 1994), and the first voided urine PSA level is not considered a useful marker to detect locally persistent or recurrent tumor (Iwakiri 1993). On the other hand, we have demonstrated that extraprostatic PSA production does not influence serum PSA levels (Elgamal et al. 1995b).

The rise in PSA or persistence of PSA above the detection level following radical prostatectomy is undoubtedly related to tumor persistence or recurrence. Therefore in general, when PSA remains at the detection level, no additional studies are necessary (Lightner et al. 1990). Actuarial PSA relapse rates demonstrate a quite consistent relapse rate over time (Montie 1994). The time interval between PSA that becomes detectable and identification of local or systemic recurrence is commonly greater than 5 years (Partin et al. 1993a). When the PSA becomes detectable within the first postoperative year, objective evidence of tumor progression occurs earlier than when PSA becomes detectable after 2 or 3 years following surgery. Despite these considerations, it should, however, be noted that exceptionally a patient will present local or disseminated disease despite undetectable PSA levels (Goldrath et al. 1989; Takayama et al. 1992).

When PSA remains or becomes detectable after radical prostatectomy, it may be expected that residual or recurrent prostate cancer is present, initially most frequently in the pelvis. As mentioned earlier, the efficacy of the available diagnostic tools in detecting the location of the residual or recurrent cancer is very low. Since adjuvant radiation therapy to the pelvis may be beneficial in patients with local recurrence, the distinction between local and distant recurrent disease becomes important.

Knowledge of PSA doubling time and PSA velocity can help in distinguishing local and systemic recurrence. A PSA doubling time of 6 months or less is indicative of metastatic disease (Danella et al. 1993; Trapasso et al. 1994; Fowler et al. 1995), and the exponential rise in PSA that occurs early in metastatic disease has been shown to be delayed by approximately 3 years in those with local recurrence. Furthermore, a PSA velocity of 0.75 ng/ml per year or less is associated with local recurrence (Partin et al. 1993c, 1994b). Therefore, a slow PSA rise after surgery suggests the presence of local recurrence whereas a fast rise suggests the existence of systemic disease.

When the PSA level, the PSA velocity, and the PSA doubling time all suggest the presence of a local recurrence, a TRUS-guided needle biopsy of the vesicourethral anastomosis can be proposed (Lightner et al. 1990; Abi Aad et al. 1992; Kapoor et al. 1993). Sometimes benign prostatic tissue found on biopsy may have been responsible for a low PSA level; this occurs when a part of the prostatic apex was left behind during inaccurate apical dissection (Foster et al. 1993). A sampling error cannot be ruled out when the biopsy shows benign glandular structures and these patients should be closely followed. Because of this sampling error it is still a matter of debate whether every patient with detectable PSA after radical prostatectomy should undergo biopsy.

10.2.2.3 Significance and Treatment Options

Once a locally persistent or recurrent cancer is presumed or clinically or pathologically confirmed, the therapeutic options can be discussed. Some urologists will offer adjuvant radiotherapy in patients with extraprostatic disease that is confined to the pathologic specimen with negative margins and is accompanied by an undetectable PSA. Others have advocated that no further treatment be given in these patients until rising PSA and obvious local recurrence occur. We believe, at the present time, that no rationale exists for categorical adjuvant treatment in patients with extracapsular disease (pT3) when margins are negative and PSA is at detection level (Beyer et al. 1993; Ozcan and Freiha 1995). It has been shown that progression in pT3 patients is mainly determined by the tumor grade and that adjuvant radiotherapy or hormonal treatment in these patients can decrease time to progression but cannot improve survival (Cheng et al. 1993). Others, however, have reported that the patients with pT3 tumors who are most likely to benefit from postoperative radiotherapy are those with initially undetectable PSA levels (McCarthy et al. 1994).

When no immediate adjuvant treatment has been given and the PSA rises, the interval between initial elevation of PSA and the clinical detection of failure has been reported by some to range from 2 to 28 months (Frazier et al. 1993), while other investigators have cited longer intervals of 3–7 years (Montie 1994; Paulson 1994). The latter authors felt that increase in PSA alone in patients clinically free of cancer may not be sufficient to justify treatment. They stated that disease recurrence as detected by PSA increase does not predict survival outcome, probably does not differentiate between local and distant microscopic recurrence, and is not predictive of biologic tumor aggressiveness.

While an isolated PSA elevation after radical prostatectomy in a patient who has undergone radical prostatectomy for a pT3 cancer can indicate systemic failure and lead to the consideration of early or delayed hormonal treatment, in a patient of a relatively young age we feel that adjuvant local treatment by radiotherapy is warranted. Unless the patient can be included in a randomized study comparing early versus delayed radiotherapy for isolated PSA increase, we do not agree with others that one should wait until evidence of persistent disease exists before starting radiotherapy (Gilson and Parra 1995). An increase in PSA after radical prostatectomy will always be followed by tumor recurrence and there is no need to withhold effective and well-tolerated therapy for local control because the tumor recurrence could be systemic. Most patients who receive radiation therapy to the pelvis for persistent PSA levels will show a PSA decrease that reflects local tumor response (Lee and Hanks 1995). In patients with previously undetectable PSA, an increasing PSA calls for pelvic irradiation which effectively decreases PSA in half of the cases by eradicating cancer in the postoperative tumor bed (Schild et al. 1994). Many patients will fail systemically even after radiotherapy but at least local problems may be avoided. All of these considerations suggest that treating patients before the development of a palpable local recurrence may improve treatment results; in particular, it may be expected to improve quality of life.

The role of hormonal treatment for local recurrence has never been well documented. The optimal timing of this therapy remains controversial, with some authors favoring early androgen deprivation for T3 cancers and others advocating expectant management guided by either PSA relapse or clinical evidence of metastatic disease. Currently, no definitive treatment recommendations can be offered. The timing and method of hormonal manipulation after radical prostatectomy in these patients should be highly individualized (Mayer and Crawford 1994).

10.2.2.4 Conclusions

Local recurrence is a common problem after radical prostatectomy, especially in patients with pT3 cancer which is not specimen confined. Most patients with PSA elevation after initial undetectable PSA following radical prostatectomy have residual disease in the prostatic fossa. Postprostatectomy radiation therapy to the prostate bed can essentially eliminate local recurrences as a pattern of failure without influencing systemic relapse. Further randomized studies will have to demonstrate how and when a PSA persistence, a PSA increase, and a local recurrence should be managed.

10.3 Systemic Failure

10.3.1 Etiology

Systemic failure after radical prostatectomy can be due to unrecognized disseminated disease at the time of surgery. The bone scan often will not show micrometastatic disease. The presence of systemic undetectable metastasis at the time of radical prostatectomy should be suspected in patients with high PSA levels and high Gleason scores. It should be highly suspected in those with seminal vesicle or microscopic pelvic lymph node involvement (pN+). Although it is difficult to refuse radical prostatectomy to a patient in whom no distant metastases can be found, it has been demonstrated that those with a PSA above 20 ng/ml and a Gleason score above 7 in the prostate puncture biopsy are unlikely to benefit from radical prostatectomy (van den Ouden et al. 1994).

Secondly, metastatic disease can originate in locally persistent tumor after radical prostatectomy, while at the time of surgery no metastases were present. Margin-positive disease can indeed be the focus from which recurrent tumor develops with metastatic potential. Also seeding of malignant cells from the prostate or seminal vesicles (Abi Aad et al. 1993; Kassabian et al. 1993) can be responsible for local recurrence that may subsequently metastasize. This mode of dissemination could be virtually prevented by postoperative adjuvant radiotherapy.

The third origin of distant failure is unrecognized nodal disease, which is widely known to indicate a disseminated tumor stage. The nodal status has been shown to be accurately assessable by CT scan and fine-needle aspiration cytology (Van Poppel et al. 1994), or by open or laparoscopic lymphadenectomy. However, the lymph nodes are not always assessed, e.g., when a perineal radical prostatectomy is planned, when patients have a very low PSA, or when the patient has had previous vascular reconstructive surgery in the pelvis. Obviously, positive lymph nodes can be missed by incomplete lymphadenectomy (either open or laparoscopic) or because the lymph nodes involved are not localized in the ilio-obturator fossa but in the presacral or pararectal area.

10.3.2 Diagnosis

A shorter PSA doubling time and a greater PSA velocity may be suggestive of metastatic spread rather than local recurrence (Danella et al. 1993; Partin et al. 1994a), but the definitive evidence of metastatic spread after radical prostatectomy is usually provided by a positive bone scan.

The interpretation of bone scans is difficult since in the radical prostatectomy patient population degenerative changes often can be seen and they can be misdiagnosed as metastatic disease. When a preoperative bone scan is available, comparison with a subsequent scan can greatly facilitate the recognition of metastatic disease. Therefore, not performing a bone scan in patients with a low PSA before radical prostatectomy is in our opinion not always a correct action.

Metastases from prostate cancer are mostly osteoblastic, involving preferentially the pelvis and sacrum and the axial skeleton. When lesions are seen on a bone scan, they should be confirmed by radiography and possibly CT or MRI. The bone scan is accepted as being the most sensitive examination for detecting skeletal tumor spread. If the PSA after radical prostatectomy is undetectable, the bone scan will almost never provide additional information (Terris et al. 1991; Miller et al. 1992).

Therefore bone scans should not be performed after radical prostatectomy in asymptomatic patients with undetectable PSA. When the PSA rises and the patient develops skeletal symptoms, a bone scan is mandatory. The problematic situation is when the PSA rises and the patient remains completely asymptomatic. In the absence of data on when to proceed to bone scans, we tend to wait in an asymptomatic patient until the PSA reaches levels above 20 ng/ml before requesting skeletal scintigraphy. However, we have recently seen a patient with a PSA of 8.5 ng/ml, without symptoms, who presented with sudden collapse of the first lumbar vertebra with paraplegia. We are not sure how such rare events can be avoided without performing unnecessary bone scans in many patients.

Finally, it is well recognized that when adjuvant hormonal treatment is administered after radical prostatectomy, the PSA level becomes an unreliable indicator of disease status (Ferguson and Oesterling 1994).

10.4 Conclusion

Margin positivity, PSA relapse, local recurrence, and metastatic spread after radical prostatectomy have become very important challenges in routine urologic practice. For most of these different patterns of failure, reliable data, guiding the urologist towards the optimal management, are often lacking. Randomized studies are currently underway or being designed in order to optimize the treatment strategy for individual patients. In practice many different acceptable treatment options can be proposed, and they need to be individualized and thoroughly discussed with the patient. All urologists should be encouraged to participate in serious multicenter clinical trials.

Acknowledgements. Special thanks are due to Mrs. Agnes Goethuys for her motivation and help in the outline, wordprocessing, and typing of the paper.

References

Abi Aad AS, MacFarlane MT, Stein A, deKernion JB (1992) Detection of local recurrence after radical prostatectomy by prostate-specific antigen and transrectal ultrasound. J Urol 147:952–955

Abi Aad AS, Noel H, Lorge F, Wese FX, Opsomer RJ, Van Cangh PJ (1993) Do seminal or prostatic secretions play a role in local recurrence after radical prostatectomy for localized prostate cancer? Eur Urol 24:471–473

Ackerman DA, Barry JM, Wicklund RA, Olson N, Lowe BA (1993) Analysis of risk factors associated with prostate cancer extension to the surgical margin and pelvic node metastases at radical prostatectomy. J Urol 150:1845–1850

Anscher MS, Prosnitz LR (1991) Multivariate analysis of factors predicting local relapse after radical prostatectomy – possible indications for postoperative radiotherapy. Int J Radiat Oncol Biol Phys 21:941–947

Ayala AG, Ro JY, Babaian R, Troncoso P, Grignon DJ (1989) The prostate capsule: does it exist? Its importance in the staging and treatment of prostate carcinoma. Am J Surg Pathol 1:21–27

Basler J, Figenshau R, Bullock A, McCarthy J, Arcangeli C (1994) Does bladder neck sparing radical prostatectomy improve continence or compromise margins of resection? J Urol 151 (Suppl):255A, abstract no 110

Bastacky SI, Walsh P, Epstein JI (1993) Relationship between perineural tumor invasion on needle biopsy and radical prostatectomy capsular penetration in clinical stage B adenocarcinoma of the prostate. Am J Surg Pathol 17:336–341

Bentvelsen FM, van den Ouden D, Schröder FH (1993) PSA in screening for recurrence following radical prostatectomy for localized prostatic cancer. Br J Urol 72:88–91

Beyer A, Leitenberger A, Altwein JE (1993) Adjuvant hormonal therapy following radical prostatectomy. Eur Urol 24 (Suppl):51–56

Bolla M, Gonzalez D, Van Tienhoven G et al. (1994) External irradiation and adjuvant hormonal treatment, and postoperative irradiation in prostatic carcinoma revisited. Rationale, trial design, eligibility criteria, statistical considerations. Contrib Oncol 47:111–123

Catalona WJ (1993) Editorial comment. J Urol 150:147–148

Catalona WJ, Smith DS (1994) 5 year tumor recurrence rates after anatomical radical retropubic prostatectomy for prostate cancer. J Urol 152:1837–1842

Catalona WJ, Miller DR, Kavoussi LR (1988) Intermediate term survival results in clinically understaged prostate cancer patients following radical prostatectomy. J Urol 140:540–543

Cheng WS, Frydenberg M, Bergstralh EJ, Larson-Keller JJ, Zincke H (1993) Radical prostatectomy for pathologic stage C prostate cancer: influence of pathologic variables and adjuvant treatment on disease outcome. Urology 42:283–295

Coetzee LJ, Paulson DF (1995) Does early adjuvant radiotherapy after radical prostatectomy in patients with margin positive disease hold any advantage over delayed radiotherapy at the first sign of treatment failure? J Urol 153 (Suppl):502A, abstract no 1093

Cohen MB, Soloway MS, Murphy WM (1994) Sampling of radical prostatectomy specimens. How much is adequate? Am J Clin Pathol 101:250–252

D'Amico AV, Whittington R, Malkowicz SB, Schnall M, Tomaszewski JE, Schultz D, Wein A (1995) A multivariate analysis of clinical and pathological factors which predict for PSA failure after radical prostatectomy for prostate cancer. J Urol 153 (Suppl):430A, abstract no 805

Danella J, Steckel J, Dorey F, Smith RB, deKernion JB (1993) Detectable PSA levels following radical prostatectomy: relationship of doubling time to clinical outcome. J Urol 149 (Suppl):447A, abstract no 938

Eggleston JC, Walsh PC (1985) Radical prostatectomy with preservation of sexual function: pathological findings in the first 100 cases. J Urol 134:1146–1148

Eisbruch A, Perez CA, Roessler EH, Locket MA (1994) Adjuvant irradiation after prostatectomy for a carcinoma of the prostate with positive surgical margins. Cancer 73:384–387

Elgamal AA, Van de Voorde WM, Van Poppel H, Lauweryns JM, Baert L (1994) Immunohistochemical localization of prostate specific markers within the accessory male sex glands of Cowper, Littré and Morgagni. Urology 44:84–90

Elgamal AA, Van de Voorde WM, Van Poppel H, Lauweryns JM, Baert L (1995a) Selective zonal distribution of tumor volume versus grade in T1c prostate cancer. J Urol 153 (Suppl):484A, abstract no 1024

Elgamal AA, Billen J, Van de Voorde WM, Van Poppel H, Blanckaert N, De Roo M, Baert LV (1995b) Extraprostatic sources of PSA, does it infer the subjective biochemical recurrence after radical prostatectomy? J Urol 153 (Suppl):518A, abstract no 1157

Epstein JI (1990) Evaluation of radical prostatectomy capsular margins of resection. The significance of margin designated as negative, closely approaching and positive. Am J Surg Pathol 14:626–632

Epstein JI, Carmichael M, Walsh PC (1993a) Adenocarcinoma of the prostate invading the seminal vesicle: definition and relation of tumor volume, grade and margins of resection to prognosis. J Urol 149:1040–1045

Epstein JI, Carmichael M, Partin AW, Walsh PC (1993b) Is tumor volume an independent predictor of progression following radical prostatectomy? J Urol 149:1478–1481

Epstein JI, Carmichael MJ, Pizov G, Walsh PC (1993c) Influence of capsular penetration on progression following radical prostatectomy: a study of 196 cases with long-term follow-up. J Urol 150:135–141

Epstein JI, Pizov G, Walsh PC (1993d) Correlation of pathologic findings with progression after radical retropubic prostatectomy. Cancer 71:3582–3593

Fair WR, Wang Y, Cohen D et al. (1995) Neoadjuvant androgen deprivation therapy in patients with clinically localized prostate cancer. Effect on positive margins and postoperative PSA. J Urol 153 (Suppl):313A, abstract no 337

Fendler J-P, Perrin P (1994) Positive margins and residual disease following radical prostatectomy: prediction and therapy. Curr Opin Urol 4:251–255

Ferguson JK, Oesterling JE (1994) Patient evaluation if PSA becomes elevated following radical prostatectomy or radiation therapy. Urol Clin North Am 21:677–685

Fesseha T, Pontes JE, Montie JM, Haas GP, Powell I, Crignon D, Sakr W (1995) Prognostic significance of a positive apical margin in radical prostatectomy specimens. J Urol 153 (Suppl):430A, abstract no 808

Foster LS, Jajodia P, Fournier G, Shinohara K, Carroll P, Narrayan P (1993) The value of PSA and TRUS guided biopsy in detecting prostate fossa recurrences following radical prostatectomy. J Urol 149:1024–1028

Fowler JE, Brooks J, Pandey P, Seaver LE (1995) Variable histology of anastomotic biopsies with detectable PSA after radical prostatectomy. J Urol 153:1011–1014

Frazier HA, Robertson JE, Paulson DF (1992) Radical prostatectomy. The pros and cons of the perineal versus retrograde approach. J Urol 147:888–890

Frazier HA, Robertson JE, Humphrey PA, Paulson DF (1993) Is prostate specific antigen of clinical importance in evaluating outcome after radical prostatectomy. J Urol 149:516–518

Gilson PG, Parra RO (1995) Prognosis of men with stage T3 prostate cancer: impact of early versus delayed adjuvant therapy. J Urol 153 (Suppl):239A, abstract no 44

Goldenberg SL, Carter M, Dashefsky S, Cooperberg PL (1992) Sonographic characteristics of the urethrovesical anastomosis in the early post-radical prostatectomy patient. J Urol 147:1307–1309

Goldrath DE, Messing EM (1989) PSA: not detectable despite tumor progression after radical prostatectomy. J Urol 142:1082–1084

Huland H, Hübner D, Henke RP (1994) Systematic biopsies and digital rectal examination to identify the nerve-sparing side for radical prostatectomy without risk of positive margin in patients with clinical stage T2,N0 prostatic carcinoma. Urology 44:211–214

Iwakiri J, Granbois K, Wehner N, Graves HC, Stamey T (1993) An analysis of urinary PSA before and after radical prostatectomy: evidence of secretion of PSA by periurethral glands. J Urol 149:783–786

Jones EC (1990) Resection margin status in radical retropubic prostatectomy specimens: relationship to type of operation, tumor size, tumor grade and local tumor extension. J Urol 144:89–93

Kapoor DA, Wasserman NF, Zhang G, Reddy PK (1993) Value of transrectal ultrasound in identifying local disease after radical prostatectomy. Urology 41:594–597

Kassabian VS, Bottles K, Weaver R, Williams RD, Paulson DF, Scardino PT (1993) Possible mechanism for seeding of tumor during radical prostatectomy. J Urol 150:1169–1171

Keetch DW, Catalona WJ, Smith DS (1994) Serial prostatic biopsies in men with persistently elevated serum prostate specific antigen values. J Urol 151:1571–1574

Killeen KP, Libertino JA, Sughayer MA, Lee AK, Watkins E (1991) Pathologic review of consecutive radical prostatectomy specimens. Urology 38:212–215

Lange PH, Ercole CJ, Lightner DJ, Fraley EE, Vessella R (1989) The value of serum PSA determination before and after radical prostatectomy. J Urol 141:873–879

Lee WR, Hanks GE (1995) Radiation therapy following radical prostatectomy. Cancer 75:1909–1913

Lerner SE, Blute ML, Eickholt JT, Bergstralh EJ (1995) Analysis of risk factors for progression in patients with pathologically confined prostate cancers after radical retropubic prostatectomy. J Urol 153 (Suppl):390A, abstract no 648

Licht MR, Klein EA, Tuason L, Levin H (1994) Impact of bladder neck preservation during radical prostatectomy on continence and cancer control. Urology 44:883–887

Lightner DJ, Lange PH, Reddy RK, Moore L (1990) PSA and local recurrence after radical prostatectomy. J Urol 144:921–926

Mayer FJ, Crawford ED (1994) The role of endocrine therapy in the management of local and distant recurrence of prostate cancer following radical prostatectomy or radiation therapy. Urol Clin North Am 21:707–715

McCarthy JF, Catalona WJ, Hudson MA (1994) Effect of radiation therapy on detectable serum PSA levels following radical prostatectomy: early versus delayed treatment. J Urol 151:1575–1578

McNeal JE, Villers AA, Redwine EA, Freiha SS, Stamey TA (1990) Capsular penetration in prostate cancer. Significance for natural history and treatment. Am J Surg Pathol 14:240–247

Miller PD, Eardley I, Kirby RJ (1992) PSA and bone scan correlation in the staging of monitoring of patients with prostate cancer. Br J Urol 70:295–298

Montie JE (1994) Follow-up after radical prostatectomy or radiation therapy for prostate cancer. Urol Clin North Am 21:673–676

Morton RA, Steiner MS, Walsh PC (1991) Cancer control following anatomical radical prostatectomy: an interim report. J Urol 145:1197–1200

Moul JW, Paulson DF (1991) The role of radical surgery in the management of radiation recurrent and large volume prostate cancer. Cancer 68:1265–1271

Myers RP, Goellner JR, Cahill DR (1987) Prostate shape, external striated urethral sphincter and radical prostatectomy: the apical dissection. J Urol 138:543–546

Ohori M, Egawa S, Shinohara K, Wheeler TM, Scardino PT (1994) Detection of microscopic extracapsular extension prior to radical prostatectomy for clinically localized prostate cancer. J Urol 74:72–79

Ohori M, Dunn JK, Wheeler TM, Goto Y, Scardino PT (1995) Is there really a difference between peripheral zone and transition zone prostate cancer? J Urol 153 (Suppl):517A, abstract no 1153

Ozcan F, Freiha F (1995) Causes of failure of radical retropubic prostatectomy. J Urol 153 (Suppl):429A, abstract no 804

Partin AW, Pound CR, Clemens JQ, Epstein JI, Walsh PC (1993a) Serum PSA after anatomic radical prostatectomy. The Johns Hopkins experience after 10 years. Urol Clin North Am 20:713–725

Partin AW, Borland RN, Epstein JI, Brendler CB (1993b) Influence of wide excision of the neurovascular bundle(s) on the prognosis in men with clinically localized prostate cancer with established capsular penetration. J Urol 150:142–148

Partin A, Pearson J, Pound C, Clemens Q, Epstein J, Chan D, Walsh P (1993c) Rate of change of serum PSA after radical prostatectomy distinguishes local recurrence from distant metastases. J Urol 149 (Suppl):447A, abstract no 937

Partin AW, Lee BR, Carmichael M, Walsh PC, Epstein JI (1994a) Radical prostatectomy for high grade disease: a reevaluation, 1994. J Urol 151:1583–1586

Partin AW, Pearson JD, Landis PK et al. (1994b) Evaluation of PSA velocity after radical prostatectomy to distinguish local recurrence from distant metastases. Urology 43:649–659

Paulson DF (1994) Impact of radical prostatectomy in the management of clinically localized disease. J Urol 152:1826–1830

Pearle MS, Oyasu R, Hidvegi D et al. (1994) Touch preparation cytological examination of radical prostatectomy. J Urol 152:124–128

Prestigiacomo AF, Stamey JA (1994) A comparison of 4 ultrasensitive PSA assays for early detection of residual cancer after radical prostatectomy. J Urol 152:1515–1519

Ramon J, Rossignol G, Leandri P, Gautier JR (1994) Morbidity after radical retropubic prostatectomy following previous prostate resection. J Surg Oncol 55:14–19

Ravery V, Boccon-Gibod LA, Dauge-Geffroy MC et al. (1994) Systematic biopsies accurately predict extracapsular extension of prostate cancer and persistent/recurrent PSA after radical prostatectomy. Urology 44:371–376

Rosen MA, Goldstone L, Lapin S, Wheeler T, Scardino PT (1992) Frequency and location of extracapsular extension and positive surgical margins in radical prostatectomy specimens. J Urol 148:331–337

Salomon CG, Flisak ME, Olson MC, Dudiak CM, Flanigan RC, Waters WB (1993) Radical prostatectomy: transrectal sonographic evaluation to assess for local recurrence. Radiology 189:713–719

Sanders WH, Cooner WH, Woodward M, Graham SD (1995) Detection of local recurrence after radical prostatectomy. J Urol 153 (Suppl):518A, abstract no 1159

Schild SE, Wong WW, Grado GL, Buskirk SJ, Robinow JS, Frick LM, Ferrigni RG (1994) Radiotherapy for isolated increases in serum PSA levels after radical prostatectomy. Mayo Clin Proc 69:613–619

Semjonow A, Hamm M, Rathert P (1993) Prediction of tumor recurrence after radical prostatectomy using elimination kinetics of PSA. World J Urol 11:218–220

Smith RC, Brendler CB, Partin AW (1995) Extended follow-up of the influence of wide excision of the neurovascular bundle(s) on prognosis in men with clinically localized prostate cancer. J Urol 153 (Suppl):392A, abstract no 654

Stamey TA, Yang N, Hay AR, McNeal JE, Freiha FS, Redwine E (1987) PSA as a serum marker for adenocarcinoma of the prostate. N Engl J Med 317:909–1002

Stamey TA, Villers AA, McNeal JE, Link PC, Freiha FS (1990) Positive surgical margins at radical prostatectomy: importance of the apical dissection. J Urol 143:1166–1173

Stamey TA, Graves HC, Wehner N, Ferrari M, Freiha FS (1993) Early detection of residual prostate cancer after radical prostatectomy by an ultrasensitive assay for prostate specific antigen. J Urol 149:787–792

Summers RM, Korobkin M, Quint LE, Ellis JE, Grossman HB, Sandler HM, Mandell SH (1993) Pelvic computer tomography findings after radical prostatectomy. J Comput Assist Tomogr 17:767–771

Takayama TK, Krieger JN, True LD, Lange PH (1992) Recurrent prostate cancer despite undetectable PSA. J Urol 148:1541–1542

Takayama TK, Vessella RL, Brawer MK, Noteboom K, Lange PH (1993a) The enhanced detection of persistent disease

after prostatectomy with a new PSA immunoassay. J Urol 150:374–378
Takayama TK, Vessella RL, Lange PH (1993b) A brief review of ultrasensitive PSA assays for the evaluation of patients after radical prostatectomy. World J Urol 11:192–195
Takayama TK, Vessella RL, Brawer MK, True LD, Noteboom J, Lange PH (1994) Urinary prostate specific antigen after radical prostatectomy. J Urol 151:82–87
Terris MK, Klonecke AS, McDougall IR, Stamey TA (1991) Utilization of bone scans in conjunction with prostate specific antigen levels in the surveillance for recurrence of adenocarcinoma after radical prostatectomy. J Nucl Med 32:1713–1717
Trapasso JG, deKernion JB, Smith RB, Dorey F (1994) The incidence and significance of detectable levels of serum prostate specific antigen after radical prostatectomy. J Urol 152:1821–1825
van den Ouden D, Bentvelsen FM, Boeve ER, Schröder FH (1993) Positive margins after radical prostatectomy: correlation with local recurrence and distant progression. Br J Urol 72:489–494
van den Ouden D, Davidson PJT, Hop W, Schröder FH (1994) Radical prostatectomy as monotherapy for locally advanced (stage T3) prostate cancer. J Urol 151:646–651
Van Poppel H, Baert L (1994) Clinical results of radical prostatectomy. Contrib Oncol 47:57–72
Van Poppel H, Ameye F, Oyen R, Van de Voorde WM, Baert L (1992) Radical prostatectomy for localized prostate cancer. Eur J Surg Oncol 18:456–462
Van Poppel H, Ameye F, Oyen R, Van de Voorde WM, Baert L (1994) Accuracy of combined computerized tomography and fine needle aspiration cytology in lymph node staging of localized prostatic carcinoma. J Urol 151:1310–1340
Van Poppel H, De Ridder D, Elgamal AA et al. (1995) Neoadjuvant hormonal therapy before radical prostatectomy decreases the number of positive surgical margins in stage T2 prostate cancer. Interim results of a prospective randomized trial. J Urol 154:429–434
Van Straalen JP, Bossems MM, de Reyke TM, Sanders GT (1994) Biological half-life of prostate specific antigen after radical prostatectomy. Eur J Clin Chem Chim Clin Biochem 32:53–55
Voges GE, McNeal JE, Redwine EA, Freiha FS, Stamey TA (1992) Morphological analysis of surgical margins with positive findings in prostatectomy for adenocarcinoma of the prostate. Cancer 69:520–526
Wahle S, Reznicek M, Fallon B, Platz C, Williams R (1990) Incidence of surgical margin involvement in various forms of radical prostatectomy. Urology 36:23–26
Walsh PC (1993) Editorial comment. J Urol 150:269
Walsh PC, Epstein JI (1993) Radical prostatectomy and positive surgical margins: when, where and what to do? In: Murphy G, Khoury S, Chatelain C, Denis L (eds) Proceedings 4th International Symposium on Recent Advances in Urological Cancer. Diagnosis and Treatment. Scientific Communication International, Jersey, pp 199–207
Walsh PC, Partin AW, Epstein JI (1994) Cancer control and quality of life following anatomical radical retropubic prostatectomy. Results at 10 years. J Urol 152:1831–1836
Wasserman NF, Kapoor DA, Hildebrandt WC, Zhang G, Born KM, Eppel SM, Reddy PK (1992) Transrectal ultrasound in evaluation of patients after radical prostatectomy. II. Transrectal ultrasound and biopsy findings in the presence of residual and early recurrent prostatic cancer. Radiology 185:367–372
Weldon VE, Tavel FR, Neuwirth H, Cohen R (1995) Patterns of positive specimen margins and detectable PSA after radical perineal prostatectomy. J Urol 153:1565–1569
Zietman AL, Shipley WU, Willet CG (1993) Residual disease after surgery or radiation therapy for prostate cancer: clinical significance and therapeutic implications. Cancer 71:959–969
Zimmern PE, Leach GE (1995) Nerve-sparing radical retropubic prostatectomy for localized prostate cancer. The pros and cons. Cancer 75:1944–1948

11 Complications of Radical Prostatectomy

L. Baert, A.A. Elgamal, and H. Van Poppel

CONTENTS

11.1 Introduction

The pattern of care of localized prostate cancer (CaP) has been undergoing a significant change in recent years, in that there has been a sharp increase in the use of radical prostatectomy for the treatment of newly diagnosed localized CaP (Mettlin et al. 1994). Innovations in surgical technique (Walsh 1992) and methods for the early detection of localized CaP (Catalona et al. 1994; Brawer et al. 1992; Stamey 1992) have led to the current low incidence of operative mortality and morbidity.

Since CaP is a disease of older men, the improvement in social and medical care during the period following the Second World War might have impacted on the number of men at risk of this disease in the United States and Western Europe. Today, CaP is an increasingly important health issue in all developed and developing countries since at least 149 000 deaths per annum throughout the world are caused by this disease (Pisani et al. 1993). It has become the most common internal cancer and the second leading cause of cancer-related death in men in the United States. It has been estimated that more than 200 000 new patients were diagnosed with CaP in the United States in 1994 and that 38 000 patients died of this disease in the same year (Boring et al. 1994).

In the European Community (EC) an estimated 85 000 new CaP cases are diagnosed every year. This incidence represents 13% of all cancers in men and has been responsible for 9% of all cancer deaths among men in the EC. The highest estimated incidence of CaP has been seen in Germany, France, Belgium, and The Netherlands (Jensen et al. 1990). In a more recent report, Esteve et al. (1993) estimated the number of new CaP cases and deaths in the EC during 1990 to be 76 100 and 44 600, respectively. In England and Wales, the most recent report showed 10 837 new cases of CaP to have been diagnosed in 1987, resulting in 8570 CaP deaths (Dearnaley 1993). This small difference between mortality rates and the estimated incidence rates of CaP in the EC as compared to the United States might reflect more efficient management of this disease in North America. This improved management of CaP has resulted in a marked improvement in the incidence of tumor control during the past 10 years in the United States (Catalona and Smith 1994; Murphy et al. 1994; Ohori et al. 1994; Walsh et al. 1994; Zincke et al. 1994). It has been widely accepted that CaP will cause the death of 3% of all men alive today who are now >50 years of age. This trend is taking place while mortality from other causes is declining. Even among those patients who do not die of CaP, many will suffer serious complications from local tumor growth or the presence of distant metastases. Therefore, as the general health of the population improves and its longevity increases, the argument for early cancer detection and the need for aggressive treatment of local disease is strengthened (Dearnaly 1993; Scardino 1995; Walsh 1994).

L. Baert, MD, PhD, Professor and Chairman Department of Urology, St. Pieter's Hospital, Catholic University of Leuven, Brusselsestraat 69, 3000 Leuven, Belgium and Clinical Professor, Department of Urology and Radiation Oncology, University of Southern California, 1441 Eastlake Avenue, Los Angeles, CA 90033, USA
A.A. Elgamal, MD, Consultant Urologist and Research Fellow, Department of Urology, St. Pieter's Hospital, Catholic University of Leuven, Brusselsestraat 69, 3000 Leuven, Belgium
H. van Poppel, MD, PhD, Professor, Department of Urology, St. Pieter's Hospital, Catholic University of Leuven, Brusselsestraat 69, 3000 Leuven, Belgium

In this chapter we address our experience with the management of complications of radical prostatectomy in patients with CaP. We strongly believe that radical prostatectomy is the gold standard treatment for patients with localized CaP who are fit for surgery and have a life expectancy of at least 10 years. We will correlate this experience with the incidence of complications of radical prostatectomy published in the recent literature.

Earlier methods used in CaP detection and older techniques of radical prostatectomy presented considerable problems (Boxer et al. 1977; Campbell et al. 1963; Jewett 1980; Middleton 1977; Veenema et al. 1977; Yong 1945). Therefore, the reports on the relatively high morbidity and mortality which were seen following radical prostatectomy in the past are only of historical value and have little relationship to the presently obtained treatment outcomes with the use of this procedure. Contemporary diagnostic modalities have been responsible for the detection of a larger proportion of patients with localized CaP who in turn are more eligible for radical surgery. Moreover, the contemporary anatomic radical retropubic prostatectomy is a better surgical technique than those used previously. Even during the past decade, each major surgical center has experienced a learning curve in mastering the techniques of radical prostatectomy. This has resulted in a significant improvement in the final surgical outcomes (Andriole et al. 1994; Walsh et al. 1994; Zincke et al. 1994).

11.2 Contemporary Mortality

In a recent analysis of 7052 Medicare claim records in the United States in patients who underwent radical prostatectomy in 1990, the 30-day mortality was 0.5% and the 1-year all-cause mortality, 1.8%. These results represented one-half of the expected mortality rates following this procedure and were close to the estimated mortality rates of elderly (65 years or older) men in excellent health who were not treated with radical prostatectomy. Such treatment outcomes clearly demonstrate the improved perioperative survival for prostatectomy-treated patients compared to the published data for prior years. Furthermore, they tend to support the use of radical prostatectomy rather than watchful waiting in healthier patients (Mark 1994). In another report which represented a 100% national sample, the mortality rates in 1059 younger men (≤65 years old) following radical prostatectomy were shown to be 0.28% at 30 and 90 days, 1.02% at 1 year, 1.95% at 2 years, 3.14% at 3 years, and 4.64% at 4 years. These were less than one-half of the expected mortality rates seen in the general population in the United States (Optenberg et al. 1995). On the other hand, the compiled data in the literature from 1980 show the 10-year disease-specific survival in clinically localized CaP treated with radical prostatectomy, external beam radiation therapy, and deferred treatment to have been 93%, 74%, and 83%, respectively. This indicates the presence of a significant mortality and marginal benefit from radical prostatectomy at 10 years posttreatment. The same data indicated an advantage of radical prostatectomy over deferred therapy at 15 years posttreatment (Adolfsson et al. 1993). Moreover, in a survey of major institutions, including Baylor College of Medicine, Johns Hopkins School of Medicine, Stanford University, and Washington University, the mortality from pelvic lymphadenectomy and radical retropubic prostatectomy in a total of 3574 patients operated on between 1982 and 1992 was just 0.1% (Scardino 1995). Recently, the 30-day mortality in a total of 3170 consecutive patients treated with radical prostatectomy at the Mayo Clinic over the past decade for clinically localized CaP was reported to be 0.3%, and the figure was in fact 0% for the 1728 patients who underwent surgery at that center in 1988 or later (Zincke et al. 1994).

11.3 Contemporary Morbidity

The introduction of an anatomic approach to radical retropubic prostatectomy has brought several important advantages over previously used operative techniques. These include a decrease in intraoperative blood loss due to better control of the dorsal vein complex and the preservation of the neurovascular bundles (Reiner and Walsh 1979; Walsh et al. 1983; Walsh 1992). Additionally, limiting pelvic lymphadenectomy to the inferior margin of the external iliac vein has decreased the early postoperative morbidity while maintaining the accuracy of nodal staging (Paulson 1980). In fact, contemporary radical retropubic prostatectomy offers the properly selected patient the greatest chance for tumor control with a low probability of major dysfunction (Andriole et al. 1994; Bahanson and Catalona 1990; Leandri et al. 1992; Scardino 1995; Seidmon 1993; Walsh 1992; Yamada et al. 1994; Zincke et al. 1994). At present there is a tendency to offer radical prostatectomy to a carefully selected group of older patients, including those in the 8th decade of life, in whom use of the procedure would, in the past, have compromised life expectancy (ANDIOLE et al. 1994; CORRAL and BAHANSON 1994; MIDDLETON 1987). Radical prostatectomy is currently being successfully performed even in patients with significant cardiovascular disease or in those who have had renal transplantation (KINAHAN et al. 1991; CIANCIO et al. 1995). Nevertheless, no optimal treatment exists, in that once CaP is diagnosed and treated, whether by surgery, irradiation, or observation, the patient's quality of life is necessarily and permanently altered. Even if he is thought to be cured, his level of functioning may be diminished due to specific complications of treatment, such as impotence, urinary incontinence, or bowel dysfunction, or negative psychological and economic consequences from having cancer (LITWIN et al. 1995). It is of importance to note, however, that clinicians managing CaP have a major responsibility to improve the outcome of the recommended treatment, which is carefully selected according to patient status.

The rationale for radical prostatectomy is based on the following observations (SCARDINO 1995; WALSH 1994):

1. CaP kills.
2. Clinically detected cancer progresses slowly, but inevitably.
3. CaP is unlikely to be cured once it extends beyond the periprostatic tissue.
4. Treatment is effective if the cancer is detected early.
5. Treatment should be safe.

The most common complications that might follow contemporary retropubic radical prostatectomy are: intraoperative bleeding, rectal injury, early postoperative pain, postoperative hemorrhage, catheter loss, urinary or lymphatic leakage, prolonged hospitalization, urethral stricture, incontinence, impotence, and infertility. There are some other general complications that are not specifically related to the type of surgical procedure used, such as: complications of anesthesia, blood transfusion-related complications, bowel dysfunction, wound and chest infection, thromboembolic disease, and cardiovascular complications.

We have analyzed our experience in 350 consecutive patients treated with radical retropubic prostatectomy between June 1989 and May 1995. Of these 350 patients, 79% had clinically localized CaP (≤T2) and 21% had locally advanced tumors (≥T3). For the purpose of this study we used the modified TNM classification (Fig. 11.1). The treatment included 57 patients who received preoperative neoadjuvant hormonal therapy, mainly in the form of oral estramustine phosphate for 6 weeks or flutamide for 3 months (for details see VAN DE

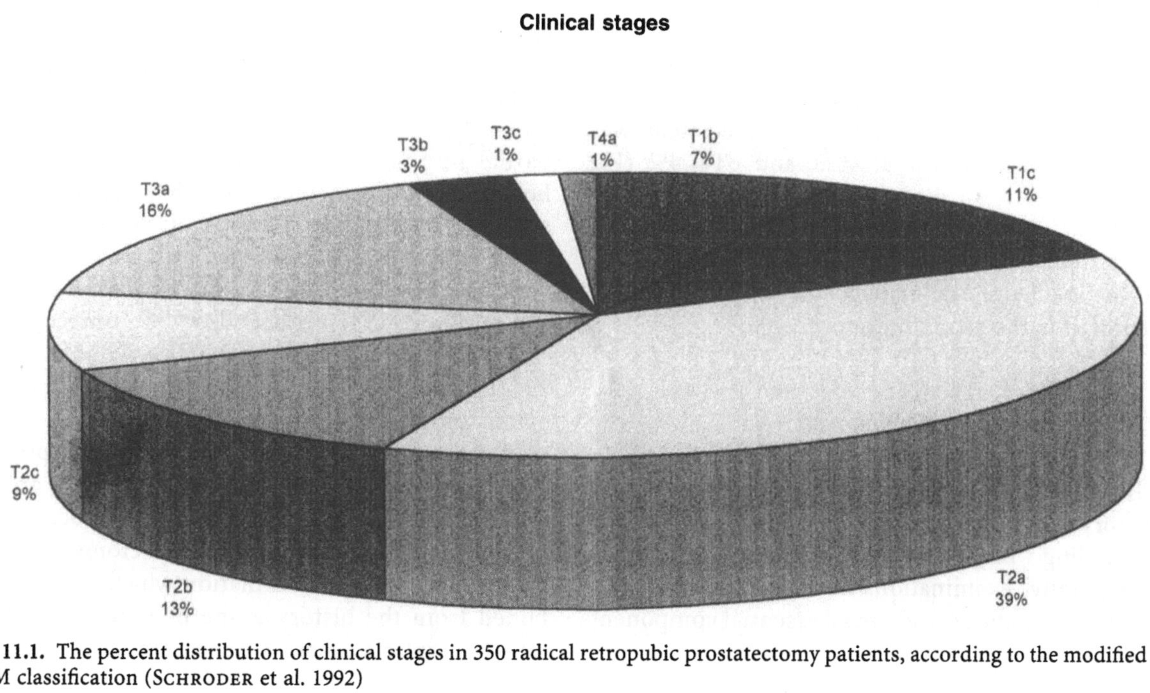

Fig. 11.1. The percent distribution of clinical stages in 350 radical retropubic prostatectomy patients, according to the modified TNM classification (SCHRODER et al. 1992)

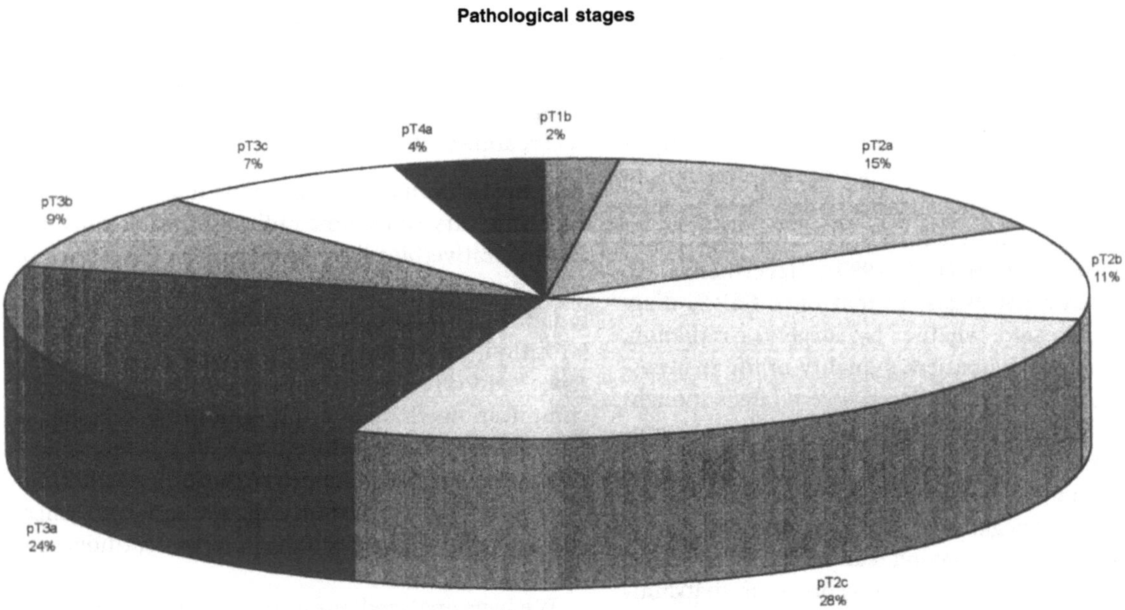

Fig. 11.2. The percent distribution of pathologic stages in radical prostatectomy specimens examined by the whole-organ multiple step sections technique

VOORDE et al. 1994). The mean age of the patients was 62.3 years, and the mean prostate specific antigen (PSA) serum level was 14.0 ng/ml with a median of 8.1 ng/ml using the Tandem-R Hybritech assay. The mean and median duration of surgical procedure was 137 and 120 min, respectively. While the mean and median duration of total hospital stay was 19 and 19 days, respectively. Beginning in 1991, all radical prostatectomy specimens have been examined by the whole-organ multiple step sections technique (for details see Chap. 4). The distribution of final pathologic stages of these specimens was: pT1, 2%; pT2, 53%; pT3, 40%; and pT4, 4% (Fig. 11.2).

Below we report on the incidence and management of each particular complication and compare it to the incidence and management of complications reported in the recent literature.

11.3.1 Preoperative Management

The patient's history, currently used medications, history of any allergy, the patient's general condition (including physical and mental status) and preoperative examinations that confirm the absence of extraprostatic spread are all essential components of preoperative evaluation.

In this series, as in other reports (VAN POPPEL et al. 1994), the clinical staging of CaP has been routinely assessed by: PSA serum level, digital rectal examination (DRE), transrectal ultrasonography (TRUS), core needle prostate puncture biopsy (PPB), whether TRUS guided or systematic, pelvic computerized axial tomography (CT) to exclude the presence of lymphadenopathy, and bone scintigraphy to exclude bone metastasis (with tomography used for equivocal lesions). Laboratory investigations have included: hemoglobin and hematocrit, complete blood count, bleeding time, prothrombin time (PT), partial thromboplastin time (PTT), and renal and hepatic profiles. In some cases this staging was assisted by image-guided selective biopsies from suspicious extraprostatic locations such as the seminal vesicles or pelvic lymph nodes. This was done to minimize the probability of unrecognized extraprostatic tumor spread (VAN POPPEL et al. 1994). Proper preoperative assessment of the tumor extent and a search for the presence of other associated prostatic or bladder lesions have an important impact on the surgical outcome. These data are essential in the planning of nerve-sparing procedure as opposed to wide excision prostatectomy. Further critically important information which may be obtained from the history is the presence of median lobe hyperplasia or prior transurethral resection of the prostate (TURP). All of these factors have a potential impact on the cephalic or caudal dissection of the prostate and result in possible positive surgical margins; they also have an influence on competent vesicourethral anastomosis. We find it quite reassuring to explain to the patient in advance by means of drawings the localization of the prostate at the bladder outlet, the postoperative placement of urethral catheter for ≥2 weeks, and the surgical impact on continence, potency, and fertility. Patients who present with manifestations of pulmonary obstructive disease or significant cardiovascular disease are usually referred to an internist for advice on whether or not they are suitable candidates for the operation from a medical point of view. Some medical conditions may require prophylactic preoperative administration of antibiotics and those on medications that increase the bleeding tendency are asked to stop them 10–14 days before the operation.

11.3.2 Perioperative Care

A systematic regimen for perioperative care may be of value in preventing common complications associated with radical retropubic prostatectomy.

11.3.2.1 Care Before Surgery

Before the surgical procedure, semen banking should be proposed to those younger patients who express an interest in having children at some time following the operation.

Patients should be encouraged to consider donating preoperatively 1–2 units of blood for autologous transfusion. It is proposed that the optimal blood replacement during radical prostatectomy consists of a combination of autologous transfusion of predonated blood and acute intraoperative hemodilution. This assures safe blood transfusion by eliminating risks of antigenic sensitization or transmission of disease (Andriole et al. 1994). Otherwise a similar volume of compatible blood should be reserved for the patient.

Mechanical bowel preparation consists of a sequential oral intake of macrogol (Kleanprep) in 5 l of saline during the evening prior to surgery. Neomycin can be added by oral intake, or in an enema on the morning of surgery to enhance bowel cleansing. Enoxaparin (Clexan) 40 mg s.c./12 h, which is a low molecular weight heparin substitute, is given in the evening before surgery. Skin preparation includes scrubbing with surgical soap and shaving the lower abdomen, pubis, scrotum, and perineum. It is important to prepare properly fitting elastic compression stockings to minimize the probability of postoperative complications.

11.3.2.2 Intraoperative Care

A single dose of a broad-spectrum antibiotic is given at the beginning of operation as prophylaxis against potential infection. Patients are placed on the operating table in the Trendelenburg position to provide adequate venous drainage of the lower extremities. Polyvidon iodum (Iso-Betadine) wash of the urethra is used prior to the catheterization.

Two 20-gauge catheters are utilized. One of the catheters is connected to a sterile closed continuous drainage that will be sacrificed at the dissection of the prostatic apex during the surgery, while the second Silastic catheter is scheduled to remain indwelling in the urethra for ≥2 weeks. It is imperative that the integrity of the catheter is tested prior to its application in order to avoid mechanical failure of the balloon. Prophylactic fixation of the urethral catheter to the penis utilizing hygienic adhesive tape, applying Tera-cortil ointment to the external urethral meatus, and connection of the catheter to sterile closed continuous drainage complete this process.

11.3.2.3 Postoperative Care

Our postoperative care protocol requires continuation of the administration of enoxaparin 40 mg 12 hourly for ca. 10 days following the surgery. Frequently repeated dorsiflexion exercises during the early postoperative period are mandatory. Early ambulation of the patient is highly recommended while avoiding a prolonged dependent position of the lower extremities. It is of importance to keep the patient properly hydrated to guard against hypercoagulability.

Continuous care of the catheter and closed sterile system for urine drainage is required while maintaining catheter fixation to the thigh, and a stand is used to support the urine sac for easier patient movements.

Oral intake is gradually increased, starting with fluids after passage of flatus. Special care is taken to avoid constipation, straining, and nausea.

11.3.2.4 Anesthetic Precautions and Pain Management

Safety and appropriate quality assurance should always be considered during catheterization, intubation, and blood transfusion. We prefer the use of combined general and lumbar epidural anesthesia to ensure better hemodynamic stability during the operation and early recovery period. This method allows for the possible use of the epidural catheter for patient-controlled analgesia (PCEA). The extra cost of analgesic medications and the pump set of the PCEA (±US $40) may be considered a disadvantage by some urologists. We believe, however, that this process is cost effective. For induction anesthesia we use the new hypnotic drug propofol, which is known to have a minimal influence on the induction of postoperative nausea and vomiting. For the epidural anesthesia we use a combination of a local anesthetic (bupivacaine 0.16%) and a very low concentration of an opioid (sufentanil 1 μg/ml).

The patient monitoring is controlled by electrocardiograph, systemic arterial catheter, central venous catheter, pulmonary artery catheter, pulse oximeter, capnograph, central body temperature probe, and measurement of urine output. In patients with postoperative nausea or vomiting, the new antiemetics alizapride and ondansetron are the drugs of choice owing to their limited adverse effect on intestinal motility.

11.3.3 Intraoperative Complications

Important intraoperative complications include bleeding, rectal injury, obturator nerve injury, and ureteral injury.

11.3.3.1 Bleeding

Considerable blood loss during radical retropubic prostatectomy is usually due to bleeding from the deep dorsal venous complex and plexus of Santorini. Such blood loss, if it is of sufficient magnitude, can be replaced by a blood transfusion. However, blood loss and transfusion requirements are expected to be markedly reduced when the deep dorsal venous complex is ligated in accordance with the reported recommendations on careful anatomic dissection (BENEVENTI and NOBACK 1949; FITZPATRICK 1974; REINER and WALSH 1979). Other useful measures which are known to reduce intraoperative blood loss include temporary hypogastric artery occlusion and the use of appropriate regional anesthesia, which may have positive effects on hemostasis (KAVOUSSI et al. 1991; WALSH 1992). More recently introduced changes in surgical techniques of radical prostatectomy allow better control of the deep dorsal venous complex, further decreasing intraoperative blood loss (HREBINKO and O'DONELL 1993).

The volume of intraoperative blood loss is estimated by subtracting the volume of irrigation fluids and potential urine leakage from the total volume of blood in the suction container and the weight of sponges used during the procedure (VAN POPPEL et al. 1992). Occasionally, bleeding during a limited pelvic lymphadenectomy may be controlled by temporary compression of the obturator fossa. Care should be taken to avoid inadvertent injury of the obturator nerve by the use of excessive coagulation. Routinely, we do not utilize temporary hypogastric artery occlusion to control intraoperative bleeding.

Other potentially important sources of bleeding include the endopelvic fascia injured during a medial incision and the superficial branch of the dorsal vein entered during division of the puboprostatic ligaments (WALSH 1992). Careful incision of the endopelvic fascia slightly lateral, followed by extension to the midline close to the prostate apex, is highly recommended; this provides good exposure of the venous complex and permits ligation of both ends of this complex if it becomes necessary to avoid retrograde bleeding. Potential retropubic bleeding after dividing the puboprostatic ligament and fulguration of the venous plexus can be controlled by an 8-shape underlying suture. Following urethral transection, we pack the distal cut edge and pelvic floor with sponges to avoid periurethral ooze while we proceed with the retrograde dissection of the posterior prostatic surface.

The estimated mean intraoperative blood loss in our recent series of radical prostatectomy patients was 1277 cc and the mean volume of transfused blood was 1000 cc (VAN POPPEL et al. 1995). These data were similar to those in other recently published series (Table 11.1).

11.3.3.2 Rectal injury

Rectal injury is uncommon when using contemporary radical prostatectomy. In general such injury occurs with significantly greater frequency in patients treated with perineal prostatectomy than in those managed with the retropubic approach

Table 11.1. Mean intraoperative blood loss and the number of transfusion units during radical retropubic prostatectomy in various medical centers

Authors	No. of patients	Mean blood loss (ml)	Mean transfusion units
HEDICAN and WALSH (1994)	100	1288	2.65
HREBRINKO and O'DONNELL (1993)	28	982	1.4
KAVOUSSI et al. (1991)	130	1513	2.2
KOCH et al. (1994a)	109	1086	2.0
VAN POPPEL et al. (1995)	130	1277	2.0

(LASSEN and KEARSE 1995). In radical retropubic prostatectomy patients, rectal injury may infrequently occur during the retrograde blunt dissection of the posterior aspect of the prostate from the rectum. The likelihood of rectal injury is higher in those who have reactive fibrosis or present with locally advanced tumors. In view of the above, preoperative mechanical bowel preparation on the evening prior to surgery has been required in all patients, with some urologists advocating additional use of neomycin. Once injury to the rectum is discovered, we start intraoperatively administration of broad-spectrum antibiotics known to control bacteria commonly found in the colon (both aerobic and anaerobic). An attempt at closure of the injured rectal wall is postponed until the radical prostatectomy has been completed. Our technique for closing rectal injuries consists in the use of primary intention two-layer sutures with an inner continuous layer and outer interrupted 2–3 zero chromic sutures, avoiding apposition of suture lines. This is followed by pelvic irrigation with saline and Refocin to provide adequate cleansing before the vesicourethral anastomosis has been completed. Systematic antibiotics are usually continued for a total period of up to 2 weeks. In one case we brought down an omental pedicle flap through a peritoneal window to cover the suture line of a wide reconstructed perforation; for the details of this technique, see Borland and Walsh (1992). It is important to place a suction drain in a dependent position close to the injury site to prevent any breakdown of the rectal repair by a potential urinary leak. Also, it is of importance to defunctionalize the anal sphincter by performance of wide digital dilatation just before the completion of radical prostatectomy.

Delayed postoperative oral intake and the use of low-residue diets and stool softeners should prevent constipation in the immediate postoperative period (30 days). Rectal injuries which are not recognized intraoperatively or postoperative complications consisting of unexplained fever and fecaluria warrant timely exploration, repair of rectal injury, and temporary diverting colostomy. Of the 350 patients who underwent radical retropubic prostatectomy at our medical center, five (1.4%) had full-thickness laceration of the anterior rectal wall due to either the presence of locally advanced tumor or preoperative administration of adjuvant hormonal therapy. All cases were identified intraoperatively and the laceration was closed by primary intention sutures without colostomy or any other morbidity. The reader is referred to Table 11.2 for a comparison of our experience with rectal injury with recent reports on complications of radical retropubic prostatectomy.

11.3.3.3 Nerve Injury

Obturator nerve injury was reported more commonly in the past when the extensive removal of lymphatic tissues from the lateral pelvic side walls was frequently attempted (BAHANSON and CATALONA 1990; SEIDMON 1993). However, with the recent staging lymph node dissection, which is limited to the inferior portion of the external iliac vein, obturator nerve injury is becoming a rare event. We have experienced three cases of obturator nerve injury (0.8%). In all three of these patients full recovery was noted at 6 months following radical surgery. These data were comparable to the recently published incidence of nerve injury of 0.2%, seen at Washington University (ANDRIOLE et al. 1994). In our series of 350 radical prostatectomy patients, we have had a single case of drop foot due to peroneal nerve injury of unknown etiology. Complete

Table 11.2. Recent reports of the incidence of rectal injury during radical retropubic prostatectomy, mostly closed by primary intention, from different institutions

Authors	No. of patients	Incidence (%)
ANDRIOLE et al. (1994)	1342	0.2%
BORLAND and WALSH (1992)	1000	1.0%
LEANDRI et al. (1992)	620	0.5%
ZINCKE et al. (1994)	3170	0.6%
Present series	350	1.4%

recovery in this case occurred within 6 months of surgery.

11.3.3.4 Ureteral Injury

Ureteral injury is a rare complication that may take place during dissection of seminal vesicles from the posterior bladder wall (BAHANSON and CATALONA 1990) or dissection at the level of bladder neck and trigone (WALSH 1992; HAUTMAN et al. 1994). The risk of ureteral injury may be increased by the presence of enlargement of the median lobe of the prostate (Fig. 11.3). In compromised cases we advocate prophylactic placement of a double J ureteral stent to avoid inadvertent early postoperative obstruction. This stent can be removed at a later date. In the early days of our series, we experienced a single case of unilateral chronic hydroureteronephrosis discovered 1 year after radical retropubic prostatectomy.

11.3.4 Early Postoperative Complications

Early postoperative complications occur in the critical period of 30 days following radical prostatectomy.

11.3.4.1 Thromboembolic Disease

Thromboembolic disease is a serious, potentially lethal complication of pelvic surgery (for a review see KIBEL and LOUGHLIN 1995). Following radical retropubic prostatectomy the risk of deep venous thrombosis and thromboembolic complications is always present; nevertheless, the clinical diagnosis

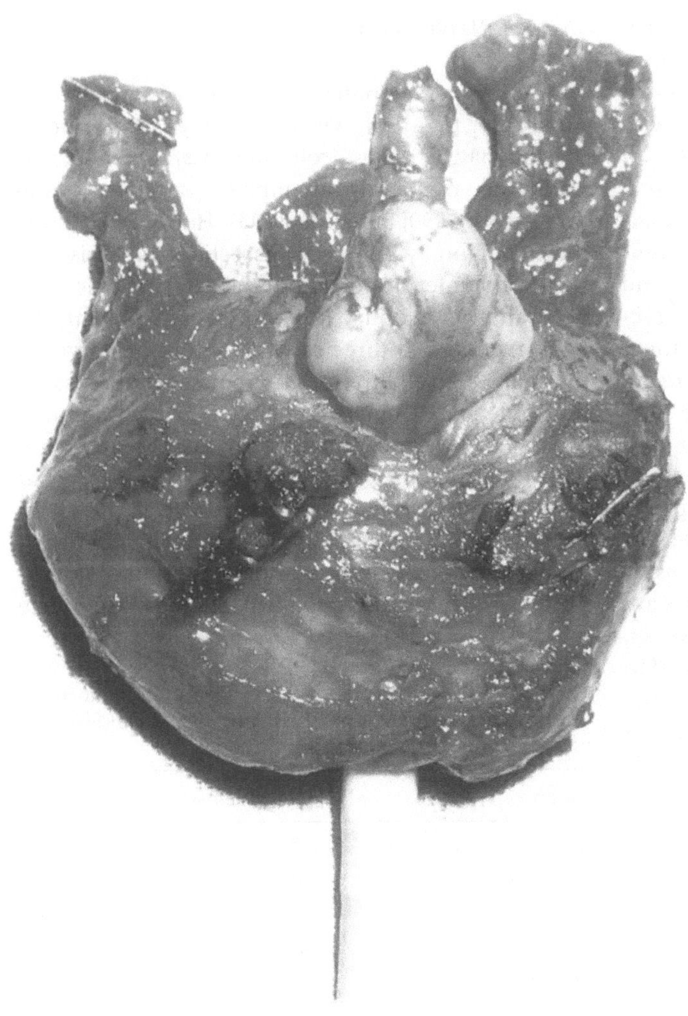

Fig. 11.3. The presence of median lobe enlargement in a radical retropubic prostatectomy specimen. This might compromise competent bladder neck dissection or induce inadvertent ureteral injury

of this complication is frequently unreliable (LEIBOVITCH et al. 1995). Earlier studies in patients who underwent pelvic surgery without thromboembolic prophylaxis had demonstrated deep venous thrombosis rates as high as 51% (MAYO et al. 1971), pulmonary embolism rates of up to 22% (ALLGOOD et al. 1970), and a fatal pulmonary embolism rate of 2.6% (COLBY 1948).

In contemporary series of cases treated by radical retropubic prostatectomy, the incidence of thromboembolic disease has significantly decreased. In the present series of 350 cases we have diagnosed and successfully treated all of the only eight patients (2.3%) with deep venous thrombosis and/or pulmonary embolism. These patients had received hormonal therapy before the radical retropubic prostatectomy; they included one who had prolonged hospitalization due to wound evisceration and another who was obese (VAN POPPEL et al. 1995).

Rates of deep venous thrombosis reported in the literature range from 1.1% to 3.0%; reported rates of pulmonary embolism are 0.4%–2.7%, and a fatal pulmonary embolism rate of 0.6% has been cited (KIBEL and LOUGHLIN 1995; ZINCKE et al. 1994). In two large published series (>1000 cases each) of anatomic radical retropubic prostatectomy, the reported incidence of thromboembolic complications has been 1.1% (WALSH 1992) and 2.6% (ANDRIOLE et al. 1994). Thromboembolic disease, although uncommon, is considered the most common early complication. Clinically apparent deep venous thrombosis may be considered the tip of the iceberg for potential thrombi that can lead to major morbidity and mortality (THOMPSON 1994). However, other authors find the clinical diagnosis of this complication inaccurate (KUMAR et al. 1993; LEIBOVICH et al. 1995).

This addresses the clinical dilemma that we frequently have to face, i.e., how to distinguish patients with subclinical deep venous thrombosis and thromboembolic disease from those with no discernible pathologic condition, in the face of clinical signs and symptoms suggestive of a thromboembolic episode. Obviously, prevention of deep venous thrombosis in the first place is preferable to treating these complications (KIBEL and LOUGHLIN 1995; MCLEOD 1995). Stasis, endothelial injury, and a hypercoagulable state are the main factors that initiate venous thrombosis following radical retropubic prostatectomy. Numerous methods of decreasing the incidence of deep venous thrombosis, pulmonary embolism, and overall surgical mortality have been explored, and various means of prophylaxis have been cited (for review see KIBEL and LOUGHLIN 1995).

We routinely start patients on low molecular weight enoxapaine (Clexan 2 × 40 mg per day), beginning on the night prior to the operation. This regimen inhibits factor Xa to a greater extent and platelet function and factor IIa to a lesser extent; therefore it decreases the bleeding complication rates without any reduction in prophylactic effect.

We routinely use elastic stockings, starting on the night prior to surgery and continuing until the patient is fully ambulatory in the early postoperative period. The application of this simple measure guards against thrombosis by increasing the velocity of venous blood flow in the lower extremities and preventing over-distention of veins. Also, adjuvant electrical calf stimulation intraoperatively might improve the efficiency of this technique. No complications have been attributed to the use of elastic stockings if they fit properly (KOCH et al. 1994a); however, their propensity to slip below the knee level and to act as tourniquets may promote thrombosis (MCLEOD 1995; SIGEL et al. 1973). Increased intraoperative blood loss is reported with the use of intermittent pneumatic compression stockings in radical prostatectomy patients due to the increased blood flow from lower extremities (STRUP et al. 1993). The main drawbacks of prophylactic minidose heparin in patients undergoing radical prostatectomy are increased intraoperative blood loss and the potential for lymphocele formation (BIGG and CATALONA 1992).

Of increasing concern is the risk of late thromboembolic complications (KIBEL and LOUGHLIN 1995). Late deep venous thrombosis is diagnosed on an average of 12–20 days postoperatively (CISEK and WALSH 1993; IGEL et al. 1987). Once prophylactic regimens are stopped, an existing nidus can propagate, since the hypercoagulable state may exist for as long as 3 weeks postoperatively. Recently, there has been a trend to decrease the duration of hospitalization following radical prostatectomy for economic reasons. This early hospital discharge may shorten the period of prophylaxis and increase the period of unprotected hypercoagulability. Therefore, it is advocated that post-discharge prophylaxis be applied in pelvic surgery patients to avoid facing increased numbers of late thromboembolic complications following early hospital discharges (KIBEL and LOUGHLIN 1995).

11.3.4.2 Bleeding

The incidence of postoperative hemorrhage requiring a second surgical intervention and the need for postoperative blood transfusion to maintain an appropriate blood pressure vary widely in the recent reports on radical prostatectomy. In the series of 1350 consecutive radical retropubic prostatectomy patients reported by HEDICAN and WALSH (1994), only seven (0.5%) developed the aforementioned complications. Of these seven, four were explored and three were managed conservatively. Both groups of patients required a comparable mean amount of blood to maintain their blood pressure. However, it has been advocated that such patients be reexplored and the pelvic hematoma evacuated to decrease the likelihood of future bladder neck contracture and incontinence.

In another series, a higher incidence of reoperation of 1.7% and of a higher incidence of conservative treatment of 5.7% were reported in 418 consecutive radical prostatectomy patients (HAUTMANN et al. 1994).

Postoperative hemorrhage is considered a separate entity from intraoperative bleeding. Potential causes include the use of medications (e.g., aspirin or nonsteroidal anti-inflammatory agents) that interfere with normal clotting), mechanical factors such as missed or poorly ligated blood vessels, and bleeding disorders; idiopathic cases also occur.

11.3.4.3 Long Hospitalization and Socioeconomic Complications

One of the main problems associated with radical prostatectomy is the high potential cost of the operation and lengthy hospitalization, which may influence medical decision-makers and potentially alter the pattern of health care delivery. Thus while there has previously been a strong belief among some surgeons that patients undergoing major abdominal surgery have to be kept under observation in the hospital for a sufficient if poorly defined period, more recently there has been a tendency to discharge patients much earlier following radical retropubic prostatectomy to avoid the financial drawbacks of lengthy hospital stay (KOCH et al. 1994b; LICHT and KLEIN 1994; WALSH 1995). The disadvantage is that early hospital discharge results in a shorter period of prophylaxis, with a reported increased risk of sequential late thromboembolic complications. It has been noted that a hypercoagulable state may exist for as long as 3 weeks postoperatively, with an increasing period of unprotected hypercoagulability as hospitalization is shortened for economic reasons (KIBEL and LOUGHLIN 1995). Indeed, thromboembolic manifestations are the most common cause for rehospitalization during the first 90 days following radical prostatectomy (OPTENBERG et al. 1995). Yet, it is estimated that more than 60% of the fatal pulmonary embolism cases are not suspected prior to the occurrence of this dramatic event (KIBEL and LOUGHLIN 1995).

KOCH et al. (1994b) have designed and implemented a broad-based program to decrease costs while maintaining quality of care for patients undergoing radical retropubic prostatectomy. They have identified nonessential procedures that contribute to the increase in costs and could safely be eliminated or sharply reduced. An overall reduction by 40% in total hospital charges has been achieved by reducing postoperative hospital stay, the operating room time, use of materials, use of antibiotics, and routine laboratory studies, as well as by refinements in postoperative pain management, without any discernible adverse effect on morbidity rates.

11.3.4.4 Excessive Drainage

Excessive drainage is defined as prolonged fluid leakage, mostly manifested by a collection of excessive volume in negative suction drains (ANDRIOLE et al. 1994). It occurs secondary to either urine leak from noncompetent neo-vesicourethral anastomosis or lymph leak from nonligated lymphatics after the lymphadenectomy. The differential diagnosis can be simply obtained by analyzing a specimen for urea and creatinine concentrations; while these can be expected to be significantly elevated in cases of urine leak, they will be similar to serum values when the leakage is due to lymph. Also, bluish discoloration following indigo carmine injection permits diagnosis of the urinary extravasation.

Management of urinary leak is usually conservative, by removal of drain suction, refinement of catheter position and its balloon capacity (±15 ml), and prolonged indwelling of the neoanastomosis until healing of the leakage. Pericatheterogram may be requested (PARIVAR et al. 1994). Lymphatic drainage can be avoided by meticulous cautery or ligation of lymphatics; however, it is managed expectantly and drains can be removed once daily leakage is ≤60 ml.

Closed lymphocele or urinoma is managed expectantly with possible image-guided percutaneous drainage once clinically manifested.

The reported incidence of excessive drainage in the contemporary series of radical retropubic prostatectomy with limited lymphadenectomy technique varies between 0.3% (LEANDRI et al. 1992; ANDRIOLE et al. 1994) and 5.5% (HAUTMAN et al. 1994).

11.3.4.5 Retention

Urinary retention is an infrequent though not rare complication of radical prostatectomy, the reported incidence being 0.5%–4.0% (BAHANSON and CATALONA 1990; OPTENBERG et al. 1995). It is one of the most common causes of early rehospitalization following discharge subsequent to radical prostatectomy.

Occasionally, urinary retention occurs shortly after removal of the urethral catheter. In such cases, it is likely to be secondary to improper circumferential mucosa to mucosa anastomosis at the neo-vesicourethral junction. Careful endoscopic resection is mandatory when one flap of bladder neck tissue is found (SEIDEMON 1993).

Infrequently, retention occurs while the urethral catheter is indwelling due to its occlusion by blood clots secondary to hemorrhage. If gentle irrigation and decreasing the balloon volume fail to control the occlusion, ultrasonography-guided suprapubic cutaneous cystostomy can be applied while the urethral catheter is left in place in order not to compromise the neoanastomosis.

11.3.4.6 Accidental Catheter Loss

Accidental catheter loss is one of the most unfavorable drawbacks that takes place due to delayed failure of the balloon, which will have been tested during the intraoperative period. Premature loss of the catheter might compromise the neoanastomosis and consequently the patient's continence. Therefore, different prophylactic methods of fixation have been suggested to avoid this event, such as passing a nylon suture through the eye of the catheter tip and external fixation over a button on the anterior abdominal wall through a small cystostomy incision (WALSH 1992). Catheter fixation to the skin of the penis by means of a pedicle suture ligated to outside the catheter distal to the glans penis is also possible. We usually apply a longitudinal flap of hygienic adhesive tape that extends from the base of the penis, enclosing its whole length and most of the external catheter segment. However, if the catheter happens to fall out prematurely, an attempt might be made to carefully pass a smaller caliber well-lubricated catheter into the bladder (BAHANSON and CATALONA 1990; WALSH 1992). This catheter can be introduced with the right hand while guided by the left hand's index finger introduced into the rectum.

We have experienced three cases (0.86%) of premature catheter loss, in which we initially commenced with abdominal ultrasonic-guided suprapubic insertion of a 14-ch cutaneous cystostomy tube (Cystofix) to avoid blunt trauma to a congested neoanastomosis. One day later, elective urethral catheter application was performed in the operating room, assisted by visual placement a of guidewire into the bladder using the urethrocystoscope.

11.3.4.7 Bowel Problems

Due to the use of the extraperitoneal approach in patients undergoing radical prostatectomy, severe bowel problems are not common complications of this surgical procedure. However, it is not uncommon to encounter a reaction that lasts 1–2 days postoperatively due to the influence of anesthetic agents and analgesic medications. Early postoperative feeding is possible by reducing the nausea associated with administration of narcotics, using Ketorolac for pain control and bisacodyl suppositories to encourage the return of normal bowel function (KOCH et al. 1994b).

11.3.4.8 Myocardial Infarction

The reported incidence of myocardial infarction in patients following radical retropubic prostatectomy is low (Table 11.3). No precise etiology for this complication in this group of patients has been identified (ANDRIOLE et al. 1994; HAUTMANN et al. 1994; LEANDRI et al. 1992; OPTENBERG et al. 1995; ZINCKE et al. 1994). Myocardial infarction is likely to be secondary to thromboembolic manifestations, atherosclerosis, myocardial insufficiency, or general cardiovascular decompensation.

Table 11.3. Incidence of myocardial infarction within the 30-day period following radical retropubic prostatectomy at various medical centers

Authors	No. of patients	Incidence
ANDRIOLE et al. (1994)	1342	0.7%
HAUTMANN et al. (1994)	418	0.7%
LEANDRI et al. (1992)	620	0.2%
OPTENBERG et al. (1995)	1059	<0.5%
ZINCKE et al. (1994)	3170	0.4%
Present series	350	0.6%

It is essential to properly evaluate the cardiovascular and pulmonary systems preoperatively, and surgery should be delayed in patients who have suffered recent myocardial infarction to avoid the high mortality of reinfarction which may occur during the perioperative period (BAHANSON and CATALONA 1990). We practise close observation of patients during the first night after the operation by monitoring each particular patient at the intensive care unit for the early and better management of unexpected events during this critical period. We advocate the preoperative use of prophylactic broad-spectrum antibiotics in patients known to have artificial cardiac valves.

11.3.4.9 Wound Infection

Wound infection is a minor and infrequently reported complication that results in delayed primary wound healing. The reported incidence of wound infection in recent series is 1.3% and 1.7% in 1342 and 418 radical retropubic prostatectomy patients, respectively (ANDRIOLE et al. 1994; HAUTMANN et al. 1994). While many authors tend to omit this complication in their reports, it is one of the two most common specific complications diagnosed as a cause for rehospitalization during the 90-day period following radical prostatectomy (OPTENBERG et al. 1995). The incidence of wound infection rate may be reduced by:

1. Strict aseptic conditions perioperatively
2. The use of systemic antibiotics perioperatively
3. Avoiding a potential urinary tract infection
4. Copious irrigation of the wound with saline and local antibiotic (Refocin)
5. Avoiding hematoma formation and minute bleeding vessels before wound closure
6. Maintenance of good care in diabetic patients

Unfortunately, wound infection has been one of the most common surgical complications seen in our practice, ten such cases (2.9%) having been identified.

11.3.5 Late Postoperative Complications

11.3.5.1 Impotence

Male erectile dysfunction is the most common complication observed following radical prostatectomy, even after identifying the neuroanatomy of the pelvic plexus and its branches that innervate the corpora cavernosa, and the modification of surgical technique in an attempt to preserve the neurovascular bundles (WALSH et al. 1983). Prior to that development, impotence was accepted as a normal and expected consequence of radical prostatectomy. Presently, there is a significantly higher probability of preserving erectile function, especially in younger patients with early-stage disease who are treated with WALSH's anatomic radical retropubic prostatectomy. The preservation of potency in patients who are sexually active preoperatively correlates well with the surgeon's experience, the patient's age, the clinical and pathologic stage, and the use of unilateral or bilateral nerve-sparing surgery. Nevertheless, the average success rate in preserving potency with the use of nerve-sparing surgery is 43% (MURPHY et al. 1994), ranging from 41% to 68% (CATALONA and BASLER 1993; QUINLAN et al. 1991). Surgical margins should not be compromised because of the use of nerve-sparing modification to radical prostatectomy. Initial histopathologic observations suggested that nerve-sparing technique achieved resected margins similar to those obtained with the standard radical retropubic prostatectomy (BAHANSON and CATALONA 1990).

Although postoperative evaluation of potency with the use of many tests is well established, preoperative evaluation of the baseline erectile function is never clearly reported in the literature (SEIDMON 1993). In the most promising patients, return of erectile activity might be anticipated within 3 months of surgery, and most patients who regain erectile function do so within 6 months postoperatively. Nevertheless, in some patients erectile function may not be regained for up to 15 months postoperatively. Patients are considered to have failed to regain erectile function if they remain impotent for 12 months or more following nerve-sparing surgery.

In the present series nerve-sparing surgery was employed in 91 patients who were potent before the operation and showed an interest in preservation of sexual function. Bilateral nerve sparing was employed in 50 cases and unilateral nerve sparing in 41. Among this group of 91 patients, spontaneous erection was achieved within 6 months postoperatively in 19 (21%), while the remaining 72 (79%) were considered candidates for adjuvant injection therapy, with a good response noted in 35. One of the patients from the impotent group has received a penile prosthesis.

Prior to radical prostatectomy, the patient and his partner should be informed about the loss of ejaculation and the probability of erectile dysfunction. Most patients will have many questions regarding their expected postoperative sexual function but frequently they may hesitate to discuss this important problem with the urologist. At this point the patient needs to be assured of the available treatment options in case of the presence of postoperative impotence. The main treatment for postoperative impotence consists in the intracavernous injections of vasoactive medications and the use of a penile prosthesis (Claes et al. 1994).

Most patients with impotence following radical prostatectomy can be successfully managed with intracavernous pharmacotherapy. The most common pharmacologic agent used in the treatment of these patients is prostaglandin E_1, alone or in combination with papaverine hydrochloride. Patients who are being considered for this treatment need to be informed of the possibility of acute complications such as priapism and the possibility of the development of long-term toxicity such as cavernous fibrosis. Informed consent must be obtained in all patients considered for this therapy. A search for an appropriate dose is done in the physician's office. The medication is injected with a tuberculin or insulin-type syringe, using a 28- or 30-gauge needle. Prostaglandin is injected along the lateral aspect of the penile shaft on one side only. There is an obvious need to avoid the neurovascular bundle dorsally and the urethra ventrally. If the patient fails to achieve a functional erection, the dose of the drug can be incrementally increased. The self-injection technique is monitored by a physician until the dose that produces a good erection lasting no longer than 1 h has been determined. Patients continue until the physician is confident that both parties have a full understanding of the nature of this treatment and have mastered the injection technique. Patients are given only a small supply of medication sufficient for 1–2 months. The frequency of the injections should be limited to twice a week.

Patients with neurogenic impotence have a high response rate to intracavernous pharmacotherapy and usually require lower doses of the drug. Their erections tend to occur more rapidly, have greater rigidity, and last longer. This is particularly the case in patients who have undergone a nerve-sparing procedure and who desire to begin their sexual function before the recovery of the nerves have taken place (usually 4–12 months). The risk of priapism in these patients is relatively high and the initial doses of prostaglandin need to be carefully titrated. In our patients, even at a dose as low as 5 μg of prostaglandin, priapism has occurred. There have been very few other complications of this therapy. The most frequent complications described in the literature – pain or hematoma formation at the site of injection, elevation of liver enzymes, dizziness, and the development of intracavernous fibrosis – have not been experienced by our patients. There is a wide selection of available inflatable prostheses. All of these have a range of diameter and lengths to enable accurate placement. Several design changes which have occurred in recent years have resulted in excellent patient and partner acceptance and satisfaction rates. We prefer to use the CX 700 or Ultrex of American Medical Systems (Minnetonka, Minnesota), both of which entail a low complication rate and provide excellent patient satisfaction. Nevertheless, because potency may gradually return over a period of 12 months postoperatively, a trial of less invasive treatment, such as intracavernous injections of vasodilators, is highly recommended for several months prior to the insertion of a penile prosthesis.

Despite the importance of erectile function one should never forget that while operating for clinically localized CaP, the main objective is total removal of the cancer rather than potency preservation. However, it is now possible with good exposure and careful dissection to provide a wide margin and complete excision of the lateral pelvic fascia and neurovascular bundle at the suspicious ipsilateral tumor site while preserving the contralateral neurovascular bundle (Walsh 1992). This might reduce the incidence of impotence in unilateral nonconfined cancer.

11.3.5.2 Incontinence

Total urinary incontinence is the most feared and disabling late complication following radical prostatectomy. Therefore, a variety of modifications to radical prostatectomy have been recommended to minimize the probability of this complication, the most important being more precise anatomic dissection (De Kernion 1995; Gomez et al. 1993; Malizia et al. 1989; Steiner et al. 1991; Steiner et al. 1993).

In a recent survey of 2122 patients treated by radical prostatectomy at 484 institutions in the United States during 1990, the reported incidence of complete incontinence was 3.6% (Murphy et al. 1994). In another European unicenter study, involving 418 standard radical retropubic prostatectomies, a total incontinence rate of 3% was reported and this was considered a suboptimal treatment outcome (Hautmann et al. 1994). On the other hand, the incidence of total incontinence was significantly lower in other single major medical centers, ranging from 0% to 0.8% (Catalona and Basler 1993; Leandri et al. 1992; Steiner et al. 1993; Zincke et al. 1994).

It has been observed (Wein 1991) that in the normal male continence is dependent upon the proximal sphincter (including smooth muscles of the bladder neck and preprostatic sphincter), the urethral supporting elements, and the distal sphincter mechanism (composed of striated urethral sphincter and periurethral levator ani fibers). Therefore, the distal sphincter mechanism per se might be insufficient to control urinary continence following radical prostatectomy.

It has now been concluded by some authors (Catalona and Basler 1993; Steiner et al. 1991) that there might be no correlation between the return of continence and the patient's age, tumor stage, nerve-sparing surgery, or prior TURP. Nevertheless, between total continence and total incontinence, a higher percentage of patients (5%–12%) present with stress incontinence, and there is considerable variability in the reported time required for return of urinary control (Table 11.4).

This wide variation in the reported results could be related to different surgical techniques and/or perceptions of the degree of return of urine control by physicians and patients. Among recent maneuvers, partial dissection (avoiding extensive division) of the puboprostatic ligaments to provide more retropubic urethral support has been suggested as a surgical modification to improve the ultimate continence and the time to recovery after radical retropubic prostatectomy (De Kernion 1995).

Catalona and Basler (1993) have reported on the recent modification of apical dissection to preserve the circumurethral sphincter muscles, this technique having yielded an incidence of continence of 53% 2–3 weeks after catheter removal. Klein (1992) reported 83% of prostatectomy patients to be dry at 3 months following incorporation of the fascia posterior to the urethra into the vesicourethral anastomosis. Steiner et al. (1993) reported an 87% continence rate at 6 months following tubularization of the anterior bladder neck after radical retropubic prostatectomy, and Gomez et al. (1993) concluded that all of their patients (ca. 100) were fully continent at a minimum follow-up of 6 months with anatomic preservation of the bladder neck and proximal urethra.

We believe that preservation of the proximal urethral (preprostatic) sphincter is beneficial for the control of continence; however, it is doomed to fail-

Table 11.4. Incidence and duration of continence control after radical retropubic prostatectomy in different medical centers

Authors	No. of patients	Continence rate	Incontinence rate	Recovery time (months)	Need for artificial sphincter
Catalona and Basler (1993)	784	94%	6%	18	2 patients
Gomez et al. (1993)	50	100%	0%	0	
Hautmann et al. (1994)	418	80.7%	15%	12	3%
Klein (1992)	60	88%	10%	4	2%
Leandri et al. (1992)	620	95%	5%	≥12	0
Murphy et al. (1994)[a]	2122	81.3%	15.3%	NA	3.6%
Steiner et al. (1991)	593	92%	8%	≥12	2 patients
Steiner et al. (1993)	69	87%	13%	6	0
Zincke et al. (1994)	3170	±93%	6.45%	NA	0.8%
Present series	350	95%	5%	4	2 patients

NA, Estimated recovery time not available; probably it was more than 12 months
[a] Data on US national patterns of treatment by radical prostatectomy in 1990 (not exclusively via the retropubic approach) from 484 different institutions

ure in patients with median lobe hypertrophy (Fig. 11.3), or after TURP (for details see surgical technique in Chap. 8).

In the present series of 350 patients treated with radical retropubic prostatectomy, we have experienced a 30%, 43%, 95%, 99%, and 99.7% incidence of continence at 15, 30, 120, 240, and 360 days after urethral catheter removal, respectively.

Treatment of urinary stress incontinence following radical retropubic prostatectomy initially can be conservative, employing pelvic floor exercises to improve the tone of the pelvic diaphragm and external sphincter. Oral imipramine (Tofranil) 25 mg tablets can reduce the associated bladder instability while improving the sphincteric function due to its anticholinergic action.

Persistent stress incontinence can be treated with periurethral injection of polytetrafluorethylene paste, collagen, silicone, or autologous fat. Better results have been obtained following coaptation of the urethra above the external sphincter, but not in or at the sphincter [for review see KABALIN (1994) and editorial comments].

The major treatment alternative to injectable therapy for patients with persistent sphincter deficiency is an artificial sphincter; this is a significantly more invasive procedure, but it offers a higher rate of continence. In our group of 350 patients we have had a single case of persistent stress incontinence (0.3%), with TURP prior to the radical prostatectomy. This case warranted a sphincter prosthesis.

11.3.5.3 Stricture

Stricture of the new vesicourethral anastomosis has also been called bladder neck contracture. It has been reported in 2.6%–23% of patients following radical retropubic prostatectomy. In most cases it is due to overzealous reconstruction of the bladder neck, previous TURP, and/or failure to achieve an accurate mucosa to mucosa apposition between the bladder neck and membranous urethra (BAHANSON and CATALONA 1990; GOMEZ et al. 1993; PARIVAR et al. 1994; WALSH 1992). Postoperative bleeding and unevacuated pelvic hematoma might also result in symptomatic bladder neck contracture (HEDICAN and WALSH 1994).

Bladder neck contracture has been reported to develop in 1%–9% of patients following anatomic radical retropubic prostatectomy (STEINER et al. 1991), while the rate is increased to 12% with a tubularized neourethra technique (STEINER et al. 1993). In a series of 119 cases, PARIVAR et al. (1994) noted a 9.3% incidence of significant bladder neck contracture at a mean of 15 weeks postoperatively previous TURP appeared to be a risk factor for its development, but there was no correlation with extravasation at the neoanastomosis after radical retropubic prostatectomy. CATALONA and BASLER (1993) have shown the importance of the learning curve in respect of avoidance of anastomotic stricture. Thus the incidence of stricture was reported to be 7.8% in their first 500 patients, as compared to 0.6% in their last 308 patients. These 308 patients were treated by preservation of circumurethral sphincter muscles during apical dissection and by refraining from closing the bladder neck too tightly around an 18 F catheter.

Anatomic dissection and preservation of the bladder neck and proximal urethra significantly diminish the likelihood of anastomotic stricture by allowing for circumferential mucosa to mucosa anastomosis. Even without the need for bladder neck reconstruction, anastomotic stricture was seen in no patient out of 100 cases who have had the bladder neck preserved (GOMEZ et al. 1993). Also, it has been reported that the preservation of the bladder neck with the creation of a wide anastomosis between the urethra and bladder neck provides a watertight closure that prevents urinary leakage and reduces the possibility of periurethral sealing and anastomotic stricture to 0.5% (LEANDRI et al. 1992). We have experienced a significant reduction in the incidence of stricture at the new anastomotic site among more recently treated patients by applying a similar technique, with preservation of the preprostatic sphincter, eversion of the bladder cuff, and mucosa to mucosa anastomosis. In the total group of 350 patients we have observed 17 (4.8%) cases of stricture, which was treated by transurethral incision at the level of the new bladder neck.

It has been advised that one should never dilate the stricture formation at the site of the urethrovesical anastomosis in post-radical prostatectomy patients who are continent, as this would incur loss of urinary control (PAULSON 1991). Some authors have noted a good response to the treatment with once-only dilatation (LEANDRI et al. 1992). Others advocate it, and if it is not successful in eliminating this problem, they proceed to incision of the bladder neck contracture followed by transurethral injection of a drug that prevents further stricture formation (BAHANSON and CATALONA

1990; WALSH 1992). Moreover, transurethral resection of the contracted bladder neck segment, with histologic examination, might be done in a sparing fashion so as not to compromise the external sphincter (SEIDMON 1993).

11.3.5.4 Orchialgia

Orchialgia is an infrequently reported complication following radical retropubic prostatectomy (BAHANSON and CATALONA 1990; WALSH 1992). This complication may be due to the ligation of the vasa deferentia at the time of dissection at the prostate base. Alternatively it may be due to excessive traction on the spermatic cord by the retractor blade during the mobilization of the peritoneum off the external iliac vessels, to the bifurcation of the common iliac artery, to perform the lymphadenectomy.

11.4 Conclusions

Contemporary radical retropubic prostatectomy provides a good opportunity for the control of organ-confined prostate cancer with minimal morbidity and virtually no mortality. Complications can be reduced by systematic preoperative management and perioperative care. Since this is a very complex operative procedure, its morbidity decreases with time in each medical center, hopefully following a steep learning curve. The application of anatomic dissection has yielded a decline in blood loss by better control of the deep dorsal vein complex. Additionally, it allows wider margins of excision when indicated and has had a favorable impact on potency by preservation of the neurovascular bundles. Anatomic dissection has also resulted in earlier and improved control of continence by preservation of the preprostatic sphincter and incorporation of the periurethral fascia into the vesicourethral anastomosis. There has been a significant decline in the incidence of rectal injury and its associated morbidity. Prevention of serious thromboembolic disease and careful cardiopulmonary observation during the perioperative period have resulted in an operation-specific mortality compatible with that of the general population of similar age. One last advantage of radical prostatectomy is the opportunity it provides for thorough histopathologic evaluation that might accurately reflect the long-term prognosis of prostate cancer.

Acknowledgement. The authors would like to thank Dr. H. Claes and Dr. B. Vanacker for providing helpful expert comments.

References

Adolfsson J, Steineck G, Whitmore WF (1993) Recent results of management of palpable clinically localized prostate cancer. Cancer 72:310–322

Allgood RJ, Cook JH, Weedn RJ et al. (1970) Prospective analysis of pulmonary embolism in the postoperative patient. Surgery 68:116

Andriole GL, Smith DS, Rao G, Goodnough L, Catalona WJ (1994) Early complications of contemporary anatomical radical retropubic prostatectomy. J Urol 152:1858–1860

Bahanson RR, Catalona WJ (1990) Complications of radical retropubic prostatectomy. In: Smith RB, Ehrlich RM (eds) Complications of urologic surgery: prevention and management. W.B. Saunders, Philadelphia, pp 386–394

Beneventi FA, Noback GJ (1949) Distribution of the blood vessels of the prostate gland and urinary bladder: application to retropubic prostatectomy. J Urol 62:663

Bigg SW, Catalona WJ (1992) Prophylactic mini-dose heparin in patients undergoing radical retropubic prostatectomy. A prospective trial. Urology 34:309–313

Boring CC, Squires TS, Tong T, Montogomery S (1994) Cancer statistics. CA Cancer J Clin 44:6–26

Borland RN, Walsh PC (1992) The management of rectal injury during radical retropubic prostatectomy. J Urol 147:905–907

Boxer RJ, Kaufman JJ, Goodwin WE (1977) Radical prostatectomy for carcinoma of the prostate: 1951–1976. A review of 329 patients. J Urol 117:208

Brawer MK, Chetner MP, Beatie J, Buchner DM, Vesela RL, Lange PH (1992) Screening for prostatic carcinoma with prostate specific antigen. J Urol 147:841–845

Campbell JL, Thomley MW, Parsons RL (1963) Complications of radical prostatic surgery. J Urol 89:253

Catalona WJ, Basler JW (1993) Return of erections and urinary continence following nerve sparing radical retropubic prostatectomy. J Urol 150:905–907

Catalona WJ, Smith DS (1994) 5-year tumor recurrence rates after anatomical radical retropubic prostatectomy for prostate cancer. J Urol 152:1837–1842

Catalona WJ, Hudson MA, Scardino PT et al. (1994) Selection of optimal prostate specific antigen cutoffs for early detection of prostate cancer: receiver operating characteristic curves. J Urol 152:2037–2042

Ciancio G, Antun RA, Norberg DG et al. (1995) Prostate cancer after heart transplantation. J Urol 153:158–160

Cisek LJ, Walsh PC (1993) Thromboembolic complications following radical retropubic prostatectomy: influence of external sequential pneumatic compression devices. Urology 42:406–408

Claes H, Van den Bogaert S, Baert L (1994) Welke medicamenten geven canleiding tot potentiestoornissen bij mannen? Tijdschr Geneeskd 50:1790–1793

Colby FH (1948) The prevention of fatal pulmonary emboli after prostatectomy. J Urol 59:920

Corral DA, Bahanson RR (1994) Survival of men with clinically localized prostate cancer detected in the eighth decade of life. J Urol 151:1326–1329

Dearnaley DP (1993) Prostate cancer: clinical overview. Lancet 342:901–905

De Kernion JB (1995) Radical prostatectomy for localized prostate cancer. AUA morning and evening seminars: early detection and treatment of prostate cancer. 23–28 April 1995, Las Vegas, Nevada. AUA Office of Education

Esteve J, Kricker A, Ferlay J, Parkin DM (1993) Facts and figures of cancer in the European Community, IARC, Lyon

Fitzpatrick TJ (1974) Venography of the deep dorsal venous and valvular systems. J Urol 111:518

Gomez CA, Soloway MS, Civantos F, Hachiya T (1993) Bladder neck preservation and its impact on positive surgical margins during radical prostatectomy. Urology 42:689–694

Hautmann RE, Sauter TW, Wenderoth UK (1994) Radical retropubic prostatectomy: morbidity and urinary continence in 418 consecutive cases. Urology 43 (Suppl):47–51

Hedican SP, Walsh PC (1994) Postoperative bleeding following radical retropubic prostatectomy. J Urol 152:1181–1183

Hrebinko RL, O'Donnell WJ (1993) Control of the deep dorsal venous complex in radical retropubic prostatectomy. J Urol 149:799–801

Igel TC, Barret DM, Segura JW, Benson RC, Rife CC (1987) Perioperative and postoperative complications form bilateral pelvic lymphadenectomy and radical retropubic prostatectomy. J Urol 137:1189–1191

Jensen OM, Estève J, Møller H, Renard H (1990) Cancer in the European Community and its member states. Eur J Cancer 26:1167–1256

Jewett JH (1980) Radical perineal prostatetomy for palpable, clinically localized, non-obstructive cancer: experience at the Johns Hopkins Hospital 1900–1963. J Urol 124:492–494

Kabalin JN (1994) Treatment of post-prostatectomy stress urinary incontinence with periurethral polytetrafluoroethylene paste injection. J Urol 152:1463–1466

Kavoussi LR, Myers JA, Catalona WJ (1991) Effect of temporary occlusion of hypogastric arteries on blood loss during radical retropubic prostatectomy. J Urol 146:362–365

Kibel AS, Loughlin KR (1995) Pathogenesis and prophylaxis of postoperative thromboembolic disease in urological pelvic surgery. J Urol 153:1763–1774

Kinahan TJ, McLoughlin MG, Manson DC (1991) Radical prostatectomy for localized prostatic carcinoma in the renal transplant patient. J Urol 146:104–107

Klein EA (1992) Early continence after radical prostatectomy. J Urol 148:92–95

Koch MO, Brandell RA, Lin D, Smith JA (1994a) The effect of sequential compression devices on intra-operative blood loss during radical prostatectomy. J Urol 152:1178–1179

Koch MO, Smith JA, Hodge EM, Brandell RA (1994b) Prospective development of a cost-efficient program for radical retropubic prostatectomy. Urology 44:311–318

Kumar R, McKinney WP, Raj G (1993) Perioperative prophylaxis of venous thromboembolism. Am J Med Sci 306:336

Lassen PM, Kearse WS (1995) Rectal injuries during radical perineal prostatectomy. Urology 45:266–269

Leandri P, Rossignol G, Gautier JR, Ramon J (1992) Radical retropubic prostatectomy: morbidity and quality of life. Experience with 620 consecutive cases. J Urol 147:883–887

Leibovitch I, Foster RS, Wass JL et al. (1995) Color doppler flow imaging for deep venous thrombosis screening in patients undergoing pelvic lymphadenectomy and radical retropublic prostatectomy for prostate cancer. J Urol 153:1866–1869

Licht MR, Klein EA (1994) Early hospital discharge after radical retropubic prostatectomy: impact on cost and complication rate. Urology 44:700–704

Litwin MS, Hays RD, Fink A et al. (1995) Quality-of-life outcomes in men treated for localized prostate cancer. JAMA 273:129–135

Malizia AA, Banks DW, Newton NE, Walton GR, Watton KN (1989) Modified radical retropubic prostatectomy: double continence technique. J Urol 141 (part 2):316A

Mark DH (1994) Mortality of patients after radical prostatectomy: analysis of recent medicare claims. J Urol 152:896–898

Mayo ME, Halil T, Browse NL (1971) The incidence of deep vein thrombosis after prostatectomy. Br J Urol 43: 738

McLeod DG (1995) Editorial: prostate cancer. J Urol 153:1873–1874

Mettlin C, Murphy GP, Menck H (1994) Trends in treatment of localized prostate cancer by radical prostatectomy: observations from the commission on cancer national cancer database, 1985–1990. Urology 43:488–492

Middleton AW Jr (1977) A comparison of the morbidity associated with radical retropubic prostatectomy with and without pubectomy. J Urol 117:202

Middleton AW Jr (1987) Radical prostatectomy for carcinoma in men more than 69 years old. J Urol 138:1185–1188

Murphy GP, Mettlin C, Menck H, Winchester DP, Davidson AM (1994) National patterns of prostate cancer treatment by radical prostatectomy: results of a survey by the American College of Surgeons Commission on Cancer. J Urol 152:1817–1819

Ohori M, Goad JR, Wheeler TM et al. (1994) Can radical prostatectomy alter the progression of poorly differentiated prostate cancer? J Urol 152:1843–1849

Optenberg SA, Wojcik BE, Thompson IM (1995) Morbidity and mortality following radical prostatectomy: a national analysis of civilian health and medical program of the Uniformed Services Beneficiaries. J Urol 153:1870–1872

Parivar F, Fournier GR, Narayan P (1994) Urethral anastomotic healing after radical retropubic prostatectomy: impact of positive urethral margin. Urology 44:705–709

Paulson DF (1980) The prognostic role of lymphadenectomy in adenocarcinoma of the prostate. Urol Clin North Am 7:615–622

Paulson DF (1991) Editorial comments on: impact of anatomical radical prostatectomy on urinary continence. J Urol 145:512–515

Pisani P, Parkin DM, Ferlay J (1993) Estimates of the worldwide mortality from eighteen major cancers in 1985. Implications for prevention and projections of future burden. Int J Cancer 55:891–903

Quinlan DM, Epstein JI, Carter BS, Walsh PC (1991) Sexual function following radical prostatectomy: influence of preservation of neurovascular bundles. J Urol 145:998–1002

Reiner WG, Walsh PC (1979) An anatomical approach to the surgical management of the dorsal vein and Santorini's plexus during radical retropubic surgery. J Urol 121:198

Scardino PT (1995) Rationale for the treatment of clinically localized prostate cancer. AUA morning and evening seminars: early detection and treatment of prostate cancer. 23–28 April 1995, Las Vegas, Nevada. AUA Office of Education

Schroder FH, Hermanek P, Denis L et al. (1992) The TNM classification of prostate cancer. Prostate (Suppl):129–138

Seidmon EJ (1993) Negotiating the complications of radical prostatectomy. Contemp Urol 5:68–78

Sigel B, Edelstein AL, Felix WR, Membardt CR (1973) Compression of the deep venous system of lower leg during inactive recumbency. Arch Surg 106:38

Stamey TA (1992) Diagnosis of prostate cancer: a personal view. J Urol 147:830–832

Steiner MS, Morton RA, Walsh PC (1991) Impact of anatomical radical prostatectomy on urinary continence. J Urol 145:512–515

Steiner MS, Burnett AL, Brooks JD et al. (1993) Tubularized neourethra following radical retropubic prostatectomy. J Urol 150:407–410

Strup SE, Gudziak M, Mulholland, Gomella LG (1993) The effect of intermittent pneumatic compression devices on intraoperative blood loss during radical prostatectomy and radical cystectomy. J Urol 150:1176–1178

Thompson IM (1994) Editorial: prostate cancer and quality of life. J Urol 152:1180

Van de Voorde WM, Elgamal AA, Van Poppel HP et al. (1994) Morphologial and immunohistochemical changes in prostate cancer after preoperative hormonal therapy. Cancer 74:3164–3175

Van Poppel H, Ameye F, Oyen R, Van de Voorde W, Baert L (1992) Neoadjuvant hormonotherapy does not facilitate radical prostatectomy. Acta Urol Belg 60:73–82

Van Poppel H, Ameye F, Oyen R, Van de Voorde W, Baert L (1994) Accuracy of combined computerized tomography and fine needle aspiration cytology in lymph node staging of localized prostatic carcinoma. J Urol 151:1310–1314

Van Poppel H, De Ridder D, Elgamal AA et al. (1995) Neoadjuvant hormonal therapy before radical prostatectomy decreases the number of positive surgical margins in stage T2 prostate cancer. Interim results of a prospective randomized trial. J Urol 154:429–434

Veenema RJ, Gursel EO, Lattimer JK (1977) Radical retropubic prostatectomy for cancer: a 20 year experience. J Urol 117:330

Walsh PC (1992) Radical retropubic prostatectomy. In: Walsh PC, Retik AB, Stamey TA, Vaughan ED (eds) Campbell's urology. Saunders, Philadelphia, pp 2865–2886

Walsh PC (1994) Prostate cancer kills: strategy to reduce deaths. Urology 44:463–466

Walsh PC (1995) Editorial: benign and malignant neoplasms of the prostate. J Urol 153:1328–1335

Walsh PC, Lepor H, Eggleston JC (1983) Radical prostatectomy with preservation of sexual function: anatomical and pathological consideration. Prostate 4:473–485

Walsh PC, Partin AW, Epstein JI (1994) Cancer control and quality of life following anatomical radical retropubic prostatectomy: results at 10 years. J Urol 152:1831–1836

Wein AJ (1991) Editorial comments on: impact of anatomical radical prostatectomy on urinary continence. J Urol 145:512–515

Yamada AH, Lieskovsky G, Petrovich Z et al. (1994) Results of radical prostatectomy and adjuvant therapy in the management of locally advanced, clinical stage TC, prostate cancer. Am J Clin Oncol 17:277–285

Yong HH (1945) The cure of cancer of the prostate by radical perineal prostatectomy (prostato-seminal vesiculectomy): history, literature and statistics of Yong's operation. J Urol 53:188–252

Zincke H, Oesterling JE, Blute ML et al. (1994) Long-term (15 years) results after radical prostatectomy for clinically localized (stage T2c or lower) prostate cancer. J Urol 152:1850–1857

12 Radical Retropubic Prostatectomy: The USC Experience

G.D. GROSSFELD, G. LIESKOVSKY, J.A. FREEMAN, S.-C. CHEN, Z. PETROVICH, and D.G. SKINNER

CONTENTS

12.1 Introduction

Adenocarcinoma of the prostate is currently the most common malignancy and second leading cause of death from cancer in men in the United States (WINGO et al. 1995). It has been estimated that 244 000 new cases of prostate cancer will be diagnosed in the United States in 1995, resulting in 40 400 prostate cancer deaths during the same period (WINGO et al. 1995). This estimate represents a 100% increase in new cases of prostate cancer when compared with 1991 (BORING et al. 1991). The discovery and subsequent routine use of serum prostate-specific antigen (PSA) is the most important factor leading to this dramatic increase in prostate cancer detection. While controversy still exists in the literature regarding the benefits of routine screening for prostate cancer, it is becoming standard practice amongst physicians to screen men over 50 years of age for prostate cancer on a yearly basis using both digital rectal examination (DRE) and serum PSA.

In addition to an increased detection of prostate cancer, the use of PSA has resulted in the discovery of prostate cancer at an earlier stage than in the pre-PSA era (CATALONA et al. 1993). Catalona et al. compared prostate cancer discovered in a group of men with abnormal DRE findings with prostate cancer discovered in a group of men initially screened with serum PSA. This study demonstrated that a larger proportion of tumors discovered in the comparison (nonscreened) group were clinically and/or pathologically advanced compared with those found in the PSA-screened group. However, even with this ability to detect prostate cancer at an earlier stage, PSA alone cannot reliably predict organ-confined disease for an individual patient (OESTERLING et al. 1988). Additionally, radiologic staging with computerized tomography, magnetic resonance imaging (MRI), or transrectal ultrasonography has added little to our ability to accurately predict organ-confined disease. As a result, studies have been reported combining PSA with clinical stage and preoperative Gleason score to better predict final pathologic stage in patients with localized prostate cancer (PARTIN et al. 1993). While the combination of all three of these variables improves the prediction of final pathologic

G.D. GROSSFELD, MD, Chief Resident in Urology, University of Southern California School of Medicine, 2025 Zonal Avenue, GH5900, Los Angeles, CA 90033, USA

G. LIESKOVSKY, MD, Professor of Urology and Radiation Oncology, University of Southern California School of Medicine, 2025 Zonal Avenue, GH5900, Los Angeles, CA 90033, USA

J.A. FREEMAN, MD, Assistant Professor of Urology, Division of Urology, University of North Carolina, Burnett-Womack Building CB#7235, Chapel Hill, NC 27599, USA

S.-C. CHEN, PhD, School of Public Health, Chung-Shan Medical and Dental School, 113 Ta-Ching Street, Section 2, Taichung, Taiwan 402

Z. PETROVICH, MD, Professor of Radiation Oncology and Urology, Chairman, Department of Radiation Oncology, University of Southern California School of Medicine, 1441 Eastlake Avenue, Los Angeles, CA 90033, USA

D.G. SKINNER, MD, Professor and Chairman, Department of Urology, University of Southern California School of Medicine, 2025 Zonal Avenue, GH5900, Los Angeles, CA 90033, USA stage over any single variable alone, one is still unable to predict for certain the final pathologic stage for any individual patient.

This clinical staging is crucial, however, as cure of a patient with prostate cancer is predicated upon removal or destruction of all viable tumor cells. Therefore, for local therapy to be effective, the tumor must be confined to the prostate gland at the time of diagnosis and treatment for the best chance of cure. Nearly 60% of the newly diagnosed cases of adenocarcinoma of the prostate per year in the United States are predicted to be organ confined; however, approximately one-third of these patients are found to have extraprostatic disease at the time of surgery (PARTIN et al. 1993; CATALONA et al. 1993; FREEMAN et al. 1993) and 10%–15% are found to have occult spread of tumor to the pelvic lymph nodes (FREEMAN et al. 1994). The continuing high mortality rates associated with prostate cancer reflect our continued inability to detect prostate cancer when it is organ confined and potentially curable.

Options for treatment of patients with clinically localized adenocarcinoma of the prostate include radical prostatectomy, definitive external beam radiotherapy, and observation. Studies from Sweden (JOHANSSON et al. 1989, 1992) reported low disease-specific mortality in patients diagnosed with early-stage prostate cancer who initially remained untreated. The conclusions from these studies have been criticized as the mean age of the study population was 72 years and the large majority of patients included in the study were found to have well-differentiated tumors. Currently, local therapy consisting of radical prostatectomy or external beam radiotherapy is offered by most physicians to patients with clinically localized prostate cancer, provided they have a 10-year life expectancy should they be cured of their prostate cancer. While controversy has existed in the literature regarding the merits of external beam radiotherapy versus radical prostatectomy for clinically localized disease, the benefits of radical prostatectomy over external beam radiotherapy now seem apparent (PAULSON et al. 1982). Patients undergoing radical prostatectomy whose tumors are confined to the prostate have an overall survival comparable to that of age-matched controls without prostate cancer (OESTERLING et al. 1987).

The philosophy at the University of Southern California has been aggressive surgical treatment of patients with clinically localized adenocarcinoma of the prostate, provided that they have a 10-year life expectancy should they be cured of disease. Adjuvant treatment, including radiotherapy to the prostate bed, chemotherapy, or androgen deprivation therapy, has been administered based on the final pathologic stage of disease. This chapter will present our 15-year experience with radical prostatectomy for patients with clinically localized adenocarcinoma of the prostate, with emphasis on our experience with adjuvant treatment for patients with extraprostatic disease.

12.2 Patient Selection

Between January 1974 and April 1989, 299 consecutive patients underwent radical retropubic prostatectomy for adenocarcinoma of the prostate at the University of Southern California affiliated hospitals. Of these patients, 243 were considered to have clinically localized prostate cancer and are the subject of this report. Patients were considered surgical candidates if they: (a) were an acceptable medical risk for major surgery with an expected 10-year survival excluding prostate cancer, and (b) had no radiographic evidence of distant metastases. An elevated prostatic acid phosphatase (PAP) by itself was not considered a contraindication to radical prostatectomy.

Patients ranged in age from 40 to 81 years, the median age being 65 years. Clinical stage was assigned preoperatively based on physical examination and/or pathologic results of tissue removed for clinically benign disease if applicable (SMITH and MIDDLETON 1987). Stage A disease is defined as malignant disease detected on pathologic examination of a gland removed for clinically benign disease. Stage A1 is defined as 5% or less of the specimen involved with prostate cancer while stage A2 is defined as greater than 5% of the specimen involved with prostate cancer. Stage B refers to clinically detected disease which is organ confined. Stage B1 refers to disease involving only one lobe of the prostate or a nodule less than 2 cm, and stage B2 refers to disease involving both lobes or a nodule larger than 2 cm. Using this staging system, preoperative clinical stage was A1 in two patients (0.8%), A2 in 32 patients (13%), B1 in 108 patients (44%), and B2 in 101 patients (42%).

12.3 Surgical Technique

Radical retropubic prostatectomy was performed in 171 patients according to the technique originally described by Campbell (LIESKOVSKY 1988) and was the procedure of choice prior to 1987. Since then an additional 72 carefully selected patients have undergone a nerve-sparing radical retropubic prostatectomy (Walsh 1988), including 14 patients in whom a unilateral nerve-sparing procedure was performed. The operation was accompanied by a bilateral pelvic lymphadenectomy including removal of the obturator, hypogastric, and external iliac lymph nodes below the level at which the ureter crosses the common iliac artery. In three patients the lymphadenectomy was omitted secondary to severe pelvic atherosclerotic disease. Early in this series a more complete pelvic lymph node dissection was carried out, but this was subsequently modified to a more limited dissection leaving the lymphatics along the lateral aspect of the external iliac artery intact. This was done to reduce the potential morbidity of the lymph node dissection, especially when accompanied by postoperative radiotherapy.

12.4 Pathologic Evaluation

Gleason scores were assigned to 240 (99%) final pathologic specimens, with the three remaining patients having no residual tumor in the final pathologic specimen. For statistical analysis, Gleason scores were divided into the following subcategories: 2–4, 5–7, and 8–10.

Direct extension beyond the prostatic capsule was subcategorized according to the schema described by Gibbons et al. (1986). Stage C1 was defined as penetration through the prostatic capsule with no tumor seen at the surgical margins and no seminal vesicle involvement. Stage C2 was defined as tumor present at any surgical margin. Stage C3 was defined as tumor invasion of the seminal vesicles, regardless of capsular penetration or surgical margin involvement. Patients with capsular invasion only, but without clear penetration, were considered pathologic stage B1 (involving only one side of the gland) or B2 (involving both sides of the gland).

Of the 240 patients undergoing simultaneous bilateral lymphadenectomy, 192 (80%) had no evidence of lymph node involvement while 48 others (20%) harbored unsuspected nodal metastases (stage D1 disease). Of these 48 patients, 31 (65%) had fewer than three positive lymph nodes identified.

12.5 Adjuvant Radiotherapy

Adjuvant radiotherapy was recommended to all patients with extracapsular extension of the primary tumor, irrespective of the status of the lymph nodes (stage PCN0 or stage PCN+ disease). Treatment was received by 111 patients and was initiated within 90 days following radical prostatectomy. These patients were treated with linear accelerator-generated photon beams. The beam energy was 4–10 MV in 67 patients (60%) and 15–25 MV in 42 patients (38%). Early in this series one patient was treated with cobalt-60 beam. In one patient radiation treatment data were not available.

Target to skin or target to axis distance was 80 or 100 cm. The volume of interest was confined to the prostatic fossa and its immediate vicinity. Radiation techniques, as expected, have been evolving during the duration of this study. Multiple radiation portals were used for the treatment of patients, with all portals treated daily. A majority of the patients [79 (71%)] were treated with the four-field "box" technique. Anterior-posterior and posterior-anterior fields with 120° lateral arcs were used in the remaining patients. All portals were shaped to optimize the protection of tissues not expected to be involved by the tumor.

Total radiation dose ranged from 42.8 to 61.8 Gy (median 45 Gy). There were 99 patients who received 42.8–50 Gy. All treatments were given daily, five times per week in 180-cGy increments. The prescribed radiation doses were to include the entire volume of interest within the 90%–95% isodose line. No more than 10% dose inhomogeneity through the volume of interest was permitted.

12.6 Follow-up

Patients were followed at 1, 2, and 6 months postoperatively, then at 6-month intervals for the first 5 years, and annually thereafter. General physical examination and DRE were performed at each follow-up visit. A chest X-ray was obtained annually. Serum acid and alkaline phosphatase levels were obtained at each visit prior to the availability of PSA beginning in 1987. Currently only PSA levels are obtained at each visit. Bone scans were obtained on the basis of bone pain or upon the discovery of a significantly elevated PSA. Biopsies were performed to document local recurrence. A clinical recurrence was defined as either a biopsy-proven local recurrence or metastatic disease confirmed by bone scan or biopsy, and was independent of PSA value.

12.7 Complications

Complications were segregated between surgical complications and those attributed to radiotherapy.

Surgical complications were further subdivided into minor and major. Incontinence and impotence were considered separately.

Radiation therapy complications were defined as mild if they required no therapy or medical therapy only. Moderate complications were defined as recurrent or those requiring minor surgery. Major complications were persistent, requiring hospitalization or major surgery, or resulting in death.

12.8 Statistical Analysis

Survival, prostate cancer-specific survival, time to any recurrence, and time to clinical recurrence were the outcomes analyzed in this study. Survival was calculated as the number of years from prostatectomy until death or last documented contact when the patient was known to be alive. For prostate cancer-specific survival, patients dying of a cause other than prostate cancer were counted as failing of a competing cause, and patients alive were censored at the date of last contact. For patients in whom disease recurred, time to any recurrence was calculated as the number of years from prostatectomy to the date of documented clinical recurrence or detectable PSA. Prior to 1 July 1994, serum PSA was determined using the Hybritech Tandem Assay. Serum PSA $\geq$ 0.4 ng/ml on two consecutive occasions was classified as detectable using this assay. Beginning July 1994, a new PSA assay with greater sensitivity was used (Tosoh AIA Pack), and subsequently a serum PSA $\geq$ 0.1 ng/ml or serum PSA $\geq$ 0.05 ng/ml on two consecutive occasions was classified as detectable. Patients who died prior to recurrence were counted as failing of a competing cause at the time of death, and patients without disease recurrence were censored at the date of last contact in which the patient was documented as free of disease. Time to clinical recurrence was calculated in a similar fashion, except that only clinical recurrence was counted as failure and the date of first elevated PSA was ignored.

Kaplan-Meier product limit estimates of overall survival were plotted (Miller 1981). Cumulative incidence curves were plotted for cause-specific survival as well as recurrence (Gaynor et al. 1993) Standard errors for the probability of surviving or not suffering recurrence were based on Greenwood's formula for the Kaplan-Meier estimates (Miller 1981) and on the delta method for the cumulative incidence curves (Gaynor et al. 1993). The log-rank test was used to compare groups of patients. All P values reported are two sided.

The survival curve based on death due to all causes was compared with an expected survival curve. The expected survival curve was constructed from the United States Decennial Life Tables for 1972–1989, matching for year of prostatectomy, age, and race based on methods described previously (Freeman 1994).

12.9 Results

12.9.1 Pathologic Findings

Organ-confined disease was confirmed pathologically in 105 patients (43%) undergoing radical prostatectomy. A total of 90 patients (37%) had pathologic evidence of extracapsular extension, without evidence of lymph node involvement. Of these patients, nine presented with clinical stage A2 disease, 40 presented with clinical stage B1 disease, and 41 presented with clinical stage B2 disease. Analysis of the prostatectomy specimen in these patients indicated 25 patients (28%) with stage C1 lesions (capsular penetration only), 40 patients (44%) with stage C2 lesions (positive margins), and 25 patients (28%) with stage C3 disease (seminal vesicle involvement). Forty-eight other patients harbored evidence of pelvic lymph node involvement on permanent section (pathologic stage D1 disease). Of these patients, two presented with clinical stage A2 disease, 14 presented with clinical stage B1 disease, and 32 presented with clinical stage B2 disease. Thirty of these patients (63%) demonstrated pathologic extension into one or both seminal vesicles. Six patients with tumor pathologically confined to the prostate were found to have microscopic extension of the tumor into the pelvic lymph nodes. Table 12.1 correlates the preoperative clinical stage with the final pathologic stage confirmed from the radical prostatectomy specimen. Three patients (one clinical stage A2, one clinical stage B1, and one clinical stage B2) did not undergo pelvic lymphadenectomy at the time of radical prostatectomy because of severe pelvic atherosclerotic vascular disease.

Analysis of the Gleason score revealed 32 patients (13%) with a Gleason score of 2–4, 172 patients (71%) with a Gleason score of 5–7, and 36 patients (15%) with a Gleason score of 8–10. Three patients (1%) with clinically localized lesions had no evidence of residual disease following analysis of the

Table 12.1. Correlation between preoperative clinical stage and final pathologic stage in 243 patients undergoing radical retropubic prostatectomy for clinically localized prostate cancer

Clinical stage	Pathologic stage							Total
	P0	B1	B2	C1	C2	C3	D1	
A1		1	1					2
A2	2	3	16[a]	2	4	3	2	32
B1	1	18	35[a]	13	19	8	14	108
B2	0	3	25	10[a]	17	14	32	101
Total	3	25	77	25	40	25	48	243

[a] Lymphadenectomy not performed in one patient

Table 12.2. Correlation between Gleason score of radical prostatectomy specimen and preoperative clinical stage

Clinical stage	Gleason score of prostatetomy specimen				Total
	P0	2–4	5–7	8–10	
A1	0	2	0	0	2
A2	2	6	23	1	32
B1	1	16	78	13	108
B2	0	8	71	22	101
Total	3	32	172	36	243

pathologic specimen (two with clinical stage A2 and one with clinical stage B1). Table 12.2 correlates preoperative clinical stage with the Gleason score.

12.9.2 Complications

There were no operative-related deaths amongst the 243 patients undergoing radical retropubic prostatectomy in this series. Minor surgical complications occurred in six patients (2.5%), while major surgical complications also occurred in six patients (2.5%). Major complications included reexploration for bleeding in three patients and one patient each with fascial dehiscence, sacral decubitus requiring myocutaneous flap, and delayed rectovesical fistula (fifth postoperative day) requiring a temporary colostomy.

Urinary continence was assessed at 1 year following surgery. Complete continence, or mild stress incontinence not requiring protection, was found in 215 patients (88%). Dampness requiring one to two pads per day occurred in 12 patients (5%) while three to four pads per day were required in five patients (2%). Total incontinence occurred in only 11 patients (5%). Postoperative adjuvant radiotherapy did not adversely affect overall continence recovery (Table 12.3). Of the 72 men undergoing nerve-sparing surgery, 70 had complete continence or only mild stress incontinence while only two patients required one to two pads per day for protection.

One hundred and sixty-five patients (68%) did not require intraoperative blood transfusion while 58 patients (24%) received 1 or 2 units of blood intraoperatively. Another 20 patients (8%) received 3 or more units of blood during surgery. Postoperatively 201 patients (83%) did not require administration of blood, while 27 patients (11%) received 1–2 units and 15 other patients (6%) required 3 or more units of blood following surgery.

12.9.3 Potency

Seventy-two patients underwent some form of nerve-sparing procedure in an attempt to preserve potency (11 patients with clinical stage A2 disease, 52 patients with clinical stage B1 disease, and nine patients with clinical stage B2 disease). Preservation of sexual function was determined 1 year following surgery. Overall potency preservation was reported in 28 patients (39%), including 5 of 26 patients (19%) who received postoperative adjuvant radiotherapy secondary to extracapsular extension of disease. Of 46 patients who did not receive postoperative radiotherapy, 23 (50%) retained potency postoperatively.

Fifty-eight of the 72 patients underwent bilateral nerve-sparing surgery, including 18 who received postoperative adjuvant radiotherapy. Twenty-six (45%) of these patients remained potent postoperatively. This is in contrast to patients who underwent unilateral nerve-sparing surgery, in whom 2 of 14 (14%) remained potent postoperatively (eight of

Table 12.3. Continence at 1 year postoperatively in 243 patients undergoing radical retropubic prostatectomy for clinically localized prostate cancer

	Entire group	No radiation	Postop radiation
Complete continence or mild stress without protection	215 (88%)	118 (89%)	97 (87%)
1–2 pads/day	12 (5%)	6 (4%)	6 (5%)
3–4 pads/day	5 (2%)	2 (2%)	3 (3%)
Incontinent	11 (5%)	6 (5%)	5 (5%)
	243	132	111

these 14 patients received adjuvant radiotherapy). Age at the time of radical prostatectomy correlated with postoperative potency recovery. Potency was preserved in four of five patients between 40 and 49, in 11 of 22 patients between 50 and 59, and in 13 of 45 patients older than 60.

Forty-one patients were found to have organ-confined disease following examination of the pathologic specimen. Potency was preserved in 20 of these 41 patients (49%).

12.9.4 Recurrence and Survival

Of the 243 patients undergoing radical retropubic prostatectomy, 130 (53.5%) currently remain alive, without clinical evidence of disease, and with an undetectable PSA at a median follow-up of 7.7 years (range 2.7–17.2 years). Of these patients, 23 (18%) were clinical stage A1 or A2, 69 (53%) clinical stage B1, and 38 (29%) clinical stage B2. In terms of pathologic stage, 71 (55%) of these patients had organ-confined disease (two of these patients did not undergo lymphadenectomy), 49 (38%) had evidence of extracapsular extension without lymph node involvement, and ten (8%) harbored pelvic nodal metastases. Of the entire group, clinical recurrence occurred in 45 patients (19%). Among these patients, the pathologic stage at the time of radical prostatectomy was stage B1 in two patients (one of these patients did not undergo lymphadenectomy), stage B2 in eight patients, stage C in 12 patients, and stage D1 in 23 patients. A palpable local mass was the first site of recurrence in nine patients, while 36 other patients presented with distant metastases as the first site of disease recurrence, resulting in 17 (7.0%) deaths from prostate cancer. Twelve patients (5%) died of other malignancies, including three patients who had elevated PSA levels at the time of their deaths. Eight other patients died during the follow-up period; seven of these patients were without evidence of disease recurrence at the time of death while one patient died of an unknown cause after having a documented clinical recurrence of prostate cancer.

An elevated PSA value without clinical evidence of recurrent disease is present in 49 patients (20.2%). The current status of all 243 patients is listed in Table 12.4.

Table 12.4. Current status of 243 patients undergoing radical retropubic prostatectomy for clinically localized prostate cancer

Current status	No. of pts	(%)
Alive, no evidence of disease (undetectable PSA)	130	53.5
Alive with elevated PSA only	49	20.2
Alive with clinical recurrence	27	11.1
Dead of prostate cancer	17	7.0
Dead of other malignancies (no recurrence)	9	3.7
Dead of other causes (no recurrence)	5	2.1
Dead of lung cancer with elevated PSA	3	1.2
Dead of unknown causes (not prostate ca., no recurrence)	2	0.8
Dead of unknown causes with clinical recurrence	1	0.4
	243	

Median follow-up 7.7 years (range 2.7–17.2 years)

For the entire group, the chance of clinical recurrence at 5 and 10 years is estimated at 12% ± 2% and 22% ± 3%, while the chance of any recurrence (clinical or PSA) at 5 and 10 years is estimated at 29% ± 3% and 47% ± 4% respectively (Fig. 12.1). By comparing pathologic stage, the chance of any recurrence (clinical or PSA) at 5 and 10 years is estimated at 17% ± 4% and 37% ± 8% for those with organ-confined disease, 29% ± 5% and 44% ± 6% for those with extracapsular extension only, and 56% ± 7% and 74% ± 7% for those with regional lymph node involvement (Fig. 12.2). For the entire group, the estimated actuarial probability of survival at 5 and 10 years is 93% ± 2% and 80% ± 3% (Fig. 12.3) while the estimated prostate cancer-specific actuarial survival at 5 and 10 years is 97% ± 1% and 90% ± 3%. For patients with organ-confined disease, the overall survival at 5 and 10 years is estimated at 97% ± 2% and 90% ± 5%. In patients with extracapsular extension only, the overall survival at 5 and 10 years is estimated at 93% ± 3% and 81% ± 5%. Finally, in patients with regional lymph node involvement, 5- and 10-year overall survival is estimated at 85% ± 5% and 61% ± 10% respectively (Fig. 12.4).

Analysis of the time to recurrence (clinical or PSA) based on the Gleason score demonstrates a significant difference in the time to recurrence between patients with Gleason scores 2–4, 5–7, and 8–10 (Fig. 12.5, $P < 0.0001$). This translates into a statistically significant improvement in overall survival between patients with Gleason scores 2–4, 5–7, and 8–10 ($P < 0.0001$). When comparing by pathologic stage, a significant difference in overall survival and probability of developing any recurrence (clinical or PSA) is seen between patients with pathologic stage B, C, and D1 disease (Figs. 12.4 and 12.2; $P = 0.0055$ for overall survival; $P < 0.0001$ for probability of any recurrence).

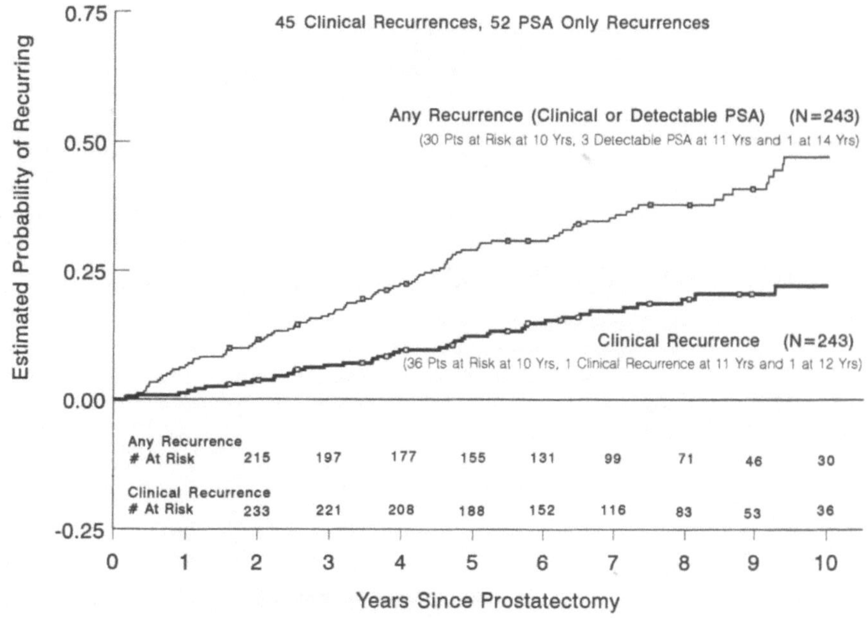

Fig. 12.1. Estimated probability of clinical recurrence and any recurrence (clinical or detectable PSA). □ indicates a patient who was dead of causes other than prostate cancer

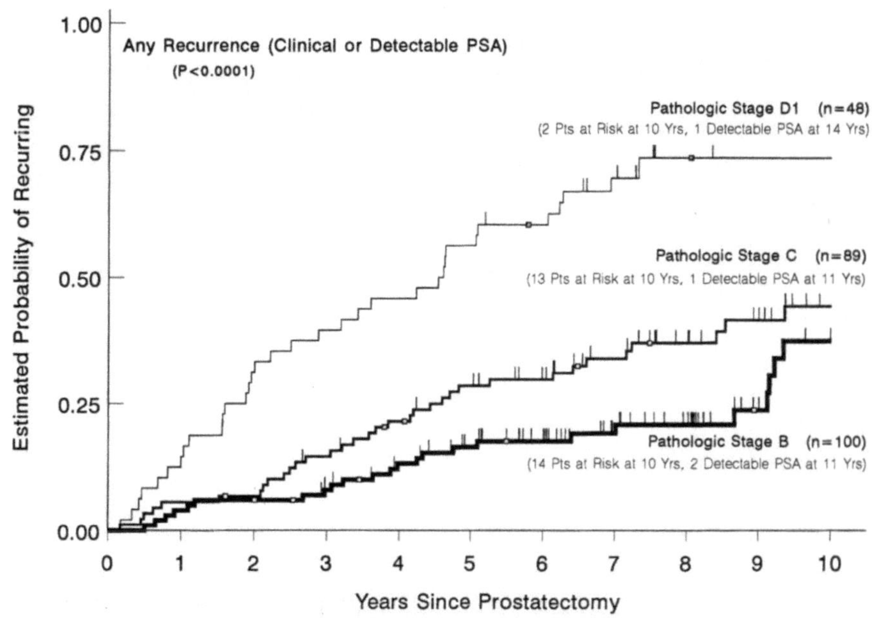

Fig. 12.2. Estimated probability of any recurrence (clinical or detectable PSA) comparing groups based on pathologic stage (excluding 3 P0 and 3 NX). Each *tick mark* represents a surviving patient who had not had a recurrence of prostate cancer at the time of last follow-up. □ indicates a patient who was dead of causes other than prostate cancer

12.9.5 PSA/PAP Values

Ninety-seven patients (40%) on careful follow-up were found to have evidence of clinical recurrence (45 patients) or an elevated PSA value only as first evidence of prostate cancer recurrence (52 patients).

For those patients with an elevated PSA only, the median time from surgery to a detectable PSA value was 50.4 months (range 5.5–173.7 months). It is our policy to biopsy the vesicourethral anastomosis and prostate bed in those patients with an elevated PSA only who have not previously received radiation

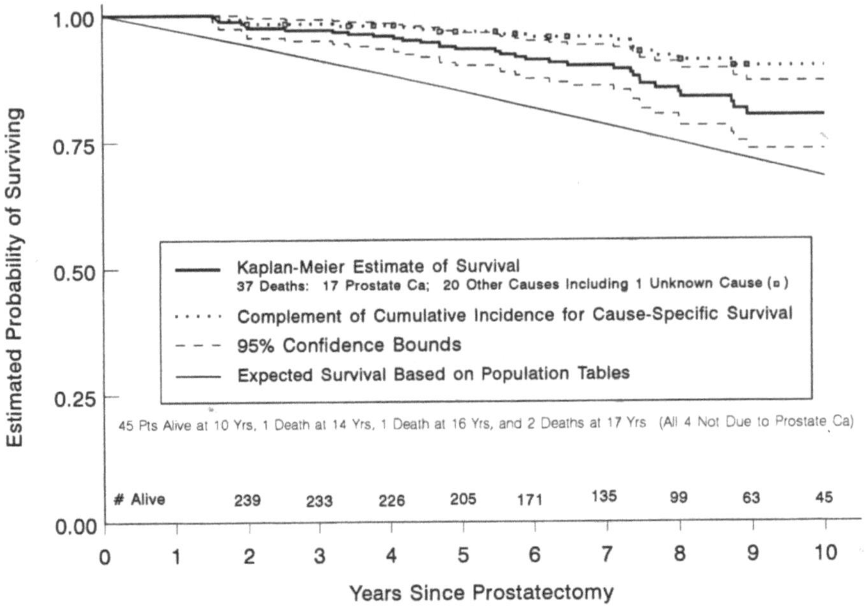

Fig. 12.3. Estimated probability of surviving from all causes and from prostate cancer, and an expected survival curve based on population tables. Bounds based on the approximate 95% point confidence intervals for overall survival are also plotted (*dashed lines*). Each *tick mark* represents a patient who was alive at the time of last follow-up. □ indicates a patient who was dead of causes other than prostate cancer

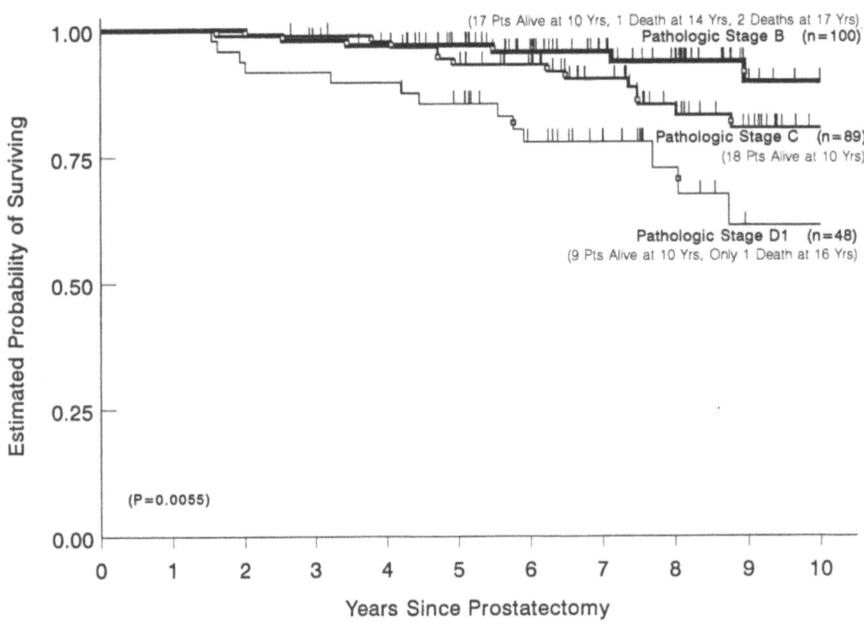

Fig. 12.4. Estimated probability of surviving from all causes comparing groups based on pathologic stage (excluding 3 P0 and 3 NX). Each *tick mark* represents a patient who was alive at the time of last follow-up. □ indicates a patient who was dead of causes other than prostate cancer

therapy in order to determine the presence or absence of local disease recurrence. In the event of a positive biopsy, radiation (60 Gy) to the prostatic fossa is recommended. All other patients with an elevated PSA only are closely monitored for signs of clinical recurrence at which time some form of androgen deprivation therapy is initiated. The nine patients who developed clinical recurrence in the absence of PSA elevation were from the era prior to the development of PSA as a diagnostic tool, which has now replaced the use of PAP at our institution. In the remaining 36 patients, clinical recurrence was associated with a simultaneous elevation of PSA.

Preoperative PSA values were available in 67 patients and were elevated (>4.0 ng/ml) in 44 (66%). Table 12.5 compares the clinical stage with the preoperative PSA values. Table 12.6 compares the pathologic stage with preoperative PSA levels. Of 29 patients with organ-confined disease, 26 (90%) had PSA values of 10 ng/ml or less. However, 16 of 28 (57%) of pathologic stage C and four of ten (40%) pathologic stage D1 patients also had PSA values under 10 ng/ml. Of patients with a PSA value less than 4.0 ng/ml, 43% had pathologic evidence of extracapsular extension or unsuspected involvement of the pelvic lymph nodes. There were 18 patients (one with clinical stage A2 disease and 17 with clinical stage B1 or B2 disease) with preoperative elevation of PAP. There was no difference in actuarial survival or time to recurrence (clinical or PSA) between patients with elevated and patients with normal preoperative PAP values.

12.10 Discussion

The number of radical prostatectomies performed for the treatment of adenocarcinoma of the prostate

Table 12.5. Relationship between clinical stage and preoperative PSA levels in 67 patients undergoing radical retropubic prostatectomy for clinically localized prostate cancer

Clinical stage	PSA range (ng/ml)				Total
	0–4	5–10	11–20	>20	
A1	1				1
A2	8	1	1		10
B1	7	14	7	2	30
B2	7	8	6	5	26
Total	23	23	14	7	67

Table 12.6. Relationship between pathologic stage and preoperative PSA levels in 67 patients undergoing radical retropubic prostatectomy for clinically localized prostate cancer

Pathologic stage	PSA range (ng/ml)				Total
	0–4	5–10	11–20	>20	
B1	4	0	0	0	4
B2	9	13	2	1	25
C1	5	0	0	1	6
C2	2	4	5	0	11
C3	2	3	3	3	11
D1	1	3	4	2	10
Total	23	23	14	7	67

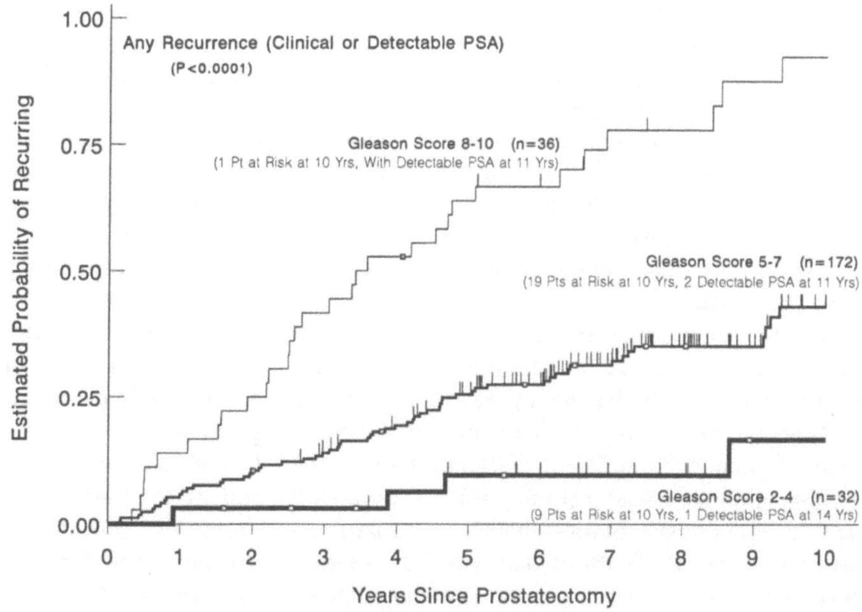

Fig. 12.5. Estimated probability of any recurrence (clinical or detectable PSA) comparing groups based on the Gleason score (excluding 3 P0). Each *tick mark* represents a surviving patient who had not had a recurrence of prostate cancer at the time of last follow-up. □ indicates a patient who was dead of causes other than prostate cancer

has increased between four- and sixfold in the United States over the last 10 years (LITWILLER et al. 1995). Data from the National Cancer Database demonstrate that the use of radical prostatectomy has been greatest in younger patients, as 69% of patients under 55 years of age diagnosed with clinically localized prostate cancer in 1990 underwent radical prostatectomy (METTLIN et al. 1994). Our 15-year experience with radical retropubic prostatectomy for clinically localized adenocarcinoma of the prostate demonstrates the safety and efficacy of this treatment for patients with prostate cancer. The overall survival in our group of 243 patients is superior to that of age-matched controls in the general population (Fig. 12.3). We have found that both overall survival and probability of any recurrence in this group of patients is significantly related to clinical stage at the time of diagnosis ($P = 0.012$ for overall survival; $P = 0.0052$ for any recurrence), final pathologic stage as determined from the prostatectomy specimen (Figs. 12.2 and 12.4), and the final Gleason score of the tumor (Fig. 12.5).

Given the continued controversy regarding the proper management of patients with clinically localized prostate cancer, the morbidity of any treatment modality must be addressed along with its efficacy. With recent advances in surgical technique, as well as advances in the perioperative management of patients undergoing major pelvic surgery, radical prostatectomy has become a procedure with minimal morbidity. No cases of operative mortality were seen in our series of 243 consecutive patients undergoing radical prostatectomy, while the morbidity of the procedure has been minimal, with only a 2.5% incidence of major postoperative complications and a 2.5% incidence of minor postoperative complications. In addition, it has recently been demonstrated that these excellent results with respect to quality of care can be obtained in a cost-efficient manner, which is important in today's economic environment (KOCH et al. 1994).

Quality of life issues are also crucial when considering a patient as a candidate for radical prostatectomy, with the postoperative continence and potency of the patient being two of the most important issues. Complete urinary continence (including minimal stress incontinence not requiring protection) has been obtained in 88% of our patients postoperatively. Only 5% of our patients reported total incontinence. These results are similar to those observed by other authors (STEIN et al. 1992b; O'DONNELL and FINAN 1989) and confirm that patients undergoing radical prostatectomy can expect an acceptable outcome with respect to urinary continence.

With the introduction of the anatomic approach to radical prostatectomy (WALSH 1988), preservation of sexual function has become possible in many patients undergoing radical prostatectomy. We have demonstrated preservation of sexual function in 45% of patients undergoing bilateral nerve-sparing radical prostatectomy. However, in patients undergoing unilateral nerve-sparing surgery, there is a marked decrease in the preservation of sexual function (14%). Data from Johns Hopkins (QUINLAN et al. 1991) demonstrated that 68% of patients were able to have an erection sufficient for vaginal penetration following nerve-sparing surgery. As with the group at Johns Hopkins, we have found that patient age at the time of surgery as well as extent of disease correlates well with preservation of sexual function after radical prostatectomy. While the exact incidence of sexual dysfunction after external beam radiotherapy is unclear, it has been estimated to be approximately 50% (WALSH and LEPOR 1987). The above results demonstrate that radical prostatectomy compares favorably with alternative treatment modalities when considering postoperative potency preservation. After reviewing these results, we began using the following criteria when considering a patient for nerve-sparing radical prostatectomy for the treatment of adenocarcinoma of the prostate: (a) age less than 65 years, (b) clinical B1 nodule, and (c) serum PSA less than 10.

12.10.1 Organ-Confined Disease (Stage B)

Patients with pathologically organ-confined disease (pathologic stage B) were found to have excellent results with respect to both disease recurrence and overall survival in our series of patients. Overall 5-year survival for this group of patients was 97% ± 2%, with prostate cancer-specific survival being 100%. Overall 10-year survival was 90% ± 5%. Recurrence data were equally impressive as the probability of clinical recurrence at 5 and 10 years in this group of patients was only 4% and 9%, respectively. Overall survival and clinical recurrence rates were similar to those found in other large series in the literature reporting on the use of radical prostatectomy for the treatment of organ-confined prostate cancer (STEIN et al. 1992b; PAULSON et al. 1990). PSA is now widely used in the follow-up of patients following radical prostatectomy. When considering an elevated serum PSA as an indicator of disease recurrence, the chance of any recurrence (clinical or PSA) increases to 17% at 5 years and 37% at 10 years in our patients with organ-confined prostate cancer. When comparing our data to the results obtained with expectant treatment of patients with clinically localized prostate cancer, one sees that patients with stage B1 or B2 disease treated expectantly have 5-year disease progression rates ranging from 23% to 54% and 10-year disease progression rates reaching 66% (WALSH 1990).

Our data clearly illustrate the efficacy of radical prostatectomy in the treatment of patients with organ-confined (pathologic stage B) disease. Excellent results can be obtained with regard to both overall survival and clinical disease-free survival. As an elevated serum PSA is considered to be indicative of residual disease, continued follow-up is crucial to determine what percentage of these patients are destined to suffer clinical recurrence and develop disease progression.

12.10.2 Pathologic Stage C (pT3N0) Disease

Ninety of our 243 patients (37%) were found to have extracapsular extension of tumor without evidence of nodal metastases. Of these 90 patients, 25 (28%) exhibited extracapsular extension only (stage C1), 40 (44%) had positive surgical margins (stage C2), and 25 (28%) had evidence of tumor present in one or both seminal vesicles. We have followed a treatment philosophy of recommending adjuvant postoperative radiotherapy following radical prostatectomy to patients with pT3 adenocarcinoma of the prostate, in the belief that residual tumor confined locally to the pelvis postoperatively can serve as the source of local and distant failure if it remains untreated. Seventy-five of the 90 patients with pT3 disease (stage C) have received the recommended postoperative adjuvant radiotherapy.

The overall 5- and 10-year survival in our patients with pathologic pT3 adenocarcinoma of the prostate in this series was 93% and 81%, respectively. The chance of clinical recurrence in this group of patients was 9% at 5 years and 16% at 10 years. If PSA recurrence is included, the chance of any recurrence at 5 and 10 years was 29% and 44%, respectively. In considering the 75 patients who received postoperative adjuvant radiotherapy, only two (3%) were found to have local disease recurrence during the follow-up period. In comparing these results with other series reported in the literature, PAULSON et al. (1990) found a 30% failure rate at 10 years in patients with extraprostatic but specimen-confined disease, and a 60% failure rate in patients with margin-positive disease at 10 years, with approximately one-third of margin-positive patients receiving postoperative adjuvant radiotherapy. PSA was not used as a marker for disease recurrence in this series. The UCLA group (STEIN et al. 1992b) also reported on patients with clinically organ-confined prostate cancer who were found to have extraprostatic disease after radical prostatectomy. Adjuvant radiotherapy was administered to 23 of 115 patients with extraprostatic disease in this series. A 90% cause-specific survival rate at 10 years was found in patients with disease spread beyond the capsule based on pathologic staging while patients with involvement of the seminal vesicles were found to have a 63% cause-specific survival rate at 10 years. With regard to disease recurrence, patients with extracapsular spread only were found to have a 21% risk of clinical recurrence at 5 years, while the patients with seminal vesicle involvement had a 42% risk of clinical recurrence at 5 years. When PSA recurrence was also included, the disease-free survival decreased substantially for the entire group of patients, including a 24% disease-free survival at 5 years for patients with seminal vesicle involvement.

As previous stated, it has been our policy to recommend postoperative adjuvant radiotherapy to our patients with pT3 adenocarcinoma of the prostate. Radiotherapy doses and techniques were designed to decrease treatment complications while maintaining tumoricidal effects. We currently recommend a dose of 45 Gy for microscopic residual disease and 54 Gy for patients with involvement of the seminal vesicles (stage C3 disease). Our experience with 95 consecutive patients with pT3 adenocarcinoma of the prostate who received postoperative adjuvant radiotherapy has been published previously (FREEMAN et al. 1993). While most of these patients presented with clinically localized disease, this series also includes patients initially presenting with clinical stage C (T3) disease (YAMADA et al. 1994). Overall 5- and 10-year actuarial survival rates in the Freeman series were found to be 94% and 70%, respectively. The chance of a clinical recurrence was estimated to be 6% at 5 years and 13% at 10 years. When PSA recurrence was also considered, the chance of any recurrence was 34% at 5 years and 46% at 10 years. Disease-specific survival and clinical recurrence-free survival in the Freeman series, as well as in our series of patients, were found to be improved over historical controls. Additionally, only 2 of 95 patients (2%) in the Freeman series developed a local recurrence during the follow-up period. This is similar to our finding of a 3% local recurrence rate in patients with pT3 adenocarcinoma of the prostate receiving postoperative adjuvant radiotherapy, and is superior to series reporting on surgery alone for pT3 disease, where local recurrence ranges from 8% to 43%. Our results have been obtained with minimal added morbidity from the radiotherapy and no change in the degree of urinary continence when compared to patients not receiving radiotherapy.

The issue of postoperative adjuvant radiotherapy for patients with pT3 adenocarcinoma of the prostate has been addressed in several other series in the literature. One of the first authors to address this issue was GIBBONS (GIBBONS et al. 1986), who found that postoperative adjuvant radiotherapy significantly decreased local recurrence in patients undergoing radical prostatectomy when compared to patients undergoing surgery alone, with a particular benefit seen in patients with positive surgical margins and/or disease in the seminal vesicles. Additionally, GIBBONS found that delayed radiotherapy for a documented local recurrence was not effective in controlling local disease. Although overall survival was not increased in the group receiving adjuvant radiotherapy in this study, the data suggested that longer follow-up might disclose such an advantage. Updated data from this group (JONSSON et al., unpublished) continue to show the benefit of adjuvant radiotherapy with regard to local recurrence, but no benefit was seen with respect to survival. Adjuvant radiotherapy given to stage C2 patients in this series (margin-positive disease), however, appeared to convey some benefit with respect to a decreased incidence of marker positivity (PSA or acid phosphatase) and an increased median time to progression that was not seen in the prior report. Other series in the literature (ZIETMAN et al. 1993; ANSCHER and PROSNITZ 1987; STEIN et al. 1992a) also confirm a benefit of adjuvant radiotherapy with regard to tumor recurrence, without proving a benefit with respect to long-term survival. Adjuvant radiotherapy has also been used for patients with a persistently elevated PSA following surgery (HUDSON and CATALONA 1990; LANGE et al. 1990). While these series demonstrate that radiation therapy can cause elevated PSA levels to decrease to undetectable levels in 29%–53% of patients, additional follow-up is needed to determine the durability of this response as well as the ultimate impact of this treatment on survival free of tumor.

In summary, postoperative adjuvant radiotherapy in patients with pT3 adenocarcinoma of the prostate at the time of radical prostatectomy remains controversial. Our data, along with those of other series in the literature, appear to confirm a benefit of adjuvant radiotherapy with regard to local disease recurrence, and in some cases, in overall clinical recurrence. The efficacy of postoperative adjuvant radiotherapy with respect to overall survival can only be evaluated by prospective, randomized trials. As the extent of capsular penetration, status of the surgical margins and seminal vesicles, and Gleason grade of the tumor all affect the risk of tumor progression (EPSTEIN et al. 1993), any clinical trial must stratify patients into groups with similar risks of progression to evaluate properly the efficacy of postoperative adjuvant radiotherapy.

12.10.3 Microscopic Lymph Node Involvement (Stage D1 Disease)

The optimal management for patients with stage D1 adenocarcinoma of the prostate remains controversial. Traditionally, patients with lymph node metastases have been thought to be unsuitable candidates for radical prostatectomy. As a result, radiation therapy or observation with delayed androgen deprivation has been utilized in the treatment of these patients with unfavorable nonprogression and survival results (FREEMAN et al. 1994; ZINCKE 1990). However, more recent studies have detailed the benefits of an aggressive approach to the management of stage D1 adenocarcinoma of the prostate utilizing radical surgery, with or without postoperative adjuvant treatment (FREEMAN et al. 1994; DEKERNION et al. 1990; ZINCKE 1989, 1990; STEINBERG et al. 1990). Forty-eight of our 243 patients with clinically localized prostate cancer were found to have microscopic involvement of the pelvic lymph nodes. Of these patients, 31 were found to have one or two involved lymph nodes, while the remaining 17 had at least three lymph nodes involved with tumor. After initial treatment with radical prostatectomy, 45 of the 48 patients received adjuvant therapy. Adjuvant treatment was delivered as follows: 29 patients received adjuvant chemotherapy and radiotherapy, seven patients received adjuvant chemotherapy only, six patients received adjuvant radiotherapy ± androgen deprivation therapy, one patient received adjuvant androgen deprivation therapy only, one patient received adjuvant radiotherapy, chemotherapy, and androgen deprivation therapy, and one patient received unknown adjuvant treatment.

The overall survival in this group of 48 patients with pathologic stage D1 disease was estimated to be 85% and 61% at 5 and 10 years, respectively. The chance of clinical recurrence only in these patients was estimated to be 34% and 63% at 5 and 10 years respectively, while the probability of any recurrence (clinical or PSA) was estimated to be 56% and 74% at 5 and 10 years, respectively. Of 33 patients who received postoperative adjuvant radiotherapy (± chemotherapy), only one (3%) developed a local recurrence during the follow-up period.

Our extended experience utilizing radical prostatectomy in the management of patients with stage D1 adenocarcinoma of the prostate has previously been reviewed (FREEMAN et al. 1994). This report includes 76 patients with a median follow-up of 7.0 years. In addition to the above 48 patients who initially presented with clinically localized disease, 28 other patients initially presenting with clinical stage C (T3) disease are included in that series (YAMADA et al. 1994). Patients received postoperative adjuvant therapy based on the pathologic stage of their primary tumor as well as the extent of nodal disease. In patients with pathologic pT3 disease, adjuvant radiotherapy was recommended. Chemotherapy with cyclophosphamide ± 5-fluorouracil was recommended for all patients to address the systemic component of disease, while androgen deprivation therapy was recommended for all patients with more than six lymph nodes positive for tumor. The overall survival was estimated to be 88% and 66% at 5 and 10 years respectively, with prostate cancer-specific survival of 88% at 5 years and 74% at 10 years. Overall survival equaled that of age- and race-matched controls. The probability of developing a clinically detectable recurrence was 29% and 62% at 5 and 10 years, respectively. When PSA was added to the detection data, the probability of any recurrence increased to 58% and 78% at 5 and 10 years, respectively. Local recurrence was seen in only five patients, with only two of these patients receiving adjuvant radiotherapy in the postoperative period. Gleason score was found to predict for both survival and recurrence (2–7 vs 8–10).

Univariate analysis in this group of patients showed there was no effect of chemotherapy or androgen deprivation therapy on time to recurrence or survival. While the use of radiotherapy had no effect on survival, it did impact on clinical recurrence ($P = 0.023$). The combination of adjuvant radiotherapy and androgen deprivation therapy significantly increased the time to clinical recurrence for all patients ($P = 0.015$) as well as the time to any recurrence (clinical or PSA, $P = 0.023$). This combination of adjuvant therapy, however, did not significantly affect survival.

The role of radical prostatectomy in the management of patients with stage D1 adenocarcinoma of the prostate has recently been the subject of a number of additional reports in the literature. In a series of 120 patients with stage D1 adenocarcinoma of the prostate treated expectantly, by radiotherapy, or by radical prostatectomy alone, local recurrence requiring an operation was noted in 23%, 24%, and 3%, respectively (STEINBERG et al. 1990). As the 5- and 10-year projected actuarial survival rates for this entire group of patients were 68% and 54%, palliation of the primary lesion with low morbidity was felt to be an important goal in patients with stage D1 adenocarcinoma of the prostate, many of whom live many years with their disease. This goal was best achieved with radical prostatectomy in this series.

The value of early endocrine therapy following radical prostatectomy has been addressed by groups at UCLA as well as at the Mayo clinic (DEKERNION et al. 1990; ZINCKE 1989, 1990). DEKERNION et al. (1990) reported that while early endocrine therapy did not increase cause-specific survival for patients with stage D1 adenocarcinoma of the prostate undergoing radical prostatectomy, survival free of disease was significantly prolonged. This was true whether or not PSA was used as an indicator for disease recurrence. Using a Cox proportional hazards model, patients in this series who did not undergo early endocrine therapy had a 3.1-fold greater risk of progression or death when compared to those receiving early endocrine therapy.

ZINCKE (1989) reported on 266 patients with stage D1 adenocarcinoma of the prostate treated with radical prostatectomy, with or without immediate androgen deprivation therapy. Overall survival rates for the entire group of patients were found to be comparable to an age-matched control population. Patients undergoing immediate adjuvant orchiectomy were found to have a significant advantage with regard to overall nonprogression rates when compared to patients undergoing radical prostatectomy alone. However, the impact of immediate orchiectomy on cause-specific survival was not found to be statistically significant. The influence of the DNA ploidy pattern of the tumor on progression and survival was also studied in this group of patients with stage D1 disease. Patients with a DNA diploid tumor were found to have a significant improvement in both nonprogression rates and disease-specific survival when compared to patients with a nondiploid tumor. A subsequent study by ZINCKE (1990) reporting on 380 patients undergoing radical prostatectomy for stage D1 adenocarcinoma of the prostate not only confirmed the above findings but also found that the impact of immediate adjuvant hormonal treatment on progression translated into a significantly improved overall survival rate for these patients. The influence of DNA ploidy and immediate adjuvant hormonal treatment was also studied in this group of patients. Adjuvant hormonal treatment resulted in a statistically significant improvement in nonprogression rates in patients with both diploid and nondiploid tumors. With regard to cause-specific survival, immediate androgen deprivation treatment significantly improved cause-specific survival in patients with DNA diploid tumors. However, the same effect on survival was not seen with nondiploid tumors.

In summary, radical prostatectomy appears to have an important role in the treatment of patients with stage D1 adenocarcinoma of the prostate. As these patients may live many years with their disease, palliation of the primary lesion is an important goal which appears to be best obtained with radical prostatectomy. Adjuvant treatment after radical prostatectomy, especially radiotherapy and/or androgen deprivation therapy, appears to be beneficial with regard to prolonging time to disease recurrence. With continued follow-up, it is possible that this benefit will translate into an improvement in overall survival in this high-risk group of patients.

12.11 Conclusion

The detection of clinically localized prostate cancer has increased dramatically over the past several years. This increase in prostate cancer detection has been accompanied by controversy regarding the benefits of routine prostate cancer screening in men over 50 years of age, as well as controversy regarding which patients with clinically localized prostate cancer should be treated aggressively.

At the University of Southern California, it has been our philosophy to recommend surgical treatment, by means of radical retropubic prostatectomy, to men with clinically localized prostate cancer and a 10-year life expectancy. Our 15-year experience with this treatment philosophy has proven that radical retropubic prostatectomy can be performed without operative mortality and with very low perioperative morbidity. The overall survival in our series of 243 patients is superior to that of age- and race-matched controls in the general population without prostate cancer. Radical retropubic prostatectomy also provides excellent results with regard to survival free of disease, especially as concerns control of the primary lesion, by preventing local disease recurrence in more than 95% of patients when coupled with appropriate adjuvant therapy.

Controversy continues to exist in the literature regarding the need for postoperative adjuvant treatment in patients with pathologically confirmed extracapsular disease extension (stage C) or microscopic lymph node metastases (stage D1). It has been our practice to recommended postoperative adjuvant radiotherapy to patients with extracapsular disease extension (stage C). Although there are no prospective, randomized trials to support the use of adjuvant radiotherapy in this setting, numerous retrospective studies strongly support its use. Our experience with a multimodal approach to the treatment of patients with stage D1 adenocarcinoma of the prostate has also been discussed, again supporting the use of radical prostatectomy with postoperative adjuvant treatment in this group of patients. Although our results are encouraging, randomized, prospective trials must be completed before the benefit of adjuvant treatment in these high-risk patients can be proven.

References

Anscher MS, Prosnitz LR (1987) Postoperative radiotherapy for patients with carcinoma of the prostate undergoing radical prostatectomy with positive surgical margins, seminal vesicle involvement and/or penetration through the capsule. J Urol 138:1407–1412

Boring CC, Squires TS, Tong T (1991) Cancer statistics, 1991. CA Cancer J Clin 41:19–36

Catalona WJ, Smith DS, Ratliff TL, Basler JW (1993) Detection of organ-confined prostate cancer is increased through prostate-specific antigen-based screening. JAMA 270:948–954

deKernion JB, Neuwirth H, Stein A, Dorey F, Stenzl A, Hannah J, Blyth B (1990) Prognosis of patients with stage D1 prostate carcinoma following radical prostatectomy with and without early endocrine therapy. J Urol 144:700–703

Epstein JI, Carmichael MJ, Pizov G, Walsh PC (1993) Influence of capsular penetration on progression following radical prostatectomy: a study of 196 cases with long-term followup. J Urol 150:135–141

Freeman JA, Lieskovsky G, Cook DW, Petrovich Z, Chen SC, Groshen S, Skinner DG (1993) Radical retropubic prostatectomy and postoperative adjuvant radiation for pathologic stage C (PCN0) prostate cancer from 1976 to 1989: intermediate findings. J Urol 149:1029–1034

Freeman JA, Lieskovsky G, Grossfeld GD et al. (1994) Adjuvant radiation, chemotherapy, and androgen deprivation

therapy for pathologic stage D1 adenocarcinoma of the prostate. Urology 44:719–725
Gaynor JJ, Feuer EJ, Tan CC et al. (1993) On the use of cause-specific failure and conditional failure probabilities: examples from clinical oncology data. J Am Stat Assoc 88:400–409
Gibbons RP, Cole BS, Richardson RG et al. (1986) Adjuvant radiotherapy following radical prostatectomy: results and complications. J Urol 135:65–68
Hudson MA, Catalona WJ (1990) Effect of adjuvant radiation therapy on prostate specific antigen following radical prostatectomy. J Urol 143:1174–1177
Johansson JE, Andersson SO, Krusemo UB, Adami HO, Bergstrom R, Kraaz W (1989) Natural history of localised prostatic cancer: a population-based study in 223 untreated patients. Lancet 8642:799–803
Johansson JE, Adami HO, Andersson SO, Bergstrom R, Holmberg L, Krusemo UB (1992) High 10-year survival rate in patients with early, untreated prostatic cancer. JAMA 267:2191–2196
Koch MO, Smith JA, Hodge EM, Brandell RA (1994) Prospective development of a cost-efficient program for radical retropubic prostatectomy. Urology 44:311–318
Lange PH, Lightner DJ, Medini E, Reddy PK, Vessella RL (1990) The effect of radiation therapy after radical prostatectomy in patients with elevated prostate specific antigen levels. J Urol 144:927–933
Lieskovsky G (1988) Technique of radical retropubic prostatectomy (Campbell's Procedure) with limited pelvic lymph node dissection. In: Skinner DG, Lieskovsky G (eds) Diagnosis and management of genitourinary cancer. Saunders, Philadelphia, p 735
Litwiller SE, Djavan B, Klopukh BV, Richier JC, Roehrborn CG (1995) Radical retropubic prostatectomy for localized carcinoma of the prostate in a large metropolitan hospital: changing trends over a 10-year period (1984–1994). Urology 45:813–822
Mettlin C, Murphy GP, Menck H (1994) Trends in treatment of localized prostate cancer by radical prostatectomy: observations from the Commission on Cancer National Cancer Database, 1985–1990. Urology 43:488–492
Miller RG (1981) Survival analysis. John Wiley, New York
O'Donnell PD, Finan BF (1989) Continence following nerve-sparing radical prostatectomy. J Urol 142:1227–1229
Oesterling JE, Brendler CB, Epstein JI, Kimball AW, Walsh PC (1987) Correlation of clinical stage, serum prostatic acid phosphatase and preoperative Gleason grade with final pathological stage in 275 patients with clinically localized adenocarcinoma of the prostate. J Urol 138:92–98
Oesterling JE, Chan DW, Epstein JI et al. (1988) Prostate specific antigen in the preoperative and postoperative evaluation of localized prostatic cancer treated with radical prostatectomy. J Urol 139:766–772
Partin AW, Yoo J, Carter HB, Pearson JD, Chan DW, Epstein JI, Walsh PC (1993) The use of prostate specific antigen, clinical stage and Gleason score to predict pathological stage in men with localized prostate cancer. J Urol 150:110–114
Paulson DF, Lin GH, Hinshaw W, Stephani S, The Uro-Oncology Research Group (1982) Radical surgery versus radiotherapy for adenocarcinoma of the prostate. J Urol 128:502–504
Paulson DF, Moul JW, Walther PJ (1990) Radical prostatectomy for clinical stage T1-2N0M0 prostatic adenocarcinoma: long-term results. J Urol 144:1180–1184
Quinlan DM, Epstein JI, Carter BS, Walsh PC (1991) Sexual function following radical prostatectomy: influence of preservation of neurovascular bundles. J Urol 145:998–1002
Smith JA, Middleton RG (1987) Clinical management of prostatic cancer. Year Book Medical Publishers, Chicago
Stein A, deKernion JB, Dorey F, Smith RB (1992a) Adjuvant radiotherapy in patients post-radical prostatectomy with tumor extending through capsule or positive seminal vesicles. Urology 39:59–62
Stein A, deKernion JB, Smith RB, Dorey F, Patel H (1992b) Prostate specific antigen levels after radical prostatectomy in patients with organ confined and locally extensive prostate cancer. J Urol 147:942–946
Steinberg GD, Epstein JI, Piantadosi S, Walsh PC (1990) Management of stage D1 adenocarcinoma of the prostate: the Johns Hopkins experience 1974 to 1987. J Urol 144:1425–1432
Walsh PC (1988) Technique of radical retropubic prostatectomy with preservation of sexual function - an anatomic approach. In: Skinner DG, Lieskovsky G (eds) Diagnosis and management of genitourinary cancer. Saunders, Philadelphia, p 753
Walsh PC (1990) Radical prostatectomy in locally confined prostatic carcinoma. In: Schroder FH (ed) EORTC genitourinary group monograph 8: treatment of prostatic cancer - facts and controversies. Wiley-Liss, New York, p 199
Walsh PC, Lepor H (1987) The role of radical prostatectomy in the management of prostatic cancer. Cancer 60:526–537
Wingo PA, Tong T, Bolden S (1995) Cancer statistics, 1995. CA Cancer J Clin 45:8–30
Yamada AH, Lieskovsky G, Petrovich Z, Chen SC, Groshen S, Skinner DG (1994) Results of Radical prostatectomy and adjuvant therapy in the management of locally advanced, clinical stage TC, prostate cancer. Am J Clin Oncol 17:277–285
Zietman AL, Coen JJ, Shipley WU, Althausen AF (1993) Adjuvant irradiation after radical prostatectomy for adenocarcinoma of the prostate: analysis of freedom from PSA failure. Urology 42:292–299
Zincke H (1989) Extended experience with surgical treatment of stage D1 adenocarcinoma of prostate: significant influences of immediate adjuvant hormonal treatment (orchiectomy) on outcome. Urology (Suppl) 33:27–36
Zincke H (1990) Combined surgery and immediate adjuvant hormonal treatment for stage D1 adenocarcinoma of the prostate: Mayo Clinic experience. Semin Urol 8:175–183

13 Surgical Salvage Options in Patients with Recurrent Tumor Following Radiotherapy

T.E. Ahlering and B. Norouzi

CONTENTS

13.1 Introduction

Radiation therapy has been effectively utilized in the management of prostate cancer since the early 1900s. Initially, techniques to apply radiotherapy to the prostate utilized implanted radium either transurethrally, transperineally, or transrectally. Although tumor shrinkage occurred, side-effects on adjacent organs limited its benefit. In the 1950s, high-energy supervoltage external beam therapy was introduced by Bagshaw et al. (1965) to the treatment armamentarium. Supervoltage external beam radiotherapy produced marked improvements in tumor control and survival rates without the previously limiting side-effects. Today, radiotherapy continues to play a central role in the management of prostate cancer along with observation, radical prostatectomy and hormonal therapy. As with surgery and other forms of therapy presently available, controversy exists about the long-term efficacy. Prostate cancer is rather unusual in that the disease process is so protracted it is often difficult to ascertain whether a specified therapy has been effective or whether the disease process was not destined to be aggressive.

Historically, patients treated definitively with radiotherapy who suffered tumor recurrence were managed with hormonal therapy. For the most part, patients treated with radiotherapy did well for a number of years, frequently 7–12 years, before recurrent disease became clinically evident. The first evidence of disease recurrence in most patients was the development of painful skeletal metastases. Because clinically evident local tumor recurrence was generally not the first event to occur with recurrence, treatment was almost uniformly palliative in nature. Since the late 1970s, increasing attention has been focused on the long-term results of radical surgery and radiotherapy, in patients followed up for 10–15 years. During the same period patients have become generally healthier and have lived longer, exposing them to greater morbidity and mortality due to prostate cancer than was previously seen. Over the last 10 years, technology and our knowledge of prostate cancer have advanced so that we can determine much earlier in the disease process, before skeletal metastases, that the tumor has not been controlled locally by the radiation treatment. The focus of this chapter is to discuss surgical options in patients whose tumor has not responded to radiation therapy or has failed following the application of pelvic irradiation.

13.2 Evaluation of Tumor Recurrence

The role of surgical salvage following radiotherapy has been slow to develop because of difficulties in defining the presence of local tumor recurrence and its significance for survival. First, we know that prostate cancer is very slow growing. Stamey (1983) estimated the doubling time for prostate cancer to be 60–120 days. Second, the mechanism of cell death with radiotherapy is slow. It is believed that radiotherapy produces free radicals in the nucleus that damage the DNA. The DNA polymerase is unable to read the DNA and the cell is unable to replicate. The cells die during mitosis; hence the term "mitotic death" was coined. In the 1970s and early 1980s, Cox and Stoffel (1977), Scardino (1983), and others

T.E. Ahlering, MD, Associate Professor of Surgery, Division of Urology, University of California, Irvine, 101 The City Drive, Orange, CA 92668, USA
B. Norouzi, MD, Division of Urology, University of California, Irvine, 101 The City Drive, Orange, CA 92668, USA

demonstrated that serial prostate biopsies following definitive radiotherapy reveal gradual resolution of malignant cells over the first 18–24 months post-treatment. These two factors further retarded the process of understanding postradiotherapy tumor recurrence.

The significance of a postradiotherapy prostate biopsy was very controversial as late as the early 1980s. Many radiation oncologists and urologists reported that a postradiotherapy prostate biopsy that demonstrated cancer was of no significance Cox and Kline (1983), Kagan et al. (1977), and Perez et al. (1980). There were a number of reasons that led to this controversy, including inaccurate preradiotherapy staging, poorly timed or uncontrolled application of hormonal therapy, and inadequate length of follow-up. By 1985 there were at least three studies, by Freiha and Bagshaw (1984), Scardino (1983), and Schellhammer et al. (1985), that had definitive preradiotherapy surgical staging, no uncontrolled concomitant hormonal therapy exposure, and accurate survival data based on follow-up of adequate duration. All of these reports demonstrated a superior survival advantage among patients with a negative postirradiation prostate biopsy. For the first time there was an intermediate end point that could be used to evaluate whether radiotherapy had been successful in eradicating the cancer. Around the same time, a number of articles were published on the feasibility of surgical salvage after radiotherapy but evaluation of survival advantage in these patients was clearly premature.

As our knowledge of prostate cancer has improved over the past decade, it has become accepted that use of the 5-year overall survival as the only end point is not adequate. With the advent of PSA, radiation oncologists and urologists are now better equipped to predict and detect tumor recurrence. Russell et al. (1991) and Zietman et al. (1994) have shown that an abnormal preradiotherapy (>4× normal or >15 ng/ml) PSA profoundly reduces the chances of a complete response to therapy. Following radiotherapy, responders should experience a rapid and dramatic reduction in their PSA levels. The exact PSA nadir that one should expect remains to be completely defined, but the works of Willett et al. (1994), Zietman et al. (1994), and Ritter et al. (1992) lend very convincing evidence that an acceptable nadir following definitive radiotherapy should be less than 1.0 ng/ml. Numerous studies have shown that a rising PSA following radiotherapy is highly indicative of tumor recurrence. A few studies have evaluated the time between progressive elevation of the PSA and development of clinical recurrence. Kaplan et al. (1993) found that among 29 patients with a rising post-radiotherapy PSA the mean time before clinical evidence of recurrence was 156 ± 46 days. This was very similar to the median time to clinical recurrence of 4.5–7 months reported by Ritter et al. (1992). The longest mean time to clinical recurrence of 12 months was reported by Killian et al. (1985). All of these studies showed clinical evidence of recurrence within 1 year of recorded PSA elevation.

For most patients treated with radiotherapy, tumor recurrence and progression are asymptomatic until the development of painful skeletal metastases. When patients develop progression the treatment most frequently offered is hormonal ablation. In general, approximately 50% of patients with a positive biopsy will have died of metastatic prostate cancer 7–8 years following the administration of radiotherapy as reported by Freiha and Bagshaw (1984). Patients with evidence of persistent disease or local recurrence should be considered for surgical salvage.

13.3 Historical Perspective on the Surgical Treatment of Postradiation Recurrent Tumor

Reports on surgical resection to cure postradiation recurrent disease have been infrequent and date to the late 1970s. At that time, Spaulding and Whitmore (1978) reported the experience at the Memorial Sloan Kettering Medical Center with extended total excision in a highly mixed population of patients with locally extensive disease. Six of these patients ostensibly had locally recurrent tumors. All of the patients, however, had extensive local disease that was out of control and not surprisingly the surgical results were unsatisfactory. By 1985, enough evidence existed that positive prostate biopsies were tantamount to disease recurrence and attempts to surgically resect these prostates were undertaken. Mador et al. (1985) were the first to report on treatment outcomes in a group of patients treated surgically for salvage after failure of local radiotherapy. This report focused on the technical difficulty associated with postradiotherapy surgical intervention and did not address survival issues. Presently, two major areas of concern continue to exist with surgical intervention for radiotherapy failures: surgical complications and improved survival. Salvage options presently under investigation include salvage prostatectomy and cystoprostatectomy, and more recently cryoablation of the prostate.

13.4 Salvage Prostatectomy and Cystoprostatectomy

If radiotherapy fails to control cancer in the prostate, ideally a patient could be salvaged by surgical removal of the prostate. The reality of the situation unfortunately is not that simple. As discussed previously, it remains controversial when one should consider a patient as a treatment failure. If one decides this too early, salvage might not have been necessary; if one decides it too late, salvage may not be curative. Other important questions remain that are difficult to answer, such as whether debulking improves survival or aids in a significant fashion with local tumor control. These questions remain unanswered at this time but an attempt to cover the major issues follows.

MADOR et al. (1985) reported on the feasibility of performing salvage radical prostatectomies following radiotherapy. They reported on five patients who were operated on with the intent of removing the prostate only. One of the five was not amenable to prostatectomy and required a total cystoprostatectomy because of severe fibrosis identified at the time of surgery. One of the four prostatectomy patients died postoperatively of pulmonary complications. Of the remaining three, only two regained urinary continence. THOMPSON et al. (1988) reported no significant postoperative complications in five patients; however, two (40%) were incontinent. Subsequently, investigators at the University of Southern California (USC), Baylor University, and the Mayo Clinic reported acceptable operative mortality but significant morbidity with salvage prostatectomy. The combined surgical salvage experience was reported by AHLERING et al. (1992), NEERHUT et al. (1988), and ZINCKE (1992). In the 59 patients treated there were no postoperative deaths; five (8.5%) had rectal injuries, all successfully managed conservatively, 13 (22%) had bladder neck contractures, and 16 (27%) had incontinence.

The indication for cystoprostatectomy varied among the authors who have reported their experience with salvage surgery. MADOR et al. (1985) and ZINCKE (1992) performed more extensive surgery for more locally advanced disease, whereas AHLERING et al. (1992) were more concerned with the probability of complications associated with salvage prostatectomy. If more extensive surgery is offered to patients with more extensive disease, then marginal results will not be unexpected. ZINCKE (1992) noted a dramatic difference in median time to tumor progression between prostatectomy and cystoprostatectomy treated patients of 7.5 versus 1.3 years, respectively. However, in the cystoprostatectomy group just 2 out of 30 (7%) patients had organ-confined disease compared to 11 of 32 (34%) patients in the prostatectomy group. By contrast, AHLERING et al. (1992) reported no significant difference in tumor progression rates between the two groups and concomitantly reported similar pathologic stage distribution. The primary difference between the two reports was the difference in the treatment philosophy: AHLERING et al. (1992) felt that incontinence and the risk of local recurrence made cystoprostatectomy a better alternative than salvage prostatectomy.

The survival benefit of surgically excising locally persistent disease following radiotherapy remains unanswered and controversial. If surgical salvage is to be accepted as beneficial, there needs to be evidence that patients are either cured or their survival is prolonged. A review of the pathologic findings after surgical resection in three studies is listed in Table 13.1. Of the 120 patients treated, only 27% had disease confined to the prostate; the remaining 73% had extraprostatic disease and thus were probably not curable. Unfortunately, PSA in these patients has not been helpful in predicting the status of disease confinement. YOUNES et al. (1993) noted that preoperative PSA levels failed to predict the presence or absence or extracapsular extension, seminal vesicle involvement, or lymph node metastasis. It appears the primary benefit of surgical intervention is in prolonging survival. AHLERING et al. (1992) compared their survival data on surgically treated patients to survival data on similar patients who received hormonal therapy without surgical intervention as reported by FREIHA and BAGSHAW (1984). The surgical group had 34 patients, of whom 27

Table 13.1. Summary of pathologic findings after surgical resection

Authors	No. of patients	Organ confined	Not organ confined
YOUNES et al. (1993)	24	7 (29%)	17 (71%)
AHLERING et al. (1992)	34	12 (35%)	22 (65%)
ZINCKE (1992)	62	13 (21%)	49 (79%)
	120	32 (27%)	88 (73%)

(79%) were managed concurrently with hormonal deprivation therapy; the nonsurgical group had 39 patients (biopsy-proven recurrent disease), of whom 35 (90%) were treated with androgen deprivation therapy. With a mean follow-up of 109 months postradiotherapy in the surgical group, 24 (71%) were alive and free of radiographically evident disease. The nonsurgical group had a mean postradiotherapy follow-up of 96 months and only 11 (28%) were alive without radiographic evidence of disease recurrence. Further, only seven (21%) patients in the surgical group had died of disease compared to 18 (46%) in the nonsurgical group. Although firm conclusions are not possible, a survival advantage in surgically resected patients is strongly suggested.

Therefore, salvage prostatecomy and cystoprostatectomy are technically feasible. The procedures are more difficult following radiotherapy primarily due to fibrosis between the prostate, rectum, and genitourinary diaphram. Serious consideration must be given to the complications versus the prolongation of survival when contemplating surgical excision of postradiation persistent or recurrent prostate cancer.

13.5 Cryoablation of the Prostate

The reintroduction of cryoablation of the prostate started in the early 1990s with the report by Onik et al. (1993). These investigators applied freezing techniques to the prostate with the assistance of recent ultrasound technology. In the early 1970s, Bonney et al. (1982) at the University of Iowa worked extensively on methods to cryoablate the prostate through an open perineal approach. These authors reported their long-term follow-up of 10 years comparing cryoablation with radical prostatectomy. Although they showed very similar survival rates, cryoablation was not widely accepted because of high complication rates, particularly as regards the formation of urethrorectal and urethrocutaneous fistulae. The important limiting factor with cryotherapy initially was the small volume of tissue which could be frozen and the poor control of tissue margins. Because the authors could not control the depth of freezing, injuries resulting in rectal and cutaneous fistulae were not uncommon. Similarly, problems arose if freezing was limited in order to avoid complications.

With the advent of transrectal ultrasonography, imaging of the prostate has dramatically improved. Further, experience with the technique of percutaneous nephrolithotripsy translated well to percutaneous transperineal cryoablation of the prostate. In 1993, Onik et al. (1993) reported their initial experience with this new treatment technology. A natural extension of this treatment technique was to employ it in patients whose tumor failed to respond to radiotherapy. For patients who failed radiotherapy and their surgeons who were reluctant to consider surgical therapy, cryoablation offered a new method to potentially control local disease.

Similar to salvage prostatectomy and cystoprostatectomy, the feasibility of cryoablation of the prostate in postradiation treatment failures is central. The first preliminary results with this procedure were recently reported by von Eschenbach et al. (1994), Cohen et al. (1994), and Bales et al. (1994). Out of 140 patients reported there was just one procedure-related death. There have been no fistulae and no need for blood transfusions. The average length of hospital stay as reported by von Eschenbach et al. (1994) was just 2 days. The incidence of incontinence has ranged from 3% to 44%. The high incontinence rate described by Bales et al. (1994) was attributed to the aggressive treatment at the apex of the prostate.

Determining the efficacy of cryoablation with respect to survival presents a most difficult challenge. Follow-up is too short at this point to comment on survival. Once follow-up is long enough, comparing results from standard hormonal intervention, salvage prostatectomy and cystoprostatectomy, and cryoablation will present a formidable problem. It seems unlikely that studies randomizing between the varied treatment options hold much promise for accruing adequate patient numbers. Even establishing a survival advantage between surgical resection and cryoablation will be difficult because of the use of different means for determining intermediate results. Open surgical resection relies on the PSA becoming nondetectable. Because the prostate remains in place after cryoablation, intermediate evaluation, much like standard radiotherapy, relies on posttreatment prostate biopsies and PSA levels. A posttreatment positive biopsy probably provides reliable results; however, a negative biopsy may or may not be significant. A negative biopsy in the first posttreatment year may ultimately turn positive 2–5 years later. Similarly, the PSA nadir needs to be evaluated and defined. Certainly, if the PSA does not drop or if it falls and then rises, disease progression is most likely occurring. Utilizing available intermediate follow-up data, efficacy of cryotherapy is summarized in Table 13.2. All three groups of

Table 13.2 Summary of cryoablation results

Authors	No. of patients	Mean age (yrs)	Posttreatment biopsy (−)	Impotence	Incontinence	Reduced PSA following treatment
VON ESCHENBACH et al. (1994)	89	70	21/31 (68%)	22%	24%	46/51 (90%)
COHEN et al. (1994)	33	NR	11/17 (65%)	NR	3%	33/33 100%
BALES et al. (1994)	18	70	8/12 (67%)	44%	44%	8/11 (73%)
	140	70	40/60 (67%)	25%	21%	87/95 (92%)

investigators reported that two-thirds of the patients biopsied in the first year had no evidence of cancer. VON ESCHENBACH et al. (1994) reported retreating patients with an initial positive prostate biopsy without untoward side-effects. Preliminary PSA data were reported by two groups. VON ESCHENBACH et al. (1994) reported that 46 of 51 (90%) patients had a redution in their PSA levels, whereas, BALES et al. (1994) reported a reduction in only 8 (73%) of 11 treated patients. Longer follow-up is needed to determine whether any role exists for the use of cryoablation in the management of patients who present with postradiation local failure.

References

Ahlering TE, Lieskovsky G, Skinner DG (1992) Salvage surgery plus androgen deprivation for radioresistant prostatic adenocarcinoma. J Urol 147:900–902

Bagshaw MA, Kaplan HS, Sagerman RH (1965) Linear accelerator supervoltage radiotherapy. VII. Carcinoma of the prostate. Radiology 85:121–129

Bales GT, Williams M, Chodak GW (1994) Initial outcomes with cryosurgery in prostate cancer patients having failed radiation therapy. J Urol 151:436A

Bonney WW, Fallon B, Gerber WL et al. (1982) Cryosurgery in prostatic cancer: survival. Urology 19:37–42

Cohen JK, Miller RJ, Onik G (1994) Cryosurgical ablation of the prostate as used in the patient who has failed radiation therapy: complete destruction in the patient with clinically localized disease and palliation of local symptoms in the patient with metastatic disease. J Urol 151:237A

Cox JD, Kline RW (1983) The lack of prognostic significance of biopsies after radiotherapy for prostatic cancer. Semin Urol 1:237–242

Cox JD, Stoffel •• (1977) ••

Freiha FS, Bagshaw MA (1984) Carcinoma of the prostate: results of post-irradiation biopsy. Prostate 5:19–25

Kagan AR, Gordon J, Cooper JF et al. (1977) A clinical appraisal of post-irradiation biopsy in prostatic cancer. Cancer 39:637–641

Kaplan ID, Cox RS, Bagshaw MA (1993) Prostate specific antigen after external beam radiotherapy for prostatic cancer: follow up. J Urol 149:519–522

Killian CS, Yang N, Emrich LJ et al. (1985) Prognostic importance of prostate-specific antigen for monitoring patients with stages B2 to D1 prostate cancer. Cancer Res 45:886–891

Mador DR, Huben RP, Wajsman Z, Pontes JE (1985) Salvage surgery following radical radiotherapy for adenocarcinoma of the prostate. J Urol 133:58–60

Neerhut GJ, Wheeler T, Cantini M, Scardino PT (1988) Salvage radical prostatectomy for radiorecurrent adenocarcinoma of the prostate. J Urol 140:544–547

Onik GM, Cohen JK, Reyes GD, Rubinsky B, Chang Z, Baust J (1993) Transrectal ultrasound guided percutaneous radical cryosurgical ablation of the prostate. Cancer 72:1291–1299

Perez CA, Walz BJ, Zivnuska FR et al. (1980) Irradiation of carcinoma of the prostate localized to the pelvis: analysis of tumor response and prognosis. Int J Radiat Oncol Biol Phys 6:555–563

Ritter MA, Messing EM, Shanahan TG, Potts S, Chappell RJ, Kinsella TJ (1992) Prostate-specific antigen as a predictor of radiotherapy response and patterns of failure in localized prostate cancer. J Clin Oncol 10:1208–1217

Russell KJ, Dunatov C, Hafermann MD et al. (1991) Prostate specific antigen in the management of patients with localized adenocarcinoma of the prostate treated with primary radiation therapy. J Urol 146:1046–1052

Scardino PT (1983) The prognostic significance of biopsies after radiotherapy for prostatic cancer. Semin Urol 1:243–245

Schellhammer PF, El-Mahdi AE, Ladaga LE, Schultheiss T (1985) 125 Iodine implantation for carcinoma of the prostate: 5-year survival free of disease and incidence of local failure. J Urol 134:1140–1145

Spaulding JT, Whitmore WF (1978) Extended total excision of prostatic adenocarcinoma. J Urol 120:188–190

Stamey TA (1983) Prostate cancer. Monogr Urol 4:67–70

Thompson IM, Rounder JB, Spence CR, Rodriguez FR (1988) Salvage radical prostatectomy for adenocarcinoma of the prostate. Cancer 61:1464–1466

von Eschenbach AC, Swanson DA, Babaian RJ, Dinney CPN, Evans RB (1994) Ultrasound-guided cryoablation of recurrent prostate cancer following radiation therapy. J Urol 151:376A

Willett CG, Zietman AL, Shipley WU, Coen JJ (1994) The effect of pelvic radiation therapy on serum levels of prostate specific antigen. J Urol 151:1579–1581

Younes E, Smith JB, Haas GP, Powell IJ, Montie JE, Pontes JE (1993) Value of preoperative PSA in predicting pathologic stage of patients undergoing salvage prostatectomy. Urology 43:22–25

Zietman AJ, Coen JJ, Shipley WU, willett CG, Efird JT (1994) Radical radiation therapy in the management of prostatic adenocarcinoma: the initial prostate specific antigen value as a predictor of treatment outcome. J Urol 151:640–645

Zincke H (1992) Radical prostatectomy and exenterative procedures for local failure after radiotherapy with curative intent: comparison of outcomes. J Urol 147:894–899

14 The Role of Prostate-Specific Antigen in the Management of Prostate Cancer

A.A. Elgamal, Z. Petrovich, H. Van Poppel, and L. Baert

CONTENTS

14.1 Introduction

The prostate is the largest male excretory sex gland, secreting four major proteins primarily to the seminal ejaculate. These four proteins are: prostatic acid phosphatase (PAP), prostate-specific antigen (PSA), prostate-specific protein (PSP-94), and human kallikrein 2 (hK2) (Table 14.1). At the present time the biochemical and pathologic mechanisms for the entry of these proteins into the systemic circulation are not well understood.

Prostatic adenocarcinoma is the most commonly diagnosed human cancer of internal organs and the second most important cause of cancer mortality in males. The natural history of this tumor is characterized by a protracted course and to a large extent an unpredictable prognosis (see Chap. 2). In recent years we have learned to identify a number of important prognostic clinical and pathologic factors which help us to understand the likely prognosis in a given patient. Additionally, these important prognostic factors provide assistance in selecting optimal management in a specific clinical situation.

Currently, PSA is the most important prostate cancer marker available to clinicians. It is relatively reliable in population screening, being very sensitive and specific. It both reflects tumor burden and provides prognostic information (Cooner 1993). The use of PSA in screening for prostate cancer is less costly than the use of other markers in screening for various tumors. As an example, the use of PSA in screening for prostate cancer costs one-quarter of screening for breast cancer. It is also a very efficient tool for monitoring the response to therapy, helping to identify patients with tumor control and those with tumor progression. The use of PSA is technically simple, noninvasive, rapid, reproducible, inexpensive, and readily acceptable to patients.

In the past few years the routine use of PSA within the European Community and in the United States has helped to improve the accuracy of early detection of prostate cancer. It has also significantly contributed to rapid changes in the management of this disease, particularly in those patients presenting with localized lesions (Table 14.2).

Recent advances in the management of carcinoma of the prostate have made the use of PSA more important and even indispensable in the practice of

A.A. Elgamal, MD, Consultant Urologist and Research Fellow, Department of Urology, St. Pieter's Hospital, Catholic University of Leuven, Brusselsestraat 69, 3000 Leuven, Belgium
Z. Petrovich, MD, Professor of Radiation Oncology and Urology, Chairman, Department of Radiation Oncology, University of Southern California School of Medicine, 1441 Eastlake Avenue, Los Angeles, CA 90033, USA
H. Van Poppel, MD, PhD, Professor, Department of Urology, St. Pieter's Hospital, Catholic University of Leuven, Brusselsestraat 69, 3000 Leuven, Belgium
L. Baert, MD, PhD, Professor and Chairman, Department of Urology, St. Pieter's Hospital, Catholic University of Leuven, Brusselsestraat 69, 3000 Leuven, Belgium and Clinical Professor, Department of Urology and Radiation Oncology, University of Southern California School of Medicine, 1441 Eastlake Avenue, Los Angeles, CA 90033, USA

Table 14.1. Major excretory proteins produced by the normal prostate gland (modified from COFFEY 1992)

Protein	Activity	Mol. weight (kDa)	Conc. in seminal plasma (ng/ml)	Conc. in normal male serum (ng/ml)
PAP	Hydrolyzes monophosphate esters	102	1×10^6	±1 unit/l
PSA	Kallikrein, serine protease	30	7×10^5	0.7
hK2	Kallikrein, serine protease	30	5×10^5	NA
PSP-94	Nonspecific, also in epithelium of GIT	16	6×10^5	NA

NA, Not available; GIT, gastrointestinal tract

Table 14.2. Changes in patients of diagnosis and treatment of localized prostate cancer in the United States (data from METTLIN et al. 1994)

Year	Overall no. of reported cases	No. of localized cancers	%	Radical prostatectomies	
				No.	%
1985	16349	4531	27.7	552	12.2
1988	25028	11488	45.9	2331	20.3
1990	44750	21697	48.5	6597	30.4

uro-oncology. These advances, which are reflected in contemporary practice, may be summarized as follows:

1. Enhancement of the sensitivity and specificity of PSA in screening for prostate cancer through the supplementation of serum PSA determination by additional parameters such as: PSA density (PSAD), PSA velocity (rate of change), PSA age-specific reference range, and the selective detection of different molecular forms and ratios of PSA.
2. Improvement of the predictive power of PSA determination in prostate cancer staging by using it in combination with other important parameters such as: tumor differentiation seen in the prostate biopsy, consideration of a higher PSAD cut-off point, assessment of periprostatic tissues by selective ultrasound-guided biopsies, and detection of PSA-mRNA secreting cells in the circulation and bone marrow aspiration with the use of the RT-PCR assya.
3. Improvement of the efficiency of PSA as an indicator of cancer progression after therapy by the use of more sensitive assays and PSA-mRNA assays (which are now widely available). Additionally, PSA doubling time can help to differentiate between local and systemic failure.
4. Improvement of the technical performance of PSA assays through the use of more specific monoclonal antibody assays which help to reduce cross-reactivity. There is now better assay reproducibility with the routine use of automated, less laborious and time-consuming assays. A major international effort is under way to accomplish standardization of PSA assay methodology and correlation between different available PSA assays (STAMEY 1995).

In spite of these recent developments, however, use of PSA has yet to be fully optimized. In the past few years, a number of reports have questioned the belief that PSA is exclusively prostate-specific under androgenic regulation. The investigators at the Catholic University of Leuven have shown that PSA is also secreted by extraprostatic sources (Figs. 14.1, 14.2) and can be simply detected in urine after curative radical prostatectomy (ELGAMAL et al. 1994a, 1995a; FRAZIER et al. 1992; IWAKIRI et al. 1993; TAKAYAMA et al. 1994). Nevertheless, under nonpathologic conditions those extraprostatic sources of PSA secretion have no significant impact on the measured serum PSA levels for up to 2 years following radical prostatectomy for specimen-confined disease including pT3a or less advanced tumors (ELGAMAL et al. 1995b; OESTERLING et al. 1995).

In this context, we would also like to make reference to our recent findings of PSA in pancreatic and salivary glands independent of the patient's sex. These important data were obtained using two different commercially available monoclonal immunohistochemical assays (Fig. 14.3) and may be of major clinical significance because urologists and pathologist rely heavily on PSA staining to confirm or exclude the prostatic origin of undifferentiated

Fig. 14.1a–d. Cowper's gland. **a** Histologic appearance of Cowper's gland with dilated central duct (*D*) and mucinous acini (*A*) surrounded by skeletal muscle (*M*). **b** Acini with some individual cells positive for PSA (*arrows*). **c** Duct with PSA-staining cells (*arrows*). **d** Duct with PAP-positive cells (*arrows*). (From ELGAMAL et al. 1994a; adapted with permission from Urology). H&E, **a** ×2.5, **b** ×400, **c** ×100, **d** ×100

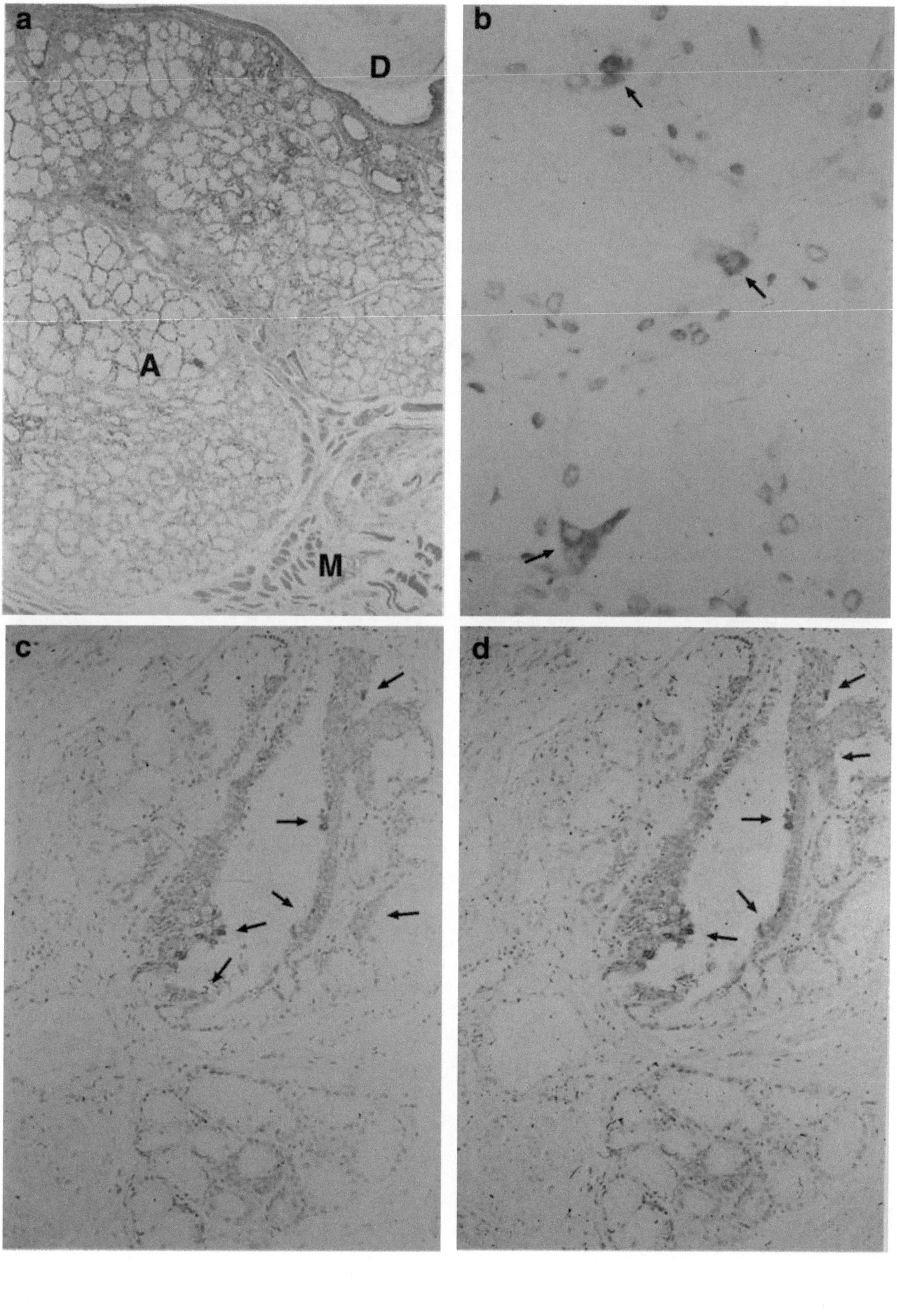
a
D
A
M
b
c
d

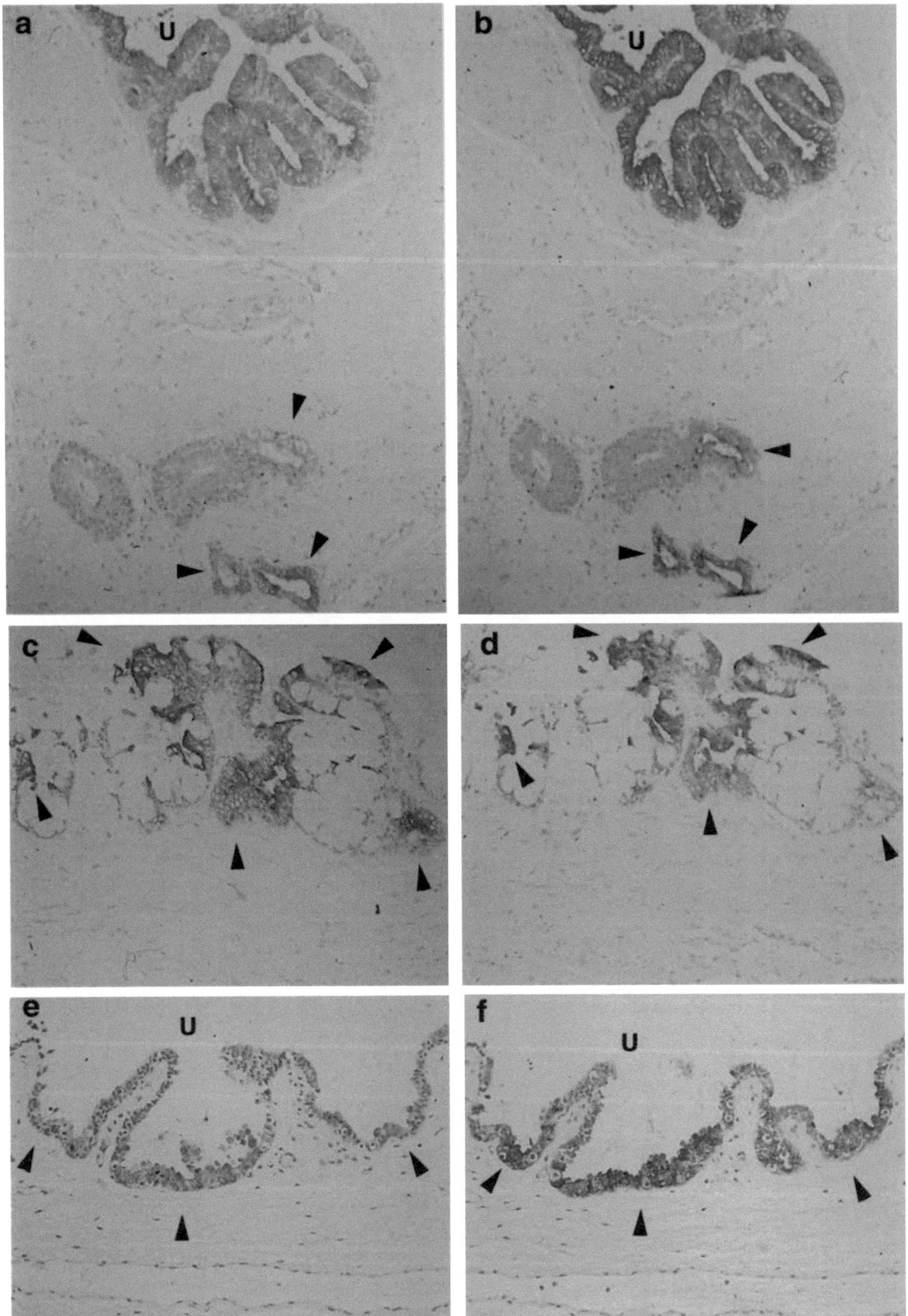

Fig. 14.2a–f. Urethral and periurethral glands. **a** Membranous urethra: PSA-positive urethral epithelium (*U*) and periurethral glands (*arrows*). **b** Membranous urethra: PAP-positive urethral epithelium (*U*) and periurethral glands (*arrows*). **c** Littre's gland with PSA-positive cells (*arrows*). **d** Littre's gland with PAP-positive cells (*arrows*). **e** Morgagni's lacunae demonstrating PSA staining (*arrows*). **f** Morgagni's lacunae demonstrating PAP staining (*arrows*). (From ELGAMAL et al. 1994a; adapted with permission from Urology) ×100

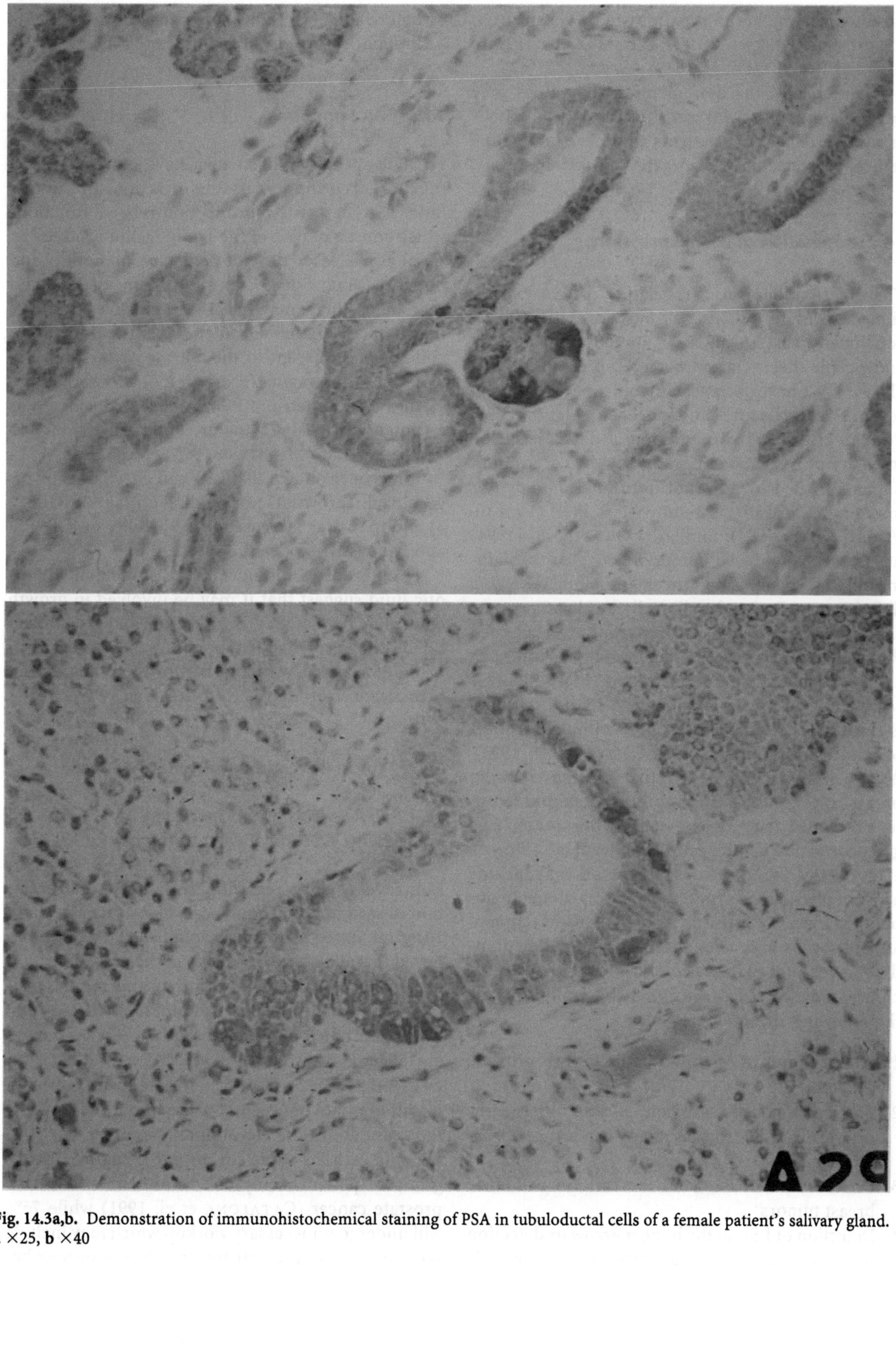

a

b

Fig. 14.3a,b. Demonstration of immunohistochemical staining of PSA in tubuloductal cells of a female patient's salivary gland. **a** ×25, **b** ×40 carcinomas, whether in proximity to or distant from the prostate (Bostwick 1994; Elgamal et al. 1994b; Epstein 1993; Lam et al. 1989).

Theoretically, the aforementioned findings may have an impact on ultrasensitive assays and RNA assays, particularly in patients who have undergone radical prostatectomy for organ-confined disease.

14.2 Regulation of PSA Expression

The exact mechanism of regulation of PSA expression in prostatic cells is still not clear. It has been concluded that PSA-mRNA is directly regulated by androgenic effects via androgen receptors (Young et al. 1991). We have observed a significant reduction in serum PSA levels after antiandrogen ablation (Van Poppel et al. 1995). In addition, a decrease in the intensity of tissue staining was noted in a group of patients treated by adjuvant hormonal therapy followed by radical prostatectomy (Fig. 14.4) (Van de Voorde et al. 1994). Similarly, Grob et al. (1994) have observed reduced immunohistochemical staining of PSA in benign and cancer epithelium following definitive irradiation for clinically localized prostate cancer. Recently, published reports have suggested PSA regulation by other nonandrogenic factors such as PSA-stimulating autocrine factor (PSAf). PSAf is secreted by androgen-independent LNCaP cells and is capable of exerting a direct PSA-stimulating effect on androgen-dependent cells (Hsieh et al. 1993). Also there is evidence of selective PSA expression in breast cancer cells bearing appropriate steroid receptors provided that cognate steroid hormones (e.g., glucocorticoids or progestin) are available (Monne et al. 1994). Other more obscure factors may include a loss of physiologic suppressor such as α_2 macroglobulin or a gene suppressor, or the agonistic action of antiandrogens and ketoconazole on modulated androgen receptors (Dawson and McLeod 1995). In clinical practice, these factors may be responsible for the following effects:

1. PSA rebound in castrated patients with prostate cancer
2. The paradoxical remission of PSA after withdrawal of antiandrogen therapy in advanced prostate cancer
3. Observations of PSA and PSA-mRNA in female breast tumors
4. Detection of PSA in the bone marrow or detection of circulating cells characterized by PSA-mRNA, before and after radical prostatectomy in patients thought to have localized prostate cancer.

14.3 PSA Function

Prostate-specific antigen may have more than one function according to its site of action. In seminal fluid PSA has two reproduction-related functions which consist of lysis of the seminogellin produed by seminal vesicles to provide better sperm motility and nutrition (Lilja 1985), and a mixture of PSA and seminal ejaculate may release a kinin-like substance that induces vaginal and uterine contractions to facilitate sperm ascent to the uterine cavity when released into the vagina (Fichtner et al. 1994).

In the endometrium PSA has been considered as a potential local regulator of uterine function (Clements and Mukhtar 1994).

It has been shown that PSA can enzymatically digest insulin growth factor binding protein-3 (IGFBP-3) and may thus increase the availability of IGFBP-2 and IGF1 (Kanety et al. 1993).

Findings of PSA in normal breast milk and amniotic fluid suggest that it may be involved in growth control by regulating growth factors and growth factor-binding proteins. This opens up the possibility of using PSA as a new biomarker for the prediction of breast cancer prognosis (Monne et al. 1994).

14.4 PSA in Detection of Prostate Cancer

14.4.1 PSA Sensitivity and Specificity in the Early Detection of Prostate Cancer

Controversy exists regarding the clinical interpretation of serum PSA at equivocal values between 4 and 10 ng/ml. Based on extensive published data, it is believed that PSA as a single test, in the early detection of prostate cancer, is superior to and more sensitive than digital rectal examination (DRE) and transrectal ultrasonography (TRUS) (Catalona et al. 1994a; Crawford et al. 1995; Ellis et al. 1994; Oesterling 1993). However, it is frequently difficult to differentiate between PSA elevation due to prostatic carcinoma and elevation due to other causes in patients with PSA levels from 4 to 10 ng/ml. In this group of patients, only one in four men will have prostate cancer (Catalona et al. 1991) while 75% will undergo unnecessary workup which may include potentially risky prostate biopsies. Some authors be-

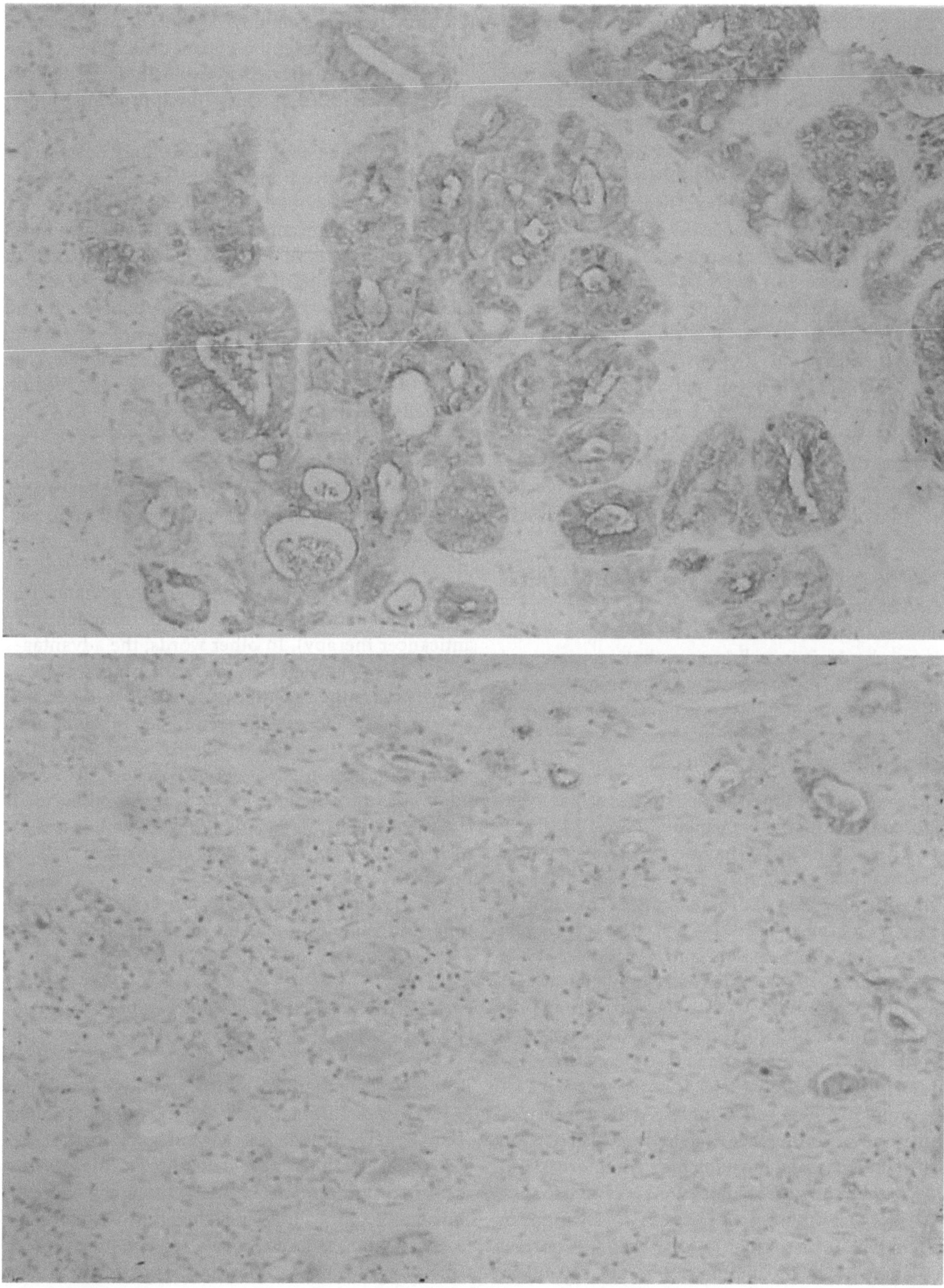

a

b

Fig. 14.4a,b. Demonstration of effect of preoperative administration of hormonal therapy on the intensity of PSA tissue staining. **a** Strong staining of PPB before hormonal therapy. **b** Impaired staining seen in radical prostatectomy specimen following a preoperative course of hormonal therapy. (From VAN DE VOORDE et al. 1994) lieve that PSA alone lacks sufficient sensitivity and specificity to detect cancer adequately in this patient group (BENSON 1994). Therefore, some investigators recommend the use of PSAD (PSA/estimated prostate volume) to differentiate benign prostate hyperplasia (BPH) from prostate cancer (BRETTON et al. 1994; NISHIYA et al. 1994; ROMMEL et al. 1994; SEAMAN et al. 1993). Other investigators have found PSAD to be unable to enhance the predictive value of PSA in the diagnosis of cancer in patients with normal DRE and a PSA level of 4–10 ng/ml (BRAWER et al. 1993a). Moreover, with respect to the early detection of prostate cancer, a 50% decrease in diagnostic sensitivity was found when using a PSAD cut-off value of 0.15 ng/ml per cc gland volume rather than the 4.0 ng/ml PSA concentration cut-off. These data were based on the receiver operating characteristic curves in 5000 men recruited from a multicenter clinical trial (CATALONA et al. 1994b). The possible reasons behind this controversy include:

1. The potential interobserver variation in estimation of the prostate volume.
2. Tumors of smaller volumes can be missed within large glands: it is well known that accurate and reproducible prostate volume determinations are difficult to obtain unless one puts in the time and effort necessary to carefully examine the prostate gland (BENSON 1994).

On the basis of longitudinal studies it has been proposed that the rate of change in PSA, PSA slope, or PSA velocity (PSAV) may be expected to follow the natural history of prostatic disease and to assist in the early detection of prostate cancer (BRAWER et al. 1993b; CARTER et al. 1992, 1995; GANN et al. 1995; SCHMID et al. 1993; SMITH and CATALONA 1994; STENMAN et al. 1994). Serial measurements of PSA on an annual basis were used in these screening programs to differentiate BPH from prostate cancer. In general, it has been accepted that a consistent increase of 20% or more, or >0.75 ng/ml, in serum PSA per annum can help to identify prostate cancer patients who warrant further evaluation. This criterion is particularly helpful in young men with normal initial PSA levels; however, it does not apply well to men >70 years or to those with initial PSA elevation. In this context it is to be noted that: (a) normal fluctuation in serum PSA levels occurs secondary to physiologic activities such as ejaculation and changes in hormonal levels, (b) there are differences in age-specific reference ranges due to concomitant obstructive symptoms due to BPH, (c) variable sampling intervals are employed, and (d) undiagnosed prostatitis has a potential impact on PSA levels (the latter may explain the negative velocity slope demonstrated in one-third of men without prostate cancer) (BENSON 1994).

In light of the above, it has been advocated that distinction between men with and men without prostate cancer should be based on a consistent PSA elevation in three consecutive PSA measurements over a relatively long period such as 2 year (CARTER et al. 1995). While it is recognized that there is a relationship between gland volume, patient age and PSA level in men without evidence of cancer (BABAIAN et al. 1992), the normal PSA reference range of up to 4.0 ng/ml does not take into account the well-known age-related differences in PSA production, PSA secretion, or prostate volume. Therefore, it has been proposed that an age-specific reference range for serum PSA would detect organ-confined prostate cancer in younger men at an earlier stage while reducing the number of cancers identified in older men harboring clinically insignificant tumors or having <10 years life expectancy (i.e. men who potentially may not benefit from definitive anticancer therapy). In other words, the advantages of the use of age-specific reference ranges are that they increase the sensitivity of PSA in younger men and increase the specificity of PSA in older men (PARTIN and OESTERLING 1995). The recommended age-specific serum PSA reference ranges are: 2.5 ng/ml or less for men of 40–49 years of age, 3.5 ng/ml or less for men 50–59 years of age, 4.5 ng/ml or less for men 60–69 years of age, and 6.5 ng/ml or less for those 70–79 years of age.

The rationale for the use of PSA in the early detection of prostate cancer is shown in Fig. 14.5.

14.4.2 PSA Detection of Clinically Inapparent Prostate Cancer

Recently, the American Joint Committee on Cancer (AJCC) and International Union Against Cancer (IUAC) have included a new category in the 1992 TNM classification for prostate cancer. This was necessary to accommodate the increasingly common impalpable and TRUS-invisible but PSA-detected prostate cancer, i.e., clinical T1c prostate cancer, which might represent an early stage of the disease where appropriate treatment would be expected to result in a high probability of tumor control. The following questions have been raised in patients with T1c:

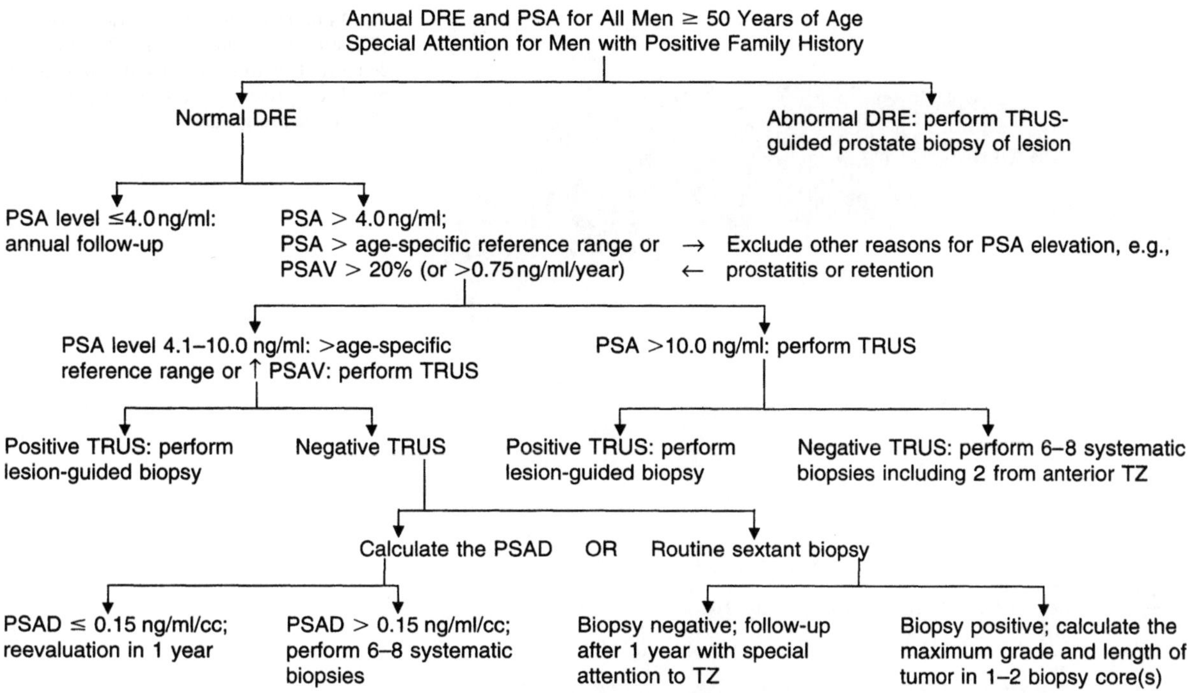

Fig. 14.5. Diagnostic algorithm demonstrating the use of PSA in the early detection of prostate cancer. *DRE*, digital rectal examination; *PSAD*, PSA density; *PSA V*, PSA velocity, slope or rate of change at annual base; *TRUS*, transrectal ultrasonography; TZ, transition zone. (Modified from OESTERLING et al. 1993)

1. Is it clinically significant cancer?
2. Why is it impalpable and invisible?
3. What is the best predictive parameter for tumor burden?
4. What are the characteristic findings and pathologic outcome?

We, like others (EPSTEIN et al. 1994; OESTERLING et al. 1993b), have tried to answer these questions by retrospective analysis of data pertaining to radical prostatectomy specimens ($n = 44$ in our study) from patients with an initial clinical diagnosis of T1c (ELGAMAL et al. 1995c). These data are summarized in Table 14.3 and Figs. 14.6 and 14.7. The following conclusions on T1c prostate cancer can be drawn from these data:

1. It currently accounts for 15%–22% of the radical prostatectomy population, and there is evidence of a progressively increasing incidence of this stage of disease.
2. There is no equivalent pathologic stage to T1c and the majority of specimens harbor significant tumors, with a much higher incidence of non-organ-confined cancers than of insignificant cancers.
3. There is a high proportion of patients with large anterior transition zone tumors (TZCa) that can be easily missed by DRE and TRUS. This supports the need for elective biopsies in patients who present with unexplained PSA elevation.
4. Patients with TZCa typically have a larger tumor volume and consequently a greater elevation of PSA than patients with peripheral zone cancer (PZCa).
5. In patients with the same tumor volume, those with PZCa will have a higher tumor grade than those with TZCa.
6. A core tumor length of 3 mm or more on one or two needle biopsies reliably predicts cancer of a clinically significant (>0.5 cm^3) volume (DIETRICK et al. 1995).

14.4.3 Cost-effectiveness of the Use of PSA in Asymptomatic Men over 50 Years of Age

The use of PSA to screen for prostate cancer is currently widespread in men over 50 years of age (BENSON 1994; BRAWER et al. 1993b; CATALONA et al. 1991, 1994a; CRAWFORD and DEANTONI 1993; GANN et al. 1995; LITTRUP et al. 1994; STENMAN et al. 1994; WALSH 1995). However, this widespread use of PSA remains controversial to certain extent, since some investigators believe that treatment of early-stage prostatic cancer may not reduce the tumor-related

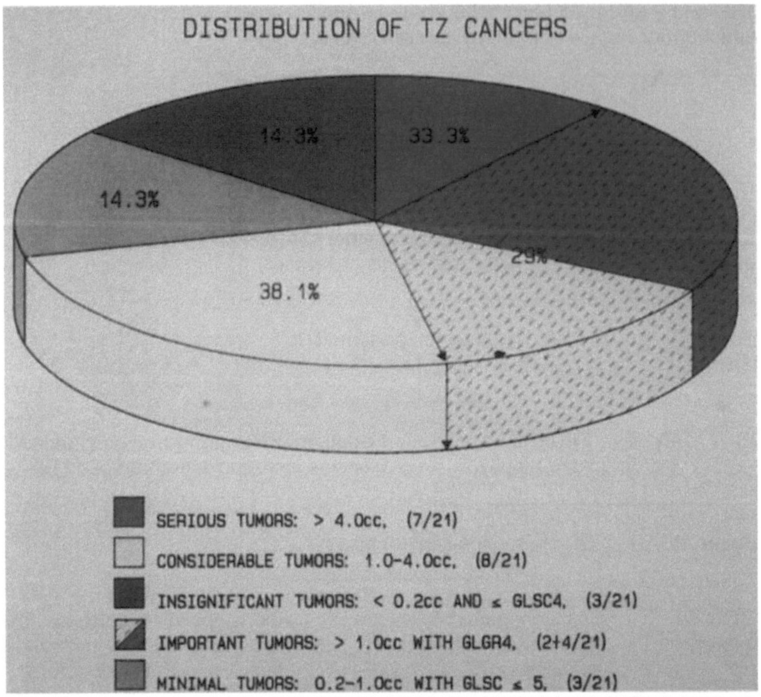

a

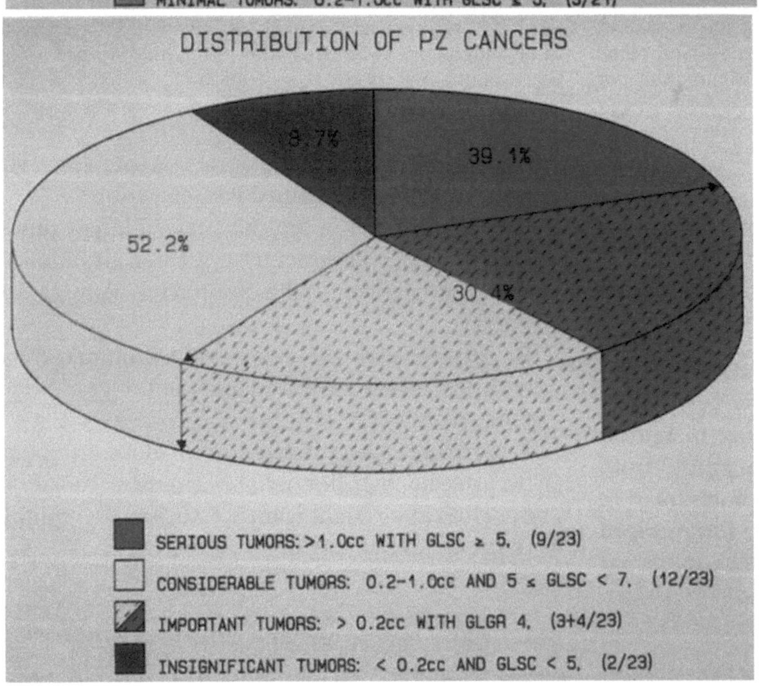

b

Fig. 14.6. Distribution of **a** transition zone (*TZ*) and **b** peripheral zone (*PZ*) tumors in 44 patients with an initial clinical diagnosis of T1c prostate cancer. *GLSC/GLGR*, Gleason score/grade

mortality at an acceptable cost in terms of treatment-related morbidity (KRAHN et al. 1994). BENOIT and NASLUND (1994) have demonstrated that breast cancer screening is 4.6 times more expensive than prostate cancer screening in terms of cost per cancer detection, in a past-middle age population including those in the 6th and 7th decades of life. This cost advantage provides a strong economic rationale for widespread prostate cancer screening and suggests that health care systems should cover the cost of this

Table 14.3. Characteristics and distribution of 44 consecutive T1c prostate cancers operated on between 1991 and 1994 (mean age of patients = 63.5 years)

Tumor location	PSA[a] (ng/ml)	No. of tumors[a]	Tumor volume[a] (cm^3)	TV %[a]	Gleason score	pT		PSM
						≤T2	≥T3	
Total (44)	12.4 ± 19.9	2.4 + 1.1	2.2 ± 3.0	5.3 ± 1.4	5.1 ± 1.4	33 (75%)	11 (25%)	11
PZCa (52%)	8.8 ± 6.7	2.2 ± 1.2	1.2 ± 1.3	3.2 ± 3.2	5.5 ± 1.0	17 (73.9%)	6 (26.1%)	6
TZCa (48%)	16.3 ± 27.8	2.6 ± 1.1	3.3 ± 3.9	7.6 ± 7.5	4.6 ± 1.6	16 (76.2%)	5 (23.8%)	5

TV%, Tumor volume/prostate volume; pT, final histologic stage according to the 1992 TNM classification; PSM, specimens with positive section margins; PZCa, primary peripheral zone cancer; TZCa, primary transition zone cancer
[a] Mean ± SD

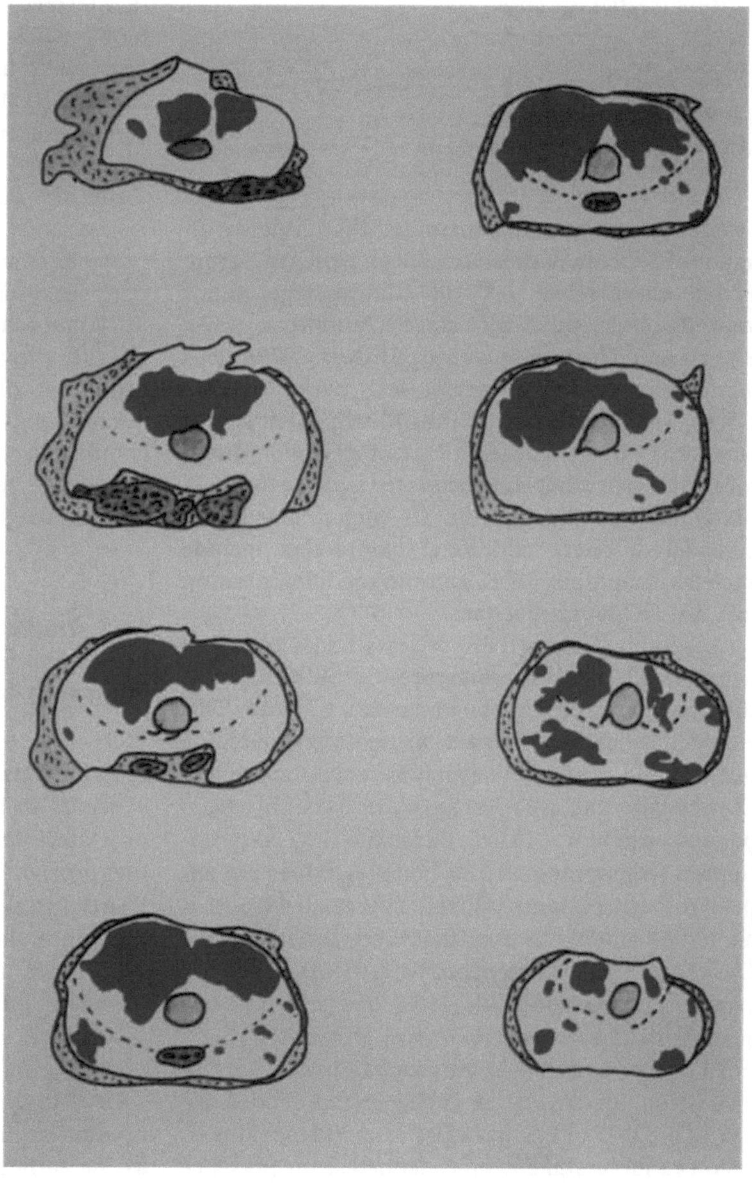

Fig. 14.7. Illustration of a case in which a T1c tumor was missed on DRE and TRUS. The whole prostate was step-sectioned from the base to the apex, at 4-mm intervals. A large bilateral anterior transition zone cancer was shown with a total tumor volume of 6.7 cc; the percentage of the total prostate volume occupied by the tumor was 16.7%. Small peripheral zone tumors are also seen

screening. It has been estimated that if the mortality due to prostate cancer were to decrease by 5.7% to 8.1%, the effectiveness of prostate cancer screening would be equal to that of breast cancer screening in terms of cancer screening's impact on patient mortality. As a result of a large increase in the incidence of organ-confined prostate cancer detected in systematic screening, it will be at least equally and possibly more effective than breast cancer screening. Recently, GUSTAFSSON et al. (1995) have found TRUS of individuals with PSA ≥4 ng/ml to be the most cost-effective strategy for early detection of prostate cancer with respect to tumors actually treated with curative intent. Population screening with the use of DRE and PSA followed by TRUS had a somewhat lower cost-effectiveness, but it detected 90% of the cancers treated for cure.

14.5 The Value of PSA in Predicting Tumor Burden

Several studies have demonstrated that in newly diagnosed untreated prostate cancer patients, serum PSA levels correlate well with clinical stage, tumor volume, and pathologic stage (BOSTWICK 1994; PARTIN and OESTERLING 1995). However, PSA level alone is insufficiently specific to provide accurate staging information for an individual patient except when it is 5.0 ng/ml or less (REES et al. 1995). Therefore, the use of other parameters to improve the PSA-predictive power in tumor staging has been considered. These additional parameters include skeletal symptoms, DRE, and tumor differentiation in a needle biopsy specimen.

A combination of PSA of less than 25.0 ng/ml, negative DRE, and Gleason score <7 could eliminate the need for a routine bone scan and CT scan. This would not have any impact on treatment outcome but it would result in a substantial economic saving (BLUESTEIN et al. 1994; REES et al. 1995). Similarly, in patients with PSA <10.0 ng/ml and no skeletal symptoms, a staging radionuclide bone scan does not appear to be necessary (OESTERLING et al. 1993a). It should be noted, however, that three patients in the OESTERLING et al. study and five patients in a study reported by MILLER et al. (1992) had positive bone scans with PSA levels <10.0 ng/ml. Obviously, this is not a common finding in the group of patients under discussion. SEAMAN et al. (1993) recommended the use of a PSAD of 0.35 ng/ml/cc as a critical value to predict a successful outcome, defined as the presence of extraprostatic spread but with capsular margins. They found that patients with a PSAD <0.35 ng/ml/cc had a 90% chance of treatment success, while those with PSAD ≥0.35 ng/ml/cc had a 66% chance of treatment failure.

Using serial PSA measurements in the follow-up of 43 untreated prostate cancer patients, SCHMID et al. (1993) found PSA doubling times to be faster in patients with higher stage and higher grade of disease.

EPSTEIN et al. (1994) found that the best model predicting insignificant tumor (<0.2 cc and <7 Gleason score) was a PSAD <0.1 ng/ml/cc and no adverse pathologic finding on needle biopsy. Similarly, an insignificant tumor can be predicted by a PSAD of 0.1–0.15 ng/ml/cc with less than 3 mm, low to intermediate grade cancer on only a single needle biopsy core. Applying the above model to radical prostatectomies performed for impalpable prostate cancer (T1c), the investigators would have been able to accurately predict 73% of insignificant tumors.

In the field of radioimmunologic imaging, ABDEL-NABI et al. (1992) have reported that staging prostate cancer using anti-PSA antibodies has shown poor sensitivity for the detection of bone and lymph node metastases. This is probably because PSA is an excretory glycoprotein, and not a transmembrane produt. Additionally, there is a high incidence of human anti-mouse antibody formation that has compromised further studies with these agents. The reader is referred to Chap. 6 for details on immunodiagnosis.

14.6 Predictive Value of PSA in Assessing Tumor Control Following Radical Prostatectomy

It is obvious to conclude that serum PSA may be expected to become undetectable following radical prostatectomy, given that it is mostly produced by the prostate (BOSTWICK 1994; OESTERLING 1991; PARTIN et al. 1993; PARTIN and OESTERLING 1995). Therefore, the most important clinical value of PSA may lie in monitoring patients following radical prostatectomy for early detection of tumor recurrence.

Except in a few cases (GOLDRATH and MESSING 1989; TAKAYAMA et al. 1992), patients with residual or recurrent tumor have detectable serum PSA levels as the earliest sign of tumor recurrence. It may be assumed that ultrasensitive immunoassays will detect PSA even earlier than the standard assays. This will provide clinicians with an additional warning period before clinical disease recurrence becomes apparent (KLEE et al. 1994; VESSELLA and LANGE 1993).

STAMEY et al. (1993), using ultrasensitive PSA assays, considered detection of a PSA level of 0.1 ng/ml per se to represent evidence of recurrence. This in turn allowed early postoperative adjuvant therapy to be offered, with a better chance of tumor control of cure of residual disease. The same investigators reported a relatively rapid PSA doubling time – less than 6 months – in patients with residual cancer after radical prostatectomy, as compared with 4 years in untreated patients. Other investigators have used the rate of change of PSA or PSA velocity after radical prostatectomy to distinguish local recurrence from distant metastasis. DANELLA et al. (1993) reported a doubling time of 6 months or less to be indicative of metastatic tumor spread, while PARTIN et al. (1994) found that a combination of several parameters, such as Gleason score, pathologic, stage and PSA velocity 1 year after surgery, to best predict the likelihood that a prospective isolated elevation in serum PSA represents a local recurrence.

Androgen provocative testing was described as another technique to improve the ability of PSA to detect microscopic residual disease after radical prostatectomy (SMITH and SCALETSKY 1993). This was based on the hypothesis that exogenous androgen administration will induce PSA release from microscopic deposits of prostate cancer cells and allow detection of residual disease earlier, thereby avoiding the potential dire consequences of late detection of more advanced disease.

ELGAMAL et al. (1995a) have hypothesized that although the periurethral glands provide a base level of urinary PSA after radical prostatectomy, longitudinal follow-up of the first stream of urine in each particular patient can detect local cancer failure according to the rate of change in urinary PSA.

This problem is rendered even more complex by the fact that various authors have found unexplained PSA elevations in some men following radical prostatectomy. These PSA elevations were found in the absence of any other clinical or pathologic sign of failure even after more than 3 years of follow-up. Based on the above findings, FRAZIER et al. (1993) have concluded that in clinically cured patients, isolated biochemical evidence of failure may not be a sufficient reason to begin a specific therapy.

14.7 New Developments to Improve PSA Sensitivity and Specificity

The prostate epithelium predominantly releases the native, enzymatically active form of PSA, which is chymotrypsin-like serine protease. This PSA is of a low molecular weight, which might facilitate its leakage to the systemic circulation; however, under nonpathologic conditions the main bulk of PSA is released into the seminal fluid via the normal anatomic pathway. The release of an enzymatically active PSA in the serum might require inactivation by the major extracellular serine protease inhibitors (serpins), namely α_1-antichymotrypsin (ACT) and α_2-macroglobulin (AMG). The equimolar complex formation with ACT increases the molecular weight and allows PSA to expose a limited number of antigenic determinants. This apparently is enough to permit detection by immunoassays. By contrast, no PSA epitope remains exposed following complex formation with AMG. Eventually, the free noncomplexed form of PSA will constitute a minor fraction of serum PSA, with unexplained failure to conjugate with the excess serpins (LILJA 1993). Recently, it has been hypothesized that measuring the proportion of different molecular forms of serum PSA may facilitate the detection of a specific lesion. Nevertheless, the exact molecular basis for this finding remains to be explained. It has been concluded that a lower proportion of uncomplexed PSA (PSA-F) or predominance of PSA-ACT can help to diagnose prostate cancer patients. This provides increased sensitivity and specificity in screening for cancer in comparison with the standard use of total PSA in screening (CATALONA et al. 1995; CHRISTENSSON et al. 1993; ELGAMAL et al. 1995d; STENEMAN et al. 1994). Increasing diagnostic sensitivity would help to select patients who warrant further management. Increasing diagnostic specificity would, on the other hand, eliminate many of the false-positive results without the potential need for use of invasive techniques such as needle biopsies (CATALONA et al. 1995; STENEMAN et al. 1994).

The main pitfall of the use of this interesting approach is that PSA-F directly correlation with the prostate volume and consequently with obstructive symptoms, rather than being lesion specific.

Inasmuch as some patients with advanced prostate cancer might have a higher PSA-F ratio than expected (ELGAMAL et al. 1995d; ZHOU et al. 1993), further investigations are needed to study the impact of cancer progression after failure of the primary therapy.

14.8 RT-PCR Enhancement Assays for the Detection of Cells That Carry Prostatic Signals

Polymerase chain reaction (PCR) is a technique that allows for in vitro amplification of a DNA segment through successive steps of denaturation, annealing, and extension of oligonucleotides under the influence of polymerase enzyme and thermal cycler. For the initiation of PCR, a complementary (c)DNA can be synthesized by the reverse-transcriptase reaction (RT). Extracted RNA (from blood cells or other tissues) and specific primers, which act as templates, are needed to direct the RT (ISRAELI et al. 1994; KATZ et al. 1995; MORENO et al. 1992; SEIDEN et al. 1994; WOOD et al. 1994). Technically, this process is feasible and noninvasive. Nevertheless, skepticism has been voiced over the sensitivity and specificity of the detected cells with the use of the RT method (WALSH 1995). The main drawbacks of RT-PCR assay include:

1. It is not a quantitative assay.
2. It has an inconsistent capacity to distinguish metastatic cancer cells, although it does detect hematogenous tumor spread in patients thought clinically to have localized cancers.
3. It fails to diagnose a high percentage of patients with otherwise well-documented advanced cancers. This is more evident in hormone-responsive extraprostatic spread and in a newly diagnosed metastatic prostate cancer using PSA-mRNA (SEIDEN et al. 1994).

It is likely that the prostate-specific membrane antigen (PSM)-mRNA, which is overexpressed in poorly differentiated prostate cancer and after androgen ablation, may be more sensitive in detecting progressive metastatic disease than PSA, especially after hormonal therapy. Unfortunately, the PSM-mRNA assay has shown a 5%–10% incidence of false-positives in a control group and a 72% incidence in patients with pT2 (organ-confined) prostate cancer following radical prostatectomy who were negative for PSA (ISRAELI et al. 1994). The clinical significance of detecting hematogenous (or bone marrow) cells which carry prostatic signals using PSA or PSM primers, and the potential application of this molecular assay merit further studies.

14.9 Extraprostatic Sources of PSA and the Potential for Contamination of Assay Results

In general PSA (with or without PAP) is a specific marker for prostatic epithelium; however, immunohistochemical detection of PSA has been reported in few normal extraprostatic tissues and few tumors of extraprostatic origin (BOSTWICK 1994; EPSTEIN 1993). We have demonstrated the presence of PSA- and PAP-producing cells in normal Cowper's glands and periurethral and intraurethral glands (Figs. 14.1, 14.2). Our findings support the previously reported data (FRAZIER et al. 1992; KAMOSHIDA and TSUTSUMI 1990) on extraprostatic sources of PSA and it may be concluded that this specific marker is not exclusively produced by the prostate gland. PSA can be detected in embryologically and physiologically related sex accessory glands. These immunohistochemical reports in periurethral glands have been verified by findings in respect of urinary PSA levels after radical prostatectomy when specimens were collected from urethral rather than bladder samples (ELGAMAL et al. 1995a; IWAKIRI et al. 1993; TAKAYAMA et al. 1994). However, the impact of nonpathologic periurethral glands on serum PSA levels following radical cysto- and/or prostatectomy has been found to be insignificant (ELGAMAL et al. 1995b; OESTERLING et al. 1995).

DODSON et al. (1994) have reported on adenocarcinoma of female paraurethral glands of Skene which demonstrated a strong positive immunohistochemical reaction for PSA with a significant increase in serum levels before operation, followed by a dramatic decrease after the surgery. This finding supports the hypothesis that Skene's glands may be considered as the homologue of the male's prostate (TEPPER et al. 1984).

LAM et al. (1989), using a polyclonal antibody assay, found positive PSA immunohistochemical staining in both mature and immature granulocytes. VAN KRIEKEN (1993), again using a polyclonal antibody assay, reported a positive PSA reaction in a male patient with primary salivary gland adenocarcinoma.

More recently, we have demonstrated PSA detection in normal as well as abnormal pancreatic and salivary gland specimens. These interesting findings were independent of the patient's sex (Fig. 14.3).

Significant serum PSA elevations with the use of a monoclonal assay have been reported in a male patient with non-Hodgkin's lymphoma of the kidney in the absence of inflammatory or malignant prostate disease. PSA level returned to normal in this patient following successful treatment with appropriate lymphoma-specific chemotherapy (DJAVAN et al. 1995).

Using an ultrasensitive immunoassay, YU and DIAMANDIS (1995) have measured detectable levels of PSA in sera of women and prostatectomized men. We had a female patient with poorly differentiated bladder cancer in whom a monoclonal assay showed unexplained PSA elevation (4.6 ng/ml). This finding was compared with those in 30 other active females who had undetectable PSA levels (unpublished data). Such cases as the above may be responsible for the reported 5% incidence of positive findings (PSA elevation) in female sera (VESSELLA and LANGE 1993).

Prostate-specific antigen has also been found in other body fluids such as saliva (BREUL et al. 1993), breast milk, and amniotic fluid (MONNE et al. 1994). Moreover, confirmed positive PSA-mRNA results have been obtained using gene-specific primers and RT-PCR in patients with breast and ovarian tumors and in some tissue samples from endometrium and kidney (CLEMENTS and MUKHTAR 1994; MONNE et al. 1994; YU et al. 1995). Similarly, SMITH et al. (1995) have found PSA-RNA in some normal blood and bone marrow cells.

Theoretically, these extraprostatic sources of PSA should be considered in the process of decision analysis in patients with carcinoma of the prostate, given that in some cases they might cause contamination of assay results obtained for diagnostic and prognostic purposes. This is particularly true under pathologic conditions that accelerate the entry of PSA or PSA-mRNA into the systemic circulation.

14.10 Conclusion

Continued efforts are being made to improve the sensitivity and specificity of detection of prostate cancer, prediction of tumor burden, and monitoring of the response to therapy. Human kallikrein 3 (hK3), prostate-specific antigen (PSA), p30, γ-seminoprotein, and E1 to a large extent represent the same substance (SENSABAUGH 1994). It has significant similarity to amino acid sequences of pancreaticorenal kallikrein (hK1) and human glandular kallikrein (hK2). Potentially, this similarity may be responsible for the infrequent cross-reactivity of some commercial PSA assays in patients with conditions unrelated to the prostate.

In addition to considering the value of measuring serum PSA levels, new investigations are assessing the clinical importance and relevance of the following studies:

1. PSA density (PSA-D)
2. PSA velocity or rate of change
3. Age-specific reference ranges
4. The ratio of different molecular forms of PSA
5. Detection of PSA-mRNA

It has now been clearly established that PSA is not exclusively of prostatic origin. Reports have been published documenting the detection of PSA in extraprostatic sites such as: bone marrow leukocytes, immature granulocytes and mature neutrophils, Cowper and periurethral glands, perianal glands, salivary glands, pancreas, breast, and endometrium. Reports on the last two of these sites have been confirmed by molecular characterization of PSA-mRNA. It is of interest that serum PSA levels decline significantly and stay at very low (or undetectable) levels for a considerable time after curative radical prostatectomy, although the aforementioned extraprostatic sources theoretically might influence the detection of PSA or PSA-carrying cells.

With all its limitations, PSA remains the most important prostate cancer marker. However, since it is not exclusively prostatic (especially after radical prostatectomy thought to be curative), important management decisions should not exclusively rely on the detection of PSA as the only evidence of treatment failure.

References

Abdel-Nabi H, Wright GL, Gulfo JV et al. (1992) Monoclonal antibodies and radioimmunoconjugates in the diagnosis and treatment of prostate cancer. Semin Urol X(1):45–54

Babaian J, Myiashita H, Evans RB (1992) The distribution of prostate specific antigen in men without clinical or pathological evidence of prostate cancer: relationship to gland volume and age. J Urol 147:837–840

Benson MC (1994) Editorial: prostate specific antigen. J Urol 152:2046–2048

Benoit RM, Naslund MJ (1994) An economic rationale for prostate cancer screening. Urology 44:795–803

Bluestein DL, Bostwick DG, Bergstrahl EJ et al. (1994) Eliminating the need for bilateral pelvic lymphadenectomy in select patients with prostate cancer. J Urol 151:1315–1320

Bostwick DG (1994) Prostate-specific antigen. Current role in diagnostic pathology of prostate cancer. Am J Clin Pathol 102(Suppl 1):S31–S37

Brawer MK, Aramburu EAG, Chen GL et al. (1993a) The inability of prostate specific antigen index to enhance the

predictive value of prostate specific antigen in the diagnosis of prostatic carcinoma. J Urol 150:369–373
Brawer MK, Beatie J, Wener MH et al. (1993b) Screening for prostatic carcinoma with prostatic specific antigen: results of the second year. J Urol 150:106–109
Bretton PR, Evans WP, Borden JD et al. (1994) The use of prostate specific antigen density to improve the sensitivity of prostate specific antigen in detecting prostate carcinoma. Cancer 74:2991–2995
Breul J, Pickl U, Hartung R (1993) Prostate specific antigen in urine and saliva. J Urol 149:302A
Carter HB, Pearson JD, Metter EJ et al. (1992) Longitudinal evaluation of prostate-specific antigen levels in men with and without disease. JAMA 267:2215–2220
Carter HB, Chan DW, Pearson JD et al. (1995) Prostate-specific antigen variability in men without prostate cancer: effect of sampling interval on prostate-specific antigen velocity. Urology 45:591–596
Catalona WJ, Smith DS, Ratliff TL et al. (1991) Measurement of prostate-specific antigen in serum as a screening test for prostate cancer. N Engl J Med 324:1156–1161
Catalona WJ, Richie JP, Ahmann FR et al. (1994a) Comparison of digital rectal examination and serum prostate specific antigen in the early detection of prostate cancer: results of a multicenter clinical trial of 6630 men. J Urol 151:1283–1290
Catalona WJ, Richie JP, deKernion JB (1994b) Comparison of prostate specific antigen concentration versus prostate specific antigen density in the early detection of prostate cancer: receiver operating characteristic curves. J Urol 152:2031–2036
Catalona WJ, Smith DS, Wolfert RL et al. (1995) Increasing specificity of PSA screening through measurement of percent free PSA in serum. J Urol 153:312A
Christensson A, Björk T, Nilsson O et al. (1993) Serum prostate specific antigen complexed to $\alpha 1$-antichymotrypsin as an indicator of prostate cancer. J Urol 150:100–105
Clements J, Mukhtar A (1994) Glandular kallikreins and prostate-specific antigen are expressed in the human endometrium. J Clin Endocrinol Metab 78:1536–1539
Coffey DS (1992) The molecular biology endocrinology and physiology of prostate and seminal vessels. In: Walsh PC, Retik AB, Stamey TA, Vaughan D (eds) Campbell's urology. Saunders, Philadelphia, pp 221–266
Cooner WH (1993) Definition of the ideal tumor marker. Urol Clin North Am 20:575–579
Crawford ED, DeAntoni EP (1993) PSA as a screening test for prostate cancer. Urol Clin North Am 20:637–646
Crawford ED, DeAntoni EP, Stone NN et al. (1995) Prostate cancer awareness week demonstrates continued value to early detection strategies. J Urol 153:312A
Danella J, Steckel J, Dorey F et al. (1993) Detectable prostate specific antigen levels following radical prostatectomy. J Urol 149:447A
Dawson NA, McLeod DG (1995) Dramatic prostate specific antigen decrease in response to discontinuation of megestrol acetate in advanced prostate cancer: expansion of the antiandrogen withdrawal syndrome. J Urol 153:1946–1947
Dietrick D, McNeal JE, Stamey TA (1995) Core cancer length in ultrasound-guided systematic sextant biopsies: a preoperative evaluation of prostate cancer volume. Urology 45:987–992
Djavan B, Keffer JH, Molberg K (1995) False-positive serum prostate-specific antigen values in a patient with non-Hodgkin lymphoma of the kidney. Urology 45:875–878
Dodson MK, Cliby WA, Keeney GL et al. (1994) Case report: Skene's gland adenocarcinoma with increased serum level of prostate-specific antigen. Gynecol Oncol 55:304–307
Elgamal AA, Van de Voorde W, Van Poppel H et al. (1994a) Immunohistochemical localization of prostate-specific markers within the accessory male sex glands of Cowper, Littre and Morgagni. Urology 44:84–90
Elgamal AA, Van de Voorde W, Van Poppel H et al. (1994b) Prostatic duct adenocarcinoma with endometrial features after TURP. Urology 43:737–742
Elgamal AA, Billen J, Van de Voorde W et al. (1995a) Verification and significance of PSA production by the periurethral glands. Proceedings of "Androgenic Hormones, Prostate Cancer and Benign Prostatic Hyperplasia", International Conference, New Orleans, March 13–15
Elgamal AA, Billen J, Van de Voorde W et al. (1995b) Extraprostatic sources of PSA, does it infer the subjective biochemical recurrence after radical prostatectomy? J Urol 153:518A
Elgamal AA, Van de Voorde WM, Van Poppel HP et al. (1995c) Selective zonal distribution of tumor volume versus grade in T1c prostate cancer. J Urol 153:484A
Elgamal AA, Cornillie F, Van Poppel H et al. (1995d) Interpretation of free/total (F/T) PSA determinations in routine clinical practice (abstract). 23rd Meeting of the International Society for Oncodevelopmental Biology and Medicine (ISOBM), Montreal, Canada. September 10–13
Ellis WJ, Chetner MP, Preston SD (1994) Diagnosis of prostatic carcinoma: the yield of serum prostate specific antigen, digital rectal examination and transrectal ultrasonography. J Urol 152:1520–1525
Epstein JI (1993) PSA and PAP as immunohistochemical markers in prostate cancer. Urol Clin North Am 20:757–770
Epstein JI, Walsh PC, Carmichael M et al. (1994) Pathologic and clinical findings to predict tumor extent of nonpalpable (stage T1c) prostate cancer. JAMA 271:368
Fichtner J, Graves H, Shortlife L et al. (1994) Prostate specific antigen releases a kinin-like substance that stimulates smooth muscle contraction. J Urol 151:313A
Frazier HA, Humphrey PA, Burchette JL et al. (1992) Immunoreactive prostatic specific antigen in male periurethral glands. J Urol 147:246–248
Frazier HA, Robertson JE, Humphrey PA et al. (1993) Is prostate specific antigen of clinical importance in evaluating outcome after radical prostatectomy? J Urol 149:516–518
Gann PH, Hennekens CH, Stampfer MJ (1995) A prospective evaluation of plasma prostate-specific antigen for detection of prostatic cancer. JAMA 273:289–294
Goldrath DE, Messing EM (1989) Prostate specific antigen: not detectable despite tumor progression after radical prostatectomy. J Urol 142:1082–1084
Graves HCB (1993) Standardization of immunoassays for prostate-specific antigen. Cancer 72:3141–3144
Grob BM, Schellhammer PF, Brassil DN et al. (1994) Changes in immunohistochemical staining of PSA, PAP and TURP-27 following irradiation therapy for clinically localized prostate cancer. Urology 44:525–529
Gustafsson O, Carlsson P, Norming U (1995) Cost-effectiveness analysis in early detection of prostate cancer: an evaluation of six screening strategies in a randomly selected population of 2000 men. Prostate 26:299–309
Hsieh J-T, Wu H-C, Gleave ME (1993) Autocrine regulation of prostate-specific antigen gene expression in a human prostatic cnacer (LNCaP) subline. Cancer Res 53:2852–2857

Israeli RS, Miller WH, Su SL (1994) Sensitive nested reverse transcription polymerase chain reaction detection of circulating prostatic tumor cells: comparison of prostate-specific membrane antigen and prostate-specific antigen-based assays. Cancer Res 54:6306–6310

Iwakiri J, Gransboris K, Wehner N et al. (1993) An analysis of urinary prostate specific antigen before and after radical prostatectomy: evidence of secretion of prostate specific antigen by the periurethral glands. J Urol 149:783–786

Jacobsen SJ, Wright GL, Lilja H et al. (1994) Comparability of the tandem-R and Imx assays for the measurement of serum prostate-specific antigen. Urology 44:512–518

Kamoshida S, Tsutsumi Y (1990) Extraprostatic localization of prostatic acid phosphatase and prostate-specific antigen: distribution of cloacogenic glandular epithelium and sex-dependent expression in human anal gland. Hum Pathol 21:1108–1111

Kanety H, Madjar Y, Dagen Y et al. (1993) Serum insuline-like growth factor-binding protein-2 (IGFBR2) is increased and IGFBR3 is decreased in patients with prostate cancer: correlation with serum prostate-specific antigen. J Clin Endocrinol Metab 77:229–233

Katz AE, de Vries GM, Begg MD et al. (1995) Enhanced reverse transcriptase-polymerase chain reaction for prostate-specific antigen as an indicator of true pathologic stage in patients with prostate cancer. Cancer 75:1642–1648

Klee GG, Dodge LA, Zincke H et al. (1994) Measurement of serum prostate specific antigen using Imx prostate specific antigen assay. J Urol 151:94–98

Krahn MD, Mahoney JE, Eckman MH (1994) Screening for prostate cancer. JAMA 272:773–780

Lam K-W, Li C-Y, Yam LT (1989) Improved immunohistochemical detection of prostatic acid phosphatase by a monoclonal antibody. Prostate 15:13–21

Lilja H (1985) A kallikrein-like serine protease in prostatic fluid cleaves the predominant seminal vesicle protein. J Clin Invest 76:1899–1903

Lilja H (1993) Significance of different molecular forms of serum PSA. The free, noncomplexed form of PSA versus that complexed to α_1-antichymotrypsin. Urol Clin North Am 20:681–686

Littrup PJ, Kane RA, Mettlin CJ et al. (1994) Cost-effective prostate cancer detection: reduction of low-yield biopsies. Cancer 74:3146–3158

Mettlin C, Murphy GP, Menck H (1994) Trends in treatment of localized prostate cancer by radical prostatectomy: observations from the commission on cancer national cancer database, 1985–1990. Urology 43:488–492

Miller PD, Eandley I, Kirby S (1992) Prostate specific antigen and bone scan correlation in the staging and monitoring of patients with prostatic cancer. Br J Urol 70:295–298

Monne M, Croce CM, Yu H et al. (1994) Molecular characterization of prostate-specific antigen messenger RNA expressed in breast tumors. Cancer Res 54:6344–6347

Moreno JG, Croce CM, Fischer R et al. (1992) Detection of hematogenous micrometastasis in patients with prostate cancer. Cancer Res 52:6110–6112

Neal DE, Clejan S, Sarma D (1992) Prostate specific antigen and prostatitis. I. Effect of prostatitis on serum PSA in the human and nonhuman primate. Prostate 20:105–111

Nishiya M, Miller GJ, Lookner DH et al. (1994) Prostate specific antigen density in patients with histologically proven prostate carcinoma. Cancer 74:3002–3009

Oesterling JE (1991) Prostate specific antigen: a critical assessment of the most useful tumor marker for adenocarcinoma of the prostate. J Urol 145:907–923

Oesterling JE (1993) PSA leads the way for detecting and following prostate cancer. Contemp Urol 5:60–81

Oesterling JE, Martin SK, Bergstrath EJ et al. (1993a) The use of prostate specific antigen in staging patients with newly diagnosed prostate cancer. JAMA 269:57–60

Oesterling JE, Suman VJ, Zincke H et al. (1993b) PSA-detected (clinical stage T1c or B0) prostate cancer. Pathologically significant tumors. Urol Clin North Am 20:687–693

Oesterling JE, Martin SK, Bergstrath EJ et al. (1995) The periurethral glands do not have a clinically significant effect on the serum PSA concentration. J Urol 153:518A

Partin AW, Oesterling JE (1995) The clinical usefulness of prostate specific antigen: update 1994. J Urol 152:1358–1368

Partin AW, Pound CR, Clemens JQ et al. (1993) Serum PSA after anatomic radical prostatectomy. The Johns Hopkins experience after 10 years. Urol Clin North Am 20:713–725

Partin AW, Pearson JD, Landis PK (1994) Evaluation of serum prostate-specific antigen velocity after radical prostatectomy to distinguish local recurrence from distant metastases. Urology 43:649–659

Rees MA, McHugh TA, Dorr RP et al. (1995) Assessment of the utility of bone scan, CT scan and lymph node dissection in staging patients with newly diagnosed prostate cancer. J Urol 153:352A

Rommel FM, Agusta VE, Breslin JA et al. (1994) The use of prostate specific antigen and prostate specific antigen density in the diagnosis of prostate cancer in a community based urology practice. J Urol 151:88–93

Schmid H-P, McNeal JE, Stamey TA (1993) Observations on the doubling time of prostate cancer. Cancer 71:2031–2040

Seaman E, Whang M, Olsson CA (1993) PSA density (PSAD). Role in patient evaluation and management. Urol Clin North Am 20:653–663

Seiden MMV, Kantoff PW, Krithivas K (1994) Detection of circulating tumor cells in men with localized prostate cancer. J Clin Oncol 12:2634–2639

Sensabaugh GF (1994) Response to Wang et al. (1994) Prostate-specific antigen, p30, γ-seminoprotein and E1. Prostate 24:109–110

Smith DS, Catalona WJ (1994) Rate of change in serum prostate speific antigen levels as a method of prostate cancer detection. J Urol 152:1163–1167

Smith JA, Scaletsky R (1993) Future directions in tumor marker technology for prostate cancer. Urol Clin North Am 20:771–777

Smith MR, Biggar S, Hussain M (1995) Prostate-specific antigen messenger RNA is expressed in non-prostate cells: implications for detection of micrometastases. Cancer Res 55:2640–2644

Stamey TA (1995) Second Stanford conference on international standardization of prostate-specific antigen immunoassays: September 1–2, 1994. Urology 45:173–184

Stamey TA, Graves HCB, Wehner N (1993) Early detection of residual prostate cancer after radical prostatectomy by an ultrasensitive assay for prostate specific antigen. J Urol 149:787–792

Stein AVI, deKernion JB, Smith RB (1992) Prostate specific antigen levels after radical prostatectomy in patients with organ confined and locally extensive prostate cancer. J Urol 147:942–946

Stenman U-H, Hakama M, Knekt P et al. (1994) Serum concentrations of prostate specific antigen and its complex with α1-antichymotrypsin before diagnosis of prostate cancer. Lancet 344:1594–1598

Takayama TK, Krieger JN, True LD et al. (1992) Recurrent prostate cancer despite undetectable prostate specific antigen. J Urol 148:1541–1542
Takayama TK, Vessella RL, Brawer MK et al. (1994) Urinary prostate specific antigen levels after radical prostatectomy. J Urol 151:82–87
Tepper SL, Jagirdar J, Heath D et al. (1984) Homology between the female paraurethral (Skene's) glands and the prostate. Arch Pathol Lab Med 108:423–425
Van de Voorde WM, Elgamal AA, Van Poppel HP et al. (1994) Morphologic and immunohistochemical changes in prostate cancer after preoperative hormonal therapy. Cancer 74:3164–3175
van Krieken JHJM (1993) Prostate marker immunoreactivity in salivary gland neoplasms. Am J Surg Pathol 17:410–414
Van Poppel H, De Ridder D, Elgamal AA (1995) Neoadjuvant hormonal therapy before radical prostatectomy decreases the number of positive surgical margins in stage T2 prostate cancer: interim results of a prospective randomized trial. J Urol 154:429–434
Vessella RL, Lange PH (1993) Issues in the assessment of PSA immunoassays. Urol Clin North AM 20:607–619
Walsh PC (1995) Editorial comments. J Urol 154:304–308
Wood DP, Banks ER, Humphreys S et al. (1994) Identification of bone marrow micrometastases in patients with prostate cancer. Cancer 74:2533–2540
Young CY, Montgomery BT, Andrews et al. (1991) Hormone regulation of prostatespecific antigen messenger RNA in human prostatic adenocarcinoma cell line LNCaP. Cancer Res 51:3748–3752
Yu HE, Diamandis EP (1995) Measurement of serum prostate specific antigen levels in women and in prostatectomized men with an ultrasensitive immunoassay technique. J Urol 153:1004–1008
Yu HE, Diamandis EP, Levesque M et al. (1995) Expression of prostate specific antigen gene in a primary ovarian carcinoma. Clin Chem 41:S219
Zhou AM, Tewari PC, Bluestein BI et al. (1993) Multiple forms of prostate specific antigen in serum: difference in immunorecognition by monoclonal and polyclonal assays. Clin Chem 39:2483–2491

15 Treatment Results with External Beam Radiation Therapy for Localized Carcinoma of the Prostate (Stages T1b, T2, and T3)

C.A. Perez, J. Michalski, and M.A. Lockett

CONTENTS

15.1 Introduction

Optimal treatment for patients with localized carcinoma of the prostate is controversial. Radiation therapy is an established modality in the management of these patients, and several reports indicate that clinical results are comparable to those achieved with radical prostatectomy (Bagshaw et al. 1990; Culp 1967; Hanks 1993; Partin et al. 1993b; Perez et al. 1993b; Zincke et al. 1991). Recently, efficacy of therapy for carcinoma of the prostate is being evaluated in the light of posttreatment prostate specific antigen (PSA) determinations (Benson et al. 1992; Catalona et al. 1991; Oesterling et al. 1988; Oesterling 1991; Pisansky et al. 1993).

A review was carried out of multiple publications and data from our institution on the management of carcinoma of the prostate. Survival data were analyzed, as well as preliminary data on postirradiation PSA levels. Factors that have an impact on the outcome of therapy and relevant clinical trials are discussed.

Effectiveness of any therapy in localized carcinoma of the prostate is always scrutinized against the background of what many describe as a fairly indolent clinical course of the disease. Whitmore (1988) pointed out that the end results of treatment in these patients may be a combined consequence of host factors, tumor natural history and behavior, and therapy efficacy; he also stated that there is no best treatment for all patients but rather a variety of methods, one of which is best for a particular patient and his tumor.

Fleming et al. (1993) described a decision analysis model based on published data of therapy results and concluded that observation is reasonable management for patients over 75 years of age, whereas, using optimistic assumptions, either radical prostatectomy or radiation therapy offers the same therapeutic benefits to patients 60–65 years old with moderately or poorly differentiated tumors.

Chodak et al. (1994), in a pooled analysis of 828 patients in six nonrandomized studies treated with watchful waiting and delayed hormone therapy for clinically localized prostate cancer, reported a 10-year disease-specific survival rate of 87% for men with grade 1 or 2 tumors and 34% for men with grade 3 tumors. They concluded that initial conservative management and delayed hormone therapy is a reasonable choice for some men with grade 1 or 2 clinically localized prostate cancer and that new treatment strategies are needed for grade 3 tumors.

C.A. Perez, MD, FACR, Professor of Radiation Oncology, Director, Radiation Oncology Center, Mallinckrodt Institute of Radiology, Washington University School of Medicine, 4511 Forest Park, St. Louis, MO 63108, USA

J. Michalski, MD, Radiation Oncology Center, Mallinckrodt Institute of Radiology, Washington University School of Medicine, 4939 Children's Place, St. Louis, MO 63110, USA

M.A. Lockett, MBA, Radiation Oncology Center, Mallinckrodt Institute of Radiology, Washington University School of Medicine, 4939 Children's Place, St. Louis, MO 63110, USA

In an editorial, WHITMORE (1993) pointed out that the conclusions of FLEMING et al. (1993) challenge prevailing conceptions of many urologists and radiation oncologists regarding the effectiveness of their respective modalities in the treatment of some patients. He noted that the optimal management of clinically localized prostate cancer may be more a matter of opinion than a fact. Similarly, MOORE et al. (1988) provided evidence that urologists and oncologists recommend treatment consistent with their respective disciplines (surgery, irradiation, or chemotherapy), thus making analysis of therapy results even more complex.

15.2 Definitive External Beam Irradiation

External beam irradiation is used as definitive therapy in a large proportion of patients with clinical stage A and B carcinoma of the prostate and, in most institutions, in the majority of patients with stage C or more locally extensive tumors. Tumor doses have ranged from 60 to 64 Gy for stage A1 (T1a), 65 to 70 Gy for A2 (T1b) and B (T2), and 66 to 72 Gy for stage C (T3) tumors. Several retrospective studies indicate that dose has a strong impact on local tumor control; PEREZ et al. (1986, 1993b) noted improved local control rates with doses greater than 65 Gy, particularly in stage C patients. HANKS et al. (1988b) reported actuarial 5-year local recurrence rates of 36% for patients with stage C tumors treated with doses below 64.9 Gy, 29% for those treated with 65–69.9 Gy, and 19% for those receiving 70 Gy or more.

The impact of elective pelvic lymph node irradiation on survival is controversial. MCGOWAN (1981) reported better survival and fewer pelvic failures in patients with stage B2 or C tumors treated with larger fields encompassing the pelvic lymph nodes compared with patients treated to the prostate and periprostatic tissues only. PLOYSONGSANG et al. (1992) described, in 126 patients treated to the prostate and whole pelvis, a 5-year survival rate of 92% in stage B and 72% in stage C patients compared with 70% and 40%, respectively, in 116 patients irradiated to the prostatic area only. BAGSHAW (1984) noted a trend toward improved survival in patients with stage B1 tumors with negative staging lymphadenectomy when the lymph nodes were irradiated; these results were superior to those observed in patients with positive nodes. However, in a later report SPAAS et al. (1988) showed no significant advantage for pelvic lymph node irradiation over prostatic field irradiation in pathologically staged patients. Likewise, ASBELL et al. (1988) reported no difference in survival or patterns of failure in a randomized study of 445 patients with stage A2 or B carcinoma of the prostate treated to the pelvic lymph nodes (45 Gy) and the prostate (additional 20 Gy) or to the prostate and adjacent tissues only (65 Gy).

In an analysis of 963 patients receiving definitive irradiation at our institution, we observed no significant difference in pelvic tumor control or survival in patients with clinical stage A2 or B tumors, whether the prostate volume only or the pelvic lymph nodes and prostate were irradiated. In clinical stage C patients, the pelvic tumor control rate was 72% when the pelvic lymph nodes were treated with 50 Gy or higher, in contrast to 60% with lower doses ($P < 0.01$); however, no correlation between irradiated volume and survival was demonstrated (PEREZ et al., to be published).

The importance of adequate radiation therapy techniques to achieve optimal tumor control in the pelvis has been emphasized (PEREZ et al. 1993a). Furthermore, a lower incidence of distant metastases and improved survival have been reported by KAPLAN et al. (1992) and PEREZ et al. (1993a) in patients with locoregional tumor control compared with patients developing pelvic failure subsequent to external beam irradiation and by KUBAN et al. (1987, 1995) in patients treated with either external beam or interstitial irradiation.

15.3 Impact of Surgical Staging on Outcome of External Beam Irradiation

Most series of radical (including nerve-sparing) prostatectomy have the advantage of patient selection (younger than 70 years, good medical condition) in addition to the practice of most urologists of not performing prostatectomy on patients with demonstrated metastatic lymph nodes at the time of staging lymphadenectomy or with gross extracapsular tumor extension. In contrast, patients treated with irradiation are older, are in less-than-ideal medical condition, and frequently have more extensive local tumors (ADOLFSSON 1993). The impact of surgical staging on outcome of irradiation was documented by ASBELL et al. (1989) in patients with clinical stage A2 and B carcinoma of the prostate. The 5-year disease-free survival was 76% in patients with negative pelvic lymph nodes at lymphadenectomy and 63% in those staged by radiographic imaging ($P = 0.008$), suggesting that in the latter group some patients had pathologically positive lymph nodes. This observation was corroborated by HANKS et al. (1992b) in an analysis of RTOG protocols 77-06 and 75-06. The 5-year disease-free survival rates in stage T2 (B) disease were 72% for pathologically negative and 63% for radiographically negative lymph nodes and in stage T3,4 (C), 64% and 44%, respectively. More importantly, the overall and disease-free survival or metastatic rates were similar in patients with positive or negative radiographically assessed nodes, indicating the limitations of this procedure in correctly evaluating lymph node status in these patients (Fig. 15.1). The authors concluded that radiographic determination of lymph node status had no prognostic value and should not be used for stratification of patients in clinical trials. Thus, for a true comparison of results of radical prostatectomy or radiation therapy, all patients treated with either modality should be surgically staged or all patients should be randomized before treatment and receive therapy based on the findings of various staging procedures.

15.4 Results of Treatment with External Beam Irradiation

15.4.1 Survival

In 963 patients treated with definitive irradiation for localized carcinoma of the prostate at our institution between January 1967 and December 1992, we reported 10-year survival rates similar to those of other published series (Fig. 15.2).

The 5-year disease-free survival rates with external irradiation reported in multiple series are approximately 95%–100% for clinical stage A1 (T1a),

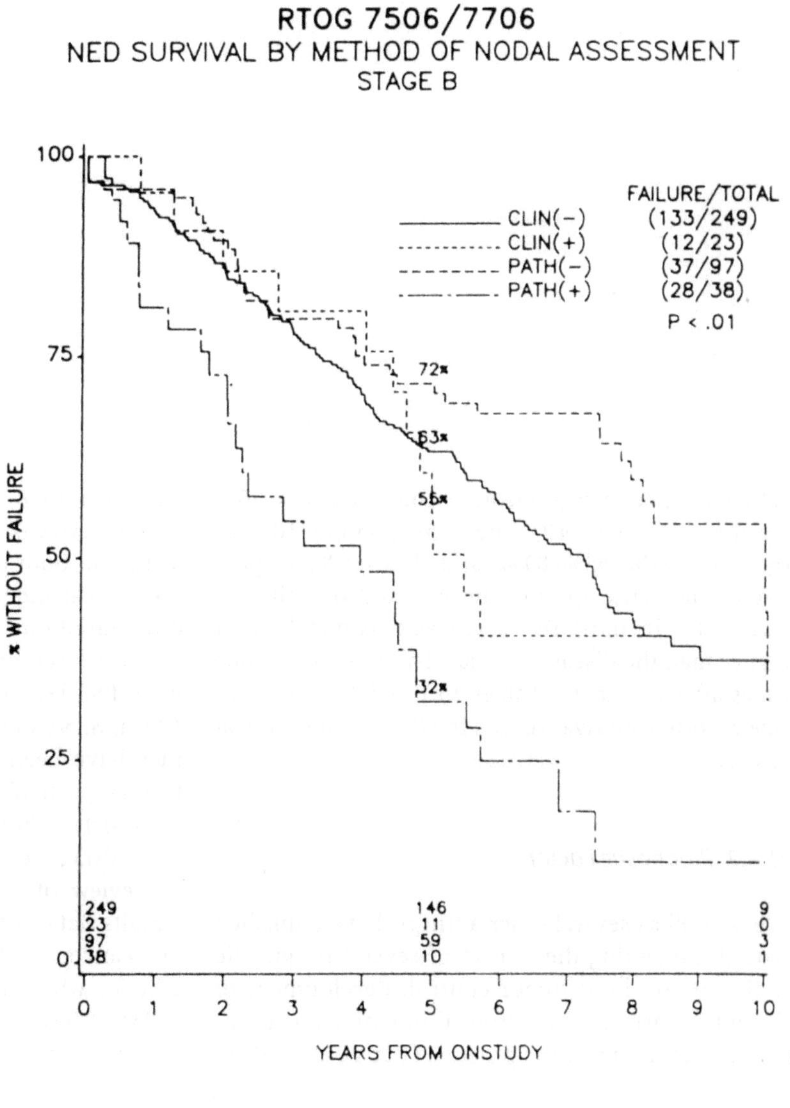

Fig. 15.1a,b. Disease-free survival correlated with method of nodal assessment for patients with T2 (**a**) or T3,4 (**b**) prostate cancer (from HANKS et al. 1992b)

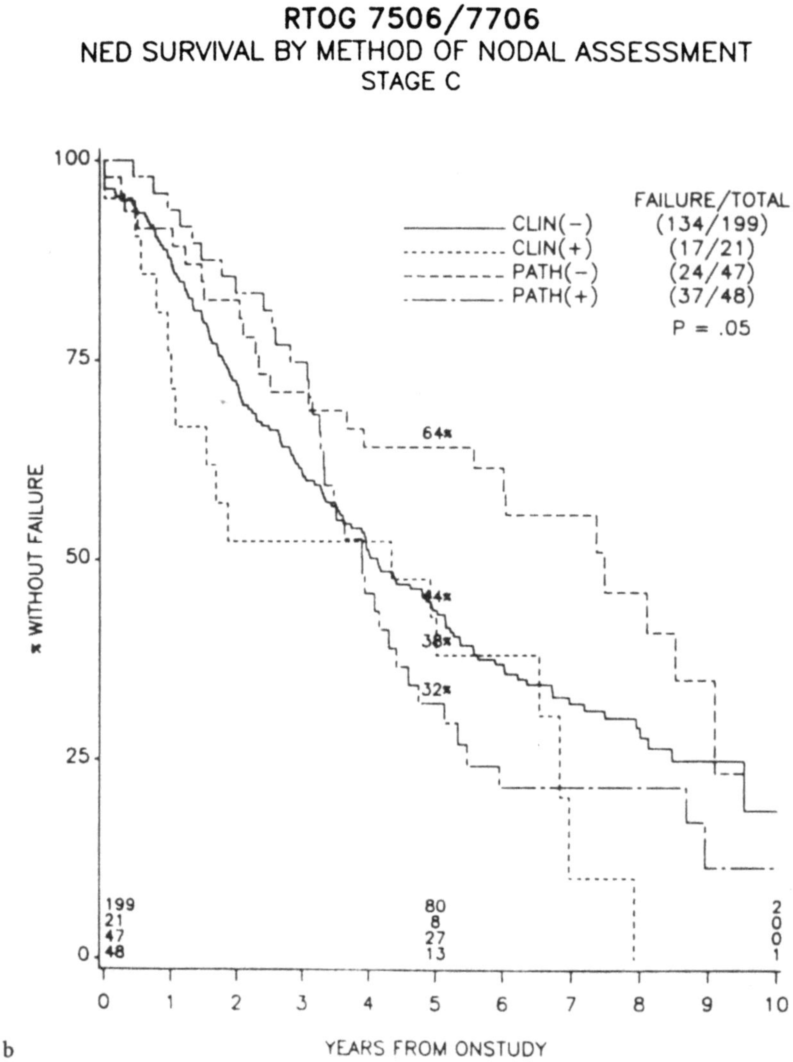

Fig. 15.1b

80%–90% for clinical stage A2 (T1b,c), and 50%–70% for clinical stage C (T2). The corresponding 10-year rates are 95%, 65%–80%, and 40%–50%, respectively. The cause-specific survival and overall survival rates in most series are approximately 10% higher than the disease-free survival rates at various times after treatment. Tables 15.1 and 15.2 summarize reported survival results for the various clinical stages.

15.4.2 Prognostic Factors

We, as well as several other authors, have published data documenting the impact of several prognostic indicators on local tumor control, development of distant metastases, and survival in patients with localized carcinoma of the prostate (Blute et al. 1989; Gleason 1988; Perez et al. 1989; Pilepich et al. 1987d; Zagars et al. 1993). Important prognostic factors in both univariate and multivariate analyses are clinical and pathologic stage, histologic degree of differentiation, elevation of prostatic acid phosphatase level, and, in more recent years, pretreatment PSA level (Bluestein et al. 1994; Partin et al. 1993a; Sands et al. 1994). In some studies age and race have been found to be significant prognostic factors, particularly for survival, although this is not a consistent finding (Brawn et al. 1993; Kim et al. 1995; Roach et al. 1992).

Review of the Surveillance, Epidemiology, End Results data in the United States showed that prostate cancer mortality for black men was 50.7 versus 23.1 for white men per 100 000 men (Miller et al. 1993). Roach et al. (1992), in three Radiation Therapy Oncology Group (RTOG) trials, noted that

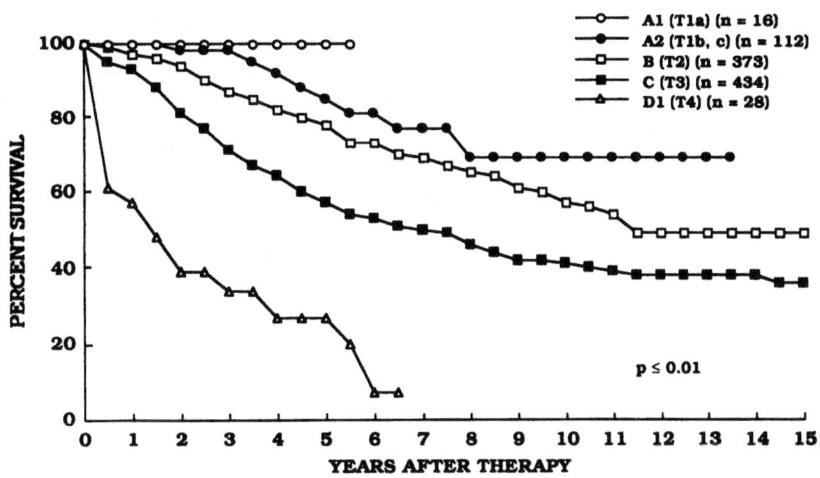

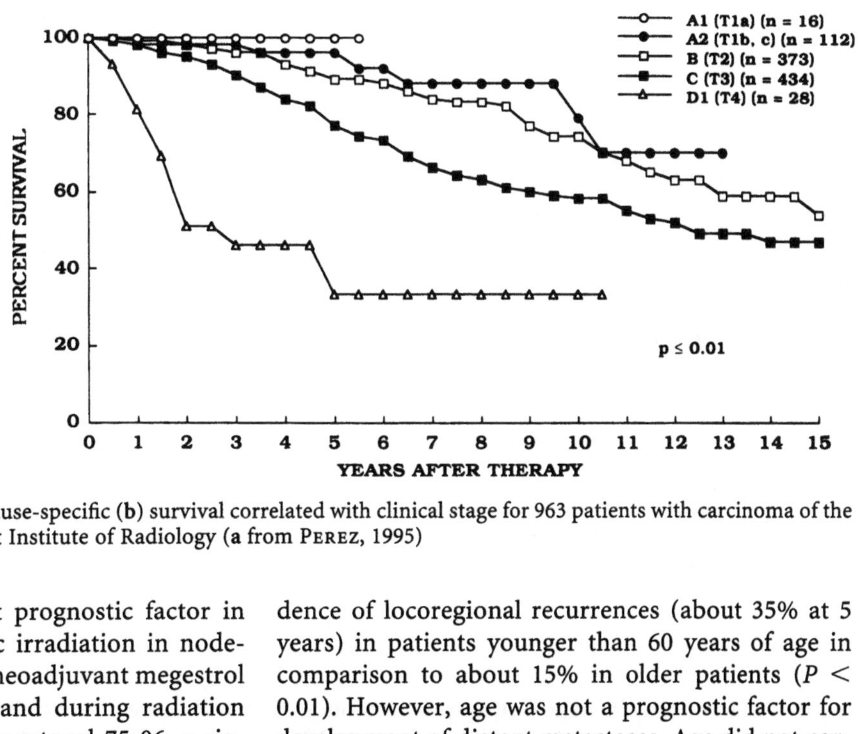

Fig. 15.2a,b. Disease-free (**a**) and cause-specific (**b**) survival correlated with clinical stage for 963 patients with carcinoma of the prostate treated at the Mallinckrodt Institute of Radiology (**a** from PEREZ, 1995)

race was not an independent prognostic factor in RTOG protocols 77-06 (pelvic irradiation in node-negative patients) and 83-07 (neoadjuvant megestrol and diethylstilbestrol before and during radiation therapy). However, in RTOG protocol 75-06, a significantly higher percentage of black patients had elevated serum acid phosphatase, and this was associated with lower disease-free survival and shorter interval to development of distant metastases. BRAWN et al. (1993), in an analysis of patients treated at the Veterans Administration Medical Center, pointed to more advanced tumor stage at diagnosis as a cause of poorer survival among black men with prostate cancer. Similar results were reported by KIM et al. (1995) in 157 black patients compared with 489 white men treated with radiation therapy for localized carcinoma of the prostate.

PILEPICH et al. (1987d), in an analysis of 566 patients in RTOG study 75-06, observed a higher incidence of locoregional recurrences (about 35% at 5 years) in patients younger than 60 years of age in comparison to about 15% in older patients ($P < 0.01$). However, age was not a prognostic factor for development of distant metastases. Age did not correlate with disease-free or overall survival. On multivariate analysis, age showed a correlation only with locoregional recurrences. GLEASON (1988) pointed out that age at time of diagnosis and histologic tumor grade are closely interdependent prognostic factors significantly affecting prognosis. A Gleason score 5 tumor in a 75-year-old man does not increase his mortality drastically in comparison with normal life expectancy, but the same tumor in a 45-year-old doubles his mortality. Alternatively, a Gleason score 7 tumor is associated with an ominous prognosis at any age.

Performance of a transurethral resection of the prostate has also been reported to be an important

Table 15.1. Survival with external beam irradiation: stage A2 (T1b) and B (T2) carcinoma of the prostate (modified from PEREZ 1992)

Study	Number of patients			Survival (%)		
	Stage T1b	Stage T2	Stages T1b and 2	5-year	10-year	15-year
ARISTIZABAL et al. (1984)	17			100	(100)	
		101		82	(65)	
ASBELL et al. (1988)	84	361		79 (66)	60 (45)	
BAGSHAW et al. (1990)	308			85 (90)	65 (70)	40 (65)
		218		83 (87)	55 (65)	35 (50)
FORMAN et al. (1986)			113	(63)		
HANKS (1993)	116			85 (74)	63 (52)	
HANKS (1993)		415		75 (53)	46 (34)	
HANKS (1993)			60	84 (76)	54 (53)	41 (39)
HANKS et al. (1988a)	84			86	64	
HANKS (1993)		312		74 (56)	43 (27)	22 (15)
HANKS et al. (1991)			104[a]	87 (96)	63 (86)	
HARISIASDIS et al. (1978)		25		87		
	13			88		
KURUP et al. (1984)	24			(95)		
		65			(76)	
PEREZ et al. (1993b)	48			85 (78)	70 (60)	
		252		82 (76)	65 (56)	
RANGALA et al. (1982)	10			100 (56)		
		25		90 (59)		
ROSEN et al. (1984)	25			96 (84)	80 (68)	
		85		77 (68)	43 (60)	
ROUNSAVILLE et al. (1987)	37			81 (82)	67 (69)	
		50		84 (71)	53 (52)	
SAGERMAN et al. (1989)	34			91 (77)		
		100			86 (72)	
SHIPLEY et al. (1988)	307[b]			85 (85)	66 (70)	50
VAN DER WERF-MESSING et al. (1984)		24		78 (61)	78 (61)	
ZAGARS et al. (1993)	104			74 (92)	68 (72)	
		168		93 (82)	70 (59)	
ZIETMAN et al. (1993b)		164		94 (92)	66 (70)	(52)

Open numbers, overall survival; *numbers in parentheses*, disease-free survival
[a] Surgically staged patients
[b] Includes T2a tumors

prognostic factor only in stage C tumors with moderate or poor differentiation (PILEPICH et al. 1987d).

At our institution, patients with stage A2 and B (T1b,c and T2) well-differentiated (Gleason score of 4 or less) or moderately differentiated (Gleason score of 5–7) carcinoma had 10-year survival rates of 72% and 60%, respectively, in contrast to 38% for patients with poorly differentiated lesions (Gleason score of 8–10) ($P \leq 0.01$) (Fig. 15.3a). In patients with clinical stage C (T3) tumors, the corresponding values were 65%, 40%, and 24% ($P \leq 0.01$) (Fig. 15.3b). In patients with stage A2 and B (T1b,c and T2) disease, the 10-year disease-free survival rates were equivalent (60%) whether diagnosis was made by needle biopsy or transurethral resection of the prostate (TURP) (Fig. 15.4a). However, among stage C (T3) patients, those diagnosed with needle biopsy had a 48% 10-year disease-free survival rate compared with 30% if diagnosis was by TURP ($P \leq 0.01$) (Fig. 15.4b).

Contrary to other reports, in our analysis race had no significant impact on disease-free survival rates in the various stages (Fig. 15.5). Patient age at diagnosis had a negative impact in patients with stage A2 and B disease; those younger than 60 years of age had a 40% 10-year survival rate compared with 55%–65% for older patients ($P = 0.04$). Among patients with clinical stage C2 (T3b) disease (involvement of the seminal vesicles), those younger than 60 years of age exhibited a 10-year disease-free survival rate of 25% compared with 40%–55% in older patients ($P \leq 0.01$) (Fig. 15.6). Multivariate analysis of the 963 patients treated at our institution shows that clinical stage, histologic grade of the tumor, age younger than 60 years, and performance of TURP (in patients with

Table 15.2. Survival with external beam irradiation: stage C (T3) carcinoma of the prostate (modified from PEREZ 1992)

Study	No. of patients	Survival (%)		
		5-year	10-year	15-year
ARISTIZABAL et al. (1984)	82	60	–	–
BAGSHAW et al. (1990)	385	68 (70)	38 (50)	20 (35)
DEL REGATO et al. (1993)	372	66 (77)	38 (63)	17 (50)
FORMAN et al. (1986)	125	(45)	–	–
HANKS (1993)	296	56 (38)	32 (26)	23 (17)
	228	65	–	
HANKS (1993)	197	66 (45)	33 (14)	
HANKS et al. (1988a)	503	70	38	
HARISIASDIS et al. (1978)	112	58	35	–
NEGLIA et al. (1977)	97 (C1)	72	–	–
	53 (C2)	59	–	–
PEREZ et al. (1993b)	412	65 (58)	42 (38)	–
RANGALA et al. (1982)	93	78 (69)	–	–
ROSEN et al. (1984)	88	61 (53)	35 (35)	–
ROUNSAVILLE et al. (1987)	140 (C1)	63 (67)	42 (44)	
	12 (C2)	32 (0)	11 (0)	
VAN DER WERF-MESSING et al. (1984)	247	62 (52)	61 (25)	
ZAGARS et al. (1993)	602	72 (59)	47 (44)	27 (30)

Open numbers, overall survival; *numbers in parentheses*, disease-free survival

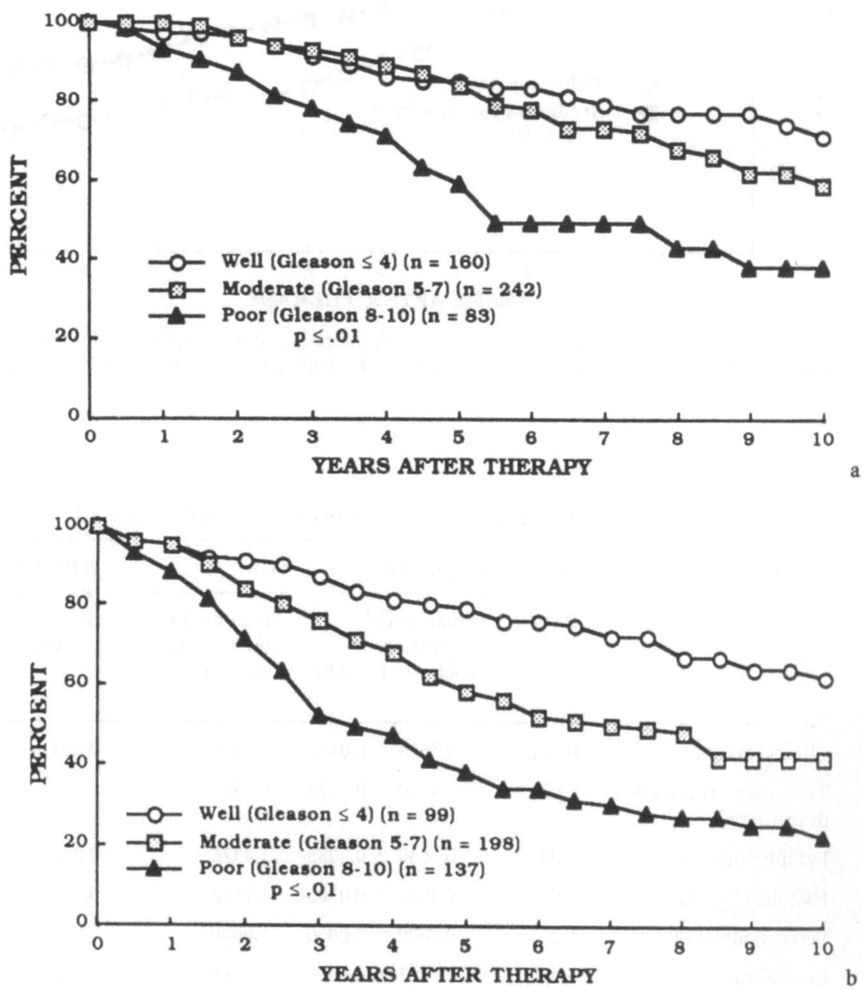

Fig. 15.3a,b. Disease-free survival correlated with histologic grade for patients with **(a)** stage A2–B (T1b,c and T2) and **(b)** stage C (T3) carcinoma of the prostate in patients treated at the Mallinckrodt Institute of Radiology

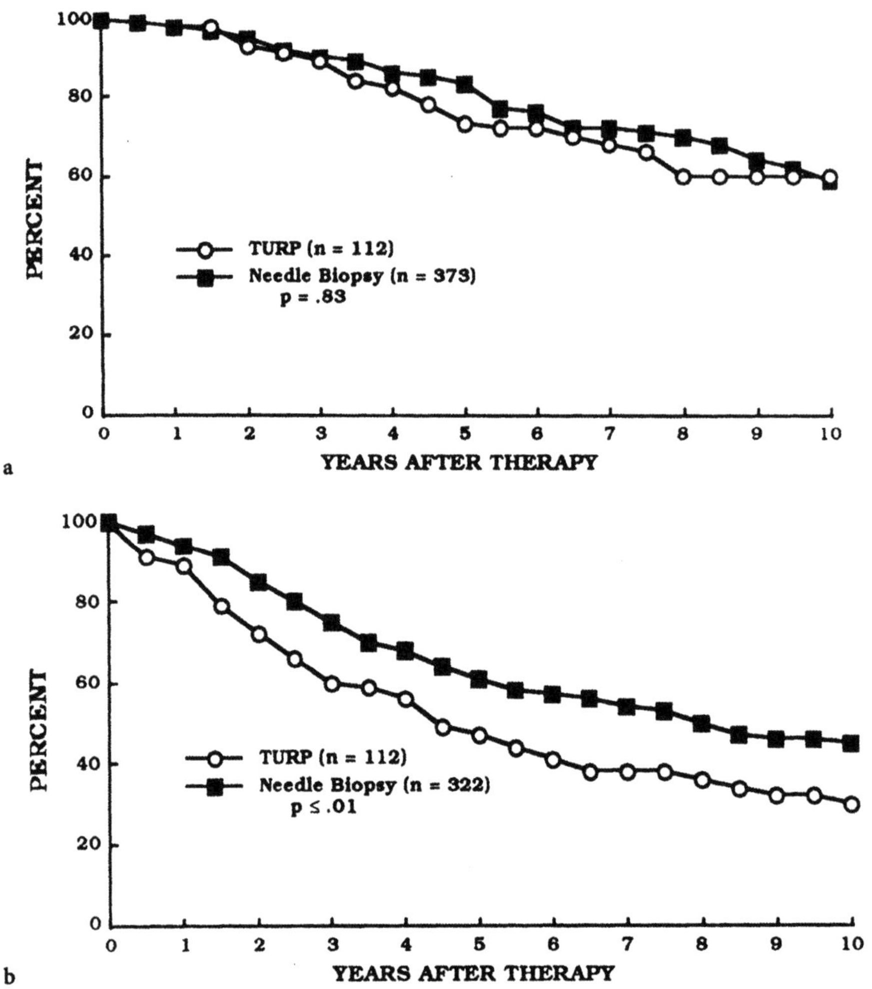

Fig. 15.4a,b. Disease-free survival correlated with method of diagnosis for patients with (**a**) stage A2–B (T1b,c and T2) and (**b**) stage C (T3) carcinoma of the prostate treated at the Mallinckrodt Institute of Radiology

Table 15.3. Carcinoma of the prostate: multivariate analysis disease-free survival

Variable	Total patient population (n = 963)			Patients with preradiation therapy PSA (n = 299)		
	P value	Final model regression coefficient (±SE)	Exponent of the regression coefficient	*P* value	Final model regression coefficient (±SE)	Exponent of the regression coefficient
Clinical stage	0.001	0.3654 ± 0.0452	1.4410	0.063	0.0056 ± 0.0078	1.056
Transurethral resection of prostate	0.001	−0.4169 ± 0.1178	0.6591			
Lymph node status	0.043	0.3630 ± 0.2085	1.4376	0.094	−0.0005 ± 0.0003	0.9995
Histologic grade	0.001	0.1962 ± 0.0383	1.2168	0.165	0.2977 ± 0.1749	1.3468
Pelvic node dose	0.221	0.0000 ± 0.0000	1.0000			
Central axis dose	0.453	0.0001 ± 0.0001	0.9999	0.702	0.9996 ± 0.0019	1.0006
PSA value				0.531	0.0056 ± 0.0078	1.0056

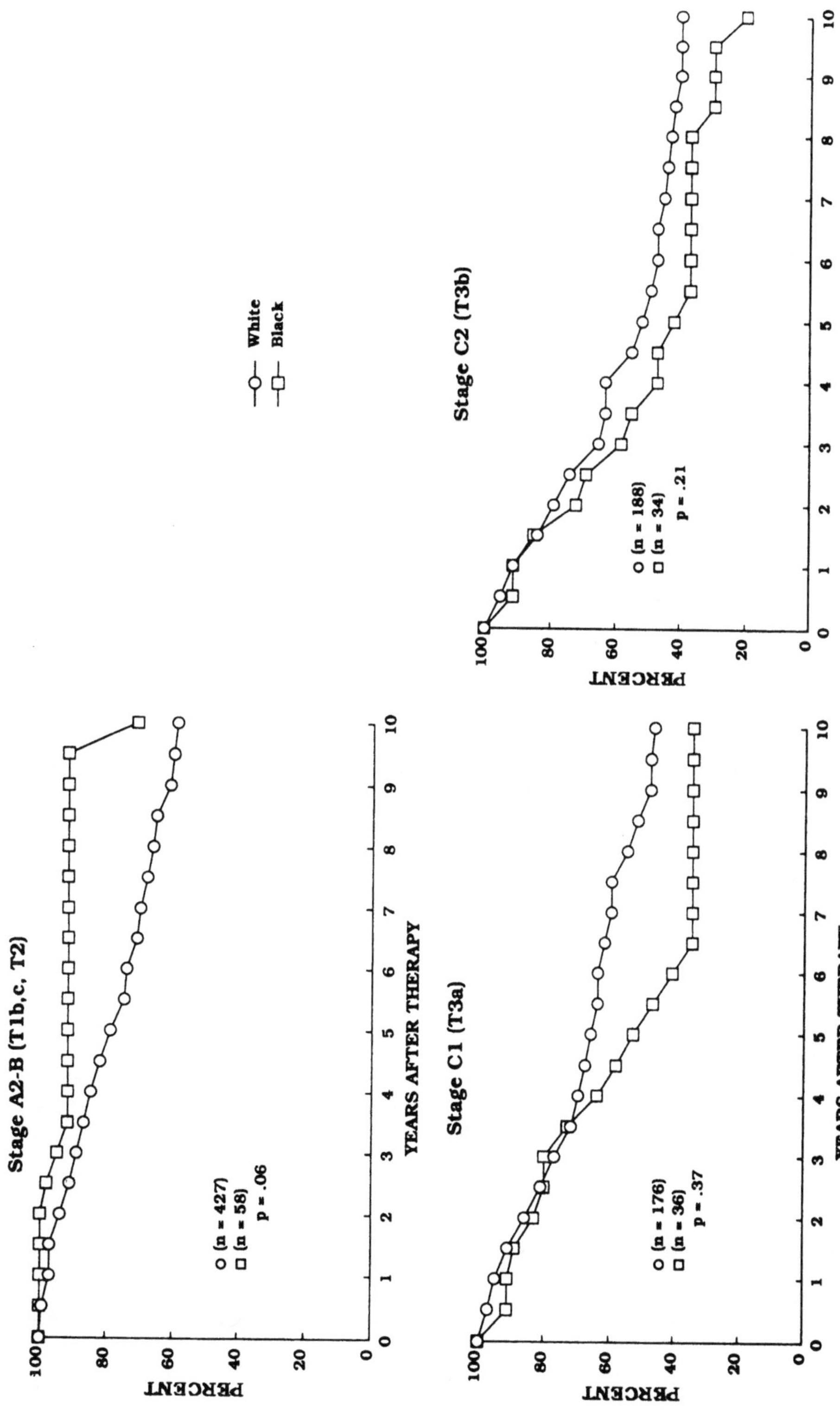

Fig. 15.5. Disease-free survival correlated with race in patients with carcinoma of the prostate treated at the Mallinckrodt Institute of Radiology

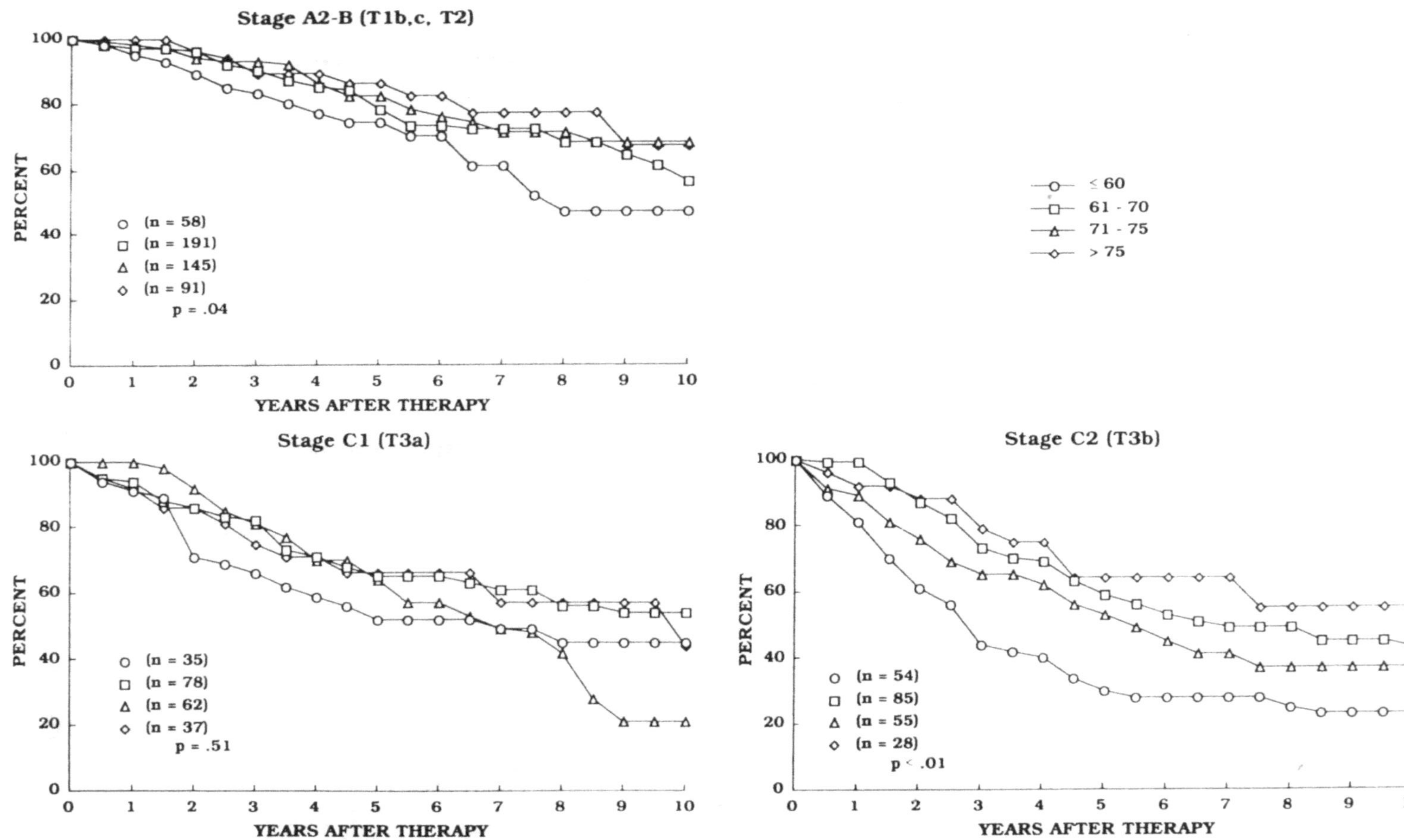

Fig. 15.6. Disease-free survival correlated with age at diagnosis in patients with carcinoma of the prostate treated at the Mallinckrodt Institute of Radiology

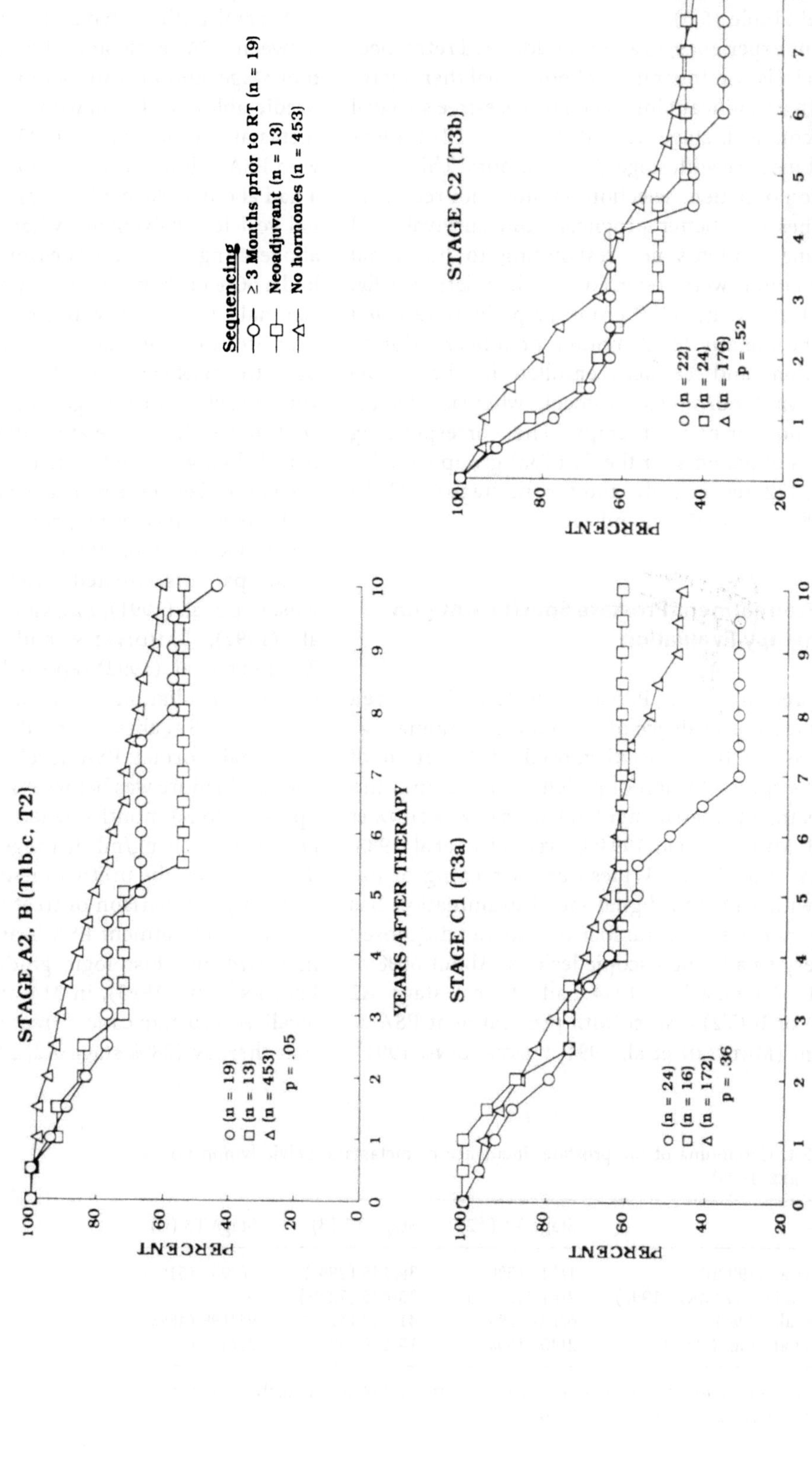

Fig. 15.7. Disease-free survival correlated with hormonal therapy in patients with carcinoma of the prostate treated at the Mallinckrodt Institute of Radiology

stage C tumors) strongly correlate with disease-free survival. A separate analysis of the subpopulation of 299 patients in whom pretreatment prostate specific antigen (PSA) levels were available documents a strong correlation of this parameter with disease-free survival (Table 15.3).

In our experience, in a nonrandomized retrospective analysis administration of hormonal therapy resulted in a significant impact on disease-free survival in patients with stage A2 and B (T1b,c, T2) tumors but not in those with stage T3 (C) tumors. This was a reflection of patient selection, as those not receiving hormones had better prognosis and survival, and sometimes patients not responding to hormonal manipulation were referred for irradiation (Fig. 15.7). In the stage A2–B group 19 patients received hormone therapy for 3 months or longer prior to irradiation, and 13 were enrolled in the RTOG neoadjuvant hormonal protocol, whereas 453 received no hormonal therapy. The corresponding numbers of patients for the C1 (T3a) group were 24, 16, and 172, respectively, and for the stage C2 (T3b) group they were 22, 24, and 176.

15.5 Pretreatment Prostate Specific Antigen and Therapy Evaluation

The increasing use of PSA has substantially altered the apparent prevalence of prostatic carcinoma, age at which the tumor is diagnosed, distribution of clinical stages, selection of patients for therapy, and posttreatment assessment of outcome (CATALONA et al. 1991; METTLIN et al. 1994; OESTERLING et al. 1988; STAMEY et al. 1987). Widespread screening of patients with PSA and digital rectal examination has greatly increased the number of patients diagnosed with very small, microscopic lesions. About 60% of patients diagnosed in 1994 had clinical stage A2 (T1b,c) or B (T2) disease with pretreatment PSA $\leq$ 10 ng/ml (METTLIN et al. 1994; OESTERLING 1991). Table 15.4 contrasts the low incidence of positive nodes in patients with stage T2 tumors diagnosed by PSA determinations with the incidence in patients in RTOG protocols who were surgically or radiographically staged without PSA assessment (PEREZ 1995).

Several authors have shown a close correlation between PSA levels and clinical and pathologic tumor stage, and in conjunction with Gleason score, a predictable correlation with incidence of lymph node metastasis. PARTIN et al. (1993a) noted that patients with PSA below 2.8 ng/ml and a Gleason score below 4 had about a 1% incidence of nodal disease or seminal vesicle involvement, whereas patients with PSA above 40 ng/ml and a Gleason score higher than 8 had a 60% probability of lymph node metastasis and seminal vesicle involvement at the time of prostatectomy. Similar findings have been described by BLUESTEIN et al. (1994). Although PSA levels vary within each clinical stage and overlap in some adjacent stages, they correlate with tumor volume (number of clonogenic cells). In an effort to integrate PSA levels and size of the prostate gland, the PSA index or PSA density has been proposed (ANDRIOLE et al. 1992; BENSON et al. 1992).

In patients treated with radiation therapy, RUSSELL et al. (1991), ZAGARS et al. (1991), FIJUTH et al. (1992), LANDMANN and HUNIG (1989), and ZENTNER et al. (1992) reported worse outcome after external irradiation in patients with elevated pretreatment PSA, above normal levels. In patients with an initial normal PSA level, the probability of a chemical failure was below 5% with a median follow-up of up to 30 months, whereas with an initial PSA greater than 10 ng/ml, it ranged from 20% to 90%, depending on the pretreatment PSA level.

In any comparison of treatment series, stratification for pretreatment PSA is as important as for tumor size and histologic grade. ZAGARS and VON ESCHENBACH (1993), in 314 patients with clinically localized prostate cancer treated by definitive radiation therapy (28% stage A2, 34% stage B, and 38%

Table 15.4. Carcinoma of the prostate: incidence of metastatic pelvic lymph nodes (from PEREZ, 1995)

Authors	Stage T1 (A2)	Stage T2 (B)	Stage T3 (C)
HANKS et al. (1992b)	1/21 (5%)	38/135 (28%)	48/95 (51%)
PETROS and CATALONA (1992)	2/61 (3.3%)	33/425 (7.8%)	0
SANDS et al. (1994)	6/127 (5%)	41/243 (17%)	95/199 (48%)
VAN POPPEL et al. (1994)	2/40 (5%)	18/199 (9%)	25/46 (54%)

HANKS et al.'s patients were treated before pretreatment PSA was available; patients in other series were diagnosed with PSA determinations stage C), reported that the 4-year risk of chemical failure was closely related to the initial PSA level: 5%, <4 ng/ml; 20%, 4 to <10 ng/ml; 60%, 10 to 30 ng/ml; and 80%, >30 ng/ml.

"Gold standard" PSA values after irradiation have not been established (RUSSELL and BOILEAU 1993). Because the prostate gland remains in place and it is possible that some nonclonogenic cells may continue to produce PSA, it is not expected that values will decline to postprostatectomy levels (less than 0.3 ng/ml) in many patients. The "normal" postirradiation PSA may be defined as that value associated with long-term disease-free survival (RUSSELL and BOILEAU 1993); ZAGARS et al. (1991) observed a median of 1.2 ng/ml (normal 0–4 ng/ml), and RITTER et al. (1992) a mean value of 1.1 ng/ml (normal 0–3.2 ng/ml). KAPLAN et al. (1990, 1991) described mathematical methods for estimating disease recurrence in patients treated with radiation therapy based on the absolute value, rates of decline posttreatment, and subsequent rise of PSA. In a report of 179 patients by CHAUVET et al. (1994), patients with normal PSA values at 6 months after irradiation had a greater probability of chemical disease-free survival (84%) than patients with higher PSA values (60%).

External irradiation can produce sustained, long-term "chemical cures" (sustained low PSA) as demonstrated by HANKS et al. (1994) in a group of 28 long-term survivors (9–13 years) in two RTOG protocols. In this analysis, 15 of 17 patients with PSA values available had levels less than 3.5 ng/ml and 11, levels less than 1.5 ng/ml. The results are similar to those reported with radical prostatectomy. HANKS et al. (1992a) reported a correlation of PSA rise doubling time and clinical behavior, including outcome with radiation therapy.

The chemical failure precedes a clinical recurrence by several years; even among patients with an initial PSA of 4–30 ng/ml, 80% were clinically tumor free 4 years after treatment. Others have reported a shorter lead time from rising PSA to clinical evidence of relapse (approximately 6 months on the average) (KAPLAN et al. 1993; RITTER et al. 1992). Patients with elevated pretreatment PSA levels, stable posttreatment levels, and subsequent elevation have a 33%–44% risk of subsequent distant metastasis in less than 3 years (KAPLAN et al. 1990).

Chemical disease-free survival in 299 patients treated at the Mallinckrodt Institute of Radiology (minimum follow-up of 18 months and mean of 2.3 years) is shown in Fig. 15.8. Patients are considered chemically free of disease if the posttreatment PSA level is less than 2 ng/ml, in any of the posttreatment determinations. This value is somewhat higher than that reported by WILLETT et al. (1994) in 36 patients

Table 15.5. Comparison of reported clinical or chemical disease-free survival after definitive external irradiation (from PEREZ, 1995)

Study	No. of patients	Clinical DFS (%)	Chemical DFS according to initial PSA level (%)				Follow-up
			≤4	4.1–10	10.1–20	20.1–≥40	
FIJUTH et al. (1992)	146			100	60		28 mo median
PEREZ et al., unpublished data	317	87		92	83	61	3.6 yr median
PISANSKY et al. (1993)	241	90		91	60		2 yr median
ZAGARS and VON ESCHENBACH (1993)	314	88[a]	95		85	63	1.5 yr median
ZIETMAN et al. (1994)	161	90		83	35	10	4 yr actuarial
HANKS et al., unpublished data							
T1	15				84[b]		5 yr actuarial
T2	96				55[b]		
T3	65				41[b]		

PSA, Prostate specific antigen; DFS, disease-free survival
[a] Approximate, for all stages (A2, B, and C)
[b] Initial PSA levels unknown

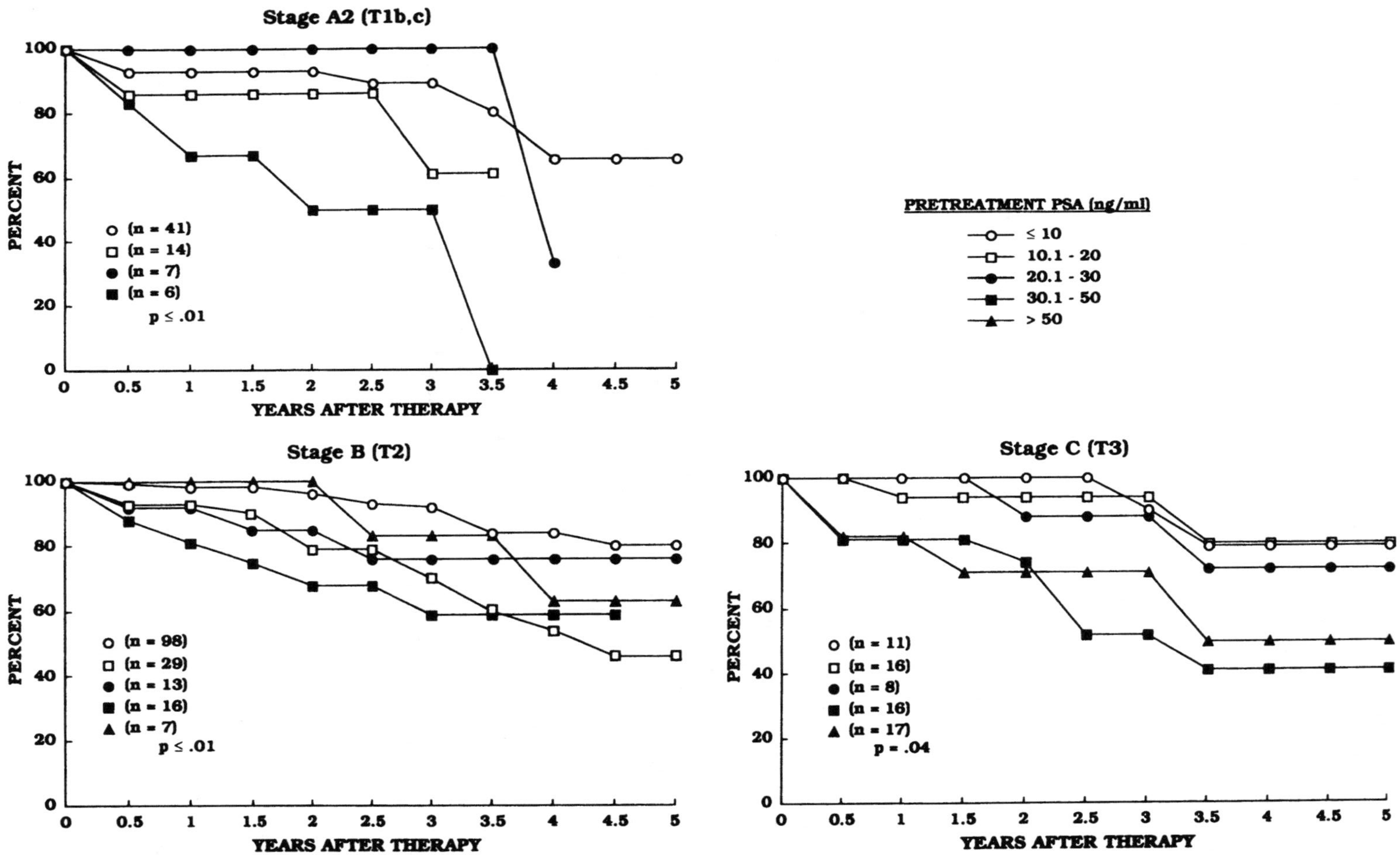

Fig. 15.8. Disease-free survival correlated with initial PSA level in patients with carcinoma of the prostate treated at the Mallinckrodt Institute of Radiology

treated for pelvic malignancies without carcinoma of the prostate, in whom the median PSA level was 0.65 ng/ml (Tandem R, Hybretech assay); 70% of the patients had PSA levels of 1 ng/ml or less, and 80% had 1.5 ng/ml or lower. A greater decrease in PSA level was observed in 27 patients irradiated for prostate cancer (median, 0.5 ng/ml).

For patients with clinical stage A2 and B (T1b,c and T2) tumors and pretreatment PSA levels of ≤10 ng/ml, 5-year actuarial chemical disease-free survival was 60%–70%, in contrast to 40%–50% with higher PSA levels. For stage C patients with PSA levels of ≤10 ng/ml, the 5-year survival was 75%–80%, and with higher PSA levels, 40%–45%. These results are comparable to those reported by Partin et al. (1993b), Stein et al. (1992), and Zietman et al. (1993a) in patients treated with radical prostatectomy.

Table 15.5 summarizes results published by several authors on chemical failure-free survival after irradiation according to initial PSA level.

15.6 Time/Dose

In an analysis of 780 patients treated with radiation therapy (65 Gy minimal tumor dose) and no endocrine therapy, Lai et al. (1991) observed no significant impact of overall treatment time (less than 7 weeks, 8–9 weeks, or greater than 9 weeks) on the outcome of definitive irradiation. They hypothesized that prostatic carcinoma behaves as late-reacting tissue in which little, if any, accelerated repopulation of clonogenic tumor cells occurs during the later half of a protracted course of irradiation. In contrast, Amdur et al. (1990), in an analysis of 167 patients in which 10% of the patients received split-course irradiation (doses of 65 Gy or higher), noted lower local tumor control in patients with stage B2, C1, or C2 prostatic carcinoma treated in periods longer than 8 weeks. In their view, the data suggest tumor repopulation during excessively protracted treatment. Thus, additional studies are needed to better define the possible role of time–dose factors in irradiation of carcinoma of the prostate. Fowler and Ritter (1995) recently reviewed the rationale for fractionated irradiation in carcinoma of the prostate, taking into consideration the slow growth rate of the tumor. The authors stated that in the absence of tumor kinetic measurements, we might consider low-grade tumors for prolonged fractionation schedules, whereas high-grade tumors would be more suitable for 1.2 Gy b.i.d. with no prolongation, or for dose escalation using conventional fraction doses and conformal radiation therapy.

15.7 Morbidity of External Beam Irradiation

As reported by Lawton et al. (1991) and Perez et al. (1994a), the incidence of fatal complications in localized carcinoma of the prostate treated with external irradiation is about 0.2%, demonstrating the low risk of this therapy. The overall incidence of severe urinary or rectosigmoid sequelae is approximately 3% and that of moderate sequelae, 7%–10% (Bagshaw et al. 1990; Hanks et al. 1985; Lawton et al. 1991; Perez et al. 1994a; Pilepich et al. 1987a,c; Shipley et al. 1988). The most frequent urinary sequelae are urethral stricture and cystitis with intermittent hematuria (3%–6%). Bladder fistula, hemorrhagic cystitis, or ureteral stricture occurs in fewer than 0.5% of patients. A higher incidence of urethral stricture (about 5%) has been described in patients irradiated after TURP versus 3% in patients without such a history. Some degree of urinary incontinence, in some cases related to stress, is noted in about 2% of patients, more frequently after TURP. The incidence of severe anal or rectal injury requiring colostomy is less than 1%; Perez et al. (1994a) reported one rectovesical and one vesicosigmoid fistula in 738 patients (0.27%), and Lawton et al. (1991) recorded 11 (1%) grade 4 and 5 rectal injuries in 1020 patients. The incidence of proctitis or rectal ulcer causing bleeding is approximately 5%; occasionally a perianal abscess or anal stricture is noted.

Perez et al. (1993a) initially described a 10% actuarial incidence of grade 2 rectosigmoid sequelae at 10 years in patients treated to the pelvic lymph nodes and the prostate compared with 4% in patients treated to the prostate volume only. An updated analysis showed that in patients with clinical stage A2 and B tumors, the urinary and rectosigmoid morbidity was similar with pelvic and prostate or prostatic bed only irradiation. In stage C patients only, rectosigmoid grade 2 morbidity was greater (10%) when the pelvic lymph nodes were irradiated to doses of 50–55 Gy (Fig. 15.9).

Mameghan et al. (1990) noted a significantly increased risk of complications with larger irradiated volumes (14% for prostate only, 24% for true pelvis, and 38% for whole pelvis) in 218 patients treated with 10-MV photons for carcinoma of the prostate; only 1.8% of the sequelae were grade 3 or 4. They observed no significant correlation between the total dose of irradiation and the incidence of morbidity.

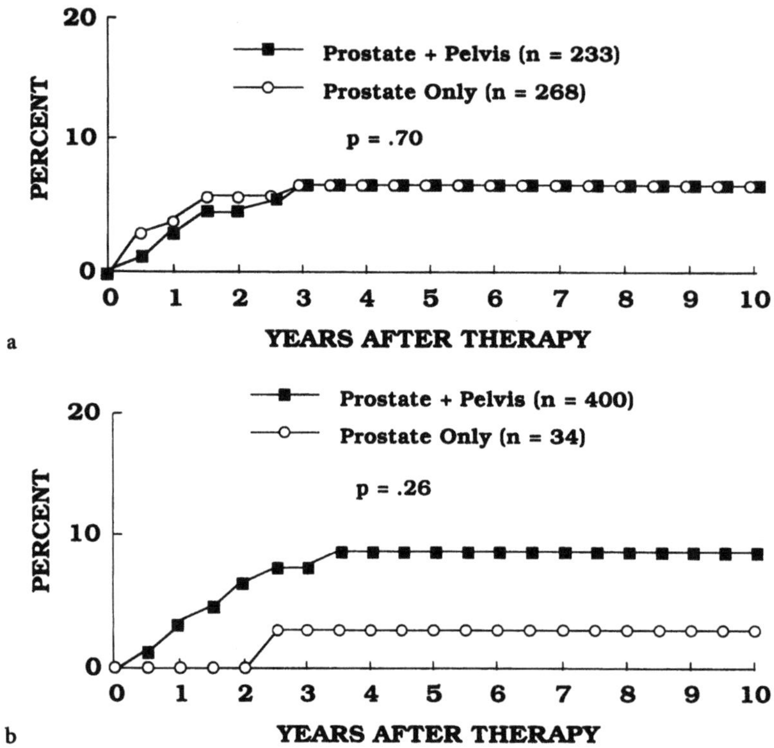

Fig. 15.9a,b. Incidence of grade 2 recto-sigmoid sequelae correlated with irradiation to the pelvis and prostate or to the prostate only. (**a**) Stages A and B (T1a,b,c, T2). (**b**) Stage C (T3). (From PEREZ et al., to be published)

However, the integral dose significantly correlated with the incidence of complications.

ROSEN et al. (1985) reported, in 229 patients treated with definitive irradiation, an incidence of urinary or bowel complications similar to ours. The authors described a higher incidence of significant complications with fields larger than 150 cm^2 (8.7% vs 1.6%). For fields 150 cm^2 or smaller, treatment with bilateral arcs was associated with a lower complication rate than with opposed anterior-posterior or other rotational field.

PILEPICH et al. (1987a) noted no increase in the incidence of proctitis or other late rectal injuries with doses up to 70 Gy. Similar lack of correlation was reported by PEREZ et al. (1994a) in 738 patients (Fig. 15.10). On the other hand, SMIT et al. (1990) described a 2-year 22% actuarial incidence of moderate or severe proctitis in patients receiving less than 70 Gy to the anterior rectal wall, 20% with 70–75 Gy, and 60% with doses higher than 75 Gy. HANKS et al. (1985) and LAWTON et al. (1991) also observed a significantly increased incidence of grade 3, 4, and 5 urinary toxicity in patients receiving more than 70 Gy (7% vs 35% with lower doses) ($P = 0.03$). These findings are highly relevant in light of recent attempts to increase the dose of irradiation delivered to the prostate using three-dimensional treatment planning and conformal delivery techniques.

Leg, scrotal, or penile edema is extremely rare in patients treated with irradiation alone (less than 1%), but its incidence ranges from 10% to 3% in patients undergoing lymph node dissection, depending on the extent of this procedure (PILEPICH et al. 1987a). Erectile dysfunction, a significant treatment sequela affecting quality of life, particularly in younger men, has been described in 14%–50% of patients, depending on patient age and techniques of irradiation. However, prospective, well-documented quantitative assessment of this sequela is lacking (ZINREICH et al. 1990).

Morbidity in 963 patients treated at our institution is shown in Table 15.6.

15.8 New Approaches to External Beam Irradiation (Three-Dimensional Treatment Planning and Conformal Therapy)

The concept of "conformal irradiation" was introduced by BUSSE (1956) and FRIEDMAN et al. (1955) in the 1950s and PROIMOS (1960) and TAKAHASHI et al. (1961) in the early 1960s. With the advent of three-dimensional (3-D) treatment planning and conformal radiation therapy, it is feasible to deliver higher tumor doses to selected (conformed) target volumes while relatively sparing adjacent normal tissues, thus

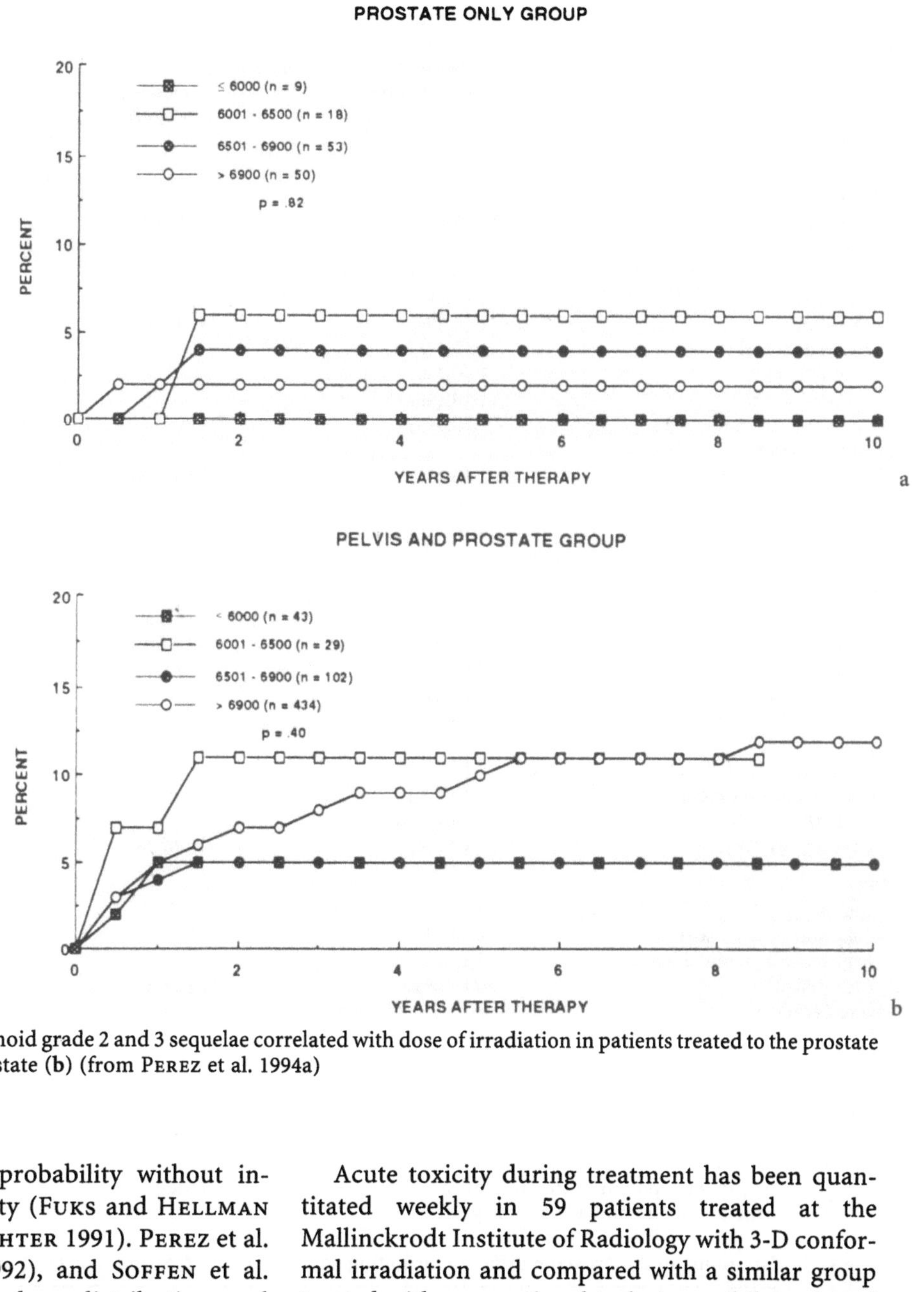

Fig. 15.10. Incidence of rectosigmoid grade 2 and 3 sequelae correlated with dose of irradiation in patients treated to the prostate only (**a**) or to the pelvis and prostate (**b**) (from PEREZ et al. 1994a)

improving tumor control probability without increasing treatment morbidity (FUKS and HELLMAN 1993; LEIBEL et al. 1991; LICHTER 1991). PEREZ et al. (1995), SANDLER et al. (1992), and SOFFEN et al. (1991) reported improved dose distribution and smaller volumes of rectum and bladder receiving higher doses with conformal than with conventional techniques in the treatment of prostate cancer.

SOFFEN et al. (1992) described fewer acute urinary and rectal sequelae (27%) in 26 patients treated using 3-D treatment planning and conformal therapy than in 20 patients irradiated with conventional techniques (55%). HANKS et al. (1995) reported a 34% incidence of grade 2 morbidity in 247 patients treated with conformal therapy for prostate cancer in comparison with 57% in 162 patients treated with standard treatment.

Acute toxicity during treatment has been quantitated weekly in 59 patients treated at the Mallinckrodt Institute of Radiology with 3-D conformal irradiation and compared with a similar group treated with conventional techniques (bilateral 120° arc rotation). Urinary symptoms (difficulty urinating) were reported as minimal by 15%–20% of patients and moderate by 12%–15% of patients with standard therapy in contrast to 3%–8% of patients treated with conformal therapy (Table 15.7). Moderate dysuria and nocturia were reported by 25%–35% of patients treated with standard technique and a similar number in the conformal therapy group.

Moderate diarrhea was noted in 11%–22% of patients in the standard therapy group, depending on the week in which it was evaluated, in contrast to 5%–12% of the conformal therapy patients (Table

Table 15.6. Carcinoma of the prostate (1967–1992): sequelae correlated with pelvic node irradiation (from PEREZ et al., to be published)

	Prostate and pelvis (n = 658)	Prostate only (n = 305)
Rectosigmoid and small bowel		
Moderate (grade 2)		
Proctitis	39 (6%)	13 (4%)
Enteritis	9 (1%)	
Rectal fibrosis	2 (0.3%)	
Anal stricture	2 (0.3%)	
Rectal ulcer	1 (0.1%)	3 (1%)
Rectal stricture	1 (0.1%)	
Anal fissure	1 (0.1%)	
Perianal abscess	1 (0.1%)	
Anorectal telangiectasia	1 (0.1%)	
Severe (grade 3)		
Perianal abscess	1 (0.1%)	1 (0.3%)
Proctitis	1 (0.1%)	
Small bowel obstruction	3 (0.5%)	
Urinary		
Moderate (grade 2)		
Urethral stricture	22 (3%)	4 (1%)
Hematuria	4 (0.6%)	1 (0.3%)
Cystitis	7 (1%)	4 (1%)
Urinary incontinence	4 (0.6%)	1 (0.3%)
Ureteral stricture	1 (0.1%)	
Severe (grade 3)		
Vesicosigmoid fistula[a]	1 (0.1%)	
Rectovesical fistula	1 (0.1%)	
Cystitis	1 (0.1%)	
Ureteral stricture	2 (0.3%)	1 (0.3%)
Other		
Moderate (grade 2)		
Subcutaneous fibrosis	2 (0.3%)	
Leg, scrotal, penile edema	9 (1%)	
Impotence[b]	66 (18%)	19 (16%)
Severe (grade 3)		
Pubic bone necrosis	1 (0.1%)	
Pelvic soft tissue necrosis	1 (0.1%)	
Fatal (grade 4)		
Radiation-induced ileitis[c]	1 (0.1%)	

[a] Sigmoid diverticulitis
[b] Only patients who were potent at the time of radiation therapy were included
[c] History of aortic aneurysm and aorta-iliac graft

Table 15.7. Carcinoma of the prostate: difficulty urinating correlated with treatment technique

Grade	Week							
	1	2	3	4	5	6	7	8
Standard therapy (bilateral arcs)								
None	39 (95)	37 (90)	33 (80)	30 (77)	28 (74)	23 (74)	9 (69)	8 (61)
Minimal	2 (5)	2 (5)	4 (10)	6 (15)	7 (18)	5 (16)	1 (8)	2 (15)
Moderate	0	2 (5)	4 (10)	3 (8)	3 (8)	3 (10)	3 (23)	3 (23)
Total	41	41	41	39	38	31	13	13
3-D conformal therapy								
None	40 (98)	32 (78)	29 (73)	27 (69)	24 (67)	17 (68)	3 (50)	1 (17)
Minimal	1 (2)	9 (22)	10 (25)	11 (28)	9 (25)	7 (28)	3 (50)	3 (50)
Moderate	0	0	1 (2)	1 (3)	3 (8)	1 (4)	0	2 (33)
Total	41	41	40	39	36	25	6	6

Numbers in parentheses indicate percent

Table 15.8. Carcinoma of the prostate: incidence of diarrhea correlated with treatment technique

Grade	Week 1	2	3	4	5	6	7	8
Standard therapy (bilateral arcs)								
None	38 (93)	24 (58)	18 (44)	12 (30)	11 (29)	19 (50)	13 (42)	4 (31)
Minimal	3 (7)	13 (32)	20 (49)	19 (48)	20 (53)	17 (45)	13 (42)	7 (54)
Moderate	0	4 (10)	3 (7)	9 (22)	7 (18)	2 (5)	5 (16)	1 (8)
Severe	0	0	0	0	0	0	0	1 (8)
Total	41	41	41	40	38	38	31	13
3-D conformal therapy								
None	31 (76)	21 (51)	14 (34)	16 (39)	16 (40)	16 (43)	12 (46)	4 (67)
Minimal	7 (17)	16 (39)	22 (54)	23 (56)	21 (53)	18 (49)	12 (46)	2 (33)
Moderate	2 (5)	4 (10)	5 (12)	1 (2)	2 (5)	2 (5)	2 (8)	0
Severe	1 (2)	0	0	1 (2)	1 (3)	1 (3)	0	0
Total	41	41	41	41	40	37	26	6

Numbers in parentheses indicate percent

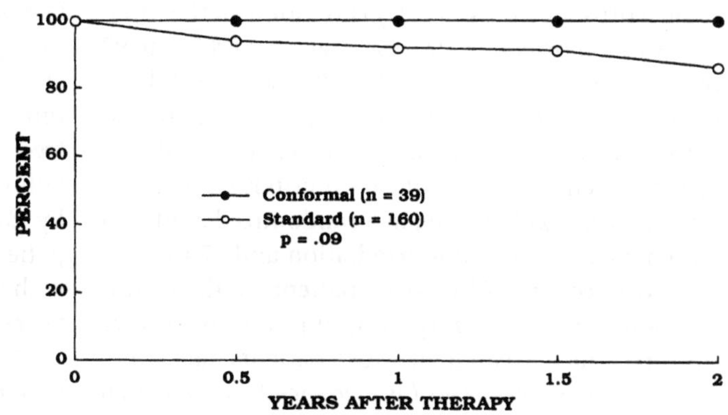

Fig. 15.11. Chemical disease-free survival correlated with treatment technique; initial PSA ≤ 20 ng/ml; stage A2–B (T1b,c, T2)

15.8). Moderate anorectal discomfort was observed in about 20% of patients in both groups. Rectal bleeding, usually of no clinical significance, was recorded in 4%–8% of patients in the standard therapy and 2% of those in the conformal group.

Follow-up is too short to assess local tumor control or late toxicity in our patients. At 2 years no chemical failures have been observed in 39 patients with clinical stage A2 and B (T1b,c and T2) disease in contrast with 86% chemical disease-free survival in 160 patients treated during the same period (1991–1993) with standard bilateral 120° arc rotation (Fig. 15.11). Leibel et al. (1994b) updated preliminary results on 324 patients with carcinoma of the prostate (48 with stage T1c, 39 with stage T2a, 135 with stage T2b,c, and 102 with stage C) irradiated with a 1-cm margin around the identifiable prostate gland (except at the interface with the rectum, where a 0.6 cm margin was used) on a dose-escalation protocol (64.8–66.6 Gy in 70 patients, 70.2 Gy in 102, 75.6 Gy in 57, and 81 Gy in 25 patients). Only 15% of patients had grade 2 or 3 rectal acute morbidity, and 34% exhibited urinary sequelae requiring short-term medication; only one patient (0.4%) has so far developed a severe grade 3 late complication. The overall 3-year actuarial PSA normalization rate was 97% in patients with stage T1c–T2a, 86% with T2b tumors, 60% with stage T2c tumors, and 43% with stage C tumors. Hanks et al. (unpublished data, 1993) observed, in 176 patients treated with conformal irradiation, 93% normal PSA levels 12 months after treatment in contrast to only 38% in 77 patients treated with conventional techniques ($P = 0.003$).

It should be possible to increase the dose of irradiation with 3-D treatment planning conformal therapy techniques to at least 75 Gy without a substantial increase in morbidity, but extreme caution must be exercised as we design dose-escalation studies. It must be recognized that it will be impossible to substantially spare the bladder trigone or the anterior rectal wall, since they are in close proximity to the prostate, without severely compromising adequate coverage of the target volume with a margin for position error. Nevertheless, more precise treatment planning and better immobilization techniques, such as with an alpha cradle, should decrease systematic errors in repositioning and improve dose distribution in the volume of interest.

Preliminary analysis shows that daily treatment times for 3-D conformal irradiation are somewhat longer (19 min for six fields) than with conventional techniques (10 min) if Cerrobend blocks are used to delineate the treatment portals; however, treatment time with multileaf collimation is similar to that of conventional techniques (10 min for six-field treatment) (PEREZ et al. 1995).

15.9 Comparison of Outcome with Irradiation or Radical Prostatectomy

A randomized comparison of radiation therapy and radical prostatectomy in early carcinoma of the prostate was reported by PAULSON et al. (1982) in 97 patients with clinical stage A2 or B disease. While 56 patients received radiation therapy, 41 were treated with radical prostatectomy. The authors did not specify whether any stratification criteria existed or satisfactorily explain why, in a randomized study, 59 patients were assigned to irradiation and 47 to radical prostatectomy. Also, seven patients in the irradiated and nine in the surgical group did not receive the prescribed treatment. Most patients failed because of bone metastases (as evidenced by abnormal bone scan) or other distant metastases. PAULSON (1988b) updated the results of the study; a better actuarial tumor-free survival was noted in the prostatectomy patients (76% vs 57% at 80 months). This difference did not reflect the direct effect of the local treatment and may be related to the initial distribution of the patients and tumor characteristics in the two study groups. Furthermore, serious reservations regarding the statistical analysis and validity of the data have been raised (HANKS 1988). For a more thorough discussion of the merits of this trial, the reader is referred to correspondence between HANKS (1988) and PAULSON (1988a). A prospective clinical trial to compare these two modalities was in progress, but unfortunately it was terminated because of poor patient accrual (ZIETMAN and SHIPLEY 1993). The results obtained with radiation therapy in this series are substantially inferior to those reported by other authors (PILEPICH et al. 1987b) and in the present review.

The impact of surgical staging on therapeutic outcome and the implications of comparing reported survival with radiation therapy or radical prostatectomy are illustrated in a report by HANKS et al. (1991) on 104 patients with clinical stage T1b or T2 carcinoma of the prostate who were surgically staged, had negative lymph nodes, and were treated with definitive radiation therapy. The disease-free survival rates at 5 and 10 years were 85% and 67%, respectively. The corresponding overall survival rates were 87% and 63%, respectively. The probability of clinical control of the tumor in the prostate was 96% at 5 years and 87% at 10 years. These results are similar to those obtained with radical prostatectomy (CULP 1967).

In a comparison of surgically staged patients treated with radiation therapy at Stanford University (KAPLAN et al., 1994) and a group of patients treated with prostatectomy at the Mayo Clinic (BLUTE et al. 1989) and in recent reports of patients treated surgically by STEIN et al. (1992) and ZIETMAN et al. (1993a), relapse rates were similar for radiation therapy and surgical patients. In the report by STEIN et al. (1992), of 230 patients with stage A and B tumors treated with prostatectomy, only 25% were free from chemical failure 12 years after treatment, although 60% were clinically tumor free. In a report by ZINCKE et al. (1991), of 148 surgically treated patients, 95% with clinical stage A1 but less than 40% with stage A2 had no evidence of chemical failure 15 years after surgery.

PARTIN et al. (1993b) reported on 955 patients with clinical stage T1 or T2 tumors treated with anatomic radical retropubic prostatectomy. Seven percent (66 patients) and seminal vesicle involvement, and 7.4% (71 patients) had lymph node metastases. PSA data were available for 894 patients within the first 3 years after surgery. Progression-free survival was 83% at 5 years and 70% at 10 years. With an average follow-up of 53 months, 21 patients (2.2%) had local clinical progression only, 57 patients (6%) had distant metastases with or without local recurrence, and 107 (11.2%) had postoperative serum PSA levels greater than 0.2 ng/ml. There was a close correlation between pretreatment PSA levels and chemical disease-free survival (Fig. 15.12). At 7.5 years, the actuarial chemical disease-free survival rate was 90% in patients with preoperative PSA of 4 ng/ml or less, 70% for 4.1–10 ng/ml, and 56% for 10.1–20 ng/ml. Results are similar to those observed in 299 patients treated at our institution with definitive radiation therapy.

The disease-free and cause-specific (or overall) survival reported in many radiation therapy series are comparable to those obtained with radical prostatectomy, as illustrated in Fig. 15.13.

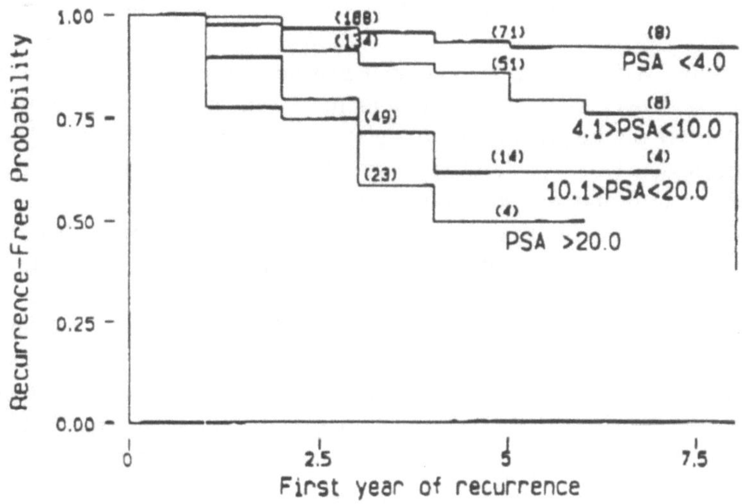

Fig. 15.12. Kaplan-Meier actuarial likelihood of PSA relapse correlated with preoperative serum PSA levels (ng/ml). *Numbers in parentheses* represent number of men in analysis at time interval. (From PARTIN et al. 1993b)

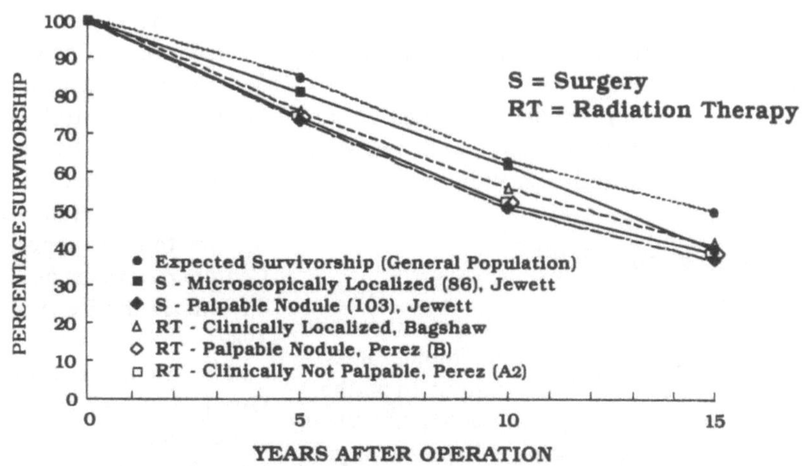

Survivorship of patients with cancer histologically localized to the prostate and of those with nonlocalized disease.

a

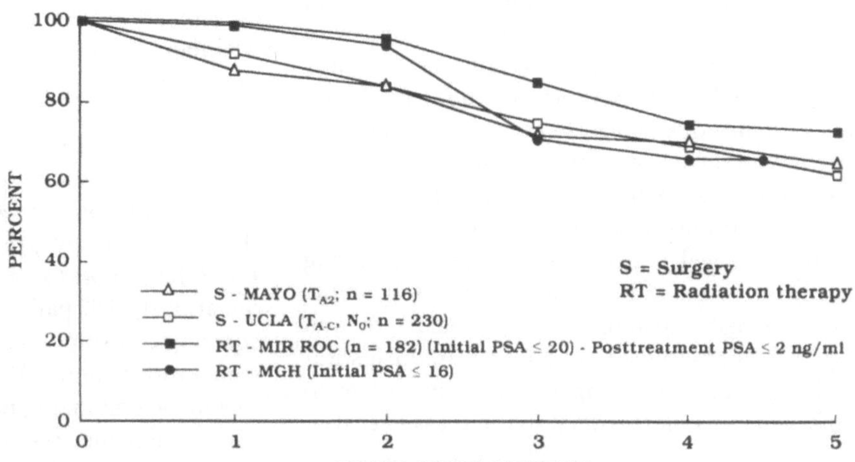

b

Fig. 15.13a,b. Comparison of survival (**a**) and chemical disease-free survival (**b**) with surgery or irradiation in patients with localized and nonlocalized prostate cancer. In this analysis, patients treated at the Mallinckrodt Institute of Radiology with posttreatment PSA of 2 ng/ml are considered disease-free. (From PEREZ, 1995)

15.10 New Directions and Future Clinical Trials

Randomized trials on locoregional prostate cancer reported over the last two decades have had little influence on the practice of urologists and radiation oncologists (Zietman and Shipley 1993). This was largely a result of flawed protocol design and evaluation of treatments that, in many cases, were outmoded by the time of reporting (perineal prostatectomy or diethylstilbestrol). Patients were usually stratified by stage and grade but not by initial PSA level or ploidy, both critical prognostic indicators. Because many patients die with, but not of, their cancer, the simple survival end points of the early trials are irrelevant to some degree. Local symptom control and quality of life issues were largely ignored. More recent phase II and III studies have avoided many of these pitfalls and, more importantly, are employing more rigorous failure criteria including prostate rebiopsies and serum PSA levels (Perez et al. 1993a).

Three areas currently under investigation are dose escalation, particle therapy, and radiation therapy combined with androgen suppression.

15.10.1 Dose-Escalation Studies

Dose escalation is possible without an increase in morbidity using 3-D conformal planning or CT-guided brachytherapy (with or without hyperthermia) (Wallner 1991) or nonconventional particle beams; randomized trials testing this potential gain are in progress.

The benefit of 3-D conformal therapy hypothetically could be linked to improved local tumor control because of better coverage of the target volume with a specific dose of irradiation, less acute and late morbidity, possibility of carrying out dose-escalation studies if morbidity is held to acceptable levels, and improved survival. Several institutions (Hanks et al. 1995; Leibel et al. 1994a; Sandler 1992), the RTOG, and nine institutions under cooperative agreement with the National Cancer Institute are conducting phase I/II dose-escalation studies. Depending on the results, the cost benefit of 3-D conformal irradiation must be further evaluated in a larger, multi-institutional protocol, comparing it with standard techniques in order to justify its initial increased cost.

15.10.2 Special Particles

An important contribution to treatment techniques is the use of special particles, such as protons and heavy ions, which provide better dose distributions and some biologic advantages and in preliminary studies have been reported to yield a high probability of tumor control with relative sparing of normal tissues (Castro et al. 1989; Griffin et al. 1989; Munzenrider et al. 1989; Suit and Urie 1992).

Neutrons have potential biologic advantages over photons in killing slowly cycling or hypoxic cells.

Laramore et al. (1993) published the final report of a RTOG clinical trial of 91 patients with stage C or D1 carcinoma of the prostate randomized to receive either conventional photon irradiation (65 Gy) or equivalent doses with mixed photon and neutron beams. Ten-year analysis showed local tumor control rates of 70% in the mixed-beam treated patients and 58% in the photon group ($P = 0.03$). The corresponding survival rates were 46% and 29%, respectively ($P = 0.04$). Distant metastases developed in 49% of the mixed-beam and 55% of the photon-treated group, consistent with other studies showing fewer distant metastases in patients with improved local tumor control. A total of seven mixed-beam and five photon-treated patients suffered significant sequelae from therapy (no statistical difference). The results with photon beam therapy in this trial are inferior to those reported at M.D. Anderson Cancer Center (Zagars et al. 1987) and Washington University and in the Patterns of Care Study (Hanks et al. 1987).

The Neutron Therapy Collaborative Working Group Trial was closed in 1990; 182 T3 or T4 pelvic node-positive patients were treated with a pelvic field (50.4 Gy in the photon arm at 1.8 Gy per fraction and 13.6 nGy at 1.7 nGy per fraction in the neutron arm). The prostate was boosted with 20 Gy and 6.8 nGy, respectively. Five-year results show a significant pathologic local tumor control advantage for neutrons (82% vs 60%), but as yet no difference in disease-free or overall survival has been observed (Russell et al., 1994). If the node-positive patients are excluded, the pathologic local tumor control is 92% for neutrons and 59% for photons. Unlike in its RTOG mixed-beam predecessor study (Russell et al. 1987), there was significant morbidity in the neutron arm; 10 of 87 patients had grade 4 morbidity (six requiring colostomy) compared with only one of 85 treated with photons. Morbidity figures such as these have made embracing neutrons for the treatment of pelvic malignancy less appealing.

Shipley et al. (1995) reported on a phase I/II study of T3 and T4 prostate cancer in which, after 50.4 Gy to the pelvis delivered through four fields, 103 patients were randomized to receive a perineal conformal field proton (160 MV) boost of 25.2 CGE (cobalt Gray equivalent), and 99 to receive a 16.8-Gy boost with photons. Median follow-up was 60 months. Among the patients completing randomization, the local relapse-free survival at 7 years was 80% for the proton and 66% for the photon group ($P = 0.14$). However, the local relapse-free survival at 7 years for 58 patients with poorly differentiated tumors was 85% with protons and 37% with photons ($P = 0.001$). The incidence of grade 1 and 2 rectal bleeding (32% vs 12%) and urethral stricture (19% vs 8%) was higher in the proton-treated patients compared with the photon-treated group. Engineering refinements should make these modalities more practical for clinical use and less expensive, thus increasing their availability to more institutions (with adequate staff and resources) to expand evaluation in the treatment of representative patient populations (SLATER et al. 1992).

15.10.3 Other Developments

Other opportunities in treatment delivery include further development and evaluation of devices and techniques for intraoperative irradiation, hyperthermia, systemic radioimmunoconjugates, and photodynamic therapy. In hyperthermia, further physics and engineering developments are required to improve delivery of heat to larger or deeper tumors so that greater application of this modality will be feasible. In brachytherapy, future directions in clinical research will include better definition of indications for high dose rate, optimization of total doses, fractionation, and doses per fraction, standardization of outcome end points, quality assurance standards, and cost-effectiveness studies. To amplify the diagnostic or therapeutic use of radioimmunoconjugates, efforts are in progress to enhance antitumor specificity and the radioactivity that will more selectively deliver the prescribed irradiation dose to the tumor.

15.10.4 External Beam Irradiation and Endocrine Therapy

Endocrine therapy in conjunction with radiation therapy has been explored as adjuvant therapy following irradiation for patients at high risk for occult metastatic disease or as neoadjuvant cytoreductive therapy in patients with bulky primary tumors to enhance likelihood of local control.

RTOG protocol 8531 evaluated adjuvant goserelin acetate (Zoladex) (3.6 mg subcutaneously every 28 days indefinitely) combined with irradiation in T3 and T4 and node-positive patients or administered on relapse after identical irradiation alone. This study accrued 977 patients; results have not been reported.

Results were recently reported for RTOG protocol 8601 (PILEPICH et al. 1995) in 456 evaluable patients with large stage T2b,c (B2, B3, B4, C, D1) disease. Patients were randomized to receive irradiation alone (45 Gy to pelvic lymph nodes and an additional 20–25 Gy, depending on stage, to the prostatic area) or a combination of the same radiation therapy and adjuvant hormonal therapy consisting of Zoladex (3.6 mg subcutaneously every 4 weeks) and Eulexin (250 mg p.o. t.i.d.), both drugs started 2 months before initiation of irradiation and continued throughout the entire course of radiation therapy. With a median observation period of 3.3 years, the 4.5-year actuarial local failure rate was 46% in the study arm and 71% in the control arm. A decreasing incidence of distant metastasis was also noted in patients receiving hormonal therapy (34% vs 41%) ($P = 0.09$). The actuarial clinical disease-free survival was 38% for the study arm and 16% for the control arm ($P < 0.001$). The corresponding chemical-free (PSA < 4 ng/ml) survival rates were 36% for the study arm and 15% for the control arm ($P < 0.001$). Overall survival differences are not statistically significant.

RTOG protocol 9202 for patients with T2b–4 disease was recently closed after accessioning more than 1000 patients. Neoadjuvant total androgen suppression (Zoladex and flutamide for 2 months) was given before irradiation in both arms of the trial; one group received 2 years of maintenance adjuvant Zoladex. End points will be freedom from PSA failure, clinical disease-free survival, and local tumor control.

The value of elective pelvic irradiation and neoadjuvant hormone therapy will be better assessed in a recently activated RTOG protocol in which patients with clinical stage T2 and T3 carcinoma of the prostate are randomized to four arms: neoadjuvant total androgen suppression (Zoladex and flutamide) or not 2 months before and during irradiation and radiation therapy to the whole pelvis (50.4 Gy, 1.8-Gy fractions) and prostate (19.8 Gy boost) or the prostate volume only (70.2 Gy).

References

Adolfsson J, Steineck G, Whitmore WF Jr (1993) Recent results of management of palpable clinical localized prostate cancer. Cancer 72:310–322

Amdur RJ, Parsons JT, Fitzgerald LT, Million RR (1990) The effect of overall treatment time on local control in patients with adenocarcinoma of the prostate treated with radiation therapy. Int J Radiat Oncol Biol Phys 19:1377–1382

Andriole GL, Telle WB, Coplen DE, Catalona WJ (1992) PSA index (PSAI) as a predictor of prostate cancer (CaP) in men with persistent serum PSA elevation (Abstract). J Urol 147 (Suppl):387A

Aristizabal SA, Steinbronn D, Heusinkveld RS (1984) External beam radiotherapy in cancer of the prostate: the University of Arizona experience. Radiother Oncol 1:309–315

Asbell SO, Krall JM, Pilepich MV et al. (1988) Elective pelvic irradiation in stage A2, B carcinoma of the prostate: analysis of RTOG 77-06. Int J Radiat Oncol Biol Phys 15:1307–1316

Asbell SO, Martz ML, Pilepich MV et al. (1989) Impact of surgical staging in evaluating the radiotherapeutic outcome in RTOG III study for A2 and B prostate carcinoma. Int J Radiat Oncol Biol Phys 17:945–951

Bagshaw MA (1984) Radiotherapeutic treatment of prostatic carcinoma with pelvic node involvement. II. Urol Clin North Am 2:297–303

Bagshaw MA, Cox RS, Ramback JE (1990) Radiation therapy for localized prostate cancer: justification by long-term follow-up. Urol Clin North Am 17:787–802

Benson MC, Whang IS, Olsson CA, McMahan DJ, Conner WH (1992) The use of prostate specific antigen density to enhance the predictive value of intermediate levels of serum prostate specific antigen. J Urol 147:817–821

Bluestein DL, Bostwick DG, Bergstralh EJ, Oesterling JE (1994) Eliminating the need for bilateral pelvic lymphadenectomy in select patients with prostate cancer. J Urol 151:1315–1320

Blute ML, Nativ O, Zinke H, Farrow GM, Therneau T, Lieber MM (1989) Pattern of failure after radical retropubic prostatectomy for clinically and pathologically localized adenocarcinoma of the prostate: influence of tumor deoxyribonucleic acid ploidy. J Urol 142:1262–1265

Brawn P, Johnson E, Kuhl DL et al. (1993) Stage at presentation and survival of white and black patients with prostate carcinoma. Cancer 71:2569–2573

Busse W (1956) Einstellung und Dosisbestimmung bei der Pendelbestrahlung der Parametrien. Strahlentherapie 101:400–404

Castro JR, Collier JM, Petti PL et al. (1989) Charged particle radiotherapy for lesions encircling the brain stem or spinal cord. Int J Radiat Oncol Biol Phys 17:477–484

Catalona WJ, Smith DS, Ratliff TL et al. (1991) Measurement of prostate-specific antigen in serum as a screening test for prostate cancer. N Engl J Med 324:1156–1161

Chauvet B, Felix-Faire C, Pupsascka N et al. (1994) Prostate-specific antigen decline: a major prognostic factor for prostate cancer treated with radiation therapy. J Clin Oncol 12:1402–1407

Chodak GW, Thisted RA, Gerber GS et al. (1994) Results of conservative management of clinically localized prostate cancer. N Engl J Med 330:242–248

Culp OS (1967) Radical perineal prostatectomy: its past, present, and possible future. J Urol 98:618–627

del Regato JA, Trailins AH, Pittman DD (1993) Twenty years follow-up of patients with inoperable cancer of the prostate (stage C) treated by radiotherapy: report of a national cooperative study. Int J Radiat Oncol Biol Phys 26:197–201

Dugan TC, Shipley WU, Young RH et al. (1991) Biopsy after external beam radiation therapy for adenocarcinoma of the prostate: correlation with original histological grade and current prostate specific antigen levels. J Urol 146:1313–1316

Fijuth J, Chauvet B, Vincent P, Felix-Faure C, Reboul F (1992) Serum prostatic-specific antigen in monitoring the response of carcinoma of the prostate to radiation therapy. Radiother Oncol 23:236–240

Fleming C, Wasson JH, Albertsen PC, Barry MJ, Wennberg JE, for the Prostate Patient Outcomes Research Team (1993) A decision analysis of alternative treatment strategies for clinically localized prostate cancer. JAMA 269:2650–2659

Forman JD, Wharam MD, Lee DJ, Zinreich ES, Order SE (1986) Definitive radiotherapy following prostatectomy: results and complications. Int J Radiat Oncol Biol Phys 12:185–189

Fowler JF, Ritter MA (1995) A rationale for fractionation for slowly proliferating tumors such as prostatic adenocarcinoma. Int J Radiat Oncol Biol Phys 32:521–529

Friedman M, Hine GJ, Dresner J (1955) Principles of supervoltage (2 million volts) rotation therapy. Radiology 64:1–16

Fuks Z, Hellman S (1993) Three-dimensional conformal radiotherapy. In: DeVita VT Jr, Hellman S, Rosenberg SA (eds) Cancer: principles and practice of oncology, 4th edn. Lippincott, Philadelphia, pp 2614–2624

Gleason DF (1988) Histologic grade, clinical stage, and patient age in prostate cancer. NCI Monogr 7:15–18

Griffin TW, Pajak TF, Maor MH et al. (1989) Mixed neutron/photon irradiation of unresectable squamous cell carcinomas of the head and neck: the final report of a randomized cooperative trial. Int J Radiat Oncol Biol Phys 17:959–965

Hanks GE (1988) More on the Uro-Oncology Research Group report of radical surgery vs. radiotherapy for adenocarcinoma of the prostate (letter). Int J Radiat Oncol Biol Phys 14:1053

Hanks GE (1993) Treatment of early stage prostate cancer: radiotherapy. In: Hellman S, DeVita V, Rosenberg S, Freeman S (eds) Important advances in oncology. Lippincott, Philadelphia

Hanks GE, Leibel SA, Krall JM, Kramer S (1985) Patterns of care studies: dose-response observations for local control of adenocarcinoma of the prostate. Int J Radiat Oncol Biol Phys 11:153–157

Hanks GE, Diamond JJ, Krall JM, Martz KL, Kramer S (1987) A ten-year follow-up of 682 patients treated for prostate cancer with radiation therapy in the United States. Int J Radiat Oncol Biol Phys 13:499–505

Hanks GE, Krall JM, Martz KL, Diamond JJ, Kramer S (1988a) The outcome of treatment of 313 patients with T-1 (UICC) prostate cancer treated with external beam irradiation. Int J Radiat Oncol Biol Phys 14:243–248

Hanks GE, Martz KL, Diamond JJ (1988b) The effect of dose on local control of prostate cancer. Int J Radiat Oncol Biol Phys 15:1299–1305

Hanks GE, Asbell S, Krall JM et al. (1991) Outcome for lymph node dissection negative T1-b, T2 (A-2,B) prostate cancer treated with external beam irradiation in RTOG 77-06. Int J Radiat Oncol Biol Phys 21:1099–1103

Hanks GE, Epstein BE, Peter R, Schultheiss TE (1992a) PSA doubling times in patients with prostate cancer, a potentially useful reflection of tumor doubling time (Abstract). Int J Radiat Oncol Biol Phys 24:150

Hanks GE, Krall JM, Pilepich MV et al. (1992b) Comparison of pathologic and clinical evaluation of lymph nodes in prostate cancer: implications of RTOG data for patient management and trial design and stratification. Int J Radiat Oncol Biol Phys 23:293–298

Hanks GE, Perez CA, Kozar M, Asbell SO, Pilepich MV, Pajak TF (1994) PSA confirmation of cure at 10 years of T1B, T2,

N0, M0 prostate cancer patients treated in RTOG protocol 7706 with external beam irradiation. Int J Radiat Oncol Biol Phys 30:289–292

Hanks GE, Schultheiss TE, Hunt MA, Epstein B (1995) Factors influencing incidence of acute grade 2 morbidity in conformal and standard radiation treatment of prostate cancer. Int J Radiat Oncol Biol Phys 31:25–29

Harisiasdis L, Veenema RJ, Senyszyn JJ et al. (1978) Carcinoma of the prostate: treatment with external radiotherapy. Cancer 41:2131–2142

Kabalin JN, Hodge KK, McNeal JE, Freiha FS, Stamey TA (1989) Identification of residual cancer in the prostate following radiation therapy: role of transrectal ultrasound guided biopsy and prostate specific antigen. J Urol 142:326–331

Kaplan ID, Prestidge BR, Cox RS, Bagshaw MA (1990) Prostate specific antigen after irradiation for prostatic carcinoma. J Urol 144:1172–1175

Kaplan ID, Cox RS, Bagshaw MA (1991) A model of prostatic carcinoma tumor kinetics based on prostate specific antigen levels after radiation therapy. Cancer 68:400–405

Kaplan ID, Prestidge BR, Bagshaw MA, Cox RS (1992) The importance of local control in the treatment of prostatic cancer. J Urol 147:917–921

Kaplan ID, Cox RS, Bagshaw MA (1993) Prostate specific antigen after external beam radiotherapy for prostatic cancer: follow-up. J Urol 149:519–522

Kaplan ID, Cox RS, Bagshaw WA (1994) Radiotherapy for prostatic cancer: patient selection and the impact of local control. Urology 43:634–639

Kavadi VS, Zagars GK, Pollack A (1994) Serum prostate-specific antigen after radiation therapy for clinically localized prostate cancer: prognostic implications. Int J Radiat Oncol Biol Phys 30:279–287

Kim JA, Kuban DA, El-Mahdi AM, Schellhammer PE (1995) Carcinoma of the prostate: race as a prognostic indicator in definitive radiation therapy. Radiology 194:545–549

Kuban DA, El-Mahdi AM, Schellhammer PF (1987) Effect of local tumor control on distant metastasis and survival in prostatic adenocarcinoma. Urology 30:420–426

Kuban DA, El-Mahdi AM, Schellhammer PF (1995) Potential benefit of improved local tumor control in patients with prostate carcinoma. Cancer 75:2373–2382

Kurup P, Kramer TS, Lee MS, Philips R (1984) External beam irradiation of prostate cancer: experience in 163 patients. Cancer 53:37–43

Lai PP, Pilepich MV, Krall JM et al. (1991) The effect of overall treatment time on the outcome of definitive radiotherapy for localized prostate carcinoma: the Radiation Therapy Oncology Group 75-06 and 77-06 experience. Int J Radiat Oncol Biol Phys 21:925–933

Landmann C, Hunig R (1989) Prostatic specific antigen as an indicator of response to radiotherapy in prostate cancer. Int J Radiat Oncol Biol Phys 17:1073–1076

Laramore GE, Krall JM, Thomas FJ (1993) Fast neutron radiotherapy for locally advanced prostate cancer: final report of a Radiation Therapy Oncology Group randomized clinical trial. Am J Clin Oncol (CCT) 16:164–167

Lawton CA, Won M, Pilepich MV et al. (1991) Long-term treatment sequelae following external beam irradiation for adenocarcinoma of the prostate: analysis of RTOG studies 7506 and 7706. Int J Radiat Oncol Biol Phys 21:935–939

Leibel SA, Ling CC, Kutcher GJ, Mohan R, Cordon-Cordo C, Fuks Z (1991) The biological basis for conformal three-dimensional radiation therapy. Int J Radiat Oncol Biol Phys 21:805–811

Leibel SA, Heimann P, Kutcher GJ et al. (1994a) Three-dimensional conformal radiation therapy in locally advanced carcinoma of the prostate: preliminary results of a phase I dose-escalation study. Int J Radiat Oncol Biol Phys 28:55–65

Leibel SA, Zeletsky MJ, Kutcher GJ, Burman CM, Kelson S, Fuks Z (1994b) Three-dimensional conformal radiation therapy in localized carcinoma of the prostate: interim report of a phase I dose escalation study. J Urol 152:1792–1798

Lichter AS (1991) Three-dimensional conformal radiation therapy: a testable hypothesis. Int J Radiat Oncol Biol Phys 21:853–855

Mameghan H, Fisher R, Mameghan J, Watt WH, Tynan A (1990) Bowel complications after radiotherapy for carcinoma of the prostate: the volume effect. Int J Radiat Oncol Biol Phys 18:315–320

McGowan DG (1981) The value of extended field radiation therapy in carcinoma of the prostate. Int J Radiat Oncol Biol Phys 7:1333–1339

Meek AG, Park TL, Oberman E, Wielopolski I (1990) A prospective study of prostate-specific antigen levels in patients receiving radiotherapy for localized carcinoma of the prostate. Int J Radiat Oncol Biol Phys 19:733–741

Mettlin C, Murphy GP, Menek H (1994) Trends in treatment of localized prostate cancer by radical prostatectomy: observations from the Commission on Cancer, National Cancer Database, 1985–1990. Urology 43:488–492

Miller BA, Gloeckler LA, Hankey BF et al. (1993) SEER Cancer Statistics Review 1983–1990. Prostate 4:1–22

Moore MJ, O'Sullivan B, Tannock IF (1988) How expert physicians would wish to be treated if they had genitourinary cancer. J Clin Oncol 6:1736–1745

Munzenrider JE, Verhey IJ, Gargouda ES et al. (1989) Conservative treatment of uveal melanoma: local recurrence after proton beam therapy. Int J Radiat Oncol Biol Phys 17:493–498

Neglia WJ, Hussey DH, Johnson DE (1977) Megavoltage radiation therapy for carcinoma of the prostate. Int J Radiat Oncol Biol Phys 2:873–882

Oesterling JE (1991) Prostate-specific antigen: a critical assessment of the most useful tumor marker for adenocarcinoma of the prostate. J Urol 145:907–923

Oesterling JE, Chan DW, Epstein JL et al. (1988) Prostate specific antigen in the preoperative and postoperative evaluation of localized prostatic cancer treated with radical prostatectomy. J Urol 139:766–772

Partin AW, Lee BR, Chan DW, Epstein AW, Walsh PC (1993a) The use of prostate specific antigen (PSA) and Gleason score to predict pathologic stage in men with localized prostate cancer. J Urol 150:110–114

Partin AW, Pound CR, Clemens JQ, Epstein JI, Walsh PC (1993b) Serum PSA after anatomic radical prostatectomy: the Johns Hopkins experience after 10 years. Urol Clin North Am 20:713–725

Paulson DF (1988a) More on the Uro-Oncology Research Group report of radical surgery vs. radiotherapy for adenocarcinoma of the prostate: rebuttal (Letter). Int J Radiat Oncol Biol Phys 14:1053–1054

Paulson DF (1988b) Randomized series of treatment with surgery versus radiation for prostate adenocarcinoma. NCI Monogr 7:127–131

Paulson DF, Lin GH, Hinshaw W, Stephani S, the Uro-Oncology Research Group (1982) Radical surgery versus radiotherapy for adenocarcinoma of the prostate. J Urol 128:502–504

Perez CA (1992) Prostate. In: Perez CA, Brady LW (eds) Principles and practice of radiation oncology, 2nd edn. Lippincott, Philadelphia, pp 1067–1116

Perez CA (1995) Carcinoma of the prostate: a model for management under impending health care reform. Radiology 196:309–322

Perez CA, Pilepich MV, Zivnuska F (1986) Tumor control in definitive irradiation of localized carcinoma of the prostate. Int J Radiat Oncol Biol Phys 12:523–531

Perez CA, Garcia D, Simpson JR, Zivnuska F, Lockett MA (1989) Factors influencing outcome of definitive radiotherapy for localized carcinoma of the prostate. Radiother Oncol 16:1–21

Perez CA, Hanks GE, Leibel SA, Zietman AL, Fuks Z, Lee WR (1993a) Localized carcinoma of the prostate (stages T1B, T1C, T2, and T3): review of management with external beam radiation therapy. Cancer 72:3156–3173

Perez CA, Lee HK, Georgiou A, Logsdon MD, Lai PP, Lockett MA (1993b) Technical and tumor-related factors affecting outcome of definitive irradiation for localized carcinoma of the prostate. Int J Radiat Oncol Biol Phys 26:581–591

Perez CA, Lee HK, Georgiou A, Lockett MA (1994a) Technical factors affecting morbidity in definitive irradiation for localized carcinoma of the prostate. Int J Radiat Oncol Biol Phys 28:811–819

Perez CA, Purdy JA, Harms W et al. (1994b) Design of a fully integrated three-dimensional computed tomography simulator and preliminary clinical evaluation. Int J Radiat Oncol Biol Phys 30:887–897

Perez CA, Purdy JA, Harms W et al. (1995) Three-dimensional treatment planning and conformal radiation therapy. Radiother Oncol 36:32–43

Perez CA, Michalski J, Brown KC, Lockett MA (to be published) Nonrandomized evaluation of pelvic lymph node irradiation in localized carcinoma of the prostate. Int J Radiat Oncol Biol Phys ••

Petros JA, Catalona WJ (1992) Lower incidence of unsuspected lymph node metastases in 521 consecutive patients with clinically localized prostate cancer. J Urol 147:1574–1575

Pilepich MV, Asbell SO, Krall JM et al. (1987a) Correlation of radiotherapeutic parameters and treatment related morbidity: analysis of RTOG study 77-06. Int J Radiat Oncol Biol Phys 13:1007–1013

Pilepich MV, Bagshaw MA, Asbell AO et al. (1987b) Definitive radiotherapy in resectable (stage A2 and B) carcinoma of the prostate: results of a nationwide overview. Int J Radiat Oncol Biol Phys 13:659–663

Pilepich MV, Krall JM, Sause WT et al. (1987c) Correlation of radiotherapeutic parameters and treatment related morbidity in carcinoma of the prostate: analysis of RTOG study 75-06. Int J Radiat Oncol Biol Phys 13:351–357

Pilepich MV, Krall JM, Sause WT et al. (1987d) Prognostic factors in carcinoma of the prostate: analysis of RTOG study 75-06. Int J Radiat Oncol Biol Phys 13:339–349

Pilepich MV, Sause WT, Shipley WU et al. (1995) Androgen deprivation with radiation therapy compared with radiation therapy alone for locally advanced prostatic carcinoma: a randomized comparative trial of the Radiation Therapy Oncology Group. Urology 45:616–623

Pisansky TM, Cha SS, Earle JD et al. (1993) Prostate-specific antigen as a pretherapy prognostic factor in patients treated with radiation therapy for clinically localized prostate cancer. J Clin Oncol 11:2158–2166

Ploysongsang SS, Aron BS, Shehata WM (1992) Radiation therapy in prostate cancer: whole pelvis prostate boost or small field to prostate? Urology 40:18–26

Proimos BS (1960) Synchronous field shaping in rotational megavolt therapy. Radiology 74:753–757

Rangala N, Cox JD, Byhardt RW, Wilson JF, Greenberg M, Lopes da Conceicao A (1982) Local control and survival after external irradiation for adenocarcinoma of the prostate. Int J Radiat Oncol Biol Phys 8:1909–1914

Ritter MA, Messing EM, Shanahan TG et al. (1992) Prostate-specific antigen as a predictor of radiotherapy response and patterns of failure in localized prostate cancer. J Clin Oncol 10:1208–1217

Roach M III, Krall J, Keller JW et al. (1992) The prognostic significance of race and survival from prostate cancer based on patients irradiated on Radiation Therapy Oncology Group protocols (1976–1985). Int J Radiat Oncol Biol Phys 24:441–449

Rosen EM, Cassady JR, Connolly J, Chaffey JT (1984) Radiotherapy for localized prostate carcinoma. Int J Radiat Oncol Biol Phys 10:2201–2210

Rosen EM, Cassady JR, Connolly J, Chaffey JT (1985) Radiotherapy for prostate carcinoma: the JCRT experience (1968–1978). II. Factors related to tumor control and complications. Int J Radiat Oncol Biol Phys 11:725–730

Rounsaville MC, Green JP, Vaeth JM, Purdon RP, Heltzel MM (1987) Prostatic carcinoma: limited field irradiaton. Int J Radiat Oncol Biol Phys 13:1013–1020

Russell KJ, Boileau MA (1993) Current status of prostate-specific antigen in the radiotherapeutic management of prostatic cancer. Semin Radiat Oncol 3:154–168

Russell KJ, Laramore GE, Krall JM et al. (1987) Eight years experience with neutron radiotherapy in the treatment of stages C and D prostate cancer: updated results of the RTOG 7704 randomized clinical trial. Prostate 11:183–193

Russell KJ, Dunatov C, Hafermann MD et al. (1991) Prostate specific antigen in the management of patients with localized adenocarcinoma of the prostate treated with primary radiation therapy. J Urol 146:1046–1052

Russell KJ, Caplax RJ, Laramore GE et al. (1994) Photon versus fast neutron external beam radiotherapy in the treatment of locally advanced prostate cancer: results of a randomized prospective trial. Int J Radiat Oncol Biol Phys 28:47–54

Sagerman RH, Chun HC, King GA, Chung CT, Dalal PS (1989) External beam radiotherapy for carcinoma of the prostate. Cancer 63:2468–2474

Sandler HM, Perez-Tamayo C, Ten Haken RK, Lichter AS (1992) Dose escalation for stage C (T3) prostate cancer: minimal rectal toxicity observed using conformal therapy. Radiother Oncol 23:53–54

Sands ME, Zagars GK, Pollack A, von Eschenbach AC (1994) Serum prostate-specific antigen, clinical stage, pathologic grade, and the incidence of nodal metastases in prostate cancer. Urology 44:215–220

Schellhammer PF, Schlossberg SM, El-Mahdi AM, Wright GL, Brassil DN (1991) Prostate-specific antigen levels after definitive irradiation for carcinoma of the prostate. J Urol 145:1008–1011

Shipley WU, Prout GR Jr, Coachman NM et al. (1988) Radiation therapy for localized prostate carcinoma: experience at the Massachusetts General Hospital (1973–1981). NCI Monogr 7:67–73

Shipley WU, Verhey LJ, Munzenrider JE et al. (1995) Advanced prostate cancer: the results of a randomized trial of high dose irradiation boosting with conformal protons compared with conventional dose irradiation using photons alone. Int J Radiat Oncol Biol Phys 32:3–12

Slater JD, Slater JM, Wahlen S (1992) The potential for proton beam therapy in locally advanced carcinoma of the cervix. Int J Radiat Oncol Biol Phys 22:343–347

Smit WGJM, Helle PA, van Putten WLJ, Wijnmaalen AJ, Seldenrath JJ, van der Werf-Messing BHP (1990) Late radiation damage in prostate cancer patients treated by high dose external radiotherapy in relation to rectal dose. Int J Radiat Oncol Biol Phys 18:23–29

Soffen EM, Hanks GE, Hwang CC, Chu JCH (1991) Conformal static field therapy for low volume low grade prostate cancer with rigid immobilization. Int J Radiat Oncol Biol Phys 20:141–146

Soffen EM, Hanks GE, Hunt MA, Epstein BE (1992) Conformal static field radiation therapy treatment of early prostate cancer versus non-conformal techniques: a reduction in acute morbidity. Int J Radiat Oncol Biol Phys 24:485–488

Spaas PG, Bagshaw MA, Cox RS (1988) The volume of extended field irradiation in surgically staged carcinoma of the prostate. Int J Radiat Oncol Biol Phys 15 (Suppl 1):133

Stamey TA, Yang N, Hay AR, McNeal JE, Freiha FS, Redwine E (1987) Prostate-specific antigen as a serum marker for adenocarcinoma of the prostate. N Engl J Med 317:909–916

Stamey TA, Kabalin JN, Ferrari M (1989) Prostatic specific antigen in the diagnosis and treatment of adenocarcinoma of the prostate. J Urol 141:1084–1087

Stein A, DeKernion JB, Smith RB, Dorey F, Patel H (1992) Prostate specific antigen levels after radical prostatectomy in patients with organ confined and locally extensive prostate cancer. J Urol 147:942–946

Suit HD, Urie M (1992) Proton beams in radiation therapy. J Natl Cancer Inst 84:155–164

Takahashi S, Kitabatake T, Morita K, Okajima S, Iida H (1961) Methoden zur besseren Anpassung der Dosisverteilung an tiefliegende Krankenheitsherde bei der Bewegungsbestrahlung. Strahlentherapie 115:478–488

Tepper JE, Calvo FA (1992) Intraoperative radiation therapy. In: Perez CA, Brady LW (eds) Principles and practice of radiation oncology, 2nd edn. Lippincott, Philadelphia, pp 388–395

van der Werf-Messing BHP, Menon RS, van Putten WLJ (1984) Prostatic cancer treated by external irradiation at the Rotterdam Radiotherapy Institute. Strahlentherapie 160:293–300

Van Poppel H, Ameye F, Oyen R, Van de Voorde W, Baert L (1994) Accuracy of combined computerized tomography and fine needle aspiration cytology in lymph node staging of localized prostatic carcinoma. J Urol 151:1310–1314

Vijayakumar S, Quadri SF, Karrison TG et al. (1992) Localized prostate cancer: use of serial prostate-specific antigen measurements during radiation therapy. Radiology 184:271–274

Wallner K (1991) Iodine 125 brachytherapy for early stage prostate cancer: new techniques may achieve better results. Oncology 5:115–1122

Whitmore WF (1988) Overview: historical and contemporary. NCI Monogr 7:7–11

Whitmore WF (1993) Management of clinically localized prostatic cancer: an unresolved problem. JAMA 269:2676–2677

Willett CG, Zietman AL, Shipley WU, Coen JJ (1994) The effect of pelvic radiation therapy on serum levels of prostate specific antigen. J Urol 151:1579–1581

Zagars GK, von Eschenbach AC (1993) Prostate-specific antigen: an important marker for prostate cancer treated by external beam radiation therapy. Cancer 72:538–548

Zagars GK, von Eschenbach AC, Johnson DE, Oswald MJ (1987) Stage C adenocarcinoma of the prostate: an analysis of 551 patients treated with external beam radiation. Cancer 60:1489–1499

Zagars GK, Sherman NE, Babaian RJ (1991) Prostatic-specific antigen and external beam radiation therapy in prostatic cancer. Cancer 67:412–420

Zagars GK, von Eschenbach AC, Ayala AG (1993) Prognostic factors in prostate cancer: analysis of 874 patients treated with radiation therapy. Cancer 72:1709–1725

Zentner PG, Pao LK, Benson MC, Schiff PB (1992) PSA density: a new prognostic factor for the prediction of outcome in patients with prostate cancer. Int J Radiat Oncol Biol Phys 24 (Suppl 1):150

Zietman AL, Shipley WU (1993) Randomized trials in locoregionally confined prostate cancer: past, present, and future. Semin Radiat Oncol 3:210–220

Zietman AL, Coen JJ, Shipley WU, Authausen AF (1993a) Adjuvant irradiation after radical prostatectomy in patients with organ confined and locally extensive prostate cancer. J Urol 147:942–946

Zietman AL, Shipley WU, Willett CG (1993b) Residual disease after radical surgery or radiation therapy for prostate cancer: clinical significance and therapeutic implications. Cancer 71:959–969

Zietman AL, Coen JJ, Shipley WU, Willett CG, Efird JT (1994) Radical radiation therapy in the management of prostatic adenocarcinoma: the initial PSA value as a predictor of treatment outcome. J Urol 151:640–645

Zincke H, Blute ML, Fallen MJ, Farrow GM (1991) Radical prostatectomy for stage A adenocarcinoma of the prostate: staging errors and their implications for treatment recommendations and disease outcome. J Urol 146:1053–1058

Zinreich ES, Derogatis LR, Herpst J, Auvil G, Piantadosi S, Order SE (1990) Pre and post-treatment evaluation of sexual function in patients with adenocarcinoma of the prostate. Int J Radiat Oncol Biol Phys 19:729–732

16 Localized Carcinoma of the Prostate: Patterns of Failure with External Beam Radiation Therapy

C.A. Perez and M.A. Lockett

CONTENTS

16.1 Introduction

External beam irradiation is used as definitive therapy in a large proportion of patients with clinical stage A and B carcinoma of the prostate and, in most institutions, in the majority of patients with stage C or more locally extensive tumors (Perez et al. 1993a). Tumor doses have ranged from 60 to 64 Gy for stage A1 (T1a), 65 to 70 Gy for stage A2 (T1b) and B (T2), and 66 to 72 Gy for stage C (T3) tumors. Several retrospective studies indicate that dose has an impact on the local tumor control. Perez et al. (1986, 1993c) reported improved local control rates with doses greater than 65 Gy, particularly in stage C patients. Hanks et al. (1988), in 1348 patients with stage B and C tumors, reported an actuarial 5-year local recurrence rate of 37% for patients with stage C tumors treated to doses of less than 60 Gy, 36% for 60–64.9 Gy, 29% for 65–69.9 Gy, and 19% for those receiving 70 Gy or more. By 7 years, 32% of patients receiving 65–69 Gy and 24% treated with higher doses had local recurrences.

Controversy regarding elective pelvic lymph node irradiation and its impact on survival is not settled. McGowan (1981) reported better survival and fewer pelvic failures in patients with stage B2 or C tumors treated with larger fields encompassing the pelvic lymph nodes compared with patients treated to the prostate and periprostatic tissues only. Ploysongsang et al. (1992) described, in 126 patients treated to the prostate and whole pelvis, a 5-year survival rate of 92% in stage B and 72% in stage C compared with 70% and 40%, respectively, in 116 patients irradiated to the prostatic area only. Perez et al. (1993c) noted a 20% incidence of pelvic recurrences in patients with stage C disease treated to the pelvic lymph nodes (50 Gy) compared with 37% in 137 patients treated to the pelvic area with portals smaller than 14 cm² after 40 Gy ($P < 0.01$).

The importance of adequate radiation therapy techniques to achieve optimal tumor control in the pelvis has been recently emphasized (Perez et al. 1993c). Furthermore, a lower incidence of distant metastases and improved survival have been reported in patients with locoregional tumor control compared with patients developing pelvic failure in reports by Fuks et al. (1991) in patients treated with interstitial irradiation, by Kaplan et al. (1992) and Perez et al. (1993c) with external beam irradiation, and by Kuban et al. (1987, 1995) with either treatment modality.

The complex natural history and, in many patients, slow growth rate of carcinoma of the prostate require detailed histologic classification and careful long-term follow-up to evaluate patterns of failure and results of various therapeutic modalities.

C.A. Perez, MD, FACR, Professor of Radiation Oncology, Director, Radiation Oncology Center, Mallinckrodt Institute of Radiology, Washington University School of Medicine, 4511 Forest Park, St. Louis, MO 63108, USA
M.A. Lockett, MBA, Radiation Oncology Center, Mallinckrodt Institute of Radiology, Washington University School of Medicine, 4939 Children's Place, St. Louis, MO 63110, USA

16.2 Patterns of Failure and Prognostic Factors

In 963 patients treated at our institution with definitive external beam irradiation between January 1967 and December 1992 (minimal follow-up, 2 years; median, 6 years), we analyzed patterns of failure as detected by clinical examination, radiographic or other imaging studies, and, when appropriate, biopsy of suspicious lesions. Table 16.1 shows the incidence of pelvic failures, distant metastases, or combination of both in our patients.

16.2.1 Pelvic Failures

In carcinoma of the prostate the majority of pelvic failures are in the prostate gland, but in some patients periprostatic extension is detected. Actuarial analyses are a more accurate method to report post-treatment failures, based on the number of patients at risk for any specific period. In Fig. 16.1 the 5-year pelvic failure rates in our patients are 8% for those with A2 (T1b,c), 12% for B1 (T2a,b) and B2 (T2c), 24% for C (T3), and 30% for clinical D1 (T4) tumors. The corresponding 10-year pelvic failure rates are 16%, 22%, and 25%, and at 7 years 58% for D1 (T4) tumors.

Although there is a trend toward a greater incidence of pelvic failure in patients with poorly differentiated tumors than for those with well or moderately differentiated tumors, the differences among the various groups in clinical stages A2, B, and C are not statistically different (Table 16.2).

The pelvic failure rate was similar in patients with clinical stage A2 (T1b,c) and B (T2) disease when correlated with method of diagnosis (Table 16.3). However, in patients with stage C (T3) tumors diagnosed by transurethral resection (TURP) there is a 45% 10-year incidence of pelvic recurrences compared with 27% for those diagnosed by needle biopsy ($P \leq 0.01$) (Fig. 16.2).

No significant correlation of pelvic failures with pretreatment PSA levels by clinical stage was ob-

Table 16.1. Carcinoma of the prostate: patterns of clinical failure correlated with stage

Stage	No. of patients	Sites of clinical failure		
		Pelvic	Pelvic and distant metastases	Distant metastases only
A1 (T1a)	16	0	0	0
A2 (T1b,c)	112	1 (9%)	3 (3%)	5 (4%)
B (T2)	373	30 (8%)	19 (5%)	45 (12%)
C (T3)	434	41 (9%)	54 (12%)	113 (26%)
D (T4)	28	4 (14%)	5 (18%)	12 (43%)

Table 16.2. Carcinoma of the prostate: 10-year actuarial clinical pelvic failure correlated with histologic differentiation of tumor and clinical stage

Grade	Stage		
	A2 (T1b,c)	B (T2)	C (T3)
Well	36 (10%)	124 (22%)	99 (30%)
Moderate	54 (25%)	188 (29%)	198 (26%)
Poor	22 (18%)	61 (28%)	137 (32%)
	$P = 0.35$	$P = 0.48$	$P = 0.17$

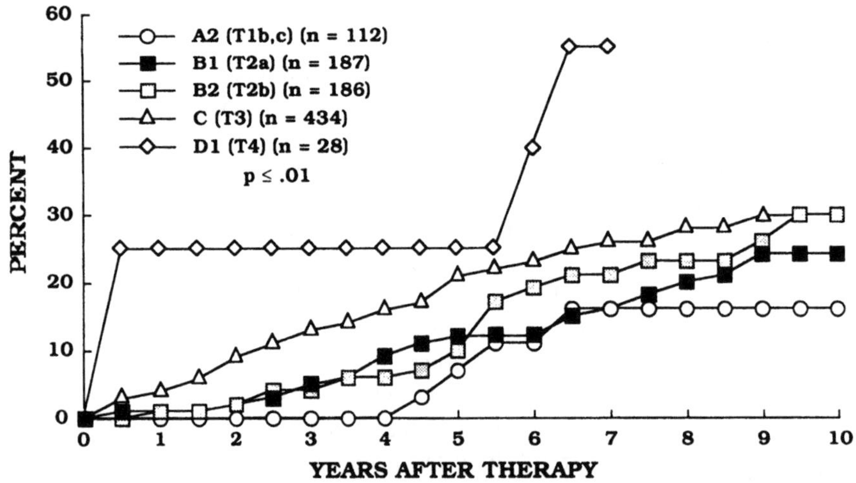

Fig. 16.1. Pelvic failure rate correlated with clinical stage for 947 patients treated at the Mallinckrodt Institute of Radiology

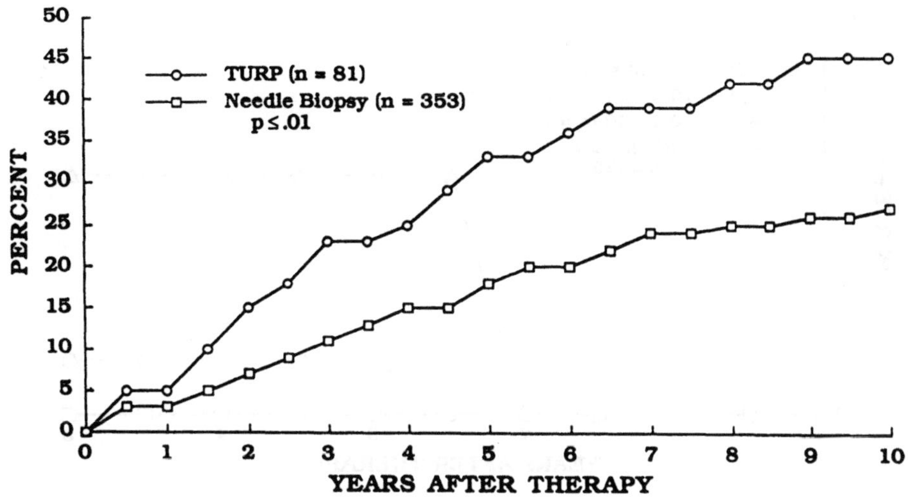

Fig. 16.2. Pelvic failure rate correlated with method of diagnosis for 434 stage C (T3) patients treated at the Mallinckrodt Institute of Radiology

Table 16.3. Carcinoma of the prostate: 10-year actuarial pelvic failure rate correlated with method of diagnosis

Clinical stage	Pelvic failure rate		
	Needle biopsy	TURP	*P* value
A2 (T1b,c)	69 (0%)	43 (17%)	0.67
B (T2)	331 (28%)	42 (15%)	0.18
C (T3)	353 (37%)	81 (55%)	≤0.01

TURP, Transurethral resection of the prostate

served (Fig. 16.3) although patients with PSA higher than 20 ng/ml had a greater incidence of local recurrences ($P = 0.2$–0.37).

In patients with stage B (T2) tumors there was a statistically significant greater pelvic failure rate in white than in black men (27% vs 8% at 10 years, $P \leq 0.01$) (Table 16.4), but there was not significant difference in the other stages.

No significant correlation was noted in the incidence of clinically detected pelvic recurrences and the age of the patient at diagnosis in stages A2 (T1b,c) and B (T2) (Table 16.5). However, in 89 patients with stage C (T3), the pelvic failure rates were 42% in those younger than 60 years of age, about 30% in the group of patients 61–75 years of age, and 16% in patients older than 75 (Fig. 16.4) ($P = 0.01$).

The incidence of clinical local recurrences after definitive irradiation reported by many authors has ranged from 0% to 20% for stage T1b, 5% to 30% for T2, and 12% to 40% for T3 tumors. These figures are comparable to the reported incidence of histologically positive routine prostate biopsies, as will be discussed later. However, when the data are analyzed using actuarial methods, the incidence of clinically detected local recurrences is somewhat higher (at 10 years, 20% for stage T1b, 24% for T2, and 30%–40% for T3 lesions) (Perez et al. 1993c; Shipley et al. 1988). Hanks et al. (1992b) found no significant correlation between the pathologic or radiographic status of the lymph nodes and incidence of local recurrences, suggesting that local tumor control studies can be carried out without knowledge of nodal status.

16.2.2 Distant Metastases

Figure 16.5 shows an increasing actuarial incidence of distant metastases with more-advanced clinical stages. Also, there is a strong correlation of incidence of distant metastases with histologic degree of tumor differentiation in all clinical stage groups (Fig. 16.6). The greatest incidence of distant metastases occurred in patients with poorly differentiated carcinoma (Gleason score 8–10). A greater incidence of distant metastases was noted only in patients with stage C tumors diagnosed with TURP compared with patients diagnosed with needle biopsy (Fig. 16.7).

There was good correlation between the incidence of distant metastases and pretreatment prostate specific antigen (PSA) in patients with clinical stage B (T2) and C (T3) tumors. Patients with PSA of ≤20 ng/

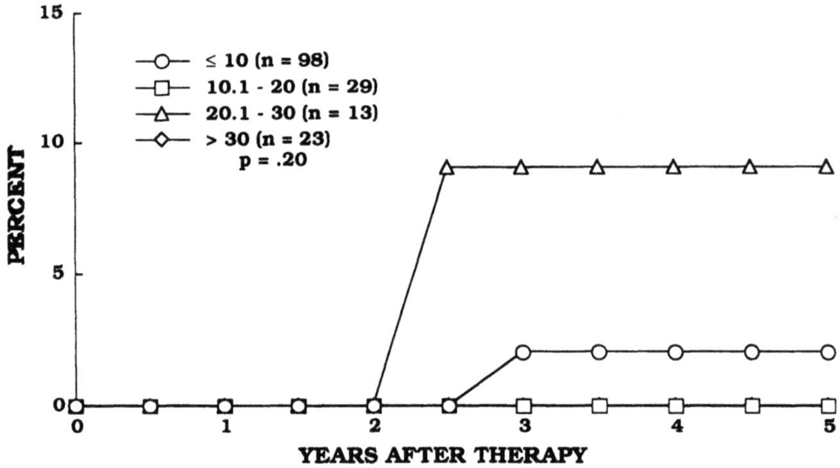

a

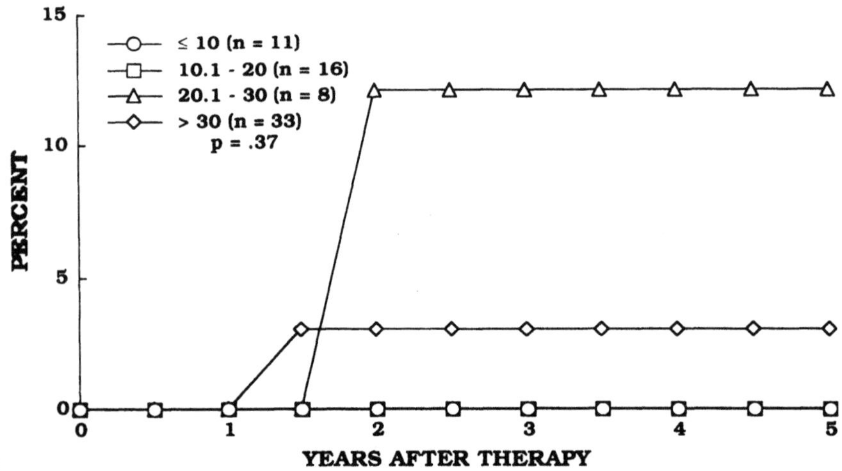

b

Fig. 16.3a,b. Pelvic failure rate correlated with initial PSA level for (**a**) stage B (T2) and (**b**) stage C (T3) patients treated at the Mallinckrodt Institute of Radiology

Table 16.4. Carcinoma of the prostate: 10-year actuarial pelvic and distant failures correlated with race

Race	No. of patients	Pelvic failure rate		Distant metastasis rate	
A2 (T1b,c)					
White	94	17%	$P = 0.67$	27%	$P = 0.35$
Black	18	0%		0%	
B (T2)					
White	333	27%	$P \leq 0.01$	28%	
Black	38	8%[a]		25%	
C (T3)					
White	364	29%	$P = 0.56$	47%	$P = 0.31$
Black	69	50%		57%	

[a] 5-year actuarial

Table 16.5. Carcinoma of the prostate: 10-year failure patterns correlated with age at diagnosis

Age at diagnosis (years)	No. of patients	Pelvic failure rate		Distant metastasis rate	
A2 (T1b,c)					
≤60	9	0		0	
61–70	46	14%		29%	
71–75	32	12%		27%	
>75	25	29%		5%	
B (T2)					
≤60	49	37%	$P = 0.23$	36%	
61–70	145	26%		32%	
71–75	113	27%	$P = 0.14$	15%	
>75	66	8%		30%	
C (T3)					
≤60	89	42%	$P = 0.01$	60%	$P \leq 0.01$
61–70	163	27%		43%	
71–75	117	32%	$P = 0.20$	50%	
≥75	65	16%		46%	

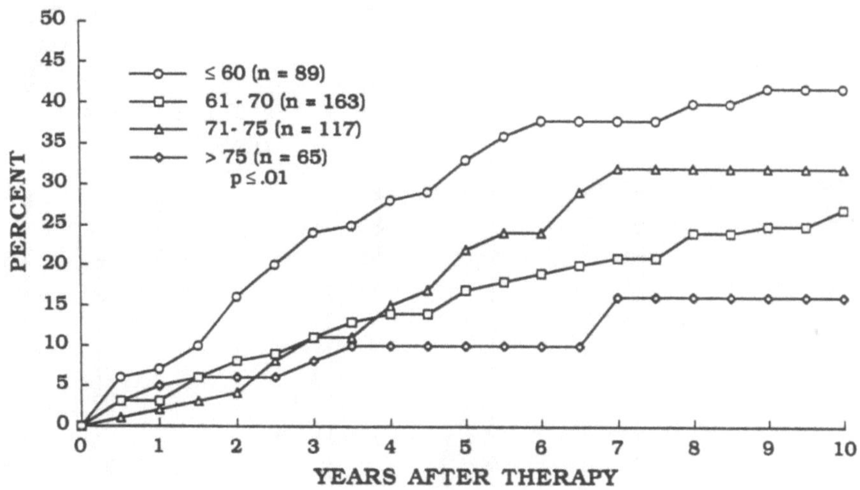

Fig. 16.4. Pelvic failure rate correlated with age for 434 stage C (T3) patients treated at the Mallinckrodt Institute of Radiology

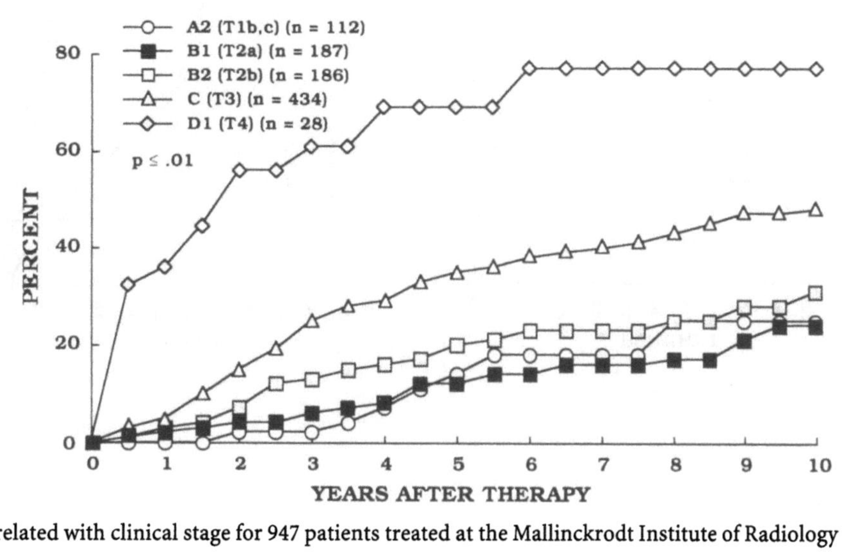

Fig. 16.5. Distant metastasis rate correlated with clinical stage for 947 patients treated at the Mallinckrodt Institute of Radiology

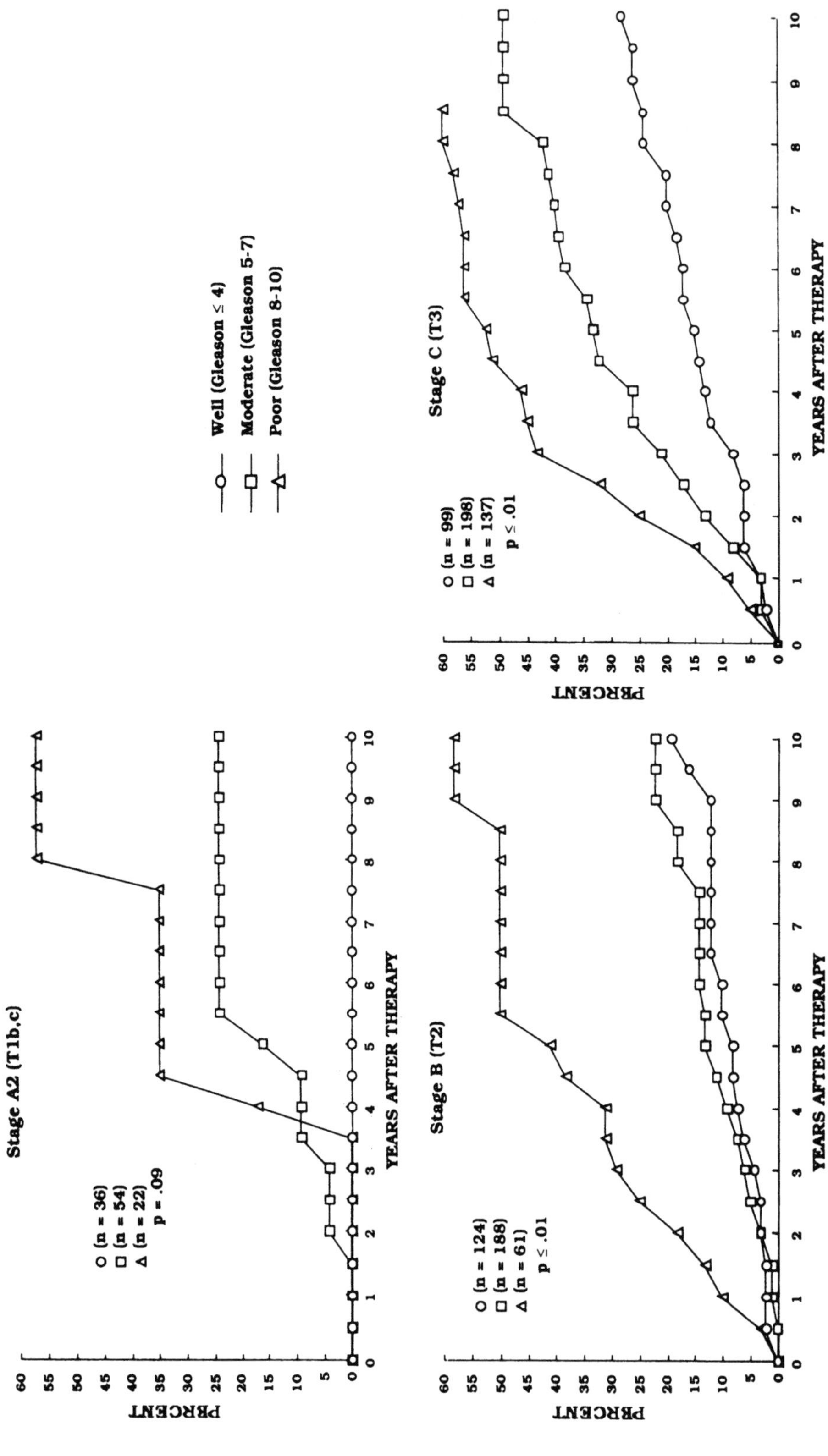

Fig. 16.6. Distant metastasis rate correlated with histologic grade for patients with stage A, B, and C tumors treated at the Mallinckrodt Institute of Radiology

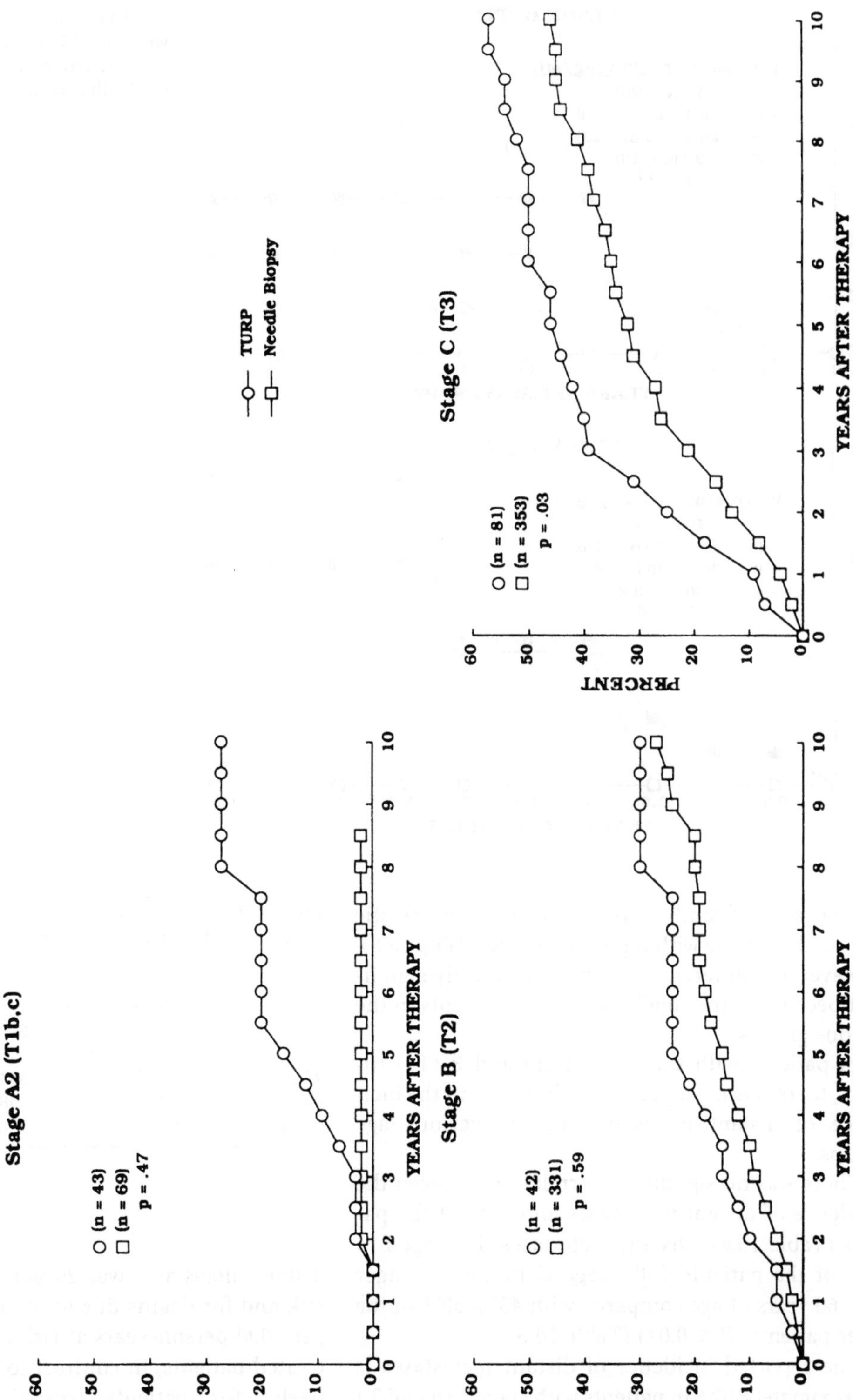

Fig. 16.7. Distant metastasis rate correlated with method of diagnosis for patients with stage A, B, and C tumors treated at the Mallinckrodt Institute of Radiology

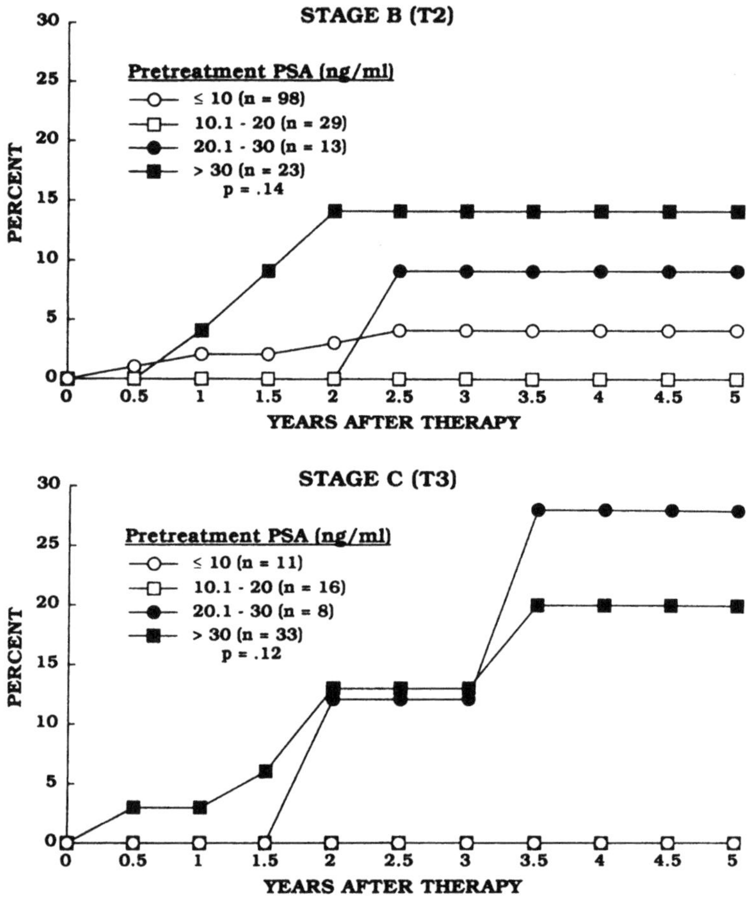

Fig. 16.8. Distant metastasis rate correlated with initial PSA level for patients with stage B and C carcinoma of the prostate treated at the Mallinckrodt Institute of Radiology

ml have a significantly lower incidence of metastatic disease than those with higher PSA levels (Fig. 16.8). However, the differences are not statistically significant because of the small numbers of patients in the various groups.

In patients with stage A (T1b,c) and B (T2) tumors, there was no appreciable difference in the incidence of distant metastases in the various age groups.

There was no significant correlation between the incidence of distant metastases and race of the patient (Table 16.6). Distant metastases developed in 60% of the patients with stage C tumors younger than 60 years of age compared with 43%–50% in the older patients ($P \leq 0.01$) (Table 16.5).

The reported incidence of distant metastases is approximately 20% in patients with stage T1b and T2 tumors and 40% in patients with T3 lesions. The incidence of local pelvic recurrence and distant metastasis described in the literature is summarized in Tables 16.7 and 16.8. In a report by Adolfsson et al. (1993), the calculated weighted mean number of distant metastases was 29 per 1000 person-years at risk and for deaths due to intercurrent disease, 36.3 per 1000 person-years at risk for radiation therapy-treated patients, in contrast to 12.6 and 9.9, respectively, for patients treated with radical prostatectomy, a strong reflection of patient selection based on prognostic factors. Distant dissemination is closely correlated with clinical/surgical stage, histologic degree of tumor differentiation (Gleason score), and pretreatment PSA level (Bagshaw et al.

Table 16.6. Carcinoma of prostate: 10-year actuarial distant metastasis rate correlated with race

Race	Clinical stage		
	A2 (T1b,c)	B (T2)	C (T3)
White	94 (27%)	333 (28%)	364 (47%)
Black	18 (0%)[a]	38 (25%)	69 (57%)
P-value	0.35	0.44	0.47

[a] 7.5 years

Table 16.7. Incidence of clinical local recurrence and distant metastases in patients with stages T1b and T2 tumors treated with external beam radiation therapy (from PEREZ et al. 1993b)

Study	Number of patients		Local recurrence (%)		Distant metastases (%)	
	T1b	T2	T1b	T2	T1b	T2
ARISTIZABAL et al. (1984)	17	101	6	5	6	19
ASBELL (1988)	84	361		11		16
BAGSHAW et al. (1990)	308		20[a]			
		218		30[a]		
HANKS (1993)	60[b]		4[b]			
HANKS (1993)	116		15[c]			
HANKS (1993)		312		35[d]		
HANKS (1993)		415		29[c]		
HANKS et al. (1991)[e]	16	88	0	15[a]	0	21[a]
KUBAN et al. (1989)	41		2			
		118		19		
KURUP et al. (1984)	24		0		0	
		65		3		9
PEREZ et al. (unpublished data)	113		16[a]		20	
		373		24[a]		24[a]
ROSEN et al. (1984)	25		0			
		85		20[a]		
ROUNSAVILLE et al. (1987)	37		5		19	
		50		20		36
SAGERMAN et al. (1989)	34		9		17	
		100		15		8
SHIPLEY et al. (1988)	307	162	16[a]	18[a]		
ZAGARS et al. (1993)	104	168	21[a]	32[a]	8[a]	27[a]

[a] 10-year actuarial
[b] Includes T2 tumors
[c] At 10 years
[d] At 15 years
[e] Surgically staged patients

Table 16.8. Incidence of clinical local recurrence and distant metastases in patients with stage T3 tumors treated with external beam radiation therapy (from PEREZ et al. 1993b)

Study	Number of patients	Locoregional recurrence (%)	Distant metastases (%)
ARISTIZABAL et al. (1984)	82	12	33
BAGSHAW et al. (1990)	385	38[a]	
DEL REGATO et al. (1993)			
HANKS (1993)	296	30[b]	
HANKS (1993)	197	42[c]	
KURUP et al. (1984)	74	12	39
PEREZ et al. (unpublished data)	434	30[a]	42
ROSEN et al. (1984)	88	30[a]	
ROUNSAVILLE (1987)	152	23	39
SAGERMAN et al. (1989)	63	23	29
ZAGARS et al. (1993)	602	24[a]	45[a]

[a] 10-year actuarial
[b] At 10 years
[c] At 15 years

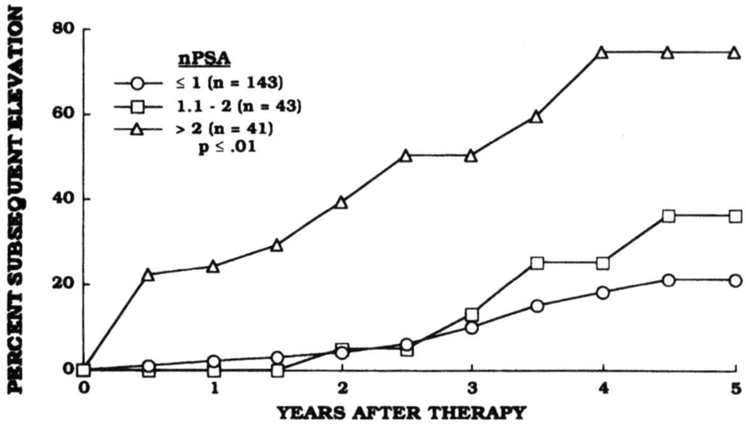

a

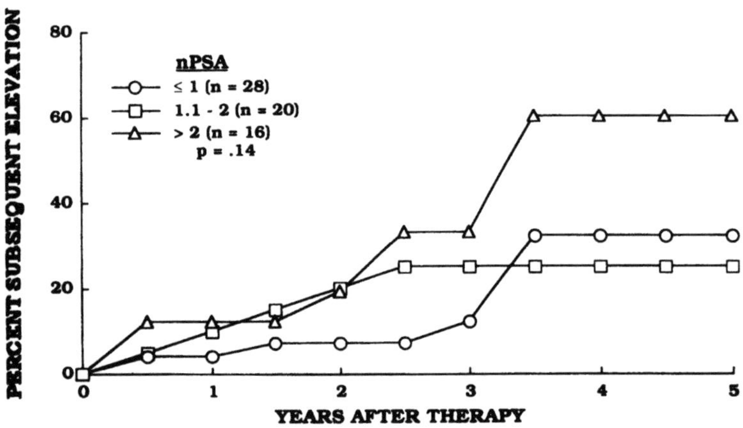

b

Fig. 16.9a,b. Probability of chemical failure as a function of postirradiation nadir PSA levels in 291 patients treated at the Mallinckrodt Institute of Radiology. (**a**) Stage A2–B (T1b, c, T2); (**b**) stage C (T3)

1990; Gleason et al. 1977; Perez et al. 1986; Stamey et al. 1989; Zagars et al. 1995).

16.2.3 Chemical Failures

As reviewed in Chap. 15, the probability of chemical relapse is closely correlated with the pretreatment PSA level and the pathologic extent of the tumor. Figure 16.9 illustrates the probability of chemical failure in 291 patients treated at our institution, as a function of postirradiation nadir PSA levels. In clinical stage A (T1b,c), B (T2), and C (T3) patients achieving a posttreatment nadir PSA (nPSA) of 1 or 2 ng/ml, the incidence of subsequent chemical failure at 5 years is 20% or less compared with more than 60% in patients with an nPSA greater than 2 ng/ml.

Our results confirm those of Kavadi et al. (1994), who noted that nPSA level after irradiation was a very reliable indicator of therapy efficacy. Patients with an nPSA ≤1 ng/ml had only a 10% (8 of 83) probability of developing a clinical relapse compared with 16.7% (19 of 114) with an nPSA of 1.1–2 ng/ml and 28% (28 of 99) with an nPSA of 2.1–3 ng/ml.

Several authors have shown a close correlation between PSA levels and clinical and pathologic tumor stage, and, in conjunction with Gleason score, a predictable correlation with incidence of lymph node metastasis (Bluestein et al. 1994; Partin et al. 1993).

Roach et al. (1993) described an equation, based on data of Partin et al. (1993), to predict risk of lymph node metastases: $N + \% = 2/3$ PSA + (Gleason score $- 6) \times 10$. Predictions were tested in 212 patients treated with radical prostatectomy; incidence of positive nodes was 6% in the low-risk and 40% in the high-risk group ($P < 0.001$).

Kaplan et al. (1990, 1991) designed mathematical methods for estimating tumor recurrence in patients treated with radiation therapy based on the absolute value, rate of decline posttreatment, and subsequent rise of PSA. Hanks et al. (1992a) reported a correlation of PSA rise doubling time and clinical behavior including outcome with radiation therapy.

In any comparison of treatment series, stratification for PSA levels is as important as stratification for tumor size and grade. ZAGARS and VON ESCHENBACH (1993), in 314 patients with clinically localized prostate cancer treated by definitive radiation therapy (28% stage A2, 34% stage B, and 38% stage C), reported a 4-year risk of chemical failure closely related to the initial PSA level: 5%, <4 ng/ml; 20%, >4 to <10 ng/ml; 60%, 10–30 ng/ml; and 80%, >30 ng/ml. The chemical failure preceded clinical recurrence by several years; even among patients with an initial PSA of 4–30 ng/ml, 80% were clinically tumor free 4 years after treatment. Others have reported a shorter lead time from rising PSA to clinical evidence of relapse (approximately 6 months on the average)(KAPLAN et al. 1993; RITTER et al. 1992). Patients with elevated pretreatment PSA levels, stable posttreatment levels, and subsequent elevation have a 33%–44% risk of subsequent distant metastasis in less than 3 years (KAPLAN et al. 1990).

ZIETMAN et al. (1994), in 161 patients treated with definitive radiation therapy for localized carcinoma of the prostate, noted that 54% achieved a postirradiation nadir of 0–1 ng/ml, and 29% had an undetectably low level (<0.5 ng/ml). As in our experience, the authors found a significant correlation between the likelihood of being free from chemical failure at 4 years and the initial PSA value (<4 ng/ml, 81%; 4.1–10 ng/ml, 43%; 10.1–20 ng/ml, 31%; 20.1–50 ng/ml, 6%; and >50 ng/ml, 0%). Survival with no clinical evidence of recurrence was significantly higher than the PSA-based (free of chemical failure) survival. Table 16.9 summarizes results published by several authors on chemical failure-free survival according to initial PSA level.

KAVADI et al. (1994) reported outcome in 427 patients with localized carcinoma of the prostate treated with external beam irradiation (30-month median follow-up); 57 patients sustained either chemical or clinical relapse. PSA levels fell 12 months after irradiation, but there was no evidence of significant decline beyond this time. Time to nPSA was 3 months in 60 patients (14.1%), 6 months in 68 patients (15.9%), 9 months in 148 patients (34.7%), and 12 months in 144 patients (33.7%); time to nadir was not a significant determinant of outcome. However, the nadir value independently correlated with increasing relapse rates with higher values. Patients with nadir levels less than 1 ng/ml had a chemical relapse rate below 10%, which was somewhat better than with 2 ng/ml (about 20% relapse rate). Patients with pretreatment PSA levels exceeding 10 ng/ml had a high failure rate regardless of nadir level.

16.2.4 Multivariate Analysis

Multivariate analysis was carried out in the total (963) patient population, excluding PSA, since data were not available on patients treated before 1987. Most important prognostic factors for local tumor control were clinical stage and age younger or older than 60 years, while for distant metastases they were clinical stage, histologic grade of tumor, performance of TURP (in patients with stage C), and age

Table 16.9. Comparison of reported clinical disease-free survival and chemical failure-free (PSA) survival after definitive external beam irradiation (from PEREZ et al. 1993b)

Study	No. of patients	Clinical disease-free survival (%)	Disease-free survival according to initial PSA level (%)				Follow-up
			≤4	4.1–10	10.1–20	20.1–≥40	
FIJUTH et al. (1992)	146			100		60	28 mo median
PEREZ et al.[a]	147	87		92	83	61	3.6 yr median
ZAGARS et al.[a]	314	88[b]	95		85	63	1.5 yr median
ZIETMAN et al. (1994)	161	90		83	35	10	4 yr actuarial
HANKS et al.[a]							
T1	15			84[c]			
T2	96			55[c]			
T3	65			41[c]			

[a] Unpublished data
[b] Approximate, for all stages (A2, B, and C)
[c] Initial PSA levels unknown

Table 16.10. Carcinoma of the prostate: multivariate analysis of pelvic failure rate

Variable	Total patient population (n = 963)			Patients with preirradiation PSA (n = 301)		
	P value	Final model regression coefficient (±SE)	Exponent of the regression coefficient	P value	Final model regression coefficient (±SE)	Exponent of the regression coefficient
Clinical stage	0.001	0.2691 ± 0.0646	1.3067	0.063	1.1067 ± 0.6360	3.0242
Transurethral resection of prostate	0.026	−0.3451 ± 0.1713	0.7081			
Lymph node status	0.040	0.6170 ± 0.3177	1.8534	0.094	−0.0005 ± 0.0003	0.9995
Histologic grade	0.169	0.1007 ± 0.0694	1.1059	0.165	0.2977 ± 0.1749	1.3468
Pelvic node dose	0.099	−0.0001 ± 0.0000	0.9999			
Central axis dose	0.935	0.000 ± 0.0002	1.0000	0.702	0.0006 ± 0.0019	1.0006
Initial PSA level				0.531	0.0056 ± 0.0078	1.0056

Table 16.11. Carcinoma of the prostate: multivariate analysis of incidence of distant metastasis

Variable	Total patient population (n = 963)			Patients with preirradiation PSA (n = 301)		
	P value	Final model regression coefficient (±SE)	Exponent of the regression coefficient	P value	Final model regression coefficient (±SE)	Exponent of the regression coefficient
Clinical stage	0.001	0.4200 ± 0.0612	1.5220	0.009	0.5331 ± 0.2896	1.7042
Transurethral resection of prostate	0.009	−0.8249 ± 0.2891	0.4383			
Histologic grade	0.001	0.2333 ± 0.0425	1.2627	0.074	0.2266 ± 0.1017	1.2543
Pelvic node dose	0.012	0.5205 ± 0.2928	1.6829			
Lymph node status	0.379	−0.0001 ± 0.0001	0.9999	0.099	−0.0002 ± 0.0001	0.9998
Central axis dose	0.950	0.001 ± 0.0002	1.0000	0.099	0.0006 ± 0.0010	1.0006
Initial PSA level				0.125	0.0083 ± 0.0042	1.0084

younger or older than 60 years (Tables 16.10, 16.11). Multivariate analysis in 301 patients with pretreatment PSA levels demonstrated a weak impact of this parameter on incidence of distant metastases (P = 0.15) and no correlation with pelvic failure rate (P = 0.53). Results of multivariate analysis in our patients are similar to those we reported in a smaller patient population (PEREZ et al. 1989).

ZAGARS et al. (1993) published an analysis of prognostic factors in 874 patients treated with radiation therapy. Major factors predictive of local/pelvic failure were clinical stage and histologic grade of tumor differentiation. Likewise, clinical stage and degree of tumor differentiation were significant prognostic factors for metastatic relapse. As in our experience, only in patients with stage C tumors was performance of TURP associated with an increased incidence of distant metastases. ZAGARS et al. (1993) also reported that elevation of the prostate acid phosphatase (PAP) level and age of patient (younger or older than 60 years of age) were significant prognostic factors on multivariate analysis for distant tumor dissemination.

16.3 Positive Biopsy of the Prostate After Definitive Radiation Therapy

Several authors have reported different percentages of histologic evidence of viable adenocarcinoma in the prostate at various times after completion of radiation therapy (Table 16.12). These data should be interpreted in light of radiobiologic data indicating that cell death after radiation exposure is a postmitotic event. In view of the long doubling time of many prostate tumors in early biopsies, cells that harbor lethal damage but have not had an opportunity to morphologically express it may be misinterpreted as viable cells. COX and STOFFEL (1977) noted that there was a decreasing incidence of positive biopsies as a function of time after irradiation (from

70% at 6 months to 20% after 24 months). There was no significant correlation between the status of the prostatic biopsies (positive or negative) and subsequent survival. SCARDINO (1983) confirmed this observation, reporting that 32% of his patients with a positive biopsy at 12 months had a negative pathologic specimen at 24 months.

The rate of positive specimens is also related to the initial clinical stage of the tumor; SCARDINO (1983) noted a positivity of 28% for B1, 41% for B2, and 62% for stage C lesions. Likewise, FREIHA and BAGSHAW (1984) reported no positive biopsies in patients with stages A2 and B, but rates of 38%, 59%, and 74% for small stage B2, large B2, and stage C tumors, respectively.

In the analysis by KUBAN and EL-MAHDI (1993) of 94 patients with clinically negative digital examination of the prostate who did not receive hormonal therapy until documented evidence of recurrence and on whom routine biopsies of the prostate were performed 18 months or longer after irradiation, the incidence of positive biopsies was also related to the initial stage: 1 of 10 (10%) for stage A2, 10 of 55 (18%) for stage B, and 6 of 29 (21%) for stage C lesions. By 10 years, 75% of patients with positive biopsies developed clinical local failure. Disease-free survival was 20% compared with 30% and 60%, respectively, in patients with negative biopsies. In a publication by SCARDINO and WHEELER (1988), the local recurrence rate was 52% at 5 years with a positive biopsy versus 12% with a negative specimen, and at 10 years the rates were 72% and 30%, respectively ($P < 0.001$). When only patients with a normal digital rectal examination were considered, the risk of local recurrence at 10 years was 50% with a positive and 25% with a negative biopsy.

These observations were corroborated by PRESTIDGE et al. (1992), who described 116 patients with localized carcinoma of the prostate who had a positive postirradiation prostatic biopsy 12 or more months after treatment; 51 patients (44%) developed distant metastases. Among 65 patients who remained free of metastases, only four have died of prostate cancer, compared with 41 of 51 patients with distant metastases ($P < 0.0001$).

Postirradiation biopsy findings were closely related to the clinical status of the prostate gland in the experience of FREIHA and BAGSHAW (1984) and SCARDINO (1983), who reported 89% and 64% incidence, respectively, of positive biopsies in patients with suspected or definite clinical evidence of tumor regrowth, whereas the same authors noted 25% and 20% positivity, respectively, in patients with negative clinical examination of the prostate.

Emerging data strongly correlate a rising PSA level with positive postirradiation prostate biopsies. KABALIN et al. (1989) reported 100% positive biopsy results in 27 patients with abnormal PSA levels after irradiation. DUGAN et al. (1991) described a significant correlation of negative postirradiation biopsies and PSA value (92% negative specimens with PSA less than 1 ng/ml, 50% with 1.1–2.5 ng/ml, and 29% with 2.5 ng/ml or higher levels). SCHELLHAMMER et al. (1991) reported that a selected group of 20 of 24 patients (83%) with a median follow-up of 87 months after irradiation had normal PSA levels and negative routine prostatic biopsies.

Timing of postirradiation biopsies and whether they are routinely performed in patients with suspected recurrence, regardless of rectal examination, transurethral ultrasonographic findings, or postirradiation PSA levels, or only in selected patients with

Table 16.12. Percentage of prostate cancer patients with positive biopsy after radiation therapy correlated with digital rectal examination (DRE) status[a] (from KUBAN et al. 1995)

Study	% Positive biopsy		
	Positive DRE	Negative DRE	All patients
COX and STOFFEL (1977)	–	–	19%
JACOBI and HOHENFELLNER (1982)	–	–	39%
NACHTSHEIM et al. (1978)	–	–	59%
KIESLING et al. (1980)	–	–	67%
FREIHA and BAGSHAW (1984)	89%	25%	61%
SCARDINO and WHEELER (1988)	64%	20%	32%
KUBAN et al. (1992)	–	18%	18%

[a] All biopsies done at ≥18 months posttherapy

abnormal findings will significantly affect the positivity of the examination and correlation with outcome.

16.4 Impact of New External Beam Irradiation Approaches on Patterns of Failure

16.4.1 Three-Dimensional Conformal Techniques

With the advent of three-dimensional (3-D) treatment planning and conformal radiation therapy, it is feasible to deliver higher tumor doses to selected target volumes, thus improving tumor control probability without increasing treatment morbidity (LICHTER et al. 1992).

The reluctance of radiation oncologists to escalate dose, despite good evidence of potential benefit (HANKS 1993; PEREZ et al. 1993c), has been illustrated by a recent survey of radiation oncology centers in the United States (METTLIN et al. 1993). The doses prescribed for prostate cancer did not increase from 1984 to 1990, with the modal dose remaining at only 60 Gy.

LEIBEL et al. (1994) updated preliminary results in 324 patients with carcinoma of the prostate who were irradiated to the prostate, seminal vesicles, and adjacent tissues with a 1-cm margin around the identifiable prostate gland, except at the interface with the rectum, where a 0.6 cm margin was used on a dose-escalation protocol. Doses of irradiation were 64.8–66.6 Gy in 70 patients, 70.2 Gy in 102, 75.6 Gy in 57, and 81 Gy in 25. With a median 18-month follow-up, 48 patients (15%) had postirradiation increasing PSA, and 29 (9%) showed clinical relapse (seven local recurrences, 22 distant metastases). Hanks and coworkers reported that, in 176 patients treated with conformal irradiation, 93% had normal PSA levels 12 months after treatment, in contrast to only 38% of 77 patients treated with conventional techniques ($P = 0.003$) (PEREZ et al. 1993b). CORN et al. (1995), who updated Hanks et al.'s experience, reported that in patients receiving only prostatic field irradiation, 12-month PSA values returned to normal in 96% and 85% of conformally and conventionally treated patients, respectively, when normalization was defined as ≤4 ng/ml ($P < 0.03$), and in 76% and 55% of patients when PSA normalization was defined as ≤1.5 ng/ml ($P < 0.02$). Among those receiving pelvic irradiation prior to prostatic conedown, PSA normalization (≤4 ng/ml) occurred in 82% and 61% ($P < 0.01$) of conformal and conventionally treated patients, respectively, and in 56% and 38% of patients when normalization was defined as ≤1.5 ng/ml ($P < 0.05$). In a multivariate analysis, pretreatment PSA level (≤15 vs >15) and the use of conformal irradiation were statistically significant prognostic discriminants of PSA normalization at 1 year while total irradiation dose, clinical stage, and the addition of pelvic fields were not significant.

A cooperative dose-escalation protocol for carcinoma of prostate is in progress at nine institutions under the aegis of the Radiation Therapy Oncology Group and National Cancer Institute.

16.4.2 Proton Boost Irradiation

The Massachusetts General Hospital recently completed a phase III comparison of perineal proton boost versus conventional photon boost for patients with localized T3 and T4 prostate cancer. In both arms the whole pelvis was treated to 50.4 Gy with photons. The standard radiation therapy arm gave a total dose of 60 Gy to the primary tumor. The experimental arm exploited the superior depth-dose characteristics of a 160-MV proton beam to bring the tumor volume to 75.5 Gy.

SHIPLEY et al. (1995) reported on a phase I/II study of T3 and T4 prostate cancer in which, after 50.4 Gy to the pelvis delivered through four fields, 103 patients were randomized to receive a perineal conformal field proton (160-MV) boost of 25.2 CGE (cobalt Gray equivalent) and 99 patients to receive a 16.8-Gy boost with photons. Median follow-up was 60 months. Among the patients completing randomization, the local relapse-free survival at 7 years was 80% for the proton and 66% for the photon group ($P = 0.14$). However, the local relapse-free survival at 7 years for 58 patients with poorly differentiated tumors was 85% with protons and 37% with photons ($P = 0.001$). The incidence of grade 1 and 2 rectal bleeding (32% vs 12%) and urethral stricture (19% vs 8%) was higher in the proton-treated patients compared with the photon-treated group.

16.4.3 Neutron Therapy

The neutron beam has potential biologic advantages over photons in killing slowly cycling or hypoxic cells. The Neutron Therapy Collaborative Working Group Trial was opened in 1985 and closed in 1990; 182 T3–4 or pelvic node-positive patients were treated with a pelvic field (50.4 Gy at 1.8 Gy per fraction in the photon arm and 13.6 nGy at 1.7 nGy per fraction in the neutron arm). The prostate was boosted with 20 Gy and 6.8 nGy, respectively. Five-year results show a significant pathologic local tumor control advantage for neutrons (82% vs 60%), but as yet no difference in disease-free or overall survival has been observed (RUSSELL et al. 1994). If the node-positive patients are excluded, the pathologic local control figures are 92% for neutrons and 59% for photons.

16.5 Impact of Endocrine Therapy on Patterns of Failure

Endocrine therapy in conjunction with radiation therapy in carcinoma of prostate has been used as adjuvant therapy following irradiation for patients at high risk for occult metastatic disease or as neoadjuvant cytoreductive therapy in patients with bulky primary tumors to enhance likelihood of local control. In 1988, ZAGARS et al. (1988) reported 15-year follow-up on a randomized trial in which 40 patients with T3–4 NxM0 tumors were randomized to receive irradiation alone and 38 received irradiation plus diethylstilbestrol until relapse or death. The 10-year disease-free survival rates were 43% and 63% ($P = 0.008$) and clinical local tumor control rates were 80% and 95%, respectively ($P = 0.09$). Overall survival was equivalent (60%) in both groups because of greater intercurrent disease in patients receiving estrogens.

Radiation Therapy Oncology Group (RTOG) protocol 8531 evaluated adjuvant goserelin acetate (Zoladex)(3.6 mg subcutaneously every 28 days indefinitely) combined with irradiation in T3–4 and node-positive patients or administered on relapse after identical irradiation alone. This study was closed in April 1992 having accrued 977 patients; outcome data have not been reported. The EORTC activated a comparable protocol in March 1990. Patients at higher risk of metastatic disease (T3–4 tumors or high-grade T1–2) are eligible provided there is no evidence of gross distant metastatic disease or involved lymph nodes at or above the common iliac. Patients in the experimental arm receive cyproterone acetate (150 mg t.i.d. for 4 weeks) starting 1 week prior to radiation therapy plus Zoladex (3.6 mg subcutaneously every 4 weeks) starting on the 1st day of irradiation and continuing for 3 years or until progression, whichever occurs sooner.

The cytoreductive role of goserelin acetate (Zoladex) and flutamide (Eulexin) in bulky primary disease (T2b, T3, T4) in RTOG protocol 8610 was reported by PILEPICH et al. (1995). Preliminary analysis was described in 455 patients with large stage T2b and T2c (B2, B3, B4, C, D1) adenocarcinoma of the prostate randomized to be treated with irradiation alone (45 Gy to pelvic lymph nodes and additional 20–25 Gy, depending on stage, to the prostatic area) or a combination of the same radiation therapy and adjuvant hormonal therapy consisting of Zoladex (3.6 mg subcutaneously every 4 weeks) and Eulexin (250 mg p.o. t.i.d.), both drugs starting 2 months before initiation of irradiation and continued throughout the entire course of radiation therapy. With a median observation period of 4.5 years the 5-year local recurrence rate (clinical assessment) was significantly lower in patients treated with neoadjuvant hormonal therapy and radiation therapy (46%) in comparison with the control group (71%). A decreasing incidence of distant metastasis was also noted in patients receiving hormonal therapy (34% vs 41%) ($P = 0.09$). The corresponding chemical-free (PSA $>$ 4 ng/ml) recurrence survival rates were 36% for the study arm and 15% for the control arm ($P \leq 0.001$).

In RTOG protocol 9202, more than 1000 patients with T2b–4 disease were registered. Neoadjuvant total androgen suppression (2 months, of goserelin acetate and flutamide) was given in both arms of the trial before and during irradiation; one group received 2 years of maintenance monthly Zoladex. Results have not been analyzed because of short follow-up.

The value of elective pelvic irradiation and neoadjuvant hormone therapy will be better assessed in a recently activated RTOG protocol in which patients with clinical stage T2 and T3 carcinoma of the prostate are randomized to four arms: neoadjuvant total androgen suppression (Zoladex and flutamide) or not 2 months before and during irradiation and radiation therapy to the whole pelvis (50.4 Gy, 1.8-Gy fractions) and prostate (19.8 Gy boost) or to prostatic volume only (70.2 Gy).

16.6 Conclusion

Well-designed clinical trials are highly desirable to compare efficacy and specifically analyze patterns of failures with radical prostatectomy or irradiation, taking into account patient selection, staging methods, tumor characteristics, prognostic factors, etc. End points should include survival, clinical or chemical failure, locoregional tumor control, incidence of distant metastases, morbidity, and quality of life as well as cost-benefit of each therapeutic modality.

References

Adolfsson J, Steineck G, Whitmore WF Jr (1993) Recent results of management of palpable clinical localized prostate cancer. Cancer 72:310–322

Aristizabal SA, Steinbronn D, Heusinkveld RS (1984) External beam radiotherapy in cancer of the prostate: the University of Arizona experience. Radiother Oncol 1:309–315

Asbell SO, Krall JM, Pilepich MV et al. (1988) Elective pelvic irradiation in stage A2, B carcinoma of the prostate: analysis of RTOG 77-06. Int J Radiat Oncol Biol Phys 15:1307–1316

Bagshaw MA, Cox RS, Ramback JE (1990) Radiation therapy for localized prostate cancer: justification by long-term follow-up. Urol Clin North Am 17:787–802

Bluestein DL, Bostwick DG, Bergstralh EJ, Oesterling JE (1994) Eliminating the need for bilateral pelvic lymphadenectomy in select patients with prostate cancer. J Urol 151:1315–1320

Corn BW, Hanks GE, Schultheiss TE, Hunt MA, Lee WR, Coia LR (1995) Conformal treatment of prostate cancer with improved targeting: superior prostate-specific antigen response compared to standard treatment. Int J Radiat Oncol Biol Phys 32:325–330

Cox JD, Stoffel TJ (1977) The significance of needle biopsy after irradiation for stage C adenocarcinoma of the prostate. Cancer 40:156–160

del Regato JA, Trailins AH, Pittman DD (1993) Twenty years follow-up of patients with inoperable cancer of the prostate (stage C) treated by radiotherapy: report of a national cooperative study. Int J Radiat Oncol Biol Phys 26:197–201

Dugan TC, Shipley WU, Young RH, et al. (1991) Biopsy after external beam radiation therapy for adenocarcinoma of the prostate: correlation with original histological grade and current prostate specific antigen levels. J Urol 146:1313–1316

Fijuth J, Chauvet B, Vincent P, Felix-Faure C, Reboul F (1992) Serum prostatic-specific antigen in monitoring the response of carcinoma of the prostate to radiation therapy. Radiother Oncol 23:236–240

Freiha FS, Bagshaw MA (1984) Carcinoma of the prostate: results of post-irradiation biopsy. Prostate 5:19–25

Fuks Z, Leibel SA, Wallner KE et al. (1991) The effects of local control on metastatic dissemination in carcinoma of the prostate: long-term results in patients treated with ^{125}I implantation. Int J Radiat Oncol Biol Phys 21:537–547

Gleason DF, Veterans Administration Cooperative Urological Research Group (1977) Histologic grading and clinical staging of prostatic carcinoma. In: Tannenbaum M (ed) Urologic pathology: the prostate. Lippincott, Philadelphia, pp 171–198

Hanks GE (1988) External-beam radiation therapy for clinically localized prostate cancer: patterns of care studies in the United States. NCI Monogr 7:75–84

Hanks GE (1993) Treatment of early stage prostate cancer: radiotherapy. In: Hellman S, DeVita V, Rosenberg S, Freeman S (eds) Important advances in oncology. Lippincott, Philadelphia

Hanks GE, Martz KL, Diamond JJ (1988) The effect of dose on local control of prostate cancer. Int J Radiat Oncol Biol Phys 15:1299–1305

Hanks GE, Asbell S, Krall JM et al. (1991) Outcome for lymph node dissection negative T1-b, T2 (A-2,B) prostate cancer treated with external beam irradiation in RTOG 77-06. Int J Radiat Oncol Biol Phys 21:1099–1103

Hanks GE, Epstein BE, Peter R, Schultheiss TE (1992a) PSA doubling times in patients with prostate cancer, a potentially useful reflection of tumor doubling time (abstract). Int J Radiat Oncol Biol Phys 24:150

Hanks GE, Krall JM, Pilepich MV et al. (1992b) Comparison of pathologic and clinical evaluation of lymph nodes in prostate cancer: implications of RTOG data for patient management and trial design and stratification. Int J Radiat Oncol Biol Phys 23:293–298

Jacobi GH, Hohenfellner R (1982) Staging, management and pre-treatment re-evaluation of prostate cancer: dogma questioned. In: Jacobi GH, Hohenfellner R (eds) Prostate cancer. Williams & Wilkins, Baltimore, pp 31–56

Kabalin JN, Hodge KK, McNeal JE, Freiha FS, Stamey TA (1989) Identification of residual cancer in the prostate following radiation therapy: role of transrectal ultrasound guided biopsy and prostate specific antigen. J Urol 142:326–331

Kaplan ID, Prestidge BR, Cox RS, Bagshaw MA (1990) Prostate specific antigen after irradiation for prostatic carcinoma. J Urol 144:1172–1175

Kaplan ID, Cox RS, Bagshaw MA (1991) A model of prostatic carcinoma tumor kinetics based on prostate specific antigen levels after radiation therapy. Cancer 68:400–405

Kaplan ID, Prestidge BR, Bagshaw MA, Cox RS (1992) The importance of local control in the treatment of prostatic cancer. J Urol 147:917–921

Kaplan ID, Cox RS, Bagshaw MA (1993) Prostate specific antigen after external beam radiotherapy for prostatic cancer: followup. J Urol 149:519–522

Kavadi VS, Zagars GK, Pollack A (1994) Serum prostate-specific antigen after radiation therapy for clinically localized prostate cancer: progostic implications. Int J Radiat Oncol Biol Phys 30:279–287

Kiesling VJ, McAninch JW, Goebel JL et al. (1980) External beam radiotherapy for adenocarcinoma of the prostate: a clinical follow-up. J Urol 124:851–854

Kuban DA, El-Mahdi AM (1993) Prognostic significance of post-irradiation prostate biopsies. Oncology 7:29–38

Kuban DA, El-Mahdi AM, Schellhammer PF (1987) Effect of local tumor control on distant metastasis and survival in prostatic adenocarcinoma. Urology 30:420–426

Kuban DA, El-Mahdi AM, Schellhammer PF (1989) Prognosis in patients with local recurrence after definitive irradiation for prostatic carcinoma. Cancer 63:2421–2425

Kuban DA, El-Mahdi AM, Schellhammer PF (1992) The significance of post-irradiation prostate biospy with long-term follow-up. Int J Radiat Oncol Biol Phys 24:409–414

Kuban DA, El-Mahdi AM, Schellhammer PF (1995) Potential benefit of improved local tumor control in patients with prostate carcinoma. Cancer 75:2373–2382

Kurup P, Kramer TS, Lee MS, Philips R (1984) External beam irradiation of prostate cancer: experience in 163 patients. Cancer 53:37–43

Leibel SA, Zelefsky MJ, Kutcher GJ, Burman CM, Kelson S, Fuks Z (1994) Three-dimensional conformal radiation therapy in localized carcinoma of the prostate: interim report of a phase I dose-escalation study. J Urol 152:1792–1798

Lichter AS, Sandler HM, Robertson JM et al. (1992) Clinical experience with three-dimensional treatment planning. Semin Radiat Oncol 2:257–266

McGowan DG (1981) The value of extended field radiation therapy in carcinoma of the prostate. Int J Radiat Oncol Biol Phys 7:1333–1339

Mettlin C, Jones GW, Murphy GP (1993) Trends in prostate cancer care in the United States, 1974–1990: observations from the patient care evaluation studies of the American College of Surgeons Commission on Cancer. CA Cancer J Clin 143:83–91

Nachtsheim DA Jr, McAninch JW, Stutzman RE et al. (1978) Latent residual tumor following external radiotherapy for prostate adenocarcinoma. J Urol 120:312–314

Partin AW, Yoo J, Carter H et al. (1993) The use of prostate specific antigen, clinical stage, and Gleason score to predict pathological stage in men with localized prostate cancer. J Urol 150:110–114

Perez CA, Pilepich MV, Zivnuska F (1986) Tumor control in definitive irradiation of localized carcinoma of the prostate. Int J Radiat Oncol Biol Phys 12:523–531

Perez CA, Garcia D, Simpson JR, Zivnuska F, Lockett MA (1989) Factors influencing outcome of definitive radiotherapy for localized carcinoma of the prostate. Radiother Oncol 16:1–21

Perez CA, Cosmatos D, Garcia DM, Eisbruch A, Poulter CA (1993a) Irradiation in relapsing carcinoma of the prostate. Cancer 71:1110–1122

Perez CA, Hanks GE, Leibel SA, Zietman AL, Fuks Z, Lee WR (1993b) Localized carcinoma of the prostate (stages T1B, T1C, T2, and T3): review of management with external beam radiation therapy. Cancer 72:3156–3173

Perez CA, Lee HK, Georgiou A, Logsdon MD, Lai PP, Lockett MA (1993c) Technical and tumor-related factors affecting outcome of definitive irradiation for localized carcinoma of the prostate. Int J Radiat Oncol Biol Phys 26:581–591

Pilepich MV, Krall JM, Al-Sarraf M et al. (1995) Androgen deprivation with radiation therapy compared with radiation therapy alone for locally advanced prostatic carcinoma: a randomized comparative trial of the Radiation Therapy Oncology Group. Urology 45:616–623

Ploysongsang SS, Aron BS, Shehata WM (1992) Radiation therapy in prostate cancer: whole pelvis with prostate boost or small field to prostate? Urology 40:18–26

Prestidge B, Kaplan I, Cox RS, Bagshaw MA (1992) Predictors of survival after a positive post-irradiation prostate biospy (abstract). Int J Radiat Oncol Biol Phys 24 (Suppl 1):151

Ritter MA, Messing EM, Shanahan TG et al. (1992) Prostate-specific antigen as a predictor of radiotherapy response and patterns of failure in localized prostate cancer. J Clin Oncol 10:1208–1217

Roach M III, Marquez C, Yuo H-S et al. (1993) Predicting the risk of lymph node involvement using the pre-treatment prostate specific antigen and Gleason score in men with clinically localized prostate cancer. Int J Radiat Oncol Biol Phys 28:33–37

Rosen EM, Cassady JR, Connolly J, Chaffey JT (1984) Radiotherapy for localized prostate carcinoma. Int J Radiat Oncol Biol Phys 10:2201–2210

Rounsaville MC, Green JP, Vaeth JM, Purdon RP, Heltzel MM (1987) Prostatic carcinoma: limited field irradiation. Int J Radiat Oncol Biol Phys 13:1013–1020

Russell KJ, Caplan RJ, Laramore GE et al. (1994) Photon versus fast neutron external beam radiotherapy in the treatment of locally advanced prostate cancer: results of a randomized prospective trial. Int J Radiat Oncol Biol Phys 28:47–54

Sagerman RH, Chun HC, King GA, Chung CT, Dalal PS (1989) External beam radiotherapy for carcinoma of the prostate. Cancer 63:2468–2474

Scardino PT (1983) The prognostic significance of biopsies after radiotherapy for prostatic cancer. Semin Urol 1:243–252

Scardino PT, Wheeler TM (1988) Local control of prostate cancer with radiotherapy: frequency and prognostic significance of positive results of post-irradiation prostate biopsy. NCI Monogr 7:95–103

Schellhammer PF, Schlossberg SM, El-Mahdi AM, Wright GL, Brassil DN (1991) Prostate-specific antigen levels after definitive irradiation for carcinoma of the prostate. J Urol 145:1008–1011

Shipley WU, Prout GR Jr, Coachman NM et al. (1988) Radiation therapy for localized prostate carcinoma: experience at the Massachusetts General Hospital (1973–1981). NCI Monogr 7:67–73

Shipley WU, Verhey LJ, Munzenrider JE et al. (1995) Advanced prostate cancer: the results of a randomized comparative trial of high dose irradiation boosting with conformal protons compared with conventional dose irradiation using photons alone. Int J Radiat Oncol Biol Phys 32:3–12

Stamey TA, Kabalin JN, Ferrari M (1989) Prostatic specific antigen in the diagnosis and treatment of adenocarcinoma of the prostate. J Urol 141:1084–1087

Zagars GK, von Eschenbach AC (1993) Prostate-specific antigen: an important marker for prostate cancer treated by external beam radiation therapy. Cancer 72:538–548

Zagars GK, Johnson DE, von Eschenbach AC, Hussey DH (1988) Adjuvant estrogen following radiation therapy for stage C adenocarcinoma of the prostate: long-term results of a prospective randomized study. Int J Radiat Oncol Biol Phys 14:1085–1091

Zagars GK, von Eschenbach AC, Ayala AG (1993) Prognostic factors in prostate cancer: analysis of 874 patients treated with radiation therapy. Cancer 72:1709–1725

Zagars GK, Pollack A, Kavadi VS, von Eschenbach AC (1995) Prostate-specific antigen and radiation therapy for clinically localized prostate cancer. Int J Radiat Oncol Biol Phys 32:293–306

Zietman AL, Coen JJ, Shipley WU, Authausen AF (1993a) Adjuvant irradiation after radical prostatectomy for adenocarcinoma of prostate: an analysis of freedom from PSA failure. Urology 42:292–298

Zietman AL, Shipley WU, Willett CG (1993b) Residual disease after radical surgery or radiation therapy for prostate cancer: clinical significance and therapeutic implications. Cancer 71:959–969

Zietman AL, Coen JJ, Shipley WU, Willett CG, Efird JT (1994) Radical radiation therapy in the management of prostatic adenocarcinoma: the initial PSA value as a predictor of treatment outcome. J Urol 151:640–645

17 External Beam Radiotherapy for Localized Prostatic Cancer at Stanford: Update at the 38th Year

M.A. BAGSHAW, R.S. COX, and S.L. HANCOCK

CONTENTS

17.1 Introduction

It has been 85 years since PASTEAU (1911) in France, and PASCHKIS and TITTINGER (1910) in Austria introduced gamma irradiation through intraurethral radium sources for the treatment of prostatic cancer. Since then, a wide variety of radiation sources have been used in the treatment of this neoplasm (Table 17.1) (BAGSHAW 1993). Currently, external beam x-irradiation derived from mid- to high-energy linear accelerators (6–25 MV) is the most widely employed modality, although ultrasound-guided interstitial irradiation is also used. External beam irradiation at 4, 6, and 15 MV has been utilized at Stanford since 1956 in the treatment of 1318 patients with prostatic cancer treated through December 1994. These cases provide the major database for this report.

M.A. BAGSHAW, MD, FACR, Professor of Radiation Oncology, Emeritus, Department of Radiation Oncology (A-097), Stanford University Medical Center, Stanford, CA 94305-5105, USA

R.S. COX, PhD, Senior Scientist, Radiation Oncology, Department of Radiation Oncology, Room S-044, Stanford University Medical Center, Stanford, CA 94305-5105, USA

S.L. HANCOCK, MD, Associate Professor of Radiation Oncology, Department of Radiation Oncology (A-097), Stanford University Medical Center, Stanford, CA 94305-5105, USA

17.1.1 The Stanford Series

Radiation therapy for prostatic cancer was initiated at Stanford in 1956 and a tabulation of the disposition of all patients with prostatic cancer evaluated in the Department of Radiation Oncology since then is shown in Table 17.2 (BAGSHAW et al. 1962). The first 300 patients were treated in a standing position with a 6-MV horizontal x-ray beam, produced by the Stanford medical linear accelerator (BAGSHAW et al. 1965). Patients were placed on a rotational platform which permitted 360° rotational and left or right 120° arc therapy. For these early treatments, the beam cross-section was confined to the prostate and was usually 6 × 6 cm measured at the prostate. Between 1970 and 1972, patients were transitioned to the supine position and treated with a 6-MV linear accelerator mounted on an isocentric gantry. Later, the treatment volumes were gradually expanded to include the first echelon lymphatic drainage of the prostate, and the beam cross-sections were shaped with lead trim blocks or cerrobend molded collimators in order to protect adjacent normal structures, such as the posterior wall of the rectum, anal canal and sphincter, uninvolved urethra, pubic bone, and bowel. Localization techniques were improved with the introduction of simulator technology and the CT scan.

Currently, a static contrast urethrogram is used to identify the urethral sphincter, and a low-volume barium enema obtained in the treatment position is used to identify the rectum, sigmoid, and anal canal. A special metallic marker is used to identify the anus. A six-slice mini CT scan, controlled by laser beams illuminating anterior and right and left lateral skin marks which define three-point position control, is obtained, with the patient in the treatment position on a flat top table, to verify the position of the prostate and seminal vesicles.

Each field is treated daily. The dose to the isodose contour, which encompasses the prostate, is carried to 26 Gy at the rate of 2 Gy per day. At this point, the radiation fields are reduced to the booster volume.

Table 17.1. Milestones in the application of radiation for the treatment of prostatic cancer

Year	Authors[a]	Treatment
1910	PASCHKIS and TITTINGER[89] (Aust)	Cystoscopic radium source
1911	PASTEAU[90] (Fr)	Catheter radium source
1915	YOUNG and FRONZ[123] (USA)	Various radium applications
1922	BARRINGER[20] (USA)	Radium needle implants
1934	WIDMANN[121] (USA)	Orthovoltage x-rays
1946	HULTBERG[60] (Swed)	Radium teletherapy gamma rays
1952	FLOCKS et al.[44] (USA)	Interstitial colloidal gold-198
1962	BAGSHAW and KAPLAN[15] (USA)	Linear accelerator x-rays
1964	BUDHRAJA and ANDERSON[23] (UK)	Cobalt-60 teletherapy gamma rays
1972	CARLTON et al.[26] (USA)	Gold-198 seeds
1972	HILARIS et al.[58] (USA)	Iodine-125 seeds
1979	SHIPLEY et al.[109] (USA)	Protons
1983	SYED et al.[107] (USA)	Iridium-192
1985	LARAMORE et al.[74] (USA)	Neutrons
1987	VON ESSEN et al.[119] (USA)	Negative Pi-mesons

[a] Superscripts indicate references as detailed in LEPOR and LAWSON (1993)

Table 17.2. Details of patients with prostatic cancer referred for radiation therapy (RT) at the Department of Radiation Oncology, Stanford University, October 1956–December 1994

Referrals	3210
Exclusions from analysis	
Consultation only	610
Metastatic disease	821
Secondary primary	108
Prostatectomy	139
Unusual primary	7
Previous RT	26
Incomplete RT	32
Questionable histology	4
Implants ± RT	145
	1892
Treated by external beam irradiation	
Disease limited to prostate: T1, T2	782
Extracapsular extension: T3, T4	536
	1318

This volume is tightly confined to the prostate and seminal vesicles, with a liberal immediate margin, but with sparing of the posterior wall of the rectum, distal urethra, anus, and pubic bone. The radiation dose to the isodose contour which surrounds the prostate is carried to 20 Gy, delivering a summated dose of 46 Gy to the prostate and 26 Gy to the first echelon lymph nodes. At this time, the radiation fields are opened to their original dimensions, and an additional 24 Gy is administered at the rate of 2 Gy per day, 5 days per week. The total dose is 70 Gy to the prostate and 50 Gy to the regional adenopathy over a period of 7 weeks. Thus, the booster dose is sandwiched in between the first full pelvic irradiation and the second full pelvic irradiation. This, in essence, permits a split course for the larger pelvic volume, allowing a rest period for the small bowel and elements of the colon for the middle 2 weeks of treatment. This regimen is well tolerated. The 2-week rest permits recovery of the bowel from the initial radiation exposure. At 26 Gy, the bowel is often just starting to show mild to modest irritation manifested by diarrhoea. Recent evidence suggests that because of the prolonged doubling time of prostatic cancer, repopulation of neoplastic cells during this 2-week split does not adversely influence outcome (LAI et al. 1991). In many instances, the booster program alone is utilized for the entire treatment. For example, it is used when it is desirable to confine the radiation dose to the prostatic region only, in patients with low-grade malignancy, i.e., Gleason pattern scores of 5 or less (MELLINGER et al. 1967). The booster program alone is also used in elderly patients (75 years or older) with low or intermediate Gleason pattern scores and in patients who have recently undergone radical prostatectomy and have either clear-cut pathologically positive surgical margins or rising prostate specific antigen (PSA) levels, if they had normal lymph nodes at the time of prostatectomy. In patients further removed in time from the radical prostatectomy who have escalating PSA values, full pelvic irradiation with a boost to the prostatic fossa is administered. An arbitrary interval post-prostatectomy of 18 months has been adopted on the assumption that by 18 months, enough time might have elapsed to permit metastasis from the surgical bed to the regional lymph nodes. A more detailed description of the current Stanford technique has been reported elsewhere (BAGSHAW 1992).

17.2 Results

The age at start of treatment ranged from 35 to 86 years with a mean of 65.5 and a median of 66 years and was distributed almost perfectly symmetrically around the median (Fig. 17.1). A TNM staging system developed at Stanford in the early 1970s related advancing stage to advancing tumor size as determined by digital rectal examination (DRE) (PISTENMA et al. 1979). Both the American Joint Committee on Cancer (AJCC) and the UICC (Union Internationale Contre le Cancer) TNM staging systems were developed later. However, by 1992 and with the adoption of the AJCC edition 4, the Stanford TNM system and the AJCC and UICC systems became nearly identical, making it possible to accurately recategorize the Stanford patients in the current AJCC-4 system (BEAHRS et al. 1992). In order to do this, the Stanford staging was reviewed in detail and reassigned on a case by case basis to the AJCC-4 system from the original clinical data. The staging presented here is in full conformity will the AJCC edition 4 rules. All treated patients except those shown in Fig. 17.17 were classified by clinical stage only and considered Nx, N0, and M0. In fact, 203 patients had staging laparotomies to evaluate lymph node involvement and 105 of these were histopathologically positive (Fig. 17.2). However, this known adenopathy appeared to have little impact on outcome in the various subcategories by stage and hence were ignored in the presentation of the survival data. This is not to say that node status is unimportant. It is vitally important, as shown in Figure 17.2, which clearly demonstrates a highly significant survival disadvantage for patients with positive lymph nodes. On the other hand, the database is so large and the number of patients evaluated for adenopathy so small that the presence of adenopathy

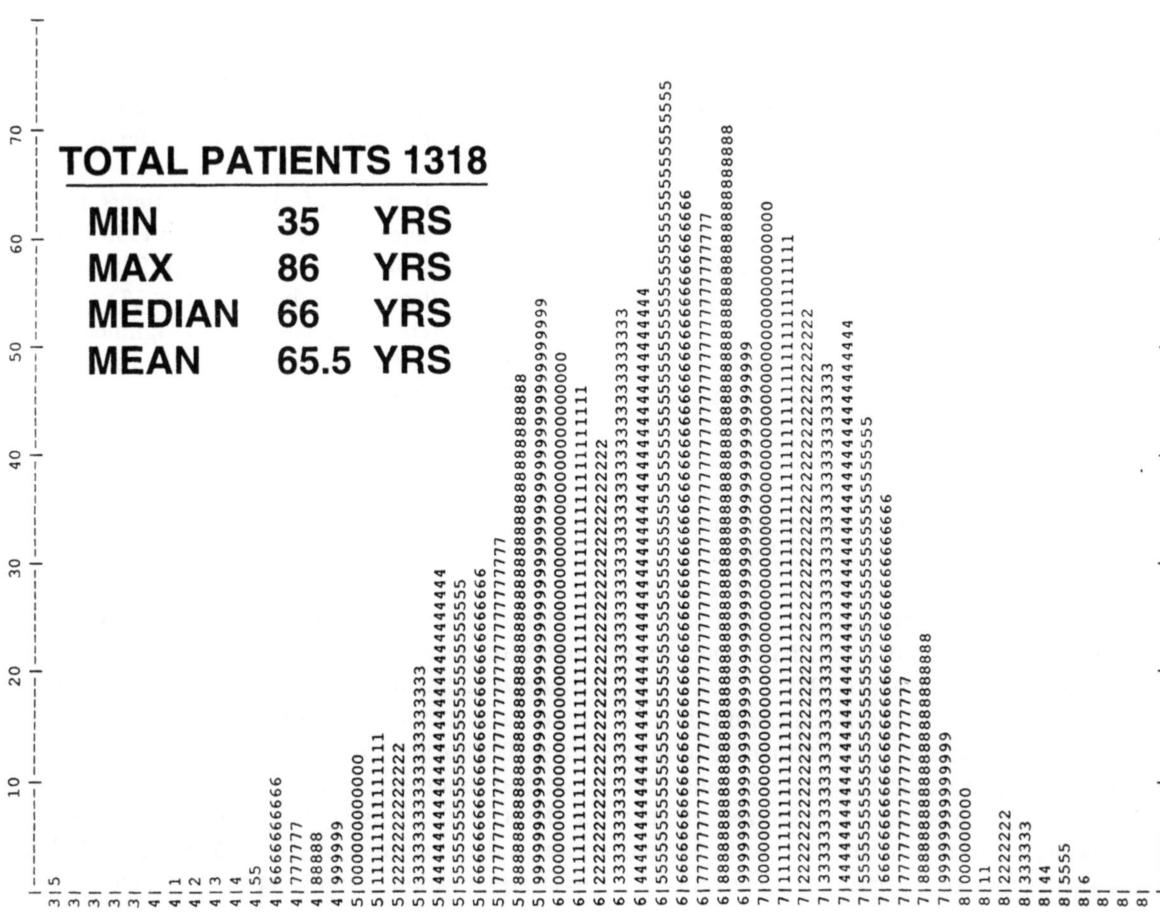

Fig. 17.1. Age distribution of patients with prostatic cancer at first radiotherapy treatment

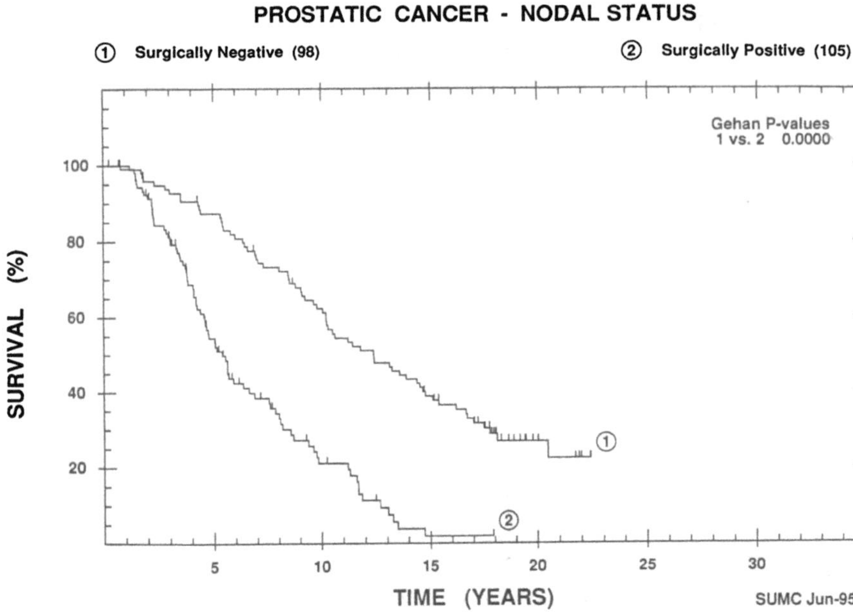

Fig. 17.2. Survival, following radiotherapy, of 203 patients who had pretreatment staging laparotomies to evaluate lymph node status

did not impact significantly on the various subgroups for which outcome data were calculated. Although only one patient with positive nodes has survived beyond 15 years, local control for the entire node positive group remained at 50% at 15 years. These data have been reported in more detail elsewhere (BAGSHAW et al. 1994). Therefore, all patients were included in the outcome calculations irrespective of the lymph node status as indicated by the very limited lymphadenopathy data.

Most of the patients in the study were followed consistently by the author. Follow-up occurred at 1, 4, 8, and 12 months post-treatment, at 6-month intervals thereafter to 5 years, and annually thereafter indefinitely. Follow-up studies consisted of a relevant history and physical examination including DRE, evaluation of the lymphatic and skeletal systems, and investigation of any complaints. Relevant x-ray examinations and/or bone scintiscans were performed as indicated and serum PSA levels have been determined routinely since 1985.

Before turning to specific long-term results by categories of stage and grade, it is worthwhile to note the relentless toll prostatic cancer takes once the metastatic process has been recognized. Figure 17.3 shows the survival pattern observed in 519 patients from the time of detection of metastatic disease. The median survival is less than 2.5 years and only seven patients have survived beyond 10 years. Since we have no untreated control patients other than the expected survival of an age-matched cohort provided by actuarial data (BAGSHAW 1993), it is worthwhile keeping Fig. 17.3 in mind while studying the outcome of treatment as shown by the following curves.

The survival status of all 1318 patients treated with external beam irradiation between 1956 and December 1994 is presented in Fig. 17.4. The median survival was 10 years and the survival at 15 years was 30%. In the remaining curves, the significance of differences between actuarial curves was assessed by the Wilcoxon test of GEHAN (1965). The "P" values between the stages are presented with each data set.

17.2.1 Survival by Major T Stage

Patients with T1 (nominal stage A) (Fig. 17.5) matched the expected survival of an age-matched cohort of California males. As might be expected, the survival systematically diminished with advancing stage. The survival at 15 years was 50% for the age-matched cohort, 45% for T1, 35% for T2, 20% for T3, and 5% for T4. Cause-specific (disease-specific) survival is demonstrated in Fig. 17.6. Figure 17.7 demonstrates freedom from relapse by T stage for the entire series and Fig. 17.8 shows metastatic control by stage. Similarly, Fig. 17.9 illustrates local control as determined by clinical examination.

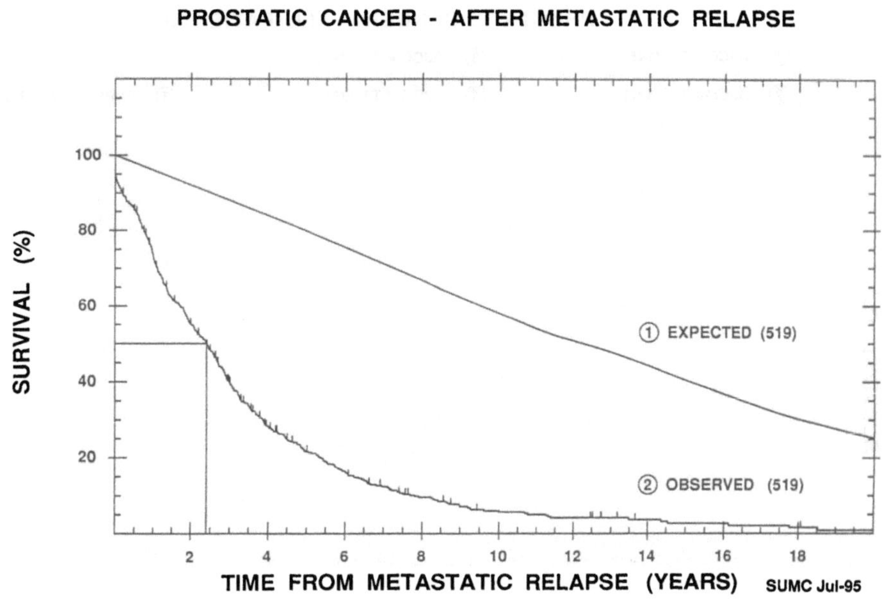

Fig. 17.3. Survival among prostatic cancer patients after detection of metastatic disease. All patients had prior definitive radiotherapy

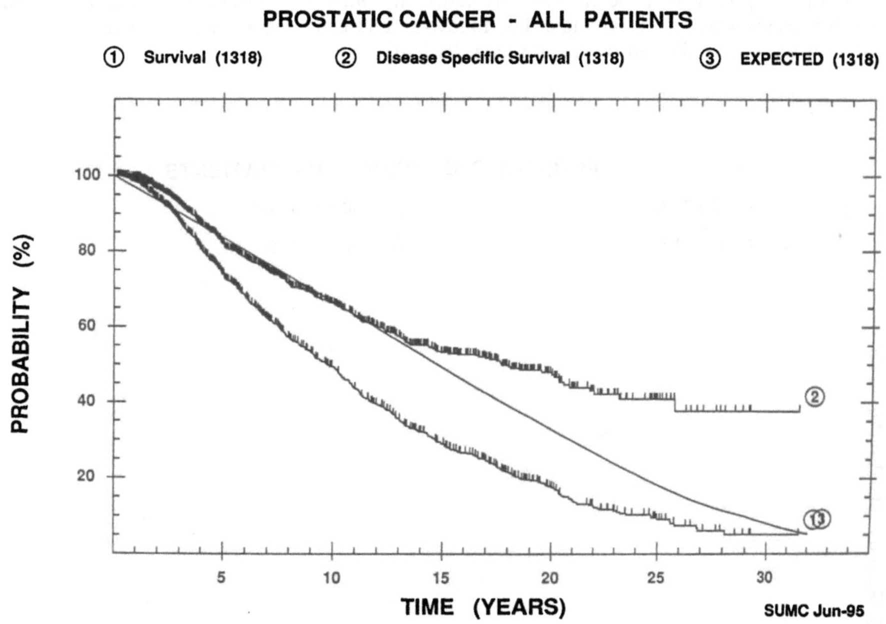

Fig. 17.4. Survival and disease-specific survival among all 1318 patients treated with external beam radiation therapy between 1956 and December 1994. All T stages and histopathologic grades by Gleason sum are included

17.2.2 T1 Category

Survival by subsets of the T1 categories is detailed in Fig. 17.10. Although the curves seem to diverge, there is no statistically significant difference in survival. Survival at 15 years was 51% for the age-matched controls, 56% for T1a, and 40% for T1b. There were only 32 T1c patients since this category was not introduced until 1992. All 32 patients are surviving. Cause-specific survival is shown in Fig. 17.11. Clinical local control for all T1 patients is shown in Fig. 17.12. A difference in outcome for T1 patients was evident only if the patients were subdivided by the Gleason sum. The 13 patients with Gleason sums of

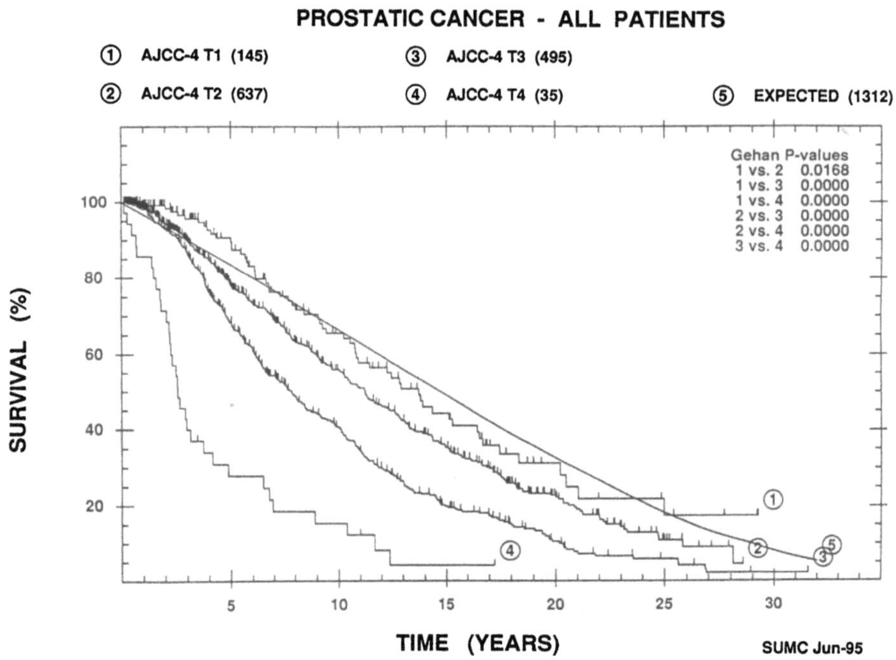

Fig. 17.5. Survival curves as a function of clinical T stage. A *downward step* represents death from any cause; an *upward tick* represents a patient surviving at last follow-up and censored at the time indicated on the abscissa. Patients may or may not have residual or metastatic cancer. *Numbers in parentheses* are the numbers of patients in each group. *Curve 5* is generated from an age-matched cohort of California males

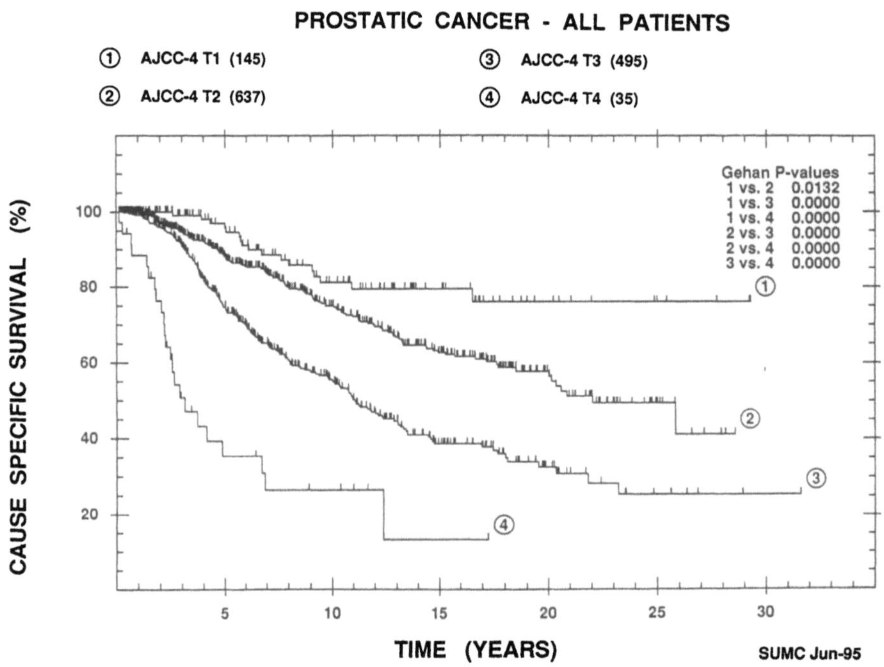

Fig. 17.6. Cause-specific survival. A *downward step* indicates death from prostatic cancer; an *upward tick* represents a patient who either died of intercurrent disease without evidence of prostatic cancer or was alive at the time of last follow-up; patients may or may not have had cancer at that time

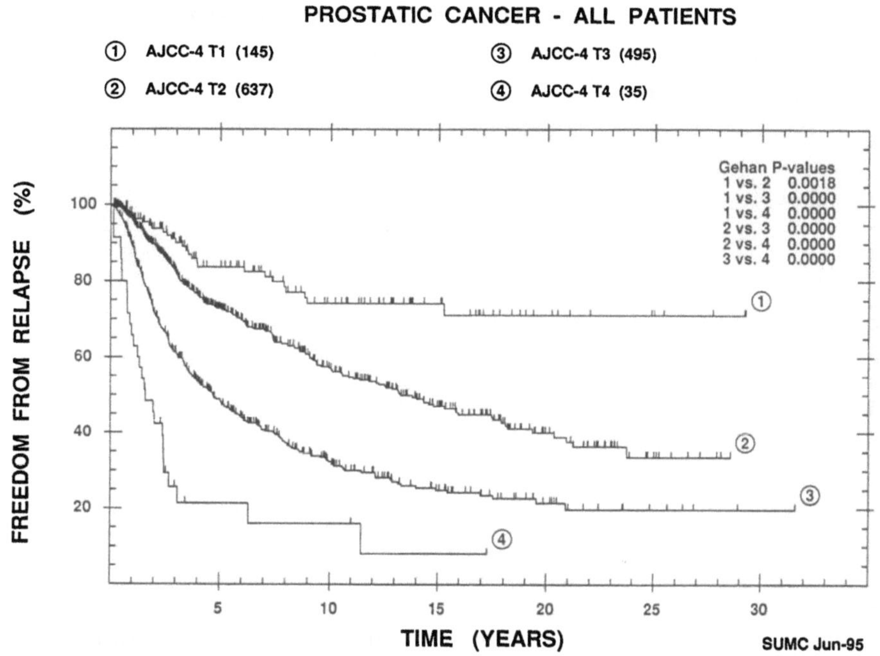

Fig. 17.7. Freedom from relapse. A *downward step* indicates the first evidence of clinical recurrence, either at the primary site or at a metastatic site as detected by clinical observation or a positive biopsy. An *upward tick* represents a patient who was either observed to be disease free or died after being disease free at the time of last observation

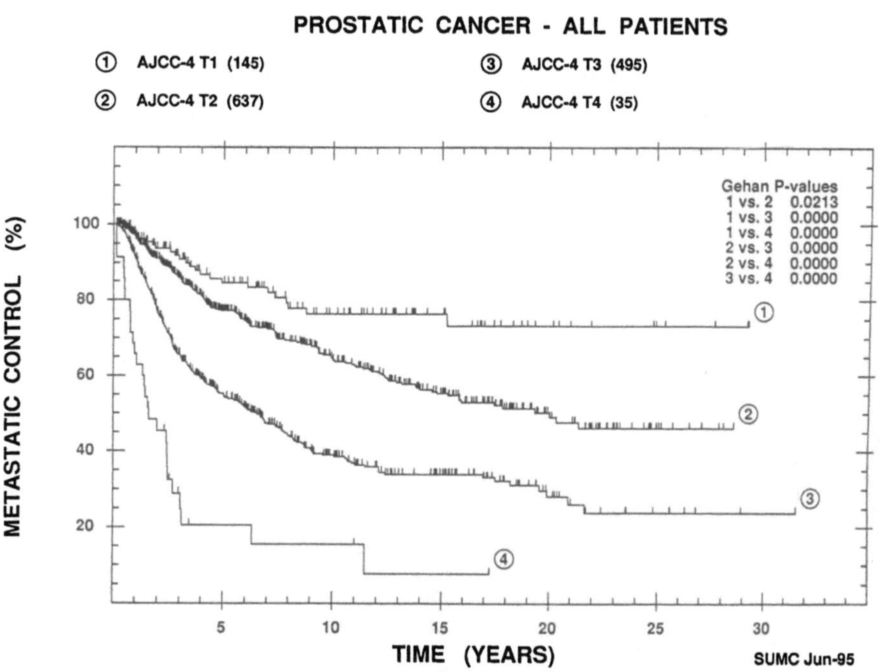

Fig. 17.8. Metastatic control. A *downward step* indicates the first evidence of recurrence at a metastatic site as detected by clinical observation, including roentgenograms or scintigrams, or a positive biopsy. An *upward tick* represents a patient who was either observed to be disease free or died after being disease free at the time of last observation

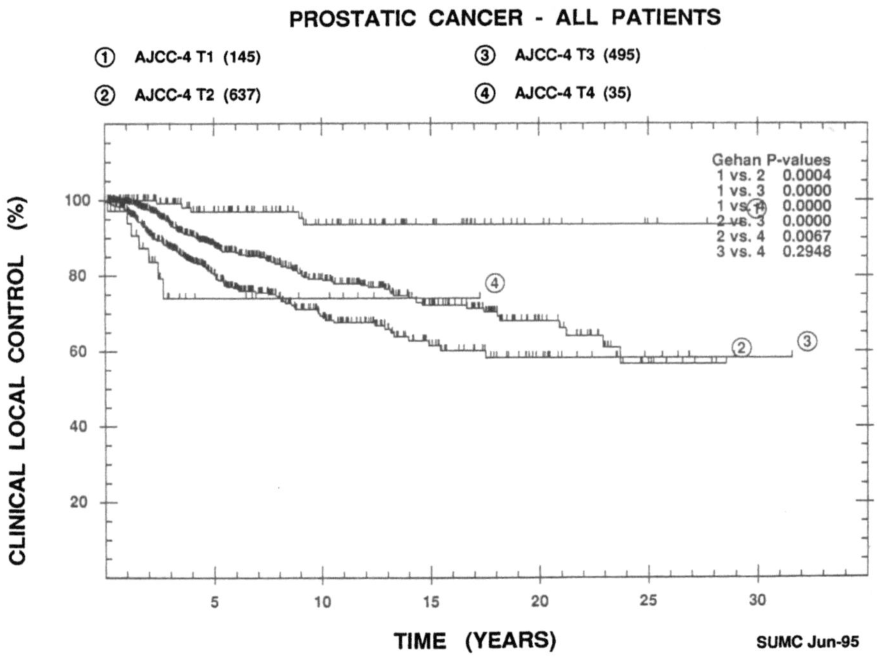

Fig. 17.9. Local control. A *downward step* indicates clinical evidence of local regrowth after initial regression of tumor or after an initial showing of no evidence of local neoplasm. An *upward tick* represents a patient who either demonstrated no clinical evidence of local tumor at last follow-up or died without clinical evidence of local neoplasm. Local control is probably a relatively "soft" observation, but it is important to have an appreciation of the efficacy of radiation therapy in the durable relief of local symptoms

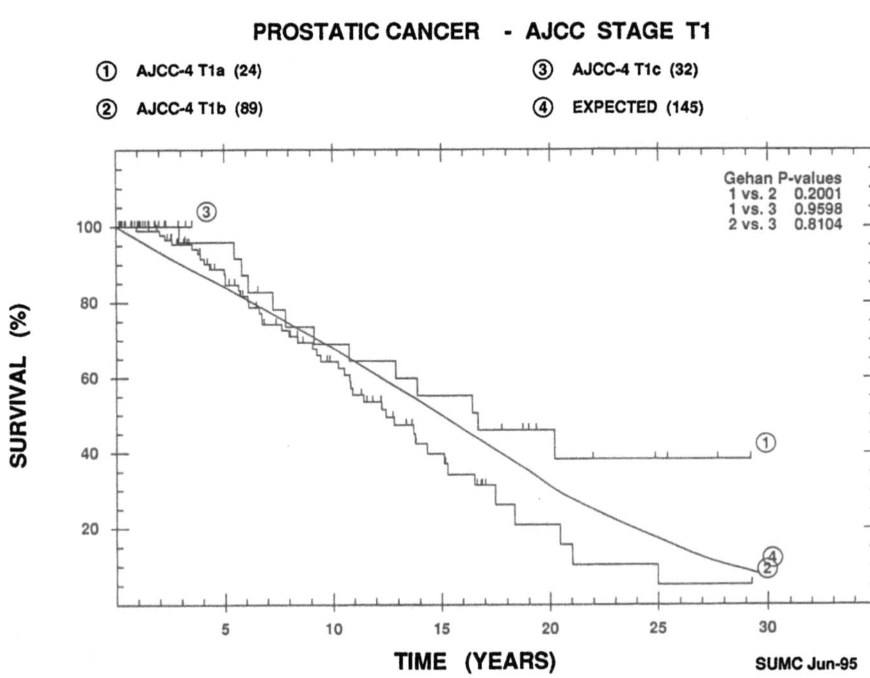

Fig. 17.10. Survival among patients with T1a, T1b, or T1c carcinoma of the prostate

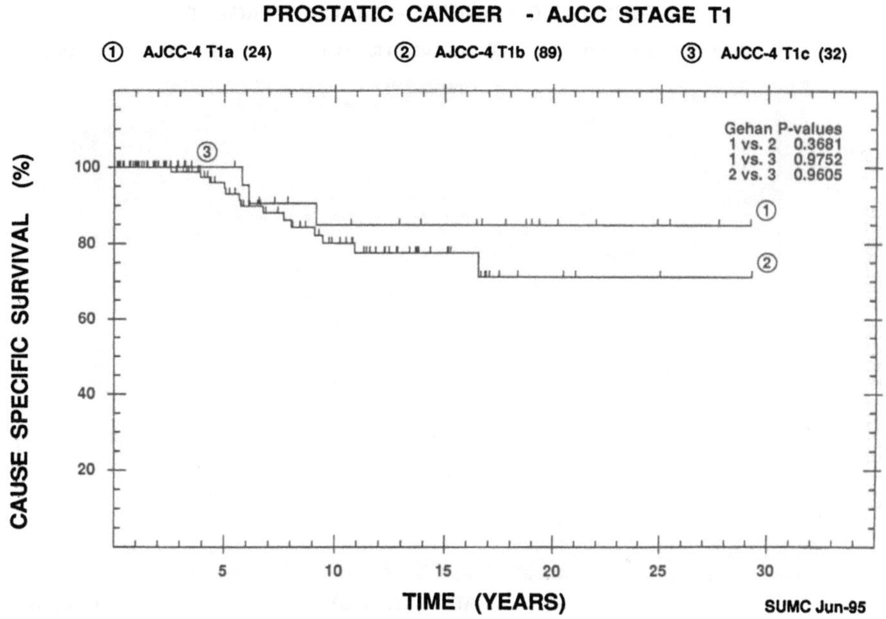

Fig. 17.11. Cause-specific survival among patients with T1a, T1b, or T1c disease

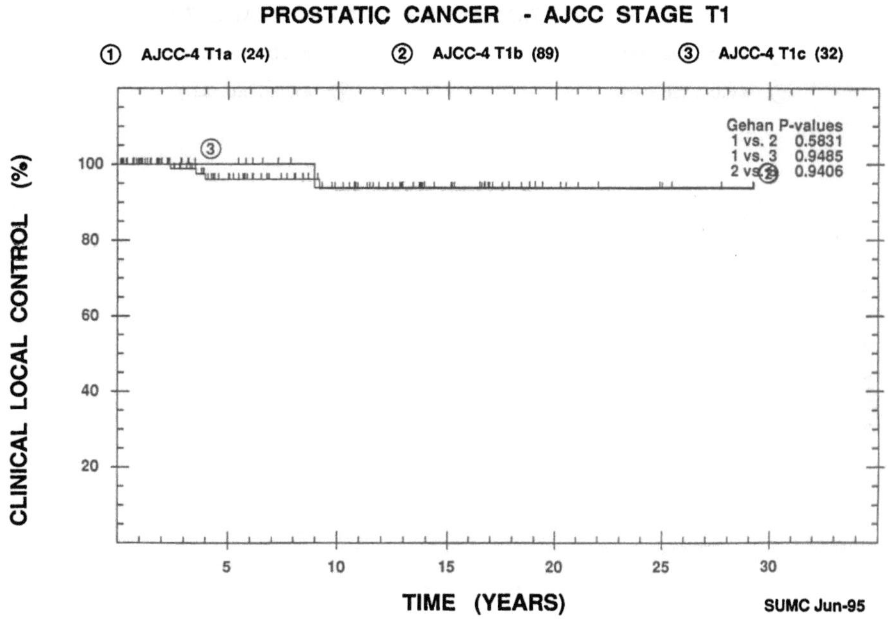

Fig. 17.12. Clinical local control among patients with T1a, T1b, or T1c disease

8–10 did poorly irrespective of endpoint and patients with Gleason sums of 6 and 7 were significantly more compromised than were those with Gleason sums of 2–5 with respect to freedom from relapse (Fig. 17.13). Curves for metastatic control are not shown, but they were nearly identical to Fig. 17.12.

17.2.3 T2 Category

Figure 17.14 demonstrates survival for subsets of T2 carcinoma of the prostate (nominal stage B). As was the case in T1 disease, the survival of T2a patients was identical to the age-matched cohort and is sig-

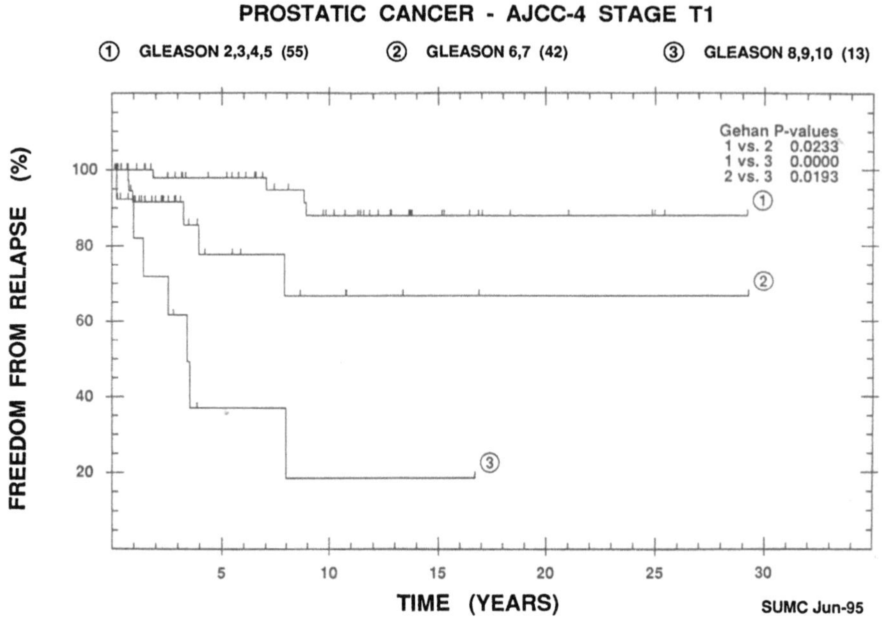

Fig. 17.13. Freedom from relapse among patients with T1 carcinoma of the prostate segregated by Gleason sums

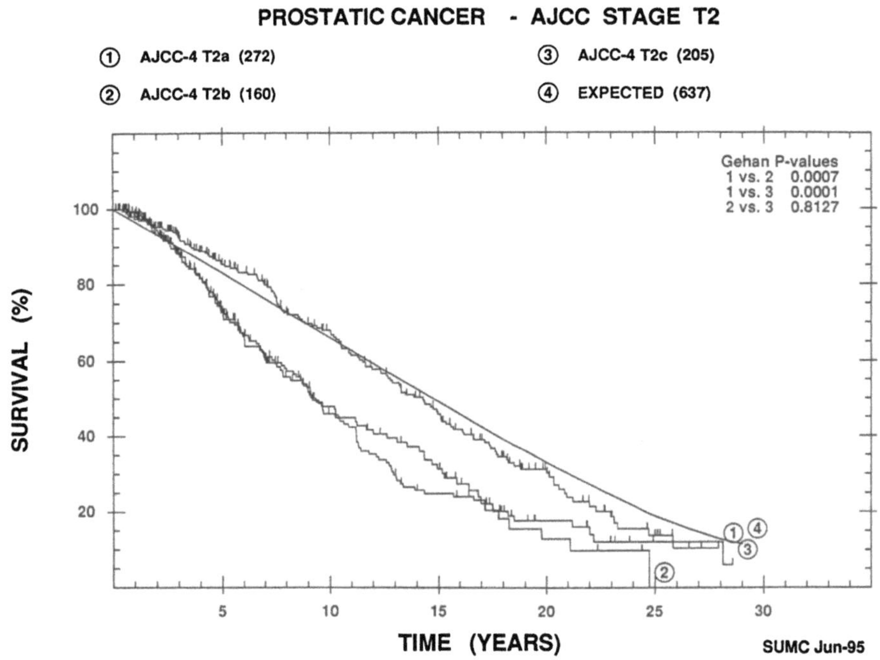

Fig. 17.14. Survival among patients with T2a, T2b, or T2c carcinoma of the prostate

nificantly better than for patients with T2b and T2c disease. Survival at 15 years was 49% for the age-matched cohort, 46% for T2a, 31% for T2b, and 25% for T2c. Cause-specific survival is shown in Figure 17.15. Relevant curves for freedom from relapse and metastatic control mimicked the survival curves.

17.2.4 T3 and T4 Categories

Figures 17.16–17.17 detail the survival parameters for T3 (nominal stage C) and T4 disease. While a substantial reduction in survival is shown for these more advanced categories, a 20% survival at 15 years was obtained in the group of 495 T3 patients. The T3a patients faired slightly better than the T3b and T3c patients with regard to survival (Fig. 17.16) and substantially better in terms of freedom from relapse (Fig. 17.17) and also metastatic control (51% at 15 years, not shown).

The median survival for T4 patients, however, was only 2.5 years (Fig. 17.5), essentially identical to that observed for patients who develop metastases (Fig. 17.3). These patients are probably best treated by androgen deprivation unless local symptoms indicate the need for palliative irradiation at the primary site.

17.2.5 Gleason Score Versus Survival

The Gleason pattern scores reflect a powerful correlation with outcome as illustrated by Figs. 17.18 and

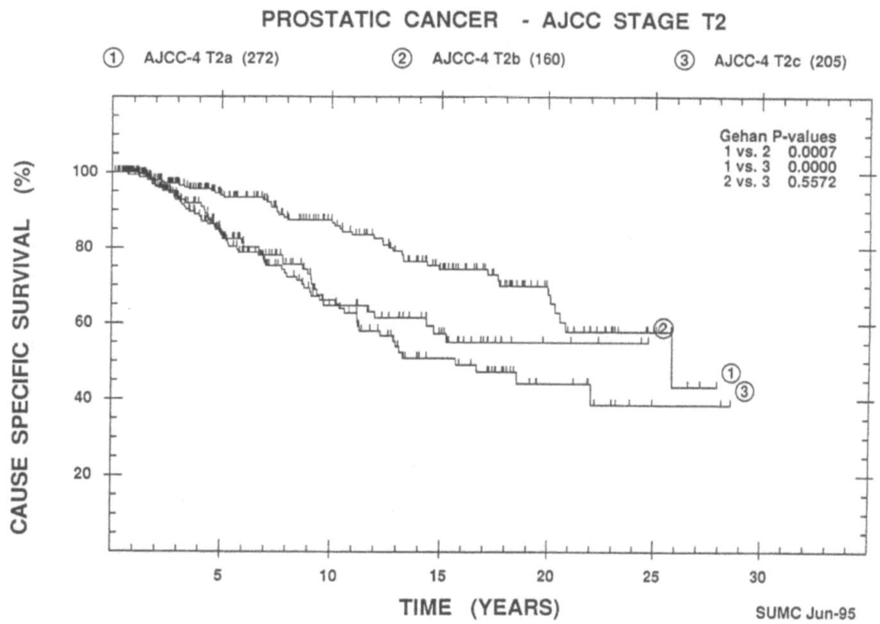

Fig. 17.15. Cause-specific survival among patients with T2a, T2b, or T2c carcinoma of the prostate

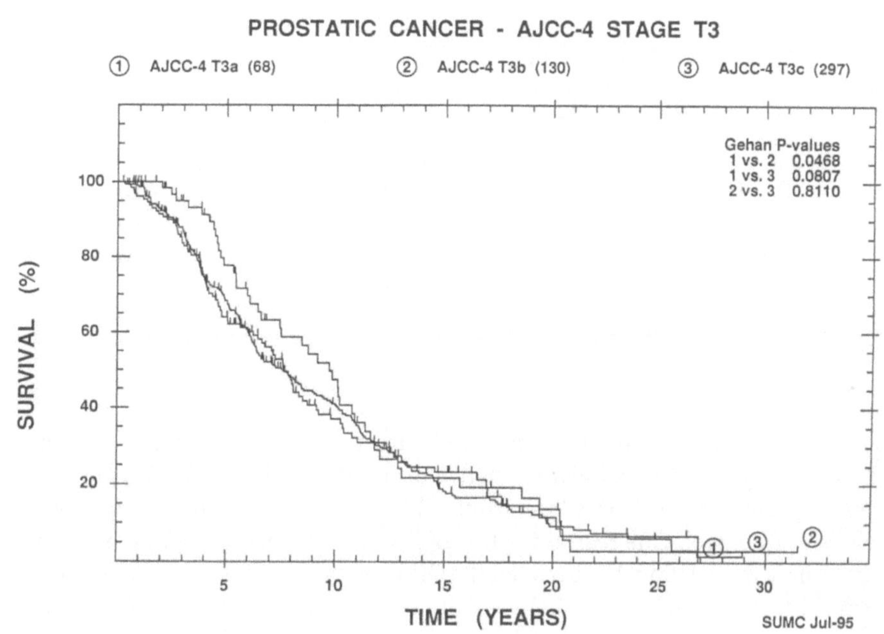

Fig. 17.16. Survival among patients with T3a, T3b, or T3c carcinoma of the prostate

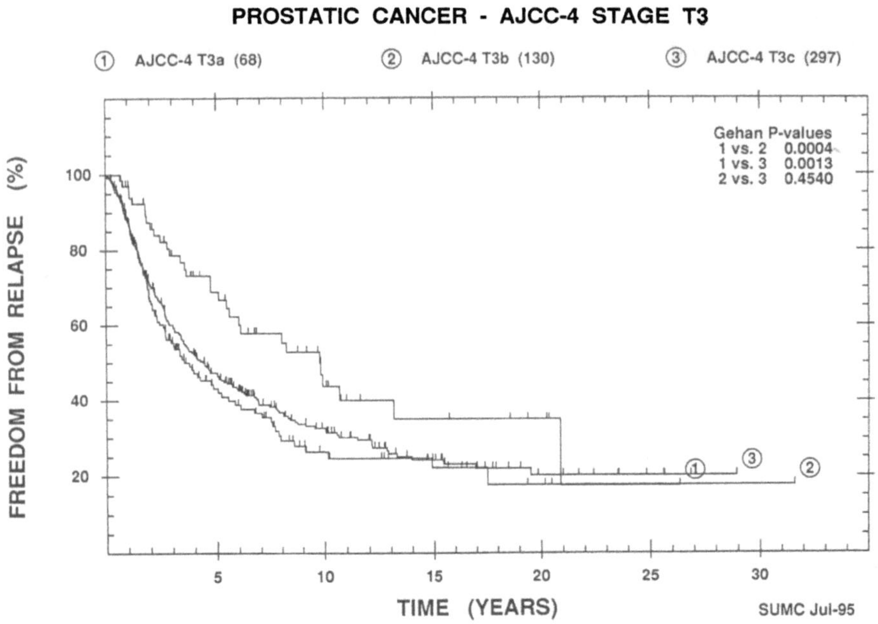

Fig. 17.17. Freedom from relapse among patients with T3a, T3b, or T3c carcinoma of the prostate

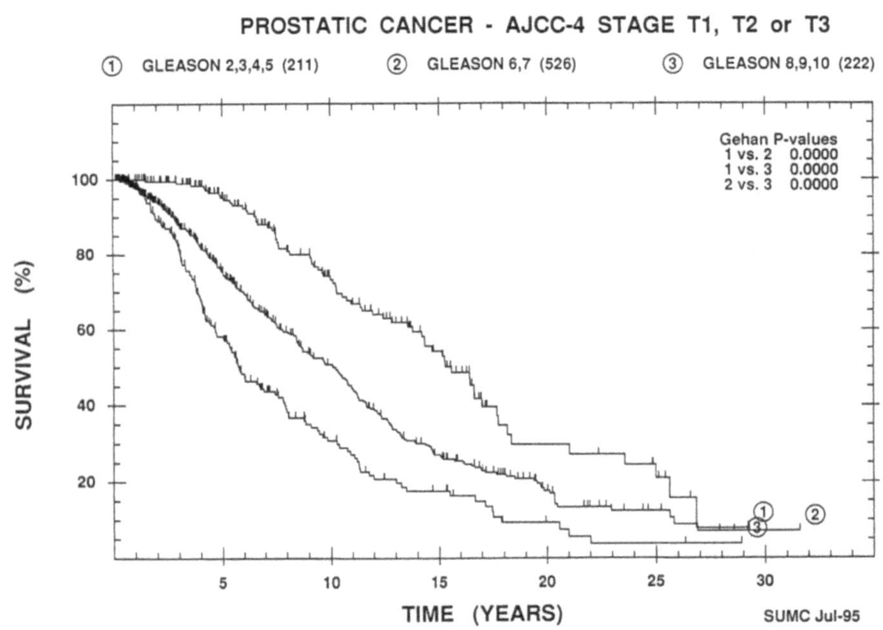

Fig. 17.18. Survival by Gleason sum among 959 patients who have been graded by the Gleason system

17.19. The Gleason sums were grouped into three distinct categories and compared relative to survival, cause-specific survival, freedom from relapse, and metastatic control. One reason for the differences in outcome is the relationship between the Gleason pattern score and lymph node involvement (PISTENMA et al. 1979). It was found that lymph nodes were rarely in involved with Gleason sums of 4 or less, but the incidence of lymph node metastases escalates 15% per Gleason unit beyond 4. Thus, the Gleason pattern score minus 4 × 15% = percentage probability of lymph node metastases (WOO et al. 1988). These data were collected and analyzed before the wide use of PSA monitoring. The predictive value of the Gleason scores has been refined by the inclusion of PSA values by ROACH et al. (1994).

17.2.6 Most Favorable Subgroup

Survival and disease-specific survival are presented for 417 patients with either T1 or T2a disease in Figure 17.20. Overall survival at 15 years was 46%, only 5% less than the 51% calculated for an age-matched cohort. The disease-specific survival for those 417 patients was 78% at 15 years. Figure 17.14 demonstrates a significant reduction in the survival parameters for T2b and T2c patients. Interestingly, selecting patients with T1 or T2a disease with surgically proven negative adenopathy (Fig. 17.21) further improved survival to 52% as compared to 56% for the age-matched cohort. These data are based on the

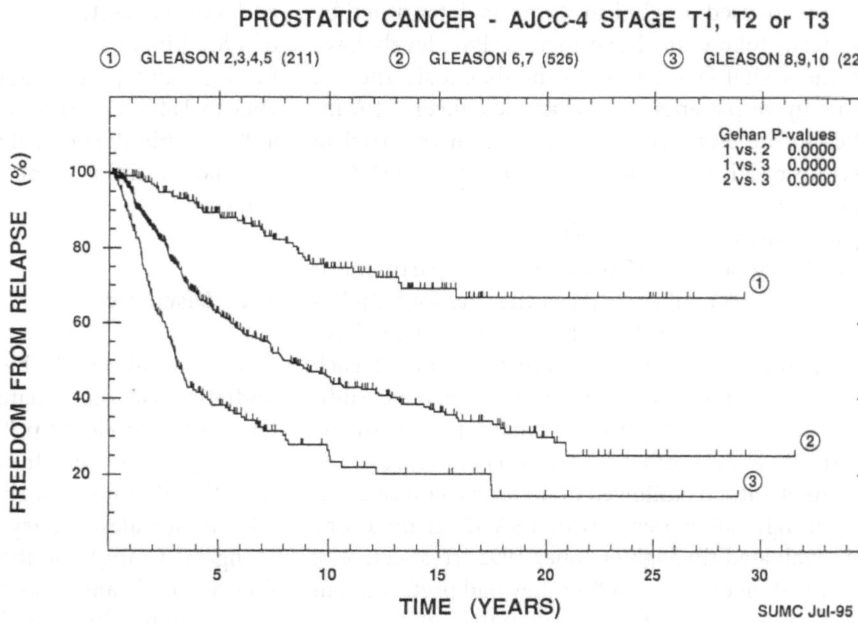

Fig. 17.19. Freedom from relapse as a function of grouped Gleason sums

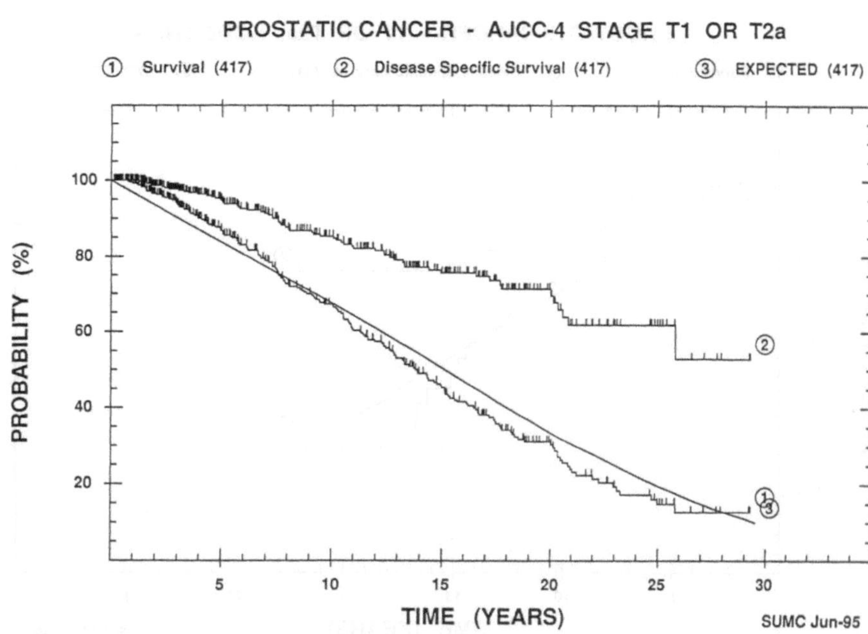

Fig. 17.20. Survival and disease (cause)-specific survival among 417 "most favorable" patients, including all T1 and T2a patients

outcome in 31 patients who had T1 or T2a disease and a staging laparotomy to evaluate lymph node status prior to irradiation.

17.2.7 PSA After Radiation Therapy

A complete examination of PSA kinetics after irradiation is beyond the scope of this presentation, which is focused on clinical status as determined by long-term follow-up. Nevertheless, PSA levels have become a vital factor in both the diagnosis and the follow-up of patients with prostatic cancer. PSA kinetics in the Stanford series have been reported in previous publications (KAPLAN et al. 1991, 1993; Cox et al. 1994).

Since the introduction of PSA testing at Stanford by the Yang polyclonal assay by the Department of Urology in 1985, all patients in the Stanford Radiation Oncology program with prostatic cancer have been evaluated at initial examination and at each post-treatment follow-up by serial PSA values. Additional PSA values have been obtained, usually by the Hybritech assay at other institutions for some of the treatment patients followed in their own community. Accordingly, all patients with PSA determinations were evaluated through October 1993 irrespective of the date of therapy or whether they had pretreatment PSA determinations. A summary of these data is presented in Table 17.3, which compares PSA data and clinical status within 2.5- and 5-year intervals between 2.5 and 25 years post-treatment. The normal range of serum PSA values is ≤4.0 with Hybritech/TOSOH assays or ≤7.4 with the Yang assay. The analysis represents a simple snapshot of the PSA values at the patient's follow-up visit closest to October 1993. One might question the wisdom of using isolated single PSA values as reflecting the patient's status at any one time. Cox et al. (1994) have done so and have presented a more sophisticated description of PSA kinetics which correlates well with clinical findings and patient outcome. Nevertheless, reference to Table 17.3 shows that 52% of the patients had a PSA within the normal range and that 78% of those with no clinical evidence of disease had normal PSA values.

17.3 Discussion

STAMEY et al. (1993) have challenged the Stanford Radiation Oncology data which are based on long-term clinical follow-up. They reviewed patients from the Department of Urology who were referred for radiation therapy (not all to Stanford) with respect to PSA values alone. They selected an upper limit of 1.7 ng/ml (Yang) for the analysis, whereas in fact, their normal range was 0–2.5 ng/ml. They identified 113 patients who were irradiated months to years before the starting date for their PSA analysis, which

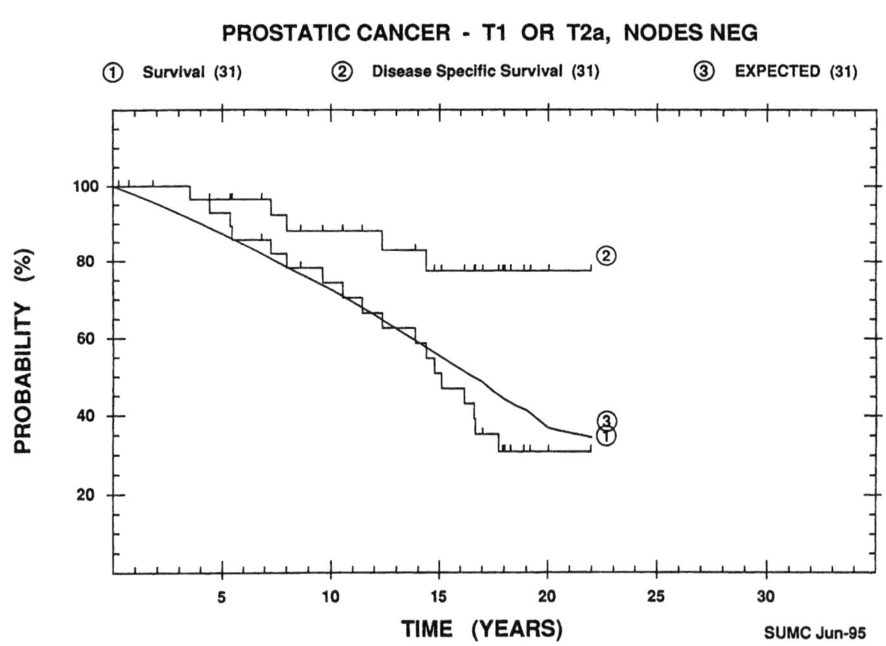

Fig. 17.21. Survival and disease (cause)-specific survival among patients included in Fig. 17.20 who also had no identifiable adenopathy as proven by pretreatment staging laparotomy

Table 17.3. Data regarding serum PSA values in patients not receiving hormonal treatment, as of October 1993

Time from RT (yrs)[a]	No. of pts.	No. without disease	No. with normal PSA[b]	% All pts. with normal PSA	% All NED pts. with normal PSA
0–2.5	176	158	122	69	77
2.5–5	114	69	57	50	83
5–10	83	46	35	42	76
10–15	73	35	24	33	69
15–20	44	23	18	41	78
20–25	14	9	8	57	89
Total	504	340	264	52	78

NED, No evidence of disease
[a] Time interval between the initiation of radiation and the last available follow-up PSA measurement
[b] Serum PSA levels ≤4.0 with Hybritech/TOSOH assays or ≤7.4 with the Yang assay

was April 1985. They reviewed the PSA values for the cohort of previously treated patients subjected to PSA testing between April 1985 and January 1988. The patients were drawn from a heterogeneous group encompassing all clinical stages and including those with known lymph node metastases (D1 patients, $n = 17$), those treated with ^{125}I implants ($n = 15$), and those treated by external beam irradiation at several different institutions. They concluded that radiotherapy cured only 20% of this group of patients and that 80% were made worse, which they attributed to clonogenic selection of more virulent cell types secondary to the radiation.

HANCOCK et al. (1995) have recently reviewed the Stanford Department of Radiation Oncology experience for the same period. They identified 110 patients treated exclusively with external beam irradiation during exactly the same period and found a 38% "cure rate." Furthermore, 42% of the patients without lymph node metastases were disease-free with stable normal PSA values at an average of 12.4 (range 4.4–24.8) years after treatment. Moreover, the authors presented compelling evidence to implicate early expression of occult metastases as the explanation for the markedly reduced doubling times. The authors suggest that STAMEY et al. (1993) underestimated the efficacy of external beam irradiation because of flawed case selection.

17.4 Conclusions

1. External beam irradiation remains a safe and effective option for the treatment of prostatic cancer.
2. Survival is strongly influenced by the extent of the primary tumor and at 15 years post-treatment remained at 45% for T1, 35% for T2, 20% for T3, and 5% for T4. The 15-year survival of an age-matched cohort was 49%.
3. The most favorable groups were T1 and T2a. Their survival at 15 years was 46% as compared to 51% for the age-matched cohort. T1 and T2a lymph node-negative patients had 52% survival at 15 years as compared to the 56% survival of an age-matched cohort.
4. While survival for T3 patients was 20%, it was slightly higher for the T3a group. Perhaps more importantly, the T3a patients achieved a freedom from relapse of 35% and metastatic control of 51% at 15 years. This strongly suggests that radiotherapy not only offered a modest 20% long-term survival in those locally advanced patients, but also substantially reduced the probability of relapse or metastatic disease.
5. Patients with T4 disease exhibited a survival pattern nearly identical to patients with known distant metastases and are probably best treated by androgen deprivation supplemented, if indicated, by local prostatic irradiation of the primary for palliation of local symptoms.

References

Bagshaw MA (1992) Carcinoma of the prostate. In: Levitt SH, Khan FM, Potish RS (eds), Levitt and Tapley's technological basis of radiation therapy: practical clinical applications. Lea & Febiger, Philadelphia, pp 300–322
Bagshaw MA (1993) The challenge of radiation treatment of carcinoma of the prostate. In: Lepor H, Lawson RK (eds) Prostate diseases. Saunders, Philadelphia, pp 326–346
Bagshaw MA, Kaplan HS (1962) Radical external radiation therapy of localized prostatic carcinom. Proceedings of Tenth International Congress of Radiology, September 1962
Bagshaw MA, Kaplan HS, Sagerman RH (1965) Linear accelerator supervoltage radiotherapy. VII. Carcinoma of the prostate. Radiology 85:121–129

Bagshaw MA, Cox RS, Hancock SL (1994) Control of prostate cancer with radiotherapy: long-term results. J Urol 152:1781–1785
Barringer BS (1922) Carcinoma of prostate. Surg Gynecol Obstet 34:168
Beahrs OH, Henson DE, Hutter RVP, Kennedy BJ (1992) Manual for staging of cancer. American Joint Committee on Cancer, 4th edn. Lippincott, Philadelphia
Budhraja SN, Anderson JC (1964) An assessment of the value of radiotherapy in the management carcinoma of the prostate. Br J Urol 36:535
Carlton CJ, Dawoud F, Hudgins P, Scott RJ (1972) Irradiation treatment of carcinoma of the prostate: a preliminary report based on 8 years of experience. J Urol 108:924–927
Cox RS, Kaplan ID, Bagshaw MA (1994) Prostate-specific antigen kinetics after external beam irradiation for carcinoma of the prostate. Int J Radiat Oncol Biol Phys 28:23–31
Flocks RH, Kerr HD, Elkins HB, Culp D (1952) Treatment of carcinoma of the prostate by interstitial radiation with radioactive gold (Au^{198}): a preliminary report. J Urol 68:510
Gehan EA (1965) A generalized Wilcoxon test for comparing arbitrarily singly-censored samples. Biometrika 52:203
Hancock SL, Cox RS, Bagshaw MA (1995) Prostate specific antigen after radiotherapy for prostate cancer: a re-evaluation of long term biochemical control and the kinetics of recurrence in patients treated at Stanford. J Urol 154:1412–1417
Hilaris BS, Whitmore WF, Grabstald H, O'Kelly PJ (1972) Radical radiation therapy of cancer the prostate: a new approach using interstitial and external sources. Clin Bull 2:94
Hultberg S (1946) Results of treatment with radiotherapy in carcinoma of the prostate. Acta Radiol 27:339
Kaplan ID, Cox RS, Bagshaw MA (1991) A model of prostatic carcinoma tumor kinetics based on prostate specific antigen levels after radiation therapy. Cancer 68:400–405
Kaplan ID, Cox RS, Bagshaw MA (1993) Prostate specific antigen after external beam radiotherapy for prostatic cancer: follow-up. J Urol 149:519–522
Lai PP, Pilepich MV, Krall JM, et al. (1991) The effect of overall treatment time on the outcome of definitive radiotherapy for localized prostate carcinoma: the Radiation Therapy Oncology Group 75-06 and 77-06 experience. Int J Radiat Oncol Biol Phys 21:925–933
Laramore GE, Krall JM, Thomas FJ, Griffin TW, Maor MH, Hendrickson FR (1985) Fast neutron radiotherapy for locally advanced prostate cancer: results of an RTOG randomized study. Int J Radiat Oncol Biol Phys 11:1621–1627
Mellinger GT, Gleason D, Bailar J, 3rd (1967) The histology and prognosis of prostatic cancer. J Urol 97:331–337
Paschkis R, Tittinger W (1910) Radiumbehandlung eines Prostatasarkoms. Wein Klin Wochenschr 48
Pasteau O (1911) Traiment du cancer de la prostate par le radium. Revue des Maladies de la Nutrition 363
Pistenma DA, Bagshaw MA, Freiha FS (1979) Extended-field radiation therapy for prostatic adenocarcinoma: status report of a limited prospective trial. In: Johnson DE, Samuels ML (eds) Cancer of the genitourinary tract. Raven Press, New York, pp 229–247
Roach M 3rd, Marquez C, Yuo HS, et al. (1994) Predicting the risk of lymph node involvement using the pretreatment prostate specific antigen and Gleason score in men with clinically localized prostate cancer. Int J Radiat Oncol Biol Phys 28:33–37
Shipley WU, Tepper JE, Prout GJ, et al. (1979) Proton radiation as boost therapy for localized prostatic carcinoma. JAMA 241:1912–1915
Stamey TA, Ferrari MK, Schmid HP (1993) The value of serial prostate specific antigen determinations 5 years after radiotherapy: steeply increasing values characterize 80% of patients. J Urol 150:1856–1859
Syed AM, Puthawala A, Tansey LA, et al. (1983) Management of prostate carcinoma. Combination of pelvic lymphadenectomy, temporary Ir-192 implantation, and external irradiation. Radiology 149:829–833
von Essen CF, Bagshaw MA, Bush SE, Smith AR, Kligerman MM (1987) Long-term results of pion therapy at Los Alamos. Int J Radiat Oncol Biol Phys 13:1389–1398
Widman BP (1934) Cancer of the prostate. The results of radium and roentgen-ray treatment. Radiology 22:153
Woo S, Kaplan I, Roach M, Bagshaw M (1988) Formula to estimate risk of pelvic lymph node metastasis from the total Gleason score for prostate cancer (letter to the editor). J Urol 140:387
Young HH, Fronz WA (1917) Some new methods in the treatment of carcinoma of the lower genitourinary tract with radium. J Urol 1:505

18 Use of Brachytherapy Techniques in the Management of Carcinoma of the Prostate

L.W. Brady, B. Micaily, C.T. Miyamoto, B.J. Costleigh, W.A. Longton, J.E. Freire, and P. Montemaggi

CONTENTS

18.1 Introduction

Prostate cancer is the most common as well as the most frequently irradiated malignancy involving the genitourinary tract. In 1995, the American Cancer Society anticipates that in the United States there will be 244 000 new cases diagnosed with 40 400 deaths due to the disease process (American Cancer Society 1995). In addition, it is among the most successfully treated cancers of the genitourinary tract in terms of both definitive outcome and metastatic presentations.

Despite these data, the appropriate treatment for this disease remains controversial. Treatment recommendations have ranged from expectant observation to radical prostatectomy, external beam radiation therapy, and brachytherapy. Brachytherapy has a long and successful history in the treatment of many malignancies, such as carcinomas of the cervix, breast, endometrium, and head and neck. Efforts to treat cancer of the prostate by interstitial implantation techniques date back to the early part of the twentieth century, with the use of interstitial implantation of radon seeds and radium needles, followed in the 1940s and 1950s by the injection of radioactive colloidal gold into the prostate in an effort to deliver radiation dosages specifically to the prostate itself.

18.2 Historical Overview

Over the past 20 years, there have been significant improvements in the technology for treatment of the prostate by brachytherapy techniques. These improvements have been stimulated by the availability of new radionuclides, innovative afterloading techniques, computer-based dosimetry, modern imaging modalities useful in determining the volume to be implanted, and better understanding of the radiobiologic characteristics associated with the different dose rates of radiation delivery.

The earliest published report of brachytherapy for treatment of cases of cancer of the prostate was by Pasteau, in 1911; the treatment entailed the simple insertion of a radium source into the prostatic urethra by way of a catheter. In 1922, Denning pub-

L.W. Brady, MD, Professor and Chairman, Department of Radiation Oncology and Nuclear Medicine, Medical College of Pennsylvania and Hahnemann University, 230 N. Broad Street, Philadelphia, PA 19102-1192, USA
B. Micaily, MD, Associate Professor, Department of Radiation Oncology and Nuclear Medicine, Medical College of Pennsylvania and Hahnemann University, 230 N. Broad Street, Philadelphia, PA 19102-1192, USA
C.T. Miyamoto, MD, Assistant Professor, Department of Radiation Oncology and Nuclear Medicine, Medical College of Pennsylvania and Hahnemann University, 230 N. Broad Street, Philadelphia, PA 19102-1192, USA
B.J. Costleigh, MD, Clinical Instructor of Radiation Oncology, Department of Radiation Oncology and Nuclear Medicine, Medical College of Pennsylvania and Hahnemann University, 230 N. Broad Street, Philadelphia, PA 19102-1192, USA
W.A. Longton, MD, Resident, Department of Radiation Oncology and Nuclear Medicine, Medical College of Pennsylvania and Hahnemann University, 230 N. Broad Street, Philadelphia, PA 19102-1192, USA
J.E. Freire, MD, Assistant Professor, Department of Radiation Oncology and Nuclear Medicine, Medical College of Pennsylvania and Hahnemann University, 230 N. Broad Street, Philadelphia, PA 19102-1192, USA
P. Montemaggi, MD, Visiting Scientist, Department of Radiation Oncology and Nuclear Medicine,, Medical College of Pennsylvania and Hahnemann University, 230 N. Broad Street, Philadelphia, PA 19102-1192, USA and Assistant Professor, Institute of Radiology, Department of Radiation Therapy, Catholic University of the Sacred Heart, Rome, Italy

lished a series of 100 cases treated by this technique and even though the follow-up was short-term, local control of the disease was surprisingly good for this rather unsophisticated technique and management. However, complications were significant, occurring in 15%–20% of patients.

Several decades later, other techniques for treatment of the prostate were introduced, stimulated by the development in 1956 of megavoltage external beam radiation therapy as a radiotherapeutic management technique for localized prostate cancer.

Although the numerous technical improvements that characterize the transperineal brachytherapy approaches are promising, no long-term data exist to confirm improved treatment results; this is particularly true when criteria for patient selection are precisely defined. Most investigators have employed the new technology of modern transperineal implantation techniques. However, technical variations are common, particularly in the use of transrectal ultrasonography, computed tomography, magnetic resonance imaging (MRI), and fluoroscopy. Because of the brevity of follow-up, most authors have relied on prostate-specific antigen (PSA) response as an indicator of treatment success or failure. Histologic evaluation by postimplant biopsy of these transperineal techniques has not been published.

Clinical and PSA responses for the studies available using iodine-125 or palladium-103 are referred to in Table 18.1. Although the relationship of early PSA normalization to long-term clinical tumor control is uncertain, these early reported treatment results appear favorable. Allowing for selection of patients suitable for iodine-125 implantation, namely those with smaller tumors, these results appear at least equivalent to those which have been observed with the use of external beam radiation therapy or radical prostatectomy.

Complications of transperineal implantation techniques have been low, with about 75% of patients who were potent before the treatment remaining potent afterwards. However, longer follow-ups are needed.

Cancer of the prostate is most commonly a disease of glandular origin; it is peripheral and multifocal in 75% of the prostatectomy specimens (Jewett 1980; Byar and Mostofi 1973). Early tumors are usually asymptomatic whereas more advanced tumors cause urinary obstructive symptoms or pain due to metastatic disease. In general, 75% of patients present with stage B, C, and D lesions (Murphy et al. 1982). A recent trend toward earlier diagnosis has been identified based primarily on the utilization of PSA screening and digital rectal examinations in asymptomatic men. The staging of prostate cancer varies among different institutions but the most common systems are shown in Table 18.2 (Brady et al. 1991). Cancer of the prostate represents the second most common cause of death from cancer in men, and about 70% of patients receive no specific treatment beyond the establishment of the diagnosis (American Cancer Society 1995). However, in 1995, there is a trend toward more patients being treated based on earlier diagnosis. It has often been stated that no treatment can effectively alter the overall survival from a disease that is often metastatic at the time of presentation (Johansson et al. 1989). However, Jewett et al. (1972) identified about 5% of all patients who would benefit from radical prostatectomy. Bagshaw (1980) identified the efficacy of definitive or curative external beam radiation therapy in achieving local control without the mor-

Table 18.1. Clinical and PSA response following transperineal brachytherapy

Reference	No. of patients	Stages	Isotope	Clinically disease-free (%)	PSA control (%)	Follow-up (years)
Blasko et al. (1995b)	197	T1b–T2b	^{125}I	95	93[a]	5
Blasko et al. (1995a)	97	T1b–T2b	^{103}Pd	95	86[a]	4
Kaye et al. (1995)	45	T1–T2	^{125}I	–	98[b]	2
Wallner et al.	62	T1b–T2b	^{125}I	90	83[c]	3
Blasko et al. (1994)	99	T2a–T3	XRT + ^{103}Pd	84	64[a]	5
Kaye et al. (1995)	31	T1–T2	XRT + ^{125}I	–	95[b]	2

XRT, external beam radiation therapy
[a] Defined as PSA <1.0 ng/ml
[b] Defined as PSA <4.0 ng/ml
[c] Defined as a lack of PSA progression, regardless of level

Table 18.2. Prostate cancer staging systems

Stage	Characteristics	TNM
A_1	Incidental finding <foci, grade I	T1A
A_2	Incidental finding >foci, grade II, III	T1B
B_1	Palpable nodule <1.5 cm	T2A
B_2	Palpable nodule >1.5 cm or diffuse involvement of gland	T2B
C_1	Extracapsular extension	T3
C_2	Seminal vesicle, bladder neck, or lateral pelvic involvement	
D_1	Extensive pelvic involvement or pelvic nodal disease	N1–2
D_2	Bone, extrapelvic node, or soft tissue metastases	M1

bidity or mortality of radical prostatectomy. The dramatic resolution of prostate cancer upon use of estrogen therapy led to enthusiasm for hormonal manipulation, but it has been shown that this treatment regimen does not affect long-term survival (WHITMORE 1956). More recent data relating to the use of gonadotropin hormone-releasing hormone analogs and/or 5× reductase inhibitors including Lupron and Eulexin, indicate that these agents have not only enhanced the overall quality of survival but also lengthened it, and have proved to be effective when used in combination with radiation therapy in curative management.

18.3 Biopsy Technique: Effect on Survival

The ideal biopsy technique to establish the diagnosis has not been found. The use of transurethral resection has been noted to increase the potential for metastatic disease, to decrease survival, and to alter the treatment outcome (McGOWAN 1980; HANKS et al. 1983; ROSEN et al. 1984). It has been postulated that this is caused by dissemination of tumor cells at the time of the transurethral resection. However, it may also represent a selection bias since patients with bulky disease or high-grade tumors are those most likely to require transurethral resection. An adverse impact of transurethral resection was noted specifically in moderately or poorly differentiated stage C tumors by HANKS et al. (1985), and it was in this group of patients that the recommendation was made for a 5 Gy tumor dose delivered to the prostate prior to the transurethral resection in order to diminish the potential for metastatic dissemination. PEREZ et al. (1980) found no adverse effect of transurethral resection in patient groups corrected for clinical stage and degree of tumor differentiation. Needle biopsy, via the transperineal or transrectal approach using ultrasonography- or MRI-guided methods, is the most commonly used technique to establish the diagnosis of adenocarcinoma of the prostate.

18.4 Pelvic Lymph Node Involvement

Involvement of regional lymph nodes is relatively common in prostatic carcinoma. The risk of positive disease is closely related to the stage and grade of the tumor. The periprostatic and obturator lymph nodes are the primary drainage sites, followed by external iliac, internal iliac, common iliac, and periaortic lymph node groups. GLEASON and MELLINGER (1974) defined a grading system based on the major and minor histologic patterns of the tumor, with the combined score accurately predicting the risk of metastatic disease in lymph nodes and survival. BAGSHAW (1986a) observed no lymph node metastases in 449 surgically staged patients with a Gleason score of 5 or less.

Since lymph node invasion correlates adversely with survival (75% distant metastases at 5 years in positive lymph node patients) it would seem important to identify those patients with occult nodal spread in order to offer them more extensive treatment (WHITMORE et al. 1979). Lymphangiographic studies are poor indicators of nodal disease due to the inconsistent visualization of the obturator lymph nodes on bipedal lymphangiograms. Laparotomy for lymph node biopsy is able to detect occult nodal disease in 40% of the localized cases; this includes 7% in stage B1 lesions, 43% in stage B2 lesions, and 60% in stage C lesions (FOWLER and WHITMORE 1981). However, staging laparotomy is associated with significant morbidity, including a 20%–25% chance of lower extremity edema (PEREZ 1983). Since lymphadenectomy is only useful as a prognostic and diagnostic procedure and not as a therapeutic procedure, it is difficult to justify this morbidity risk. Recent data indicate laparoscopic approaches to be as efficient as laparotomy in detecting occult nodal disease, but morbidity is much lower.

Among some urologists, the presence of lymph node involvement indicates an incurable disease. On the other hand, however, the utilization of whole pelvic irradiation where these lymph node groups are included within the volume being irradiated allows for the treatment of not only the local but also the regional disease process with an associated improvement in survival.

18.5 Bone Metastases

Bony metastatic disease has been postulated to reflect the venous drainage of the prostate and, therefore, to favor the vertebral bodies and pelvic bones. This hypothesis is predicated on the fact that deep pelvic veins have no valves and are in direct communication with the vertebral venous system (BATSON 1942). However, the distribution of metastases in the periphery of the body is now better appreciated due to the availability of bone scans, and the predominance of central metastatic disease may only reveal the increased regional blood flow at these sites.

18.6 Radical Prostatectomy

The chief therapeutic approaches to localized prostatic carcinoma include radical surgery, implantation of radioactive materials into the prostate itself, and external beam radiation therapy; further options include cryosurgery, the use of antitestosterone agents such as LH-RH agonists, and hyperthermia. Radical prostatectomy by either a transperineal or a retropubic approach was reported by WALSH and JEWETT (1980) to achieve a 51% 15-year survival rate in patients with stage B1 disease while patients with stage B2 disease had only a 26% 15-year survival. It is often not possible to determine accurately the stage of the cancer preoperatively. Radical prostatectomy is associated with a substantial chronic morbidity, with 5%–10% long-term incontinence, 15%–20% short-term incontinence, and nearly 100% erectile impotence (see Chaps. 9, 11, and 12 for details). It was because of these complications that WALSH (1986) described a modified technique of prostatectomy designed to preserve the neurovascular bundle that provides for erectile potency. This essentially is an intracapsular removal of the prostate tissue leaving the neurovascular bundle intact. This procedure has resulted in less morbidity in preliminary studies, with potency being maintained in 69% of 250 patients who had unilateral preservation of the neurovascular bundle and were followed up for at least 1 year (WALSH 1986). Reportedly, the incontinence rate was also decreased to 5%. However, long-term survival and local control rates are still not available. The knowledge that prostate carcinoma is a disease of the peripheral subcapsular gland and that it often involves the distal end of the gland periurethrally makes the intentional transection of the gland to preserve potency and continence a worrisome approach (BRESLOW et al. 1977). Additionally, the widespread application of a surgical technique without information on its 5-year efficacy needs further study, especially since the selection criteria for this procedure are being expanded to include patients with more advanced disease.

18.7 External Beam Irradiation

The use of external megavoltage radiation therapy was first popularized by BAGSHAW (1980). The most recent results from Stanford University as well as three other large recent reports are summarized in Table 18.3 (ROSEN et al. 1984; PEREZ et al. 1986;

Table 18.3. Definitive external beam irradiation results in patients with prostate cancer

Author/institution	Year	No.	Stage	Results			
				5 years	8 years	10 years	15 years
ROSEN et al., Harvard Jt. Ctr.	1984	198	A: 25	96%	82%		
			B: 85	77%	63%		
			C: 88	61%	38%		
PEREZ et al., Mallinckrodt	1986	327	A_2: 10	100%			
			B: 113	72%		60%	
			C_1: 107	60%		55%	
			C_2: 97	40%		35%	
BAGSHAW, Stanford	1986	898	A/B: 491	81%		60%	35%
			C: 407	61%		36%	18%
HANKS et al., Patterns of Care	1987	668	A: 60	85%		61%	
			B: 312	75%		46%	
			C: 296	58%		38%	

BAGSHAW 1986b; HANKS et al. 1987). These studies indicate that prostate cancer has a dose-response curve; in the local disease extent a dosage of at least 60–65 Gy over 6–7 weeks is required for early lesions, and 65–70 Gy over 7–8 weeks for stage C disease utilizing a shrinking field technique. Radiation doses higher than 70 Gy over 7–8 weeks have not been associated with increased local control or increased survival and are associated with increased morbidity. The morbidity associated with external beam radiation therapy of prostate cancer is shown in Table 18.4 (PILEPICH et al. 1984). Many of these patients had surgical evaluation of the lymph nodes prior to treatment, which is known to increase morbidity when combined with radiation therapy. Of those patients who had not been staged surgically, none developed genital or lower extremity edema. In the Patterns of Care review of 668 patients treated from 1973 to 1975 with a 10-year follow-up, data indicated a reduction in complications from 6% to 3% by changing from a two- to a four-field treatment technique (HANKS 1986).

The addition of concomitant hormonal therapy to radiation therapy was initially found to be of no benefit in terms of local tumor control or the delay of distant metastatic disease (PEREZ et al. 1986). However, recent studies under the aegis of the Radiation Therapy Oncology Group have shown that Zoladex administered prior to radiation therapy or concomitantly with radiation therapy improves the potential not only for local control but also for survival. Hormonal therapy, either by orchiectomy or supplemental estrogens or by LH/RH agonists, is useful in relieving bone metastatic pain and should be reserved for the treatment of metastatic disease. Strontium-89 therapy also can be used for widespread distant metastatic bone disease with efficient and effective benefit.

Table 18.4. Summary of morbidity related to external beam irradiation in 526 patients (Radiation Therapy Oncology Group 75-06)

	Grade					Total	
	1	2	3	4	5	No.	(%)
Cystitis	30	28	8			66	(12%)
Diarrhea	20	30	1			51	(9.7%)
Proctitis	14	20	6	1		41	(7.8%)
Genital and/or leg edema	7	13	5			25	(4.8%)
Melena	14	6	2		1	23	(4.4%)
Hematuria	4	4	8			16	(3.0%)
Urethral stricture			12			12	(2.3%)
Suprapubic fibrosis-edema	8	1				9	(1.7%)
Rectal-anal stricture	4	2	1			7	(1.3%)
Vesical neck contracture			2	1		3	(0.6%)
Rectal ulcer		1	2			3	(0.6%)
Bowel obstruction				2		2	(0.4%)

18.8 Iodine-125 Seed Implantation

HILARIS (1975) popularized the technique of implantation of radioactive iodine-125 seeds into the prostate following pelvic lymphadenectomy in patients with localized prostate cancer. This technique administered high-dose local radiation to the prostate only. Iodine-125 brachytherapy gained wide acceptance in the United States, with treatment results equivalent to those achieved by radical prostatectomy (HILARIS 1986; BATATA et al. 1980; GILES and BRADY 1986).

Iodine-125 seed implantation is performed at the time of a retropubic operative intervention. It is preceded by lymph node dissection or lymph node biopsy. The theoretical advantage of this technique is that it allows for the concentration of the radiation dose in the precise area that requires treatment. Higher radiation doses are obtainable than would be possible if external beam radiation therapy techniques were employed. The limitations of this brachytherapy are that it requires a surgical approach, does not irradiate the regional lymphatics, and delivers the radiation dose at a very low dose rate which may be less efficacious than that at which external beam radiation therapy is delivered. HILARIS (1986) and BATATA et al. (1980) have reported a 5-year survival rate of 96%, 76%, and 69% in patients with T1, T2, and T3 lesions, respectively. Delivering an adequate dose to the entire prostate had led to results equivalent or superior to those obtained with other therapeutic modalities. It is, however, a technically difficult procedure and it is not uniformly applicable in all medical centers. In those patients who are found to have positive lymph nodes at the time of surgery, the addition of external beam radiation therapy to iodine-125 seed implantation does not improve treatment results but does increase significantly the complications (HILARIS 1975). In the data from the Hahnemann University experience, the diagnosis of adenocarcinoma of the prostate was made by either needle biopsy or transurethral resection of the prostate (BRADY et al. 1991). A total of 983 patients were seen for evaluation of prostate cancer at Hahnemann University in the period from 1960 to

1988. The treatment outcomes in patients treated by radioactive iodine-125 implantation were compared with those in a similar group of patients treated by external beam radiation therapy. All patients had the stage of disease assessed by history, physical examination, bone scan, computerized tomography, imaging of the pelvis, and prostatic acid phosphatase studies. These data were accrued before the advent of PSA. Lymphangiograms were not performed routinely because of the disappointing diagnostic accuracy of this procedure. The clinical stage of the primary tumor and the pathologic stage of the removed lymph nodes were reported using the staging system of Whitmore, which was a modification of the American Joint Commission System. The tumors were graded according to degree of anaplasia and glandular formation into well differentiated, moderately well differentiated, and poorly differentiated (Koprowski et al. 1991).

Those individuals receiving iodine-125 implantation had no obvious evidence of disease beyond the prostate at the time of the clinical assessment. At the time of the operation, lymph node dissection or biopsies were carried out and frozen sections were obtained. If the lymph nodes were positive, the patients were rejected as candidates for iodine-125 implantation. Solely those individuals who had limited localized disease involving the prostate only were accepted for the iodine-125 implantation protocol.

The implantation procedure used was similar to that of the Memorial Sloan-Kettering Cancer Center using the Mick applicator (Hilaris 1975). The total activity of the seeds to be implanted was calculated using the dimension averaging system tables with the activity of each seed generally in the range of 0.5 mCi. The desired minimum peripheral radiation dose rate was 180 cGy per hour. Computer calculation of the achieved dose or total decay of the iodine-125 was performed after the implant using stereo-shift films. The patients were monitored following implantation by careful attention to the urine and feces for the presence of iodine seeds. One patient lost eight seeds and several patients lost less than five seeds but the remaining dosimetry was considered acceptable after recalculation. The centrally placed seeds within the higher dose area were the ones that tended to be lost.

In the early stage of the study, four patients revealed positive lymph node disease on permanent sections of the lymph nodes and had additional external beam radiation therapy as a supplemental treatment. The plan was to deliver 40 Gy over 4–5 weeks using a linear accelerator. The prostate was excluded from the high-dose area. Because of the severe complications associated with this combined radiation therapy technique, it was abandoned. In patients who did not have radioactive implantation of the prostate, because of positive lymph nodes, definitive external beam radiation therapy was given with 50 Gy to the pelvis over 5–6 weeks and an additional 20 Gy cone down to the prostate using a four-field technique (Giles and Brady 1986).

Of the 133 patients considered suitable for the iodine-125 implantation procedure, five (4%) elected to have external beam radiation therapy only, and six (5%) were referred with recurrent disease which had been previously diagnosed and treated. These 11 (8%) patients were excluded from the analysis of the Hahnemann University data. Therefore, there were 122 patients submitted to staging pelvic lymphadenectomy who had newly diagnosed localized prostate cancer. The histologic grades and pathologic stages are shown in Table 18.5 (Brady et al. 1991). Of the 122 study patients, 36 (30%) were upstaged to pathologic stage D1 (Table 18.6). A total of 15% of well-differentiated tumors and 13% of A2 tumors were upstaged to pathologic stage D1 disease. Four of the five stage C patients had pelvic lymph node disease. For the 36 stage D1 patients, various treatment options were used; 20 (56%) patients underwent implantation only, and nine (25%) received external beam radiation therapy alone. The treatment option was influenced by negative frozen section on subsequent histology (22 of 106 frozen sections were negative) and by the preference of the physician and patient as well as the extent or site of extracapsular involvement (ten had only periprostatic involvement). The patients were followed at regular intervals with history and physical examination including digital rectal examination,

Table 18.5. Distribution of histologic grade and pathologic stage in patients with carcinoma of the prostate (n = 122), treated with iodine-125 implantation

Histology	Pathologic stage							
	A1	A2	B1	B2	B	C	D1	Total
Well differentiated	7	12	18	8	4	1	9	59
Moderate	–	7	9	8	1	–	15	40
Poorly differentiated	–	–	1	1	1	–	10	13
Unspecified	–	1	6	1	–	–	2	10
Total	7	20	34	18	6	1	36	122

Table 18.6. Change in clinical stage in 36 pathologic stage D1 patients

Histology	Clinical stage at presentation						
	A1	A2	B1	B2	B	C	Total
Well differentiated	–	1	2	3	1	2	9/59 (15%)
Moderate	–	–	3	9	2	1	15/40 (37%)
Poorly differentiated	–	2	1	7	–	–	10/13 (77%)
Unspecified	–	–	1	–	–	1	2/10 (20%)
Total		3	7	19	3	4	36/122 (30%)
Percentage	13%	17%	50%	33%	80%		

Table 18.7. Clinical outcome in 114 patients (all stages) treated by implantation with iodine-125

	6 months	6–11 months	12–17 months	18–23 months	24+ months
No. of patients at risk	114	106	101	92	85
Complete resolution	22%	55%	69%	74%	
Incomplete or no change			27%	22%	
Local failure	–	1%	2%	6%	10%
Distant metastases	1%	1%	4%	5%	7%
Local and distant metastases	–	–	2%	3%	6%

biochemical studies, and bone scans. Routine biopsies were avoided unless there was clinical evidence of regrowth of tumor or progressive abnormalities in biochemical studies.

Failure of treatment was identified by:

1. An expanding nodule or increasing enlargement of the prostate on digital rectal examination
2. Positive biopsy more than 15 months after radioactive implant or positive biopsy after less than 15 months if a tumor of high histologic grade was noted at the time of primary assessment
3. Elevated biochemical studies with suspicious clinical examination
4. Bone scan or radiographic evidence of bony metastatic disease

The results from the Hahnemann University experience were analyzed by life table analysis. Additionally, multivariate statistical techniques were used to control for differences in tumor grade, stage, and the length of follow-up (Brady et al. 1991). Response to treatment and the recurrence pattern are shown in Table 18.7; there was a 22% complete response with regression of palpable tumor by 6 months posttreatment, 55% by 1 year, and 74% by 2 years. Of the 122 study patients, 22% showed no change or incomplete response. Two patients received a repeat iodine-125 implantation for local recurrence at 18 and 42 months, respectively. Both of these patients are alive, one with disease at 33 months and the other disease-free at 18 months after reimplantation. No significant short- or long-term morbidity was noted in either patient.

Figures 18.1 and 18.2 indicate overall survival, probability of freedom from relapse, and histologic differentiation for all patients. The overall 5-year probability of survival was 85% with 60% probability of no evidence of disease for all stages. Patients with well and moderately well differentiated tumors did significantly better than those with poorly differentiated tumors. Figures 18.3 and 18.4 indicate the survival and disease-free survival for different stages of disease. All patients with stage A1 lesions remain free of disease. All patients with pathologic stage A2 lesions are alive and disease-free. Of the unspecified stage B patients, one of the six patients has shown local recurrence at 52 months posttreatment. Table 18.8 shows distribution of patients by pathologic stage and local failure. Seven of the 35 stage B1 and two of the 19 stage B2 developed locally recurrent disease. None of these patients demonstrated distant metastatic disease. Of the ten patients with recurrent stage D1 lesions, only one had local failure alone, and none have developed distant metastatic disease in the absence of proved or suspicious local recurrence. There was no significant difference in survival or in the incidence of recurrence for pathologic stage D1 patients who had either a positive or a false-negative

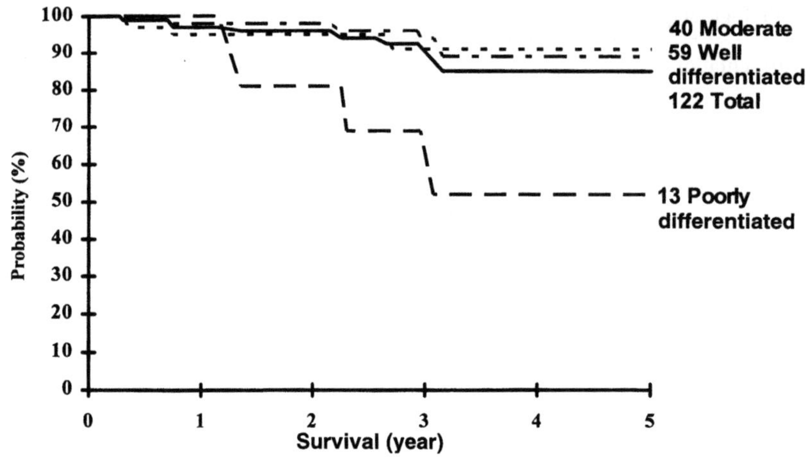

Fig. 18.1. Crude survival according to histologic differentiation in 122 patients submitted to lymphadenectomy

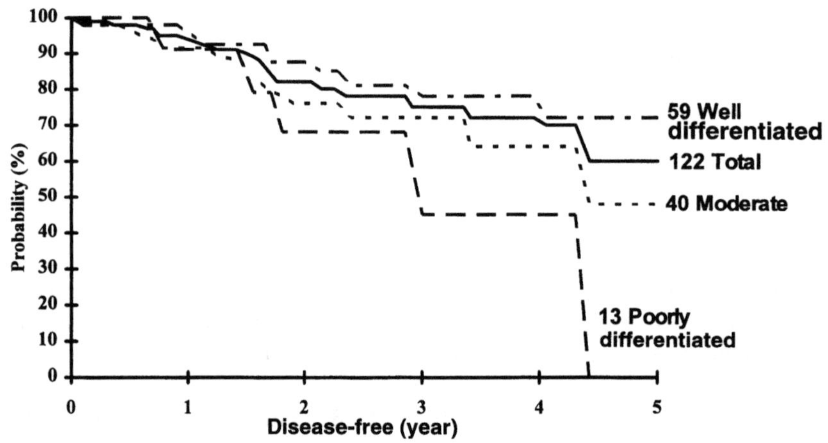

Fig. 18.2. Disease-free survival and histologic differentiation in 122 treated patients

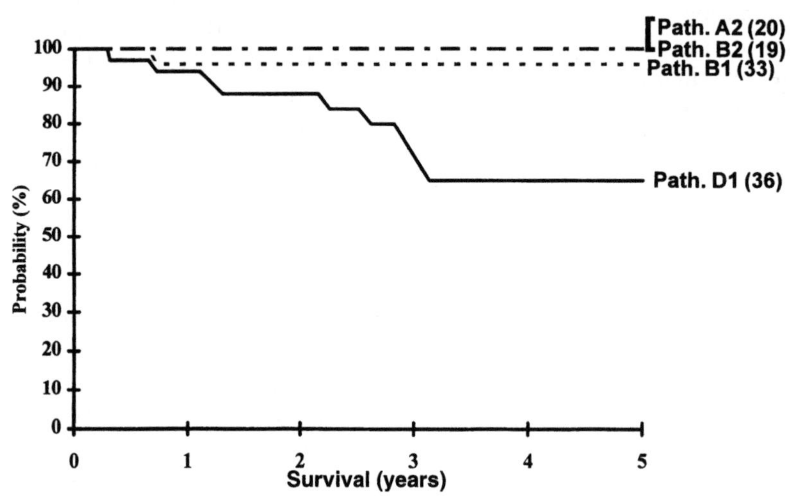

Fig. 18.3. Crude survival of 122 treated patients by stage of disease

frozen section at lymphadenectomy. The site of the metastatic disease in the pelvis (in the immediate periprostatic area or in the more distant iliac lymph nodes) did not influence survival. There was no effect of transurethral resection of the prostate versus needle biopsy for diagnosis on pattern of tumor spread or survival. Of the 122 patients treated with brachytherapy, 12 (10%) had diabetes mellitus and

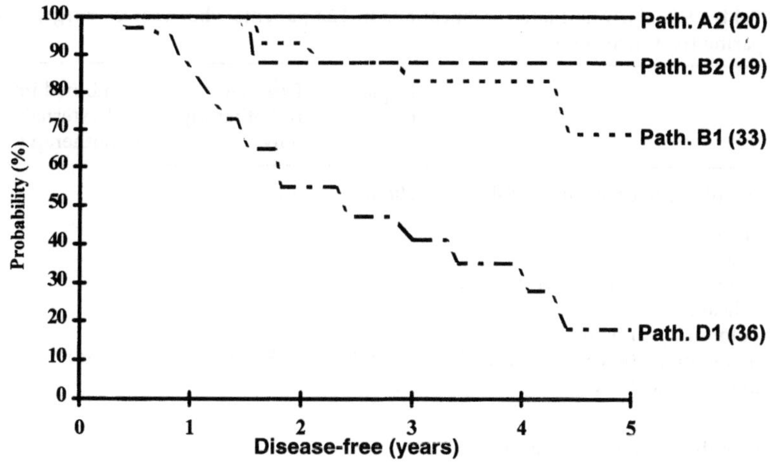

Fig. 18.4. Disease-free survival of 122 treated patients by stage of disease

Table 18.8. Latency to local failure in 114 patients treated by iodine-125 implantation, according to pathologic stage

Pathologic stage	Follow-up interval		
	<24 months	24–48 months	>48 months
A	0/27	0/21	0/10
B	4/58	2/36	3/16
D1	7/29	1/14	2/3

75 had a history of hypertension or had cardiovascular disease. There was no apparent influence of these medical problems on survival.

Early and late complications in the 122 patients treated with the implantation procedure are shown in Table 18.9 and are related to the form of definitive treatment. When external beam radiation therapy was added to lymphadenectomy and radioactive iodine-125 seed implantation, 80% of the patients experienced significant morbidity with one patient dying; this patient was disease-free following colostomy for a rectal stricture. One patient in the lymphadenectomy and implant group developed a urethral stricture, and another required a penile prosthesis for impotence. Subsequent malignancies occurred in three patients (one hepatoma, one colon, and one lung cancers). This is comparable to Reed's report that 3 of 189 patients developed subsequent rectal carcinoma after external beam radiation therapy for prostate cancer.

All patients with well-differentiated stage A1 lesions were disease-free at follow-up after implantation and lymphadenectomy. It is now recognized that such patients do not require treatment after transurethral resection other than follow-up with repeat transurethral resection 3–6 months later.

Freiha et al. (1979) reported only a 7% incidence of positive pelvic lymph nodes in patients with stage A2 and B lesions but a 90% incidence in patients with stage C lesions with elevated biochemical studies. Klein found 8%–45% positive lymph nodes in patients with stage A2 and B lesions (Klein et al. 1988). The data from several nonrandomized studies of iodine-125 implantation in clinically localized carcinomas of the prostate have shown that there is a progressive decrease in local control in the pelvis as well as distant metastatic disease with continuing decrease in probability of disease-free survival (Batata et al. 1984; El-Mahdi et al. 1985). The Hahnemann University series show equivalent patient survival rates but earlier local failure, perhaps due to more rigorous criteria for evaluation of freedom from disease.

Hilaris et al. (1978) reported survival and freedom from disease for more than 20 months in 112 patients (stages B and C). These data, however, disregarded the continuing recurrences that appeared subsequently as the series matured (Batata et al. 1984; Groosman et al. 1982). The first report from the Memorial Sloan-Kettering Cancer Center showed that the presence of minimal nodal metastasis might not adversely affect the 5-year prognosis for bone metastases or distant failure. However, this assessment was not sustained by a longer follow-up (Groosman et al. 1982). A more recent report by Whitmore (1988) provided the 10-year follow-up data on the early series from the Memorial Sloan-Kettering Cancer Center. It indicated a poor rate of survival without disease, probably influenced by less than rigorous criteria for the selection of patients during the early phases, when many with positive lymph node disease were included in the brachytherapy group, and the changing evolution of

Table 18.9. Early and late complications in 122 patients who received surgery, comparing treatments used

	Implant only	External radiotherapy only	Combined implant and external radiotherapy
No. of occurrences/no. at risk	30/106	6/7	9/9
Early			
Death	–	–	–
Wound infection and/or delayed healing	2	–	1
Pulmonary embolus	1	–	–
Moderate cystitis and/or proctitis	14 (13%)	6 (86%)	8 (90%)
Mild transient edema	2	1	–
Late			
Lymphedema of pubis, groin, or lower extremity	7	1	3
Bowel, bladder, or bleeding	1	2	3 (33%)
Transurethral prostatic resection for benign prostatism	4 (4%)	–	2 (22%)
Urethral stricture	1	–	–
Rectal stricture and colostomy Death	–	–	1

Table 18.10. Radioisotopes used for prostate brachytherapy

	Energy (keV)	Half-life (days)	Half value layer (HVL) in mm of lead	Initial dose rate (cGy/h)	Dose to infinity (Gy)
Permanent					
Iodine-125	27	60	1/40	8	160
Palladium-103	21	17	1/100	20	120
Gold-198	412	2.7	4	64	60
Ytterbium-169	93	32	1/2	13	140
Temporary					
Iridium-192	340	70	3	High, variable	Variable (30–40)

the criteria used to calculate the radiation dose. There was also an increase in the radiation dose from 140 Gy in 1965 to 238 Gy as the minimal peripheral dose in 1979 without a significant increase in morbidity or survival (Whitmore 1989). During the same period changes were introduced in the specific gamma ray constant for iodine-125 and the dosimetric methods used for calculating the radiation dose (Hilaris et al. 1978). More experience with the use of brachytherapy with newer radioisotopes is necessary before this treatment modality becomes widely accepted in selected patients with prostate cancer. Characteristics of radioisotopes used in prostate cancer patients are shown in Table 18.10.

It has been frequently stated that transurethral prostatic resection increases the incidence of treatment failure (Leibel et al. 1984; Perez 1983). This has not been found to be true in the Hahnemann University experience; this hypothesis was probably derived from those patients with more advanced stage disease and with poorly differentiated tumors.

18.9 Comparison of the Efficacy of External Beam Irradiation and Implantation Techniques

The implantation technique allows for preservation of prior sexual function in more than 90% of patients [93% according to Hilaris et al. (1978), 92% according to Schellhammer and El-Mahdi (1983), and 92% in the Hahnemann University series].

Pilepich et al. (1981) have pointed out that 65–70 Gy of external beam radiation therapy given over 6.5–7 weeks can be well tolerated although 25%

of patients developed leg or genital edema when it is combined with lymphadenectomy. There was no increased morbidity in the Radiation Therapy Oncology Group 75–06 trial in which para-aortic irradiation was added, except in the lymphadenectomy patients (PILEPICH et al. 1982).

In the most recent review of the Hahnemann University experience, 276 patients were treated definitively by external beam radiation therapy or iodine-125 implantation (KOPROWSKI et al. 1991). The patients in both groups were comparable as to the mean age and proportion diagnosed by transurethral resection. There was a mean follow-up of 5 years or longer. In the analysis of the overall survival, recurrence-free survival, incidence of local failure and complication rates, a multivariate statistical technique was used to control for differences in grade, stage, and length of follow-up. There were striking differences between the implantation patients and the external beam radiation therapy patients in local failure rates and relapse-free survival, most of the latter difference being attributable to poor local tumor control.

Of those patients treated by iodine-125 implantation, 42% developed local failure, whereas in those patients treated by external beam radiation therapy, only 10% developed local failure. Those patients treated by implantation who fared well had clinical stage A2 disease. None of these patients experienced local failure and only 18% developed distant failure. Complication rates were marginally lower in patients treated by the implantation technique (10%) than in those treated by external beam radiation therapy (16%).

This comparison of a single institution's experience has led to serious doubts about the efficacy of iodine-125 implantation in maintaining the optimum potential for local tumor control. This appears to be satisfactory only in patients with stage A2 lesions. The complication rates were not significantly different between the two treated groups. It was from these data that the current recommendation was made to limit the implantation procedure to carefully selected patients who would be treated in medical centers with experience in brachytherapy.

Other groups have used gold-198 grains and more recently transperineal temporary implantation of iridium-192 seeds in combination with external beam radiation therapy. This has been advocated in an attempt to improve local tumor control in patients with larger lesions (PUTHAWALA et al. 1985; BAGSHAW 1986b). It is too early to analyze the results for meaningful comparison with the known expected outcome in such patients. Transperineally implanted iridium-192 as a temporary interstitial treatment has been employed in many institutions as a supplement to external beam radiation therapy. The iridium-192 is implanted directly into the prostate in patients with stage C tumors after 50 Gy has been delivered to the prostate over a 5-week period using external beam treatment techniques. The implant provides a 30-Gy boost to the primary tumor. These techniques have been designed to improve the potential for local control in patients with large tumors. Other boost techniques under study include high-energy protons, neutron irradiation, negative pi meson irradiation, and heavy ion irradiation. Attempts are being made to investigate hyperthermia in combination with external beam radiation therapy or interstitial implantation to improve local control (see Chap. 23 for details).

Clinical data using palladium-103 as an implant source are limited (BLASKO et al. 1995a). BLASKO et al. (1995b) reported the use of palladium-103 with a target dose of 115 Gy in 34 patients treated with a median follow-up of 22 months. No patient has failed at this point. In 28 patients, palladium boost was used in combination with external beam radiation therapy, and the median follow-up was 24 months. Of these patients, 26 or 93% have been controlled locally and only two or 7% have had distant failure at this early time of assessment.

18.10 Conclusions

The scarcity of suitable patients for radioactive implantation techniques, the technical difficulties associated with the procedure, and the considerable doubt relative to the radiation dose delivery at the low dose rate of iodine-125 indicate that it is difficult to justify widespread use of this procedure. The results do show, however, that it gives rise to excellent long-term survival and excellent local control in those individuals who have stage A2 lesions with no evidence of extension of the disease process beyond the prostate capsule as determined by lymph node biopsy or lymphadenectomy. In patients with other stages of disease, implantation technique should be reserved to boost the local radiation dose to the prostate using temporary implantation procedures in combination with external beam radiation therapy.

The treatment of prostate carcinoma with radiation therapy is a highly successful and well-tolerated modality. In general, external beam radiation therapy techniques are the most generally applicable programs for the management of these patients. This is based upon the results that have accrued in a review of the literature as well as the high probability of microscopic disease involvement in the regional lymph node drainage of the prostate. Without question, disease in regional draining lymph nodes can be controlled by adequately designed, appropriately delivered external beam radiation therapy techniques. Permanent implantation with iodine-125 seeds and temporary transperineal implantation with iridium-192 seeds have recognizable and difficult problems in their general application and should be restricted to those patients with pathologically staged limited local disease involving the prostate.

Newer techniques of brachytherapy used in ultrasound guidance or CT-based treatment planning in addition to perineal template implantation technologies have been associated with excellent early results and a low rate of complications (Kaye et al. 1995; Blasko et al. 1994). These early results must be confirmed by others and long-term follow-up data are necessary before interstitial techniques can be accepted as a standard treatment option. At the present time, the use of interstitial techniques remains investigational and warrants further study in closely controlled clinical trials.

References

American Cancer Society. (1995) Facts and figures

Bagshaw MA (1980) External radiation therapy of carcinoma of the prostate. Cancer 45 (Suppl 2):1912–1921

Bagshaw MA (1986a) Current conflicts in the management of prostatic cancer. Int J Radiat Oncol Biol Phys 12:1721–1727

Bagshaw MA (1986b) Radiation therapy, the Stanford experience, at current controversies in the management of prostate carcinoma. American Cancer Society, Baltimore

Batata MA, Hilaris BS, Chu FCH et al. (1980) Radiation therapy in adenocarcinoma of the prostate with pelvic lymph node involvement of lymphadenectomy. Int J Radiat Oncol Biol Phys 6:149–153

Batata MA, Hilaris BS, Chu FCH, He S, Genest P, Jain P, Whitmore WF (1984) External beam versus brachytherapy in localized prostatic cancer. Int J Radiat Oncol Biol Phys 10 (Suppl 2):116

Batson OU (1942) The role of the vertebral veins in metastatic processes. Ann Intern Med 16:38–45

Blasko JC, Grimm PD, Ragde H (1994) External beam irradiation with Palladium-103 implantation for prostate carcinoma. Int J Radiat Oncol Biol Phys 30 (Suppl 1):219

Blasko JC, Ragde H, Mate T (1995a) Transperineal ultrasound guided palladium-103 brachytherapy for prostate carcinoma. (personal communication)

Blasko JC, Grimm PD, Ragde H (1995b) PSA-based disease control following ultrasound-guided I-125 implantation for stage T1/T2 prostatic carcinoma. (personal communication)

Brady LW, Koprowski C, Borofsky AM, Lightfoot DA (1991) Cancer of the prostate: brachytherapy techniques. In: Sauer R (ed) Interventional radiation therapy: techniques. Springer, Berlin Heidelberg New York, pp 245–255

Breslow N, Chan CW, Dhom G et al. (1977) Latent carcinoma of prostate at autopsy in seven areas. Int J Cancer 20:680–688

Byar DP, Mostofi FK (1973) Carcinoma of the prostate: prognostic evaluation of certain pathologic features in 208 radical prostatectomies. Cancer 30:5–13

Denning CL (1922) Results of 100 cases of cancer of the prostate and seminal vesicles treated with radium. Surg Gynecol Obstet 34:99

El-Mahdi AM, Kuban DA, Schellhammer PF (1985) The treatment of choice for localized poorly differentiated adenocarcinoma of the prostate (Abstr). 67th Meeting of the American Radium Society

Fowler JE, Whitmore WF (1981) The incidence and extent of pelvic lymph node metastases in apparently localized prostatic cancer. Cancer 47:2941–2945

Freiha S, Pistenmaa DA, Bagshaw MA (1979) Pelvic lymphadenectomy for staging prostatic carcinoma: is it always necessary? J Urol 122:176–177

Giles GM, Brady LW (1986) Iodine 125 implantation after lymphadenectomy in early carcinoma of the prostate. Int J Radiat Oncol Biol Phys 12:2117–2125

Gleason DF, Mellinger GT (1974) Veterans Administration Cooperative Urologic Research Group. Prediction of prognosis of prostatic adenocarcinoma by combined histologic grading and clinical staging. J Urol 111:58–64

Groosman HB, Batata M, Hilaris B, Whitmore WF (1982) ^{125}I implantation for carcinoma of the prostate. Urology 20:591–598

Hanks GE (1986) The RTOG patterns of care study, at current controversies in the management of prostate carcinoma. American Cancer Society, Baltimore

Hanks GE, Leibel S, Kramer S (1983) The dissemination of cancer by transurethral resection of locally advanced prostate cancer. J Urol 129:309–311

Hanks GE, Leibel SA, Krall JM et al. (1985) Patterns of care studies: dose response of observations for local control of adenocarcinoma of the prostate. Int J Radiat Oncol Biol Phys 11:153–157

Hanks GE, Diamond JJ, Krall JM et al. (1987) A 10 year follow-up of 682 patients treated for prostate cancer with radiation therapy in the United States. Int J Radiat Oncol Biol Phys 13:499–505

Hilaris BS (ed) (1975) Handbook of interstitial brachytherapy. Publishing Sciences, Boston

Hilaris BS (1986) Brachytherapy, the memorial experience, at current controversies in the management of prostate carcinoma. American Cancer Society, Baltimore

Hilaris BS, Whitmore WF, Batata MA, Barzell W, Tokita N (1978) ^{125}I implantation of prostate: dose-response considerations. Front Radiat Ther Oncol 12:82–90

Jewett HJ (1980) Radical perineal prostatectomy for palpable, clinically localized, nonobstructive cancer: experience at the Johns Hopkins Hospital 1909–1963. J Urol 124:492–494

Jewett HJ, Eggleston JC, Yawn DH (1972) Radical prostatectomy in the management of carcinoma of the prostate: probable causes of some therapeutic failures. J Urol 107:1034–1040

Johansson JE, Andersson SO, Krusemo UB, Adami HO (1989) Natural history of localized prostatic cancer. Lancet 1:799–803

Kaye KW, Olson DJ, Payne JT (1995) Detailed preliminary analysis of 125-Iodine implantation for localized prostate cancer using percutaneous approach. J Urol 153:1020–1025

Klein FA, Ali MM, Marks SE, Hacker RH (1988) Bilateral pelvic lymphadenopathy, iridium 192 template, and external beam therapy for localized prostate carcinoma: complications and results. South Med J 81:27–31

Koprowski CD, Berkenstock KG, Borofski AM, Ziegler JC, Lightfoot DA, Brady LW (1991) External beam irradiation versus iodine 125 implant in the definitive treatment of prostate carcinoma. Int J Radiat Oncol Biol Phys 21:955–960

Leibel SA, Hanks GE, Kramer S (1984) Patterns of care outcome studies: results of the national practice in adenocarcinoma of the prostate. Int J Radiat Oncol Biol Phys 10:401–409

McGowan DG (1980) The adverse influence of prior transurethral resection on prognosis in carcinoma of prostate treated by radiation therapy. Int J Radiat Oncol Biol Phys 6:1121–1126

Murphy GP, Natarjan N, Pontes JE et al. (1982) The national survey of prostate cancer in the United States by the American College of Surgeons. J Urol 127:928–934

Pasteau O (1911) Traitement du cancer de la prostate par le radium. Rev Mal Nutr 363

Perez CA (1983) Presidential address of the 24th annual meeting of the American Society of Therapeutic Radiologists: carcinoma of the prostate, a vexing biologic and clinical enigma. Int J Radiat Oncol Biol Phys 9:1427–1438

Perez CA, Walz BJ, Zivnuska FR et al. (1980) Irradiation of carcinoma of the prostate localized to the pelvis: analysis of tumor response and prognosis. Int J Radiat Oncol Biol Phys 6:555–565

Perez CA, Pilepich MV, Zivnusta F (1986) Tumor control in definitive irradiation of localized carcinoma of the prostate. Int J Radiat Oncol Biol Phys 12:523–531

Pilepich MV, Perez CA, Walz BJ, Zivnuska FR (1981) Complications of definitive radiotherapy for carcinoma of the prostate. Int J Radiat Oncol Biol Phys 7:1341–1348

Pilepich MV, Satfish MD, Prasad C, Perez CA (1982) Computed tomography in definitive radiotherapy of prostatic carcinoma. II. Definition of target volume. Int J Radiat Oncol Biol Phys 8:235–240

Pilepich MV, Krall JM, George FW et al. (1984) Treatment related morbidity in phase III RTOG studies of extended-field irradiation for carcinoma of the prostate. Int J Radiat Oncol Biol Phys 10:1861–1867

Puthawala AA, Syed AMN, Tansey LA et al. (1985) Temporary iridium 192 implant in the management of carcinoma of the prostate. Endocuriether Hyperthermia Oncol 1:25–34

Rosen EM, Cassady JR, Connolly J et al. (1984) Radiotherapy for localized prostate carcinoma. Int J Radiat Oncol Biol Phys 10:2201–2210

Schellhammer PF, El-Mahdi AM (1983) Pelvic complictions after definitive treatment of prostate cancer by interstitial or external beam radiation. Urology 21:451–457

Walsh PC (1986) Surgery. The Johns Hopkins experience, at current controversies in the management of prostate carcinoma. American Cancer Society, Baltimore

Walsh PC, Jewett HJ (1980) Radical surgery for prostatic cancer. Cancer 45:1906–1911

Whitmore WF (1956) Symposium on hormones and cancer therapy. Am J Med 21:697

Whitmore WF (1988) Clinical management of prostate cancer: an overview. In: Raymond JP, Harvey M, Ojasso T (eds) Proceedings of a satellite symposium of the 3rd International Congress on Hormones and Cancer. Raven Press, New York, pp 88–97

Whitmore WF, Butata MA, Hilaris BS (1979) Prostate irradiation; iodine 125 implantation. In: Johnson DE, Samuels ML (eds) Cancer of genitourinary tract. Raven Press, New York, pp 195–205

19 Treatment-Related Complications in Patients with Carcinoma of the Prostate: a Review

B.J. Costleigh, W.A. Longton, B.S. Hill, and L.W. Brady

CONTENTS

19.1 Introduction

Radical prostatectomy and definitive radiation therapy for prostate carcinoma have been shown to provide equal and good long-term results regarding local control and overall survival. However, with the variability of the natural history of this disease process, it is often difficult to assess the impact of the various treatment modalities on the disease course. Therefore, the optimal treatment modality remains controversial. While anticipated control and survival rates remain the main consideration in the choice of treatment for prostate carcinoma as well as other cancers, the treatment-related morbidity and subsequent quality of life are also extremely important. Therefore, with 244000 new cases of prostate carcinoma anticipated in the United States in 1995, assessment of the treatment results must take into account the morbidity of a particular therapeutic regimen.

Treatment of the prostate by external beam radiation therapy, interstitial implantation with radioactive sources, hormonal therapy, surgery, or any combination thereof may alter the bowel and bladder function, as well as sexual function. Prostatectomy exerts its effects by direct surgical manipulation and trauma of the prostate and surrounding adjacent structures. Subsequent complications or side-effects occur in 20%–30% of patients (see Chap. 11 for details). The target for limited field radiation therapy includes the prostate and, at a minimum, the immediate adjacent tissues. The adjacent tissues include periprostatic tissues and immediate draining lymph nodes (obturator, internal and external hypogastrics), but often larger pelvic fields with associated lymph nodes are incorporated. Therefore, radiation-related morbidity may represent a wide spectrum of clinical syndromes with potential injury to the prostatic urethra, bladder neck, urethral sphincters, and anterior rectal wall. However, with the larger treatment fields employed in external beam radiation therapy, potential injury may be more extensive, including damage to the remote bladder, trigone, ureteral orifices, lateral and posterior rectal wall and the bulbomembranous urethra.

The effects of radiation on normal tissues are conventionally classified as acute (early), occurring during or immediately following the course of radiation therapy (Table 19.1), or chronic (late), occurring several months to several years after completion of radiation therapy (Table 19.2). The rapidly dividing tissues such as intestinal epithelium react acutely, producing early side-effects, e.g., radiation enteritis. The pathogenesis of late effects remains controversial. Historically, late effects were thought to be due to microvascular damage and to be irreversible. It is now believed by many that the vascular changes may

B.J. Costleigh, MD, Clinical Instructor of Radiation Oncology, Medical College of Pennsylvania and Hahnemann University, 230 N. Broad Street, Philadelphia, PA 19102-1192, USA
W.A. Longton, MD, Department of Radiation Oncology, Medical College of Pennsylvania and Hahnemann University, 230 N. Broad Street, Philadelphia, PA 19102-1192, USA
B.S. Hill, MD, Department of Radiation Oncology, Medical College of Pennsylvania and Hahnemann University, 230 N. Broad Street, Philadelphia, PA 19102-1192, USA
L.W. Brady, MD, Professor and Chairman, Department of Radiation Oncology and Nuclear Medicine, Medical College of Pennsylvania and Hahnemann University, 230 N. Broad Street, Philadelphia, PA 19102-1192, USA

Table 19.1. Incidence (%) of acute complications following external beam radiation therapy (modified from Bijayakumar et al. 1993)

Authors	No. of pts.	Grades 1 and 2		Grades 3 and 4		Dose (Gy)	Technique
		GI	GU	GI	GU		
Perez	112	–	–	10	1	70	AP-PA + AP boost
Bagshaw	310	24	25	5.5	10	70–75	Four fields to 50 Gy + 20 Gy boost arcs
Shipley	121	21	23.3	–	–	64–70	Four fields

Table 19.2. Incidence (%) of chronic complications following external beam radiation therapy

Authors	No. of pts.	Grades 1 and 2		Grades 3 and 4		Dose	Technique
		GI	GU	GI	GU		
Perez et al. (1994)	594	7.7	7.7	1.1	0.9	70 Gy	AP-PA + arcs
Lawton et al. (1991)	1020	[a]	[a]	7.7	3.3 (2.3)[b]	RTOG 7706 7506 Protocol	7506 – Many pts had para-aortic treatment. 2 arms: #1 – 65 Gy to the prostatic bed area 180–200 cGy/Fx #2 – 20 Gy to prostatic bed and 45 Gy to whole pelvis
Pilepich et al. (1981)	267	8.2	10.3	1.5	0.38	65–70 Gy	AP-PA 50 Gy pelvis 2 cone-down fields
Lai et al. (1990)	542[c]	7.1	10.0	1.3	1.0	63–75 Gy	45–50 Gy + boost fields 20–25 Gy[d]
Hanks et al. (1994)	682	[a]	[a]	1.8[e]	2.5[e]	18% (60 Gy) 49% (60–70 Gy) 31% (70 Gy)	25% AP-PA alone 54% multiple fields 21% rotation component
Schellhammer and El-Mahdi (1990)	110	71	0	20.0	15.6	65 Gy	Multiple fields so rotation used

[a] Not reported
[b] Grade 5
[c] Stages B and C
[d] AP or rotational boost used
[e] Used a grading system 1–6

be secondary to destruction, atrophy, and dense fibrosis of the parenchymal and stromal cells correlating with the cell turnover kinetics of the involved tissues.

Factors which directly impact upon the complications from radiation therapy include: patient age, other co-morbid conditions, stage of the disease, volume irradiated, and radiation time–dose relationships. Additionally, the quality of both external beam irradiation and brachytherapy and the adequacy of treatment planning and simulation are other important considerations.

Although there is no standard complication scale, generally speaking a major local complication is defined as one requiring intense medical management, operation, or hospitalization.

19.2 Complications of Surgical Management

The National Medicare experience on complications after radical prostatectomy was reported by Fowler et al. (1983). Incontinence was seen in the majority of cases, with 63% of all patients complaining of this problem. Incontinence requiring pads, diapers, or clamps was seen in 30% and stress incontinence was seen in 40% of patients. With regard to sexual function, 60% of the patients reported inability to achieve erection, while 40% reported some erectile function. However, of this group of patients, only 10% reported having a functional erection. Finally, urethral stricture was reported in 20% of all patients. These figures in respect of complications appeared to be slightly higher than in the previous literature, with a recent review of the literature reporting permanent incontinence in 27% of patients and retention of sexual function in approximately 40%. However, the review did not mention the quality of erectile function in these patients. Reasons for the higher estimates than those provided in the previous reports could be related to the older patient population under the Medicare group. Also, there may have been a difference in the definition of what is meant by the degree of incontinence or sexual function. Other possible explanations for the differences include (a) less bias as compared to the other literature reports and (b) the type of prostatectomy the patient underwent (i.e., whether it was via the nerve-sparing approach, the retropubic approach, or the perineal approach). The incidence of surgical complications is expected to increase with the use of postoperative whole pelvis irradiation.

19.3 Pelvic Irradiation

An RTOG report from PILEPICH et al. (1984) reported treatment-related morbidity from extended field radiation to the pelvis for prostate cancer (Tables 19.3, 19.4). Of 526 patients evaluated, most treated-related morbidity was seen during the first several months following treatment. However, late occurrences were not uncommon such as proctitis, hematuria, and urethral stricture. The vast majority of the morbidity was grades I through III which required, at most, minor surgical or medical intervention such as urethral dilation. It was noted that certain symptoms, such as cystitis, were more likely to abate than others such as proctitis. Those who developed proctitis had a 20%–30% chance of persistence of symptoms for longer than 2 years. Hematuria and other symptoms which are secondary to urethral stricture also have a higher incidence of recurrence and/or persistence. One of the most difficult chronic complications to manage is genital and lower extremity edema.

LAWTON et al. (1991) reported long-term results from the RTOG trials and determined long-term

Table 19.3. Incidence (%) of complications of radiotherapy

Study	No. of pts.	Impotence	Stricture	Fistula	Dysuria	Cystitis	Proctitis	Edema	Obstruction	Incontinence	PE	MI	In Clammation/ abscess	Death	Dose
PILEPICH et al. (1984)	526	U	5.2	U	3	12.5	4.5	3[a]	0.4	U	U	U	U	0	Regional lymphatics 180–200 cGy/day for a total of 40–46 Gy Prostate: minimum dose of 65 Gy *or* Pelvis: 45–50 Gy. AP-PA and arcs
GRESKOVICH et al. (1991)	289	U	U	U	U	10	10	3[a]	11[b]	U	U	U	U	0	18 MV: 46 Gy + 22 Gy + 22% (65) had lymphadenectomy
MORENO and AHLERING (1992)	33	U	30	3	12	9	U	U	30	3	U	U	U	0	66.72 ± 3.88 Gy + 3 patients given implants
BOILEAU et al. (1987)	65	U	U	U	U	32	U	8	U	3	U	U	U	0	69.65 Gy + staging lymphadenectomy + gold grains – 31.67 Gy
WIDMARK et al. (1994)	181	U	U	U	U	9	18	U	U	50	U	U	U		
JONLER et al. (1984)	98	84	5	U	U	U	20	U	5[b]	40	U	U	U		

PE, pulmonary edema; MI, myocardial infarction; U, unknown
[a] Associated only with lymphadenectomy
[b] Associated with prior TURP and bladder neck contracture

Table 19.4. Incidence (%) of complications of pelvic irradiation

Study	No. of pts.	Impotence	Stricture	Fistula	Dysuria	Cystitis	Proctitis	Edema	Obstruction	Incontinence	PE	MI	Inflammation/ abscess	Death	Dose
Perez (1992)	738	11	6.3	0.4		3.4	5.2	3[a]	0.5	1.0	0	0	0.4	0.2[b]	40–45 Gy+ arcs – AP+PA + boost; 608: pelvis plus prostate 130: pelvis only
Koprowski et al. (1991)	175	U	5.0	0	0	9.0	17.0	0	0	3.0	0	0	0	0	6000–7800 cGy 4-field box technique
Lawton et al. (1991)	1020	U	5.0	0	3.1	2.6	16.0	1.6	0.6	U	0	0	0	1[c]	+ lymph-adenectomy
Pilepich et al. (1981)	267	U	7.2	0	1.9	1.5	4.5	5.2	2.0	1.5	0	0	0	1[d]	60–70 Gy
Lai et al. (1990)	653	13	4.0	0.5	0	2.0	4.0	3.0	1.0	2.0	0	0	0	0	65–70 Gy

Abbreviations as in Table 19.3
[a] 11/113 = 10% of those with lymphadenectomy
[b] Radiation-induced ileitis
[c] Fatal obstruction
[d] Fatal enteritis

complication rates after definitive treatment with radiation therapy. The incidence of gastrointestinal complications which were grade 3 or higher was 3.3%; less than 1% of patients experienced bowel obstruction or perforation. Of the 7.7% of patients with grade 3 or higher toxicity of the urinary tract, only 0.5% experienced morbidity requiring surgical intervention including laparotomy or prolonged hospitalization. It was also noted that a total radiation dose greater than 70 Gy was the only significant factor impacting on the incidence of urinary complications. On the other hand, this factor had no impact on the incidence of intestinal complications.

In a Patterns of Care study reported by Hanks et al. (1987), complications of radiation therapy to the pelvis for prostate carcinoma were infrequent, with 93% of the patients being free of serious complications at 5 years, and 89% free at 10 years. Only 2% of patients required surgical correction for their complications, and only two (0.2%) of 682 patients died from complications secondary to radiation therapy.

Complications after external beam radiation therapy were evaluated by Greskovich et al. (1991). Of the 289 patients evaluated, complications were noted in 42 (14%) patients. Of these, 60% were mild and 19% were moderate in severity. No severe complications were noted in this study. Of the 42 patients with complications, only six experienced symptoms for longer than 6 months. Additionally, it was noted that the rate of complications was not increased in those patients who had undergone prior lymph node dissection. However, this study was limited to patients who received total radiation doses of 68 Gy or less.

19.4 Comparison of Incidence of Treatment Complications

A comparison of complications after prostatectomy versus external beam radiation versus iodine-125 (^{125}I) seed implantation was reported by Schellhammer and El-Mahdi (1990) (Table 19.5). Patients with stage A2 or B1 tumors treated by any of the modalities experienced virtually no complications secondary to the treatment or treatment failure (Table 19.5). However, patients with stage C tumors had a high incidence of morbidity or death with each of the treatment modalities used in the study. An interesting item of note was that within stage B2, the incidence of complications with ^{125}I implants was statistically higher than with either external beam radiation therapy or radical prostatectomy. When the patients were analyzed by tumor grade, the well-differentiated tumors were rarely associated with post-treatment local morbidity regardless of the type of treatment. Also, among the poorly differentiated tumor group, there was no statistically significant difference in morbidity and mortality rates whether patients were treated by external beam radiation therapy, radical prostatectomy, or ^{125}I seed implantation. However, for the moderately differentiated tumors, the local morbidity was higher for the ^{125}I group.

Table 19.5. Complications (%) of ^{125}I Brachytherapy ± lymphadenectomy ± preoperative EXRT ± postoperative EXRT

Study	No. of pts.	Transfusion	Impotence	Stricture	Fistula	Dysuria	Cystitis	Proctitis	Edema	Obstruction	Incontinence	PE	MI	Abscess	Death	Dose	Lymphadenectomy	EXRT
Flanigan et al. (1983)	25	10	52	–	–	–	12	4	–	–	12	–	–	–	–	26.5 mCi	+	[a]
Gomella et al. (1991)	45	3	53	–	4	15	4	7	13	4	6	–	4	–	4	23–47 mCi	+	[b]
Kumar et al. (1990)	43	–	0	5	2	2	–	–	–	–	–	–	–	–	–	160 Gy	–	
	34	U	15	15	3	11	3	3	6	3	3	3	6	–	–	160 Gy	+	[c]
Schellhammer et al. (1989)	90	50	25	2	–	6	–	16	2	–	2	1	1	2	–	160 Gy	+	

EXRT, external beam radiation therapy; other abbreviations as in Table 19.3
[a] 10.5 Gy preoperatively and 14–40 Gy postoperatively for undertreated patients
[b] 10.5 Gy preoperatively; 8/45 received postoperative radiation from 10.5 to 33.17 Gy (undertreated patients)
[c] 3 patients: 60–70 Gy EXRT 2 yrs. previously
4 patients: 40 Gy after + pelvic lymph nodes
2 patients: received 40 Gy EXRT followed by implant for obesity

Table 19.6. Complications (%) of radical prostatectomy ± subsequent ± lymphadenectomy

Study	No. of pts.	Impotence	Transfusion	Stricture	Dysuria	Cystitis	Proctitis	Edema	Obstruction	Incontinence	PE	MI	Abscess	Death	Postop. XRT
Fowler et al. (1983)	757	89	U	20	U	U	U	U	U	63	U	U	U	0	None
Meier et al. (1982)	39	97	U	18	U	U	U	5	U	44	U	U	U	0	[a]
	19	95	U	27	U	U	U	5	U	27	U	U	U	0	[b] + 45–70 Gy
Forman et al. (1986)	34	82	U	6	0	0	9	24 LND+ 17 LND−	6	15	0	0	0	0	45 Gy + 20 Gy

XRT, radiation therapy; other abbreviations as in Table 19.3; LND, lymph node dissection
[a] Node dissection, 49%
[b] Node dissection, 89%

With regard to sexual function, Schover (1993) compared radical prostatectomy versus radiation therapy versus hormonal therapy. Historically, radical prostatectomy consisted of removal of the prostatic neuroplexus, which meant a 100% chance of impotence. However, with the advent of nerve-sparing radical prostatectomy, an improved outlook for men who wish to continue sexual activity is apparent. In the most recent case series from Johns Hopkins, 68% of patients retained their functional erections. A majority of men younger than 50 years retained functional erections; however, in men older than age 70, maintenance of sexual function was minimal. The chance of potency was superior if both neurovascular bundles were spared compared to a situation where one bundle was removed in order to obtain good clear margins. With larger tumors, there was an increased risk of impotence in all age groups. In the same report, it was mentioned that 50% of men who had definitive radiation therapy developed erectile dysfunction (in the literature, a range of 14%–46% is usually reported), while patients treated with interstitial implantation of radioactive seeds have a 7%–13% chance of erectile dysfunction. It has also been noted that erectile dysfunction is more likely to occur in those patients who have borderline erectile function prior to radiation therapy. With regard to sexual function after hormonal therapy, 80%–90% of men will lose both their libido and their ability to achieve firm erections. Again, after hormonal therapy, most of the men who do maintain functional erections are below the age of 60.

Litwin et al. (1995) evaluated the quality of life in general for men treated with radiation versus surgery versus observation. It was determined that men treated by any modality and those managed by observation experienced a similar quality of life after treatment. With regard to specific complaints, there was no difference in bowel function among the three groups; however, with regard to urinary complaints and sexual function, patients treated in the surgery – alone group were less satisfied with the treatment outcome as compared to those managed with irradiation or observation. Among the irradiation and observation groups, no difference was noted in the incidence of complaints or satisfaction.

A report by Forman et al. (1986) discussed the complications after definitive radiation therapy following prostatectomy (Table 19.6). Although there was a complication rate of 41%, this was deemed acceptable in light of the 100% local control following therapy. In this report, complications were presented by treatment modality, consisting of surgery alone versus radiotherapy alone versus surgery followed by radiotherapy. Total incidence of genitourinary complications was 24%, 8%, and 21% respectively. The incidence of gastrointestinal complications was 5%, 5%, and 9% respectively. Impotence was recorded in 90%, 43%, and 82% patients, respectively.

The complication rate following radical prostatectomy versus prostatectomy plus radiation therapy was evaluated by MEIER et al. (1982). It was determined that complications occurred in similar frequencies in both groups of patients. Impotence occurred in 97% of the prostatectomy-alone patients versus 95% of the prostatectomy plus radiation therapy group. The addition of radiation to prostatectomy did not increase the incidence of incontinence, urethral stricture, or lower extremity or genital edema as compared to prostatectomy alone. It was, however, noted that there was a substantial difference in complication rate according to whether large-field or small-field radiation therapy was performed following prostatectomy. In those patients receiving radiation to the whole pelvis, 42% developed complications, whereas only 14% of patients treated to the prostatic bed alone did so. With regard to radiation dose, those receiving greater than 65 Gy to the prostatic bed had a complication rate of 100%, while those treated to a dose of less than 65 Gy had a complication rate of only 24%.

19.5 Complications Following Local Failure

The complication rate associated with clinical local failure after definitive radiation therapy using interstitial ^{125}I implantation, external beam radiation therapy or radical prostatectomy was compared by SCHELLHAMMER et al. (1989). Complications secondary to local failure were negligible in patients with stage A2 or B1 and well-differentiated tumors regardless of treatment modality. The same was true in stage C patients with poorly differentiated tumors. However, with regard to stage B2 moderately differentiated tumors, patients treated by implantation had a statistically greater incidence of complications than those treated with external beam radiation therapy or radical prostatectomy.

19.6 Treatment of Advanced Disease

MORENO and AHLERING (1992), comparing radiotherapy and hormonal therapy for advanced disease, found that 70% of all patients who received radiotherapy developed local complications compared to 30% of those undergoing hormonal therapy alone. The most common complication in the radiotherapy patients was urethral stricture (in 30%), followed by prostatic obstruction (in 24%), while the most common complication of the hormonally treated patients was prostatic obstruction, which occurred in 21%. These results question the benefit of palliative radiation therapy for patients with advanced local disease.

19.7 Late Complications

In a report by SCHELLHAMMER and EL-MAHDI (1983) it was determined that the rate of late serious complications affecting structures adjacent to the prostate was similar in patients undergoing interstitial implantation with ^{125}I seeds (complication rate = 17%) and in those receiving external beam radiation therapy (complication rate = 20%). By contrast, late serious complications of the nonadjacent pelvic structures were significantly worse in the external beam radiation therapy group: in this group the total complication rate for these remote structures was 15.5%, as against slightly more than 1% in the ^{125}I group. With regard to early major complications, the rate was similar in the implantation group (4.5%) and the external beam group (10%). However, the minor complication rate was significantly higher for the external beam group (22% vs 8% in the ^{125}I group).

In a comparison of external beam radiation therapy and ^{125}I implants, KOPROWSKI et al. (1991) found the incidence of complications to be 11% versus 19%, respectively with 4% of patients in each group requiring surgical intervention. A total of 183 patients were evaluated in this study.

19.8 Brachytherapy

Eighty patients who underwent transrectal ultrasonography (TRUS)-guided interstitial palladium-103 implantation were reported by BROSMAN and TOKITA (1991). The major early side-effect was bladder and urethral irritation; this occurred in 90% of patients, of whom more than half required medical intervention. Seven percent of patients experienced urinary retention, though only one needed transurethral resection of the prostate (TURP) to relieve this problem. A few patients developed gross hematuria, which was intermittent in nature in the first 3–4 months; however, all cases resolved spontaneously. With regard to gastrointestinal symptomatology, two (2%) of the 80 patients developed severe diarrhea and pain; both of these patients developed rectal ulcers which again healed spontaneously within 2–3 months posttreatment. There was no evidence of impotence or incontinence in this group of patients. It was concluded that this form of therapy produces minimal systemic side-effects with few severe local side-effects and meets with good patient acceptance; all else being equal, it was felt to be preferable to external beam radiation therapy since it can be performed in a single visit, as opposed to daily treatments for several weeks.

In a report by FLANIGAN et al. (1983) on complications associated with preoperative radiation therapy followed by ^{125}I brachytherapy, there was an overall late complication rate of 48%. This appeared to be a much greater incidence than that seen in previous reports. However, it included a subgroup of patients who also received postoperative radiation therapy. These patients had a 75% late complication rate. Postoperative radiation therapy after ^{125}I seed implantation where lymph nodes were positive produced major bowel complications requiring surgical intervention in all cases (PEREZ 1992).

GOMELLA et al. (1991) also reported the complications of interstitial implantation with the use of ^{125}I seeds. The complication rate of this report was similar to that of the other reports in the literature. Overall, 61% of patients retained potency for at least 1 year, with 47% retaining potency for a longer period. However, if external beam radiation therapy was delivered as additional radiation due to poor dosimetry of the implanted seeds, there was an unacceptable incidence (82%) of lower extremity and/or penile edema.

A series of 321 patients was evaluated by KAHN et al. (1992) with regard to complications after transperineal iridium-192 seed implantation. Using the RTOG toxicity scoring system, there were found to be no grade 4 or 5 complications, with only 1% of patients showing grade 3 and 16% showing grade 2 complications. Of these complications, 55% involved the urinary tract while 40% involved the rectum. Even though external beam radiation therapy was added in the vast majority of these patients, it appeared not to change the overall complication rate.

The complications from implantation followed by pelvic lymphadenectomy in 65 patients were reported by BOILEAU et al. (1987). It was noted that complications of therapy in general were mild and limited. The most common complications included cystitis in 32% of patients, diarrhea in 31% of patients, and extremity lymphedema in 8% of patients.

Similar results of external beam radiation therapy after pelvic lymphadenectomy were reported by BABAIAN and AGUILAR (1987). It was again concluded that radiotherapy did not increase the complication rate after pelvic lymph node dissection, particularly when the radiotherapy was well planned.

KUMAR et al. (1990) reported on ^{125}I seed implantation with and without lymphadenectomy and/or adjuvant pelvic external beam radiation therapy. When seed implantation was performed alone, the major and minor complication rates were minimal, at 4.7% and 2.3% respectively. However, when it was combined with pelvic lymphadenectomy, the major and minor complication rates increased to 24% and 33%, respectively. Furthermore, when adjuvant external beam radiation therapy was added, with or without lymphadenectomy, the minor complication rate rose to 50%.

19.9 The Effects of TURP

SEYMORE et al. (1986) looked at the effect of TURP on the complication rate after radiation therapy. The overall complication rate in patients who underwent TURP was 15% versus 6% in those who underwent no prior surgery. Again, when distinguishing between external beam radiation therapy and ^{125}I therapy, there was a substantially increased risk in both groups among patients who underwent a preradiation TURP. There appeared to be no difference in the overall rate of urethral strictures, bladder neck contractures, or both whether external beam radiation therapy or ^{125}I therapy was used. One item of note was that those patients who underwent multiple preradiation TURPs had an 18% complication rate, as compared with 13% in those undergoing a single TURP prior to radiation therapy.

19.10 Conformal Radiation Therapy

HANKS et al. (1994) evaluated the factors influencing acute grade 2 morbidity in both conformal and standard radiation therapy. It was noted that the conformal technique is associated with fewer grade 2 toxicities for all patients; it was also noted that older age is associated with increased toxicity when using the standard technique though not when employing the conformal technique. The volume of tissue radiated was not significantly related to complications in patients treated with the standard modality; however, for conformal treatments, the volume treated was directly correlated with morbidity. Furthermore, the study revealed that grade II acute toxicities are more volume dependent than dose dependent.

19.11 Conclusion

Although there are differences in treatment results between individual institutions, favorable reductions in complication rates after radiation therapy are usually seen. This is particularly so with regard to impotence, which occurs in virtually no patients with radioactive implantation and in only a small number of those treated with external beam irradiation. In multi-institutional studies of large numbers of patients, such as the RTOG and Pattern of Care studies, major side-effects were seen in less than 10% of patients. Even with a broad definition of major complications, radiation therapy (whether external beam radiation therapy or implantation of radioactive seeds) appears to have a marked advantage over radical prostatectomy. Radiation therapy after pelvic lymph node dissection or laparotomy is shown to increase the risk of complications, particularly lower extremity and genital edema and bowel obstruction. Since there is no therapeutic benefit of pelvic lymph node dissection and it is used basically for staging purposes, there is little reason to perform this procedure if definitive radiation treatment is planned. However, if it is performed, the risks of lymphadenectomy can be minimized by treating with smaller radiation volumes than the whole pelvis and with doses below 68 Gy. There are conflicting reports on whether radiation after TURP will increase the complication rate, particularly the incidence of urethral strictures. Again, use of smaller treatment volumes and moderate radiation doses and application of radiation therapy at least 4–6 weeks after the surgical procedure should minimize the risk of complications.

There is a significant risk of tumor-related morbidity in patients with local recurrence after definitive therapy. With regard to the grade and stage of the tumor, low-grade and low-stage tumors have a very low biologic potential with a low risk of progression. In this case, any form of therapy may produce a higher risk of complications than observation alone. At the other end of the spectrum, high-grade and high-stage tumors are expected to progress and may cause excessive morbidity with or without subsequent therapy. Consequently, for each treatment modality there is a higher associated rate of morbidity. Whereas local control in the presence of metastasis will not increase survival, it may favorably affect quality of life. Hormonal therapy in this situation may be the answer to the problem of how to slow down local tumor progression.

The incidence of complications after radiation therapy appears to be volume and to a lesser extent, dose dependent. The differences in the complication rates between external beam radiation therapy and radioactive seed implantation can be explained by the differences in the isodose curve distribution, with rapid dose fall-off obtained with the use of radioactive seeds. As a consequence, while the morbidity for the adjacent structures will be similar with the two techniques, complications affecting remote pelvic structures will be limited to patients treated with external beam irradiation. With equal local control rates and survival reported in the literature for large- and small-field pelvic irradiation for early-stage disease, minimizing the treated volume can minimize morbidity. It has been shown that more recently accepted techniques, such as conformal treatment with or without multileaf collimators, along with three-dimensional treatment planning, allow for the administration of a 10% higher dose of radiation without increasing treatment-related morbidity.

Acute radiation complications correlate well with total dose and overall treatment time while chronic effects depend on the total radiation dose and fraction size. Therefore a treatment regimen can account for acute morbidity, late morbidity, or both.

It is imperative in the process of radiation treatment planning to determine the optimal volume and dose by paying proper attention to detail, as this will obtain the highest incidence of local tumor control while minimizing treatment morbidity. Other factors which also play a large role in radiation-related morbidity include a previous medical history of such entities as collagen vascular disease, hypertension, regional enteritis, colitis, diverticulitis, and diabetes mellitus, and multiple previous pelvic and/or abdominal surgical procedures including TURP.

Based on the above data each patient's treatment has to be highly individualized to make appropriate allowance for important host and tumor-related parameters. The use of this approach is expected to optimize the treatment outcome, maintain good quality of life, and minimize the incidence of treatment complications.

References

Babaian RJ, Aguilar OF (1987) Radiation after pelvic lymphadenectomy: effect on morbidity. J Surg Oncol 34:36–38

Bijayakumar S, Awan A, Karrison T et al. (1993) Acute toxicity during external beam radiotherapy for localized prostate cancer: comparison of different techniques. Int J Radiat Oncol Biol Phys 25:359–371

Boileau MA, Dowling RA, Gonzales M et al. (1987) Interstitial gold and external beam irradiation for prostate cancer. J Urol 139:985–988

Brosman SA, Tokita K (1991) Transrectal ultrasound guided interstitial radiation therapy for localized prostate cancer. Urol 38:372–376

Carey PO, Lippert MC, Constable WC et al. (1987) Combined gold seed implant in external radiotherapy for stage B2 or C prostate cancer. J Urol 139:989–994

Flanigan RC, Patterson J, Mediondo OA et al. (1983) Complications associated with preoperative radiation therapy in iodine 125 brachytherapy for localized prostatic carcinoma. Urol 22:123–126

Forman JD, Wharan MD, Lee DJ et al. (1986) Definitive radiotherapy following prostatectomy: resultant complications. Int J Radiat Oncol Biol Phys 12:185–189

Fowler FJ, Barry MJ, Lu-Yao G et al. (1983) Patient reported complications in follow up treatment after radical prostatectomy: National Medicare Experience:1988–1990. Urology 42:622–629

Gomella LG, Steinberg SM, Ellison MF et al. (1991) Analysis of iodine-125 interstitial therapy in the treatment of localized carcinoma of the prostate. J Surg Oncol 46:235–240

Greskovich FJ, Zagars GK, Sherman NE et al. (1991) Complications following external beam radiation therapy for prostate cancer: analysis of patients treated with and without staging pelvic lymphadenectomy. J Urol 146:798–802

Hanks GE, Diamond JJ, Krall JM et al. (1987) A ten year follow up of 682 patients treated for prostate cancer with radiation therapy in the United States. Int J Radiat Oncol Biol Phys 13:499–505

Hanks GE, Schultheiss TE, Hunt MA et al. (1994) Factors influencing the incidence of acute grade II morbidity in conformal and standard treatment of prostate cancer. Int J Radiat Oncol Biol Phys 31:25–29

Jonler M, Ritter MA, Brinmann R et al. (1984) Sequelae of definitive radiation therapy for prostate cancer localized to the pelvis. Urology 44:876–882

Khan K, Thompson W, Bush S et al. (1992) Transperineal percutaneous iridium-192 interstitial template implant of the prostate: resulting complications in 321 patients. Int J Radiat Oncol Biol Phys 22:935–939

Koprowski CD, Berkenstock KG, Borofski AM et al. (1991) External beam radiation versus iodine 125 implant in the definitive treatment of prostate carcinoma. Int J Radiat Oncol Biol Phys 21:955–960

Kumar PP, Good RR, Bartone FF (1990) Iodine 125 interstitial irradiation for localized prostate cancer. J Natl Med Assoc 82:181–193

Lai PP, Perez CA, Shapiro SJ et al. (1990) Carcinoma of the prostate stage B and C: lack of influence of duration of radiotherapy on tumor control and morbidity. Int J Radiat Oncol Biol Phys 19:561–568

Lawton CA, Won M, Pilepich NV et al. (1991) Long term treatments that correlate external beam radiation for adenocarcinoma of the prostate: analysis of RTOG studies 7506–7706. Int J Radiat Oncol Biol Phys 21:935–939

Litwin MD, Hays RD, Fink A et al. (1995) Quality of life outcomes in men treated for localized prostate cancer. JAMA 273:129–135

Meier R, Mark RR, St Royal L et al. (1982) Postoperative radiation therapy after prostatectomy for prostate carcinoma. Cancer 70:1960–1966

Moreno JG, Ahlering TE (1992) Late complications after definitive radiotherapy for prostatic adenocarcinoma. J Urol 147:926–928

Perez CA (1992) Prostate. In: Perez CA, Brady LW (eds) Principles and practice of radiation oncology. Lippincott, Philadelphia, pp 1067–1116

Perez CA, Lee HK, Georgiou A et al. (1994) Technical factors affecting morbidity in definitive irradiation for localized carcinoma of the prostate. Int J Radiat Oncol Biol Phys 28:811–819

Pilepich MV, Perez CA, Walz BJ et al. (1981) Complications of definitive radiotherapy for carcinoma of the prostate. Int J Radiat Oncol Biol Phys 7:1341–1348

Pilepich MV, Krall J, George FW et al. (1984) Treatment related morbidity in a phase II RTOG studies of extended fields irradiation for carcinoma of the prostate. Int J Radiat Oncol Biol Phys 10:1861–1867

Schellhammer PF, El-Mahdi AN (1983) Complications after definitive treatment of prostate cancer by interstitial or external beam radiation. Urology 21:451–457

Schellhammer PF, El-Mahdi AN (1990) Local failure and related complications after definitive treatment of carcinoma of the prostate by irradiation or surgery. Urol Clin North Am 17:835–848

Schellhammer PF, Whitmore RB, Kuban DA et al. (1989) Morbidity and mortality of local failure after definitive therapy for prostate cancer. J Urol 141:567–571

Schover LR (1993) Sexual rehabilitation after treatment for prostate cancer. Cancer 71:1024–1030

Seymore CH, El-Mahdi AN, Schellhammer PF (1986) Effects of prior transurethral resection of the prostate on post radiation urethral strictures and bladder neck contractures. Int J Radiat Oncol Biol Phys 12:1597–1600

Widmark A, Fransson P, Tavelin B (1994) Self assessment questionnaire for evaluating urinary and late intestinal side effects after pelvic radiotherapy in patients with prostate cancer, comparing with an age matched controlled population. Cancer 74:2520–2532 [illegible] the treatment ... quality of life, and minimize the incidence of com[illegible] ...

[illegible]

20 Adjuvant Radiotherapy Following Radical Prostatectomy in the Management of Carcinoma of the Prostate

Z. Petrovich, G. Lieskovsky, G. Luxton, L. Baert, and D.G. Skinner

CONTENTS

Z. Petrovich, MD, Professor of Radiation Oncology and Urology, Chairman, Department of Radiation Oncology, University of Southern California School of Medicine, 1441 Eastlake Avenue, Los Angeles, CA 90033, USA

G. Lieskovsky, MD, Professor of Urology and Radiation Oncology, University of Southern California School of Medicine, 2025 Zonal Avenue, GH 5900, Los Angeles, CA 90033, USA

G. Luxton, PhD, Associate Professor of Radiation Oncology, Department of Radiation Oncology, University of Southern California School of Medicine, 1441 Eastlake Avenue, Los Angeles, CA 90033, USA

L. Baert, MD, PhD, Professor and Chairman, Department of Urology, St. Pieter's Hospital, Catholic University of Leuven, Brusselsestraat 69 3000 Leuven, Belgium and Clinical Professor, Department of Urology and Radiation Oncology, University of Southern California School of Medicine, 1441 Eastlake Avenue, Los Angeles CA 90033, USA

D.G. Skinner, MD, Professor and Chairman, Department of Urology, University of Southern California School of Medicine, 2025 Zonal Avenue, GH 5900, Los Angeles, CA 90033, USA

20.1 Introduction

In the past 5 years in the United States, there has been an unprecedented growth in the incidence of adenocarcinoma of the prostate (CaP). The number of new patients diagnosed with this disease since 1989 has more than doubled. This resulted in CaP becoming the most common human cancer in the United States, representing 36% of all male cancers. In 1995, the American Cancer Society has estimated that 244 000 new patients will be diagnosed with CaP (American Cancer Society 1995). It is expected that 40 400 patients will die of CaP in the same year, making CaP the second most important cause of cancer death among American males. The rapid increase in the incidence of CaP can be explained to a large extent by the routine use of the prostate specific antigen (PSA) and by the aging of the American male population.

There has been a progressive increase in the long-term survival of patients treated for CaP. This increase in patient survival has been particularly steep when compared to the survival statistics between 1983 and 1990 (Table 20.1). Multiple factors were responsible for the increase in survival. The factors primarily affecting survival included improved imaging modalities permitting for early diagnosis and the improvements in therapy with optimization of surgical and radiotherapy techniques. The development and wide clinical application of modern imaging, particularly routine use of transrectal ultrasonography (TRUS) and PSA (Oesterling 1991; Oesterling et al. 1988; Gann et al. 1995) in patient screening and assessment of treatment outcomes, made a dramatic difference in the management of CaP patients. The use of modern imaging in the diagnosis and treatment of CaP is discussed in Chaps. 6, 7, and 21.

20.2 Trends in Therapy

Patients with tumors clinically localized to the prostate have been effectively managed with radical prostatectomy and pelvic lymphadenectomy (GITTES 1991; EPSTEIN et al. 1993b; MORTON et al. 1991). This surgical treatment was found to be safe and cost effective (KOCH et al. 1994; STEINER et al. 1991) even when applied in patients with clinical stage (CS) C disease (BOSCH et al. 1987; SCHELLHAMMER 1988; SCHELLHAMMER et al. 1990) (see Chaps. 9–12 for details on surgical therapy). Excellent long-term results have also been reported in patients treated with definitive radiotherapy (BAGSHAW et al. 1990; PEREZ et al. 1988, 1993b; SCHELLHAMMER et al. 1991; ZAGARS et al. 1987) (see Chaps. 15–21 for details on definitive radiotherapy in patients with locoregional tumors).

In the past 10 years, the management of patients with CaP has been undergoing significant evolution. In 1987, during the National Consensus Conference, the management of clinically localized prostate cancer was specifically defined (CONSENSUS CONFERENCE 1987). Appropriate candidates for radical prostatectomy were patients with CS A2, B1, and B2, while CS A2, B1, B2, and C patients were felt to be optimal candidates for definitive radiation therapy. Much has changed since the time of that consensus conference. In 1986, a report of a study assessing postradiation biopsy in patients treated with pelvic lymphadenectomy and external beam radiotherapy combined with brachytherapy showed a good correlation between positive posttreatment biopsy and subsequent clinical recurrence (SCARDINO et al. 1986). The results of a study using TRUS-guided biopsy in 27 patients treated with definitive irradiation for CS A and B ($n = 18$), C ($n = 6$), and D1 ($n = 3$) disease with a mean follow-up of 5.2 years showed positive biopsy in 25 (93%) patients (KABALIN et al. 1989). The use of routine PSA determination in 117 radiotherapy-treated patients, with a mean follow-up of 2.3 years, showed biochemical relapse in 44 (39%) patients, of whom 30 (68%) had subsequent clinical relapse (KAPLAN et al. 1993). On the other hand, STAMEY et al. (1993) reported on a routine PSA determination in 124 consecutive unselected patients treated with definitive pelvic irradiation with a mean follow-up of 5 years. Of the 113 patients with a minimum follow-up of 4 years, 88 (78%) showed biochemical relapse.

Table 20.1. Relative 5 year survival in patients with CaP (American Cancer Society 1995)

Disease status at diagnosis	% Survival 1983	% Survival 1990
Localized	58	95
Regional	15	87
Distant	16	30
All stages		81

The above reports, which suggest a high incidence of relapse in patients treated with definitive pelvic irradiation, have, to a certain extent, changed the pattern of care of patients with capsule-confined tumors. The most apparent evidence for this change in the pattern of care has been a progressive increase in the proportion of patients with localized disease treated with radical prostatectomy, thus decreasing the number of patients treated with definitive pelvic irradiation (METTLIN et al. 1994). A review of the National Cancer Data Base of the Commission on Cancer of the American College of Surgeons showed 12.2% of patients with localized CaP treated with radical prostatectomy in 1985, 20.3% in 1988, and 30.4% in 1990 (METTLIN et al. 1994). This proportion of patients with localized CaP treated with radical prostatectomy and pelvic lymphadenectomy is undoubtedly higher still in 1995. The American College of Surgeons' data (Table 20.2) have shown several interesting trends. The most obvious are the increase in the number of CaP patients reported to the National Cancer Data Base, the proportion of patients diagnosed with localized disease (27.7% in 1985 and 48.5% in 1990), and the proportion of patients under the age of 55 treated with radical prostatectomy (69.1% in 1990).

In addition to the controversy regarding the treatment of patients with localized disease, an even more important controversy exists as to the indications and timing of the treatment for at least some selected patients with this disease (ADOLFSSON 1993;

Table 20.2. Patients with CaP treated with radical prostatectomy (Rad. prost.) in the United States (modified from METTLIN et al. 1994)

Year	n, Total	n, Localized	% Localized	n, Rad. prost.	% Rad. prost.	% Rad. prost. <55 years
1985	16349	4531	27.7	552	12.2	34.8
1988	25028	11488	45.9	2331	20.3	49.5
1990	44750	21697	48.5	6597	30.4	69.1

CHODAK et al. 1994; GARNICK 1994; JOHANSSON 1994). The investigators favoring a more conservative approach to the management of selected CaP patients believe that treatment sequelae may outweigh treatment benefits, particularly in patients with tumors with a low Gleason's score and those patients with an estimated life expectancy of less than 10 years (CHODAK et al. 1994; GARNICK 1994; FLEMING et al. 1993). It is apparent that data from prospective, well-designed clinical trials will be necessary to resolve the above critical problem. The reader is referred to Chap. 8 for details on conservative management of CaP patients.

20.3 Clinical Staging and Its Accuracy

In spite of important new developments in imaging modalities and the routine use of PSA, preoperative staging in patients with localized CaP is still in need of improvement. Yet, the proportion of CaP patients diagnosed with localized disease has nearly doubled from 1985 to 1990 (Table 20.2). In a study of 178 consecutive CaP patients who had preoperative PSA determination and careful pathologic examination of the resected specimen, very good correlations were noted between PSA and capsular penetration ($P < 0.002$), PSA and seminal vesicle involvement ($P < 0.02$), and PSA and pelvic lymph node involvement ($P < 0.05$) (OESTERLING et al. 1988). The staging accuracy for individual patients, however, was low (55%) for capsular penetration and even lower (50%) for seminal vesicle and pelvic lymph node involvement. The same study found an excellent reliability of PSA determination in detecting the presence of residual disease following radical prostatectomy and pelvic lymphadenectomy. A multi-institutional trial compared the value of TRUS and magnetic resonance imaging (MRI) in the preoperative staging of 230 CaP patients presenting with clinical evidence of an early disease. The diagnostic accuracy of imaging for pathologically confirmed lesions >5 mm in diameter was 60% in MRI- and 59% in TRUS-studied patients (RIFKIN et al. 1990). This diagnostic accuracy was better in patients with more advanced disease (77% and 57%, respectively). It is of interest to note a lack of improvement in staging accuracy with the use of combined MRI and TRUS. Accurate preoperative assessment of tumor volume in the prostate is of importance since it is a good predictor of tumor behavior. In one report based on nine published studies, patients with tumors of 0.5 cc had a 10% probability of capsular penetration which increased to a 50% probability of penetration in those with tumors of 6.0 cc in volume (Table 20.3) (BOSTWICK et al. 1993). Digital rectal examination (DRE) combined with PSA was found in a study of 436 patients with clinically capsule-confined tumors to be superior to TRUS and PSA determination (BABAIAN et al. 1993). Preoperative staging in 703 patients with localized CaP, utilizing CS, PSA, and Gleason score, was good in predicting the pathologic stage (PS) of disease (PARTIN et al. 1993). Similar findings were reported in 157 consecutive patients with stage T1 c tumors (EPSTEIN et al. 1994). It is of interest to note that 84% of these patients with nonpalpable tumors were found at surgery to have significant lesions requiring aggressive management.

Table 20.3. The importance of tumor volume for extent of disease (modified from BOSTWICK et al. 1993)

Tumor volume (cc)	% Capsular penetration	% Sem. vesicle invasion	% Metastatic disease
0.5	10	4	3
1.0	21	4	3
2.0	26	6	4
4.0	37	10	7
6.0	50	18	12
10	75	46	29
20	98	96	87

An interesting study accurately assessing the status of pelvic lymph nodes prior to radical prostatectomy was recently reported by VAN POPPEL et al. 1994. These investigators preoperatively staged 285 patients with clinically localized CaP using computerized axial tomography (CT) and cytology obtained through fine-needle aspiration. The sensitivity of this staging method was 78%, the specificity was 100%, the accuracy was 96.5%, and only ten patients with minimal invasion of pelvic lymph nodes had false-negative results. A surprising finding of this study was the very high sensitivity, specificity, and accuracy (78%, 97%, and 94%, respectively) of lymph node staging with the use of CT alone. This is in contrast to other published reports on preoperative staging accuracy (OESTERLING et al. 1988; RIFKIN et al. 1990; BOSTWICK et al. 1993; BABAIAN et al. 1993). FREEMAN et al. (1993) reported a poor correlation between preoperatively established tumor extent and pathologic findings at radical prostatectomy with one-half of stage B2 patients having PS C tumors. Similar data were reported by LANGE and NARAYAN (1983).

Table 20.4. Accuracy of clinical staging in 221 radical prostatectomy patients without pelvic lymphadenopathy treated at USC between 1972 and 1989

Clinical stage	Pathologic stage						Total
	B1	B2	C1	C2	C3	P0	
A1	1	1	0	0	0	0	2
A2	3	15	2	4	3	2	29
B1	18	34	13	19	8	1	93
B2	3	24	9	17	14	0	67
C	0	5	11	2	12	0	30
Total	25	79	35	42	37	3	221

Clinical staging accuracy in 221 consecutive CaP patients with P N0 disease treated with radical prostatectomy and limited pelvic lymphadenectomy at the University of Southern California School of Medicine (USC) is shown in Table 20.4. Apparently, in these 221 patients, following pathologic examination of surgical specimens to establish the anatomic extent of disease, clinical staging underestimated PS in 65% of the patients, while it overestimated the true extent of the tumor in 5%. Based on these data the accuracy of clinical staging was only 30%. Clinical staging accuracy is of major importance since it determines treatment options in a given patient. Careful study of surgical specimens establishes the presence or absence of capsular penetration, positive surgical margins, and seminal vesicle or pelvic lymph node invasion. PSA determination following radical prostatectomy provides additional and critically important data on the presence or absence of residual disease. This information determines the need for postoperative adjuvant therapy.

20.4 Local Recurrence Following Definitive Treatment

20.4.1 Patterns of Failure Following Radical Surgery

There is a relative scarcity of detailed long-term outcome data in patients with localized CaP treated with radical prostatectomy. This is particularly true in the case of the analysis of patterns of failure in these patients. In a study of 67 prostatectomy-treated CaP patients, local failure (LF) at 5 years posttreatment was reported in one out of ten (10%) patients with CS A tumors, in four out of 41 (10%) patients with CS B tumors and in three out of four (75%) patients with CS C lesions (Schellhammer 1988). LF in 39 PS B disease was 10% and in 13 PS C tumors it was 31%. The incidence of LF at 15 posttreatment years for CS B disease was 15% (4/26), for PS B it was 17% (4/23), and for the 13 patients with PS C tumor it was 31%. The weakness of this report is due to the exclusion of patients who died of other causes or were lost to follow-up. It is of interest to note that there was a 44% incidence of LF and a 66% incidence of distant failure in patients with seminal vesicle invasion. In surgically treated with CS T3 (C) tumors, the incidence of LF was 14% (1/7) in those with positive margins and no seminal vesicle invasion and 0% (0/10) in those with negative surgical margins and no seminal vesicle involvement (Bosch et al. 1987). The incidence of LF in those with seminal vesicle invasion was 40% (2/5) and 14% (1/7), respectively.

In a study of 586 patients treated with anatomic radical prostatectomy, 25% patients with positive surgical margins had LF while, surprisingly, there was a relatively low incidence of LF in those patients with an invasion of seminal vesicles (9%) or pelvic lymph nodes (3%) (Table 20.5) (Morton et al. 1991). LF in radical prostatectomy-treated patients was reported in more than 40% of those with seminal vesicle involvement (Gibbons et al. 1986). Generally, it has been clearly established that patients with seminal vesicle invasion have a much higher incidence of tumor progression than those without such invasion (Epstein et al. 1993a). Details on patterns of failure in surgically treated patients are given in Chap. 10.

Table 20.5. Pattern of failure analysis in 586 radical prostatectomy patients (modified from Morton et al. 1991)

Tumor extent	No.	LF	%	DF	%	PSA elev.	%
Capsule confined	337	7	2	3	1	10	3
Specimen confined	122	10	8	2	2	20	16
Outside of specimen	127	10	8	38	30	52	41
Pos. margins	25	6	25	2	10	3	13
Pos. seminal vesicles	52	5	9	19	37	16	31
Pos. lymph nodes	50	2	3	15	30	42	84

LF, Local failure; DF, distant failure

20.4.2 Patterns of Failure Following Definitive Radiotherapy

Direct comparison of the incidence of LF in radiotherapy-treated patients for localized CaP and those treated with radical prostatectomy presents a difficult problem since the patient populations treated with these two modalities are very different (Bagshaw et al. 1988; Perez et al. 1993b). The radiotherapy-treated patients tend to be older, have more advanced tumors at diagnosis, and are frequently not optimal candidates for surgical therapy due to their poor general medical condition. The reported incidence of LF in patients treated with definitive irradiation, as expected, depends on the extent of the tumor. Perez et al. (1993b), in their excellent review article, reported the following incidence of LF: patients with stage A2 (T1b) tumors 0%–20%, stage B (T2) tumors 5%–30%, and stage C (T3) tumors 12%–40%. The incidence of clinically noted LF 10 years following pelvic irradiation was 20% for stage A2 patients, 24% for stage B patients, and 40% for stage C patients. The reported incidence of distant failure (DF) in this patient population ranged from 20% for patients with clinically capsule-confined tumors to 40% in those with locally advanced (CS C) tumors. Details on patterns of failure in patients treated with definitive radiotherapy are presented in Chap. 16.

20.5 Postoperative Radiotherapy

Postoperative pelvic irradiation was used as a salvage therapy in selected patients with residual or recurrent tumor following radical prostatectomy (Ray et al. 1984). The 32 study patients were treated to the prostate region up to a total dose of 70 Gy, given at 2-Gy daily increments. This included 11 patients who also received a mean dose to pelvic lymph nodes of 54 Gy. Of the 32 patients treated, 13 had incomplete tumor excision and began their radiotherapy within 4 months of radical prostatectomy. The remaining 19 patients received radiotherapy for palpable recurrent tumors. The 5- and 10-year actuarial disease-free survival (DFS) was 57% and 57% for the former group and 40% and 20%, respectively, for the latter group. Important factors adversely affecting treatment outcome included the presence of bladder neck or bladder invasion and/or elevation of total serum acid phosphatase. Local tumor control assessed with DRE was obtained in ten (77%) patients treated electively and in 11 (58%) patients treated for palpable recurrent tumors. Of the 32 treated patients, five (16%) had ten significant radiotherapy complications. These complications included: two cases of urinary incontinence, two urethral strictures, one case of fecal incontinence, three cases of radiation proctitis, one case of lymphedema, and one patient with a history of diverticulitis that required colostomy for acute intestinal obstruction. Based on these data, the authors recommended routine use of elective postoperative radiotherapy following radical prostatectomy in patients with extracapsular disease or in those with positive surgical margins.

20.6 Management of Pathologic Stage C Tumors

The effectiveness of salvage radiotherapy following radical prostatectomy was reported by Hanks and Dawson (1986). A total of 21 patients were treated, receiving a mean radiation dose of 66.3 Gy, given at 2-Gy daily fractions. Elective treatment for PS C tumors was given to 11 patients. None of the seven patients followed for a minimum of 5 years developed LF while one (9%) had DF. Of the ten patients treated for palpable recurrent disease, two (20%) developed LF, and three (30%) developed DF. Minor complications were seen in five (24%) patients, while none had severe treatment toxicity. The authors strongly recommended the use of elective postoperative radiotherapy in patients with PS C tumors. Postoperative pelvic irradiation was given to 14 patients with PS C tumors and to six patients with PS D1 tumors (Bahnson et al. 1986). The mean radiation dose was >60 Gy, with the treatment being initiated at a mean time of 2.4 months postoperatively. Radiation treatment to the whole pelvis, with an additional boost to the prostate bed, was given to 14 (70%) patients, while six (30%) received more localized therapy. It was not apparent what criteria were used for this radiation field size selection. Of the 20 patients treated, 14 (70%) were followed for at least 3 years. LF was reported in no patients with PS C tumor and in one (17%) patients with PS D tumor. The 5-year actuarial survival was 75% for the 14 patients with PS C and 41% for the six PS D1 patients. Minor complications were reported in 17 (85%) patients while major complications were seen in nine (45%). Late complications included five patients with lymphedema of the lower extremities and four patients with urethral stricture. This incidence of late complications was unusually high and could be related to surgical and/or radiotherapy techniques, which were not described in the paper thereby allowing for their assessment.

Postoperative radiotherapy was given to 28 patients who had radical prostatectomy ($n = 18$) or prostate enucleation ($n = 10$) (Pilepich et al. 1984). All patients had PS C disease. Radiotherapy, in 80% of patients, consisted of whole pelvis treatment up to a dose from 40 to 50 Gy and a boost dose to the prostatic fossa up to a total dose of >65 Gy. The duration of follow-up ranged from 1 to 10 years, with a mean of 54 months and median of 41 months. LF was reported in one (4%) patient who had prior enucleation of the prostate, and DF was seen in 14 (50%) patients. The treatment was very well tolerated, with radiotherapy not increasing the incidence of incontinence. Complications were noted in ten (36%) study patients. They included: proctatitis in four, stricture in two, cystitis in two, osteitis pubis in one, and intestinal obstruction and fistula in one.

An interesting study was reported by Gibbons et al. (1986). These authors presented their experience with 148 patients treated with radical prostatectomy for tumors clinically localized to the prostate. Of the 148 patients, 45 (30%) had PS C disease, of whom 22 (49%), based on the preference of the surgeon, were referred for postoperative radiotherapy, while 23 (51%) received no adjuvant treatment. The mean total radiation dose was 63 Gy and the mean follow-up was 9.2 years, with a minimum follow-up of 5 years. LF was seen in one (5%) of the 22 adjuvant radiotherapy-treated patients and in seven (30%) of the observation-only patients ($P < 0.05$). As expected, the highest incidence (44%) of LF was seen in the nine patients with seminal vesicle involvement. DF was reported in five (23%) patients of the former group and in eight (35%) of the latter group. Of the eight patients who developed LF, seven (87%) died of CaP. It is of importance to note that, of the seven patients with LF who did not receive postoperative irradiation, six received definitive radiotherapy upon recurrence. Of these six patients, only one was salvaged with pelvic irradiation while five died of disseminated CaP. There were 21 complications reported in the 22 patients who received elective postoperative radiotherapy, with some patients having more than one complication. Chronic proctatitis and chronic cystitis were present in six patients; three had fistulas, two had rectal incontinence, two had permanent colostomy, and two had permanent urinary diversion. These complications were likely related to the radiotherapy technique, which used relatively high radiation doses to a large pelvic volume.

An attempt to study the efficacy of postoperative irradiation in patients with PS C tumors was also performed at the University of Utah (Jacobson et al. 1987). Radical prostatectomy for clinically capsule-confined tumors was done in 50 patients, who, following surgery, were upstaged to PS C disease. Of these 50 patients, 26 received adjuvant radiotherapy, while 24 received no further postoperative treatment. Most of the 26 patients were given whole pelvic irradiation with the final boost dose delivered to the prostatic fossa. Radiation doses ranged from 54 to 70 Gy, with no mean dose being provided. A comparison between the adjuvant radiotherapy and observation-only group was made 5 years after prostatectomy. The important parameters which were compared included: DFS and the incidence of DF and LF. There was no significant difference in overall or DFS between the two groups. The overall 5-year actuarial survival and DFS for the 24 surgery-only and for the 26 postoperative radiotherapy patients were not statistically different. The 5-year DFS was 71% and 69% for the former and the latter group, respectively. The incidence of DF was 29% for the surgery-only and 35% for the adjuvant therapy patients, respectively. The most important finding of this study, however, was the incidence of LF. It was 17% for the observation-only patients, while none of the 26 patients receiving postoperative radiotherapy developed LF. The incidence of LF was particularly high (30%) in the ten surgery-alone patients who had seminal vesicle involvement. Radiotherapy was well tolerated by the 26 study patients. Complications were reported in six (23%) patients, including two with lower extremity edema, three with stress incontinence, and one with persistent rectal urgency. Additionally, three patients had incontinence following prostatectomy, which remained unchanged following radiotherapy. It is of interest to note that none of the five patients who received radiotherapy to the prostatic fossa only, as opposed to a large volume treatment which included regional lymphatics, had significant treatment sequelae. The authors concluded from this study that adjuvant radiotherapy following radical prostatectomy is an important treatment in reducing the high incidence of LF, particularly in patients with seminal vesicle involvement. Additionally, the incidence of treatment complications could be substantially reduced with the use of radiation fields limited to the prostatic fossa. Similar findings supporting a routine use of postoperative irradiation in patients with PS C were reported in a study of 16 patients who received this treatment (SHEVLIN et al. 1989). None of the 16 study patients developed LF, while of the 52 PS C patients who received no treatment following radical prostatectomy, 11 (21%) had LF ($P = 0.01$). Additional interesting findings of this study included: 100% incidence of local tumor control in patients with local recurrence following prostatectomy and treatment with definitive pelvic irradiation and minimal complications in surgically treated patients who received relatively high (>60 Gy) radiation doses.

An important finding in a study of 159 patients, treated with radical prostatectomy for tumors clinically localized to the prostate and found at operation to have more extensive (PS C) disease, was reported by ANSCHER and PROSNITZ (1987). Of these 156 patients, 46 (29%) received adjuvant postoperative pelvic irradiation and 113 (71%) received no adjuvant therapy. The patients of these two groups had a similar incidence of important prognostic parameters such as CS, histologic grade of tumor, and PS. Radiotherapy techniques consisted of whole pelvis treatment up to a dose of 45–50 Gy followed by a boost dose of 10–15 Gy, with this treatment being delivered using the four-field daily therapy. The 5-, 10-, and 15-year actuarial survival in the 46 radiotherapy-receiving patients was 96%, 90%, and 90%, respectively, while it was 82%, 62%, and 21%, respectively, in the 113 surgery-alone patients ($P = 0.02$). The 15-year actuarial cancer-specific survival was 90% for the former and 25% for the latter group ($P = 0.007$)). The 15-year actuarial DFS was 40% for the adjuvant radiotherapy-treated patients, as compared to 28% for the surgery-alone patients ($P = 0.34$). Local control at 5, 10, and 15 years for the 46 adjuvant radiotherapy patients was 96%, with only two (4%) patients diagnosed with LF. This compared with 5-, 10-, and 15-year incidences of local control in the 113 surgery-alone patients of 75%, 49%, and 32%, respectively, with 28 patients exhibiting LF ($P = 0.009$). Consistent with other reports, the highest incidence of LF was seen in patients with seminal vesicle involvement. This incidence was 2/19 (10%) in radiotherapy-treated patients and 12/32 (37%) in the surgery-alone patients. Of the 28 surgery-alone patients who developed LF, 11 received pelvic irradiation to treat their recurrent tumor, and local control was obtained in ten (91%) of these patients. The incidence of treatment complications is of some concern. Of the 46 patients who were fully continent following radical prostatectomy, ten (22%) developed various degrees of incontinence following postoperative radiotherapy, which included mild incontinence in eight (17%), moderate incontinence in one (2%), and severe incontinence in one (2%). Severe infection was reported in seven (15%) patients, urethral stricture in seven (15%), severe cystitis in three (7%), lower extremity or genital edema in four (9%), and fistula in one (2%). In addition, 27 (59%) patients had less severe complications, including mild ($n = 20$; 43%) and moderate ($n = 7$; 16%). In spite of the good results reported in this study in terms of improved local tumor control and improved overall long-term survival, the above incidence of complications together with their severity is not acceptable. In view of the USC data, these complications were very likely due to the large volume of tissue being treated up to relatively high doses of radiation in patients who had prior radical prostatectomy (CARTER et al. 1989; PETROVICH et al. 1991; FREEMAN et al. 1993).

An interesting study on 115 PS C patients who were treated with radical prostatectomy was reported by the group from University of California Los Angeles (UCLA). Of these 115 patients, 24 (21%) received postoperative radiotherapy and were compared with 91 patients who received no adjuvant postoperative treatment (STEIN et al. 1992). Mean duration of follow-up was 41 months for the 91 surgery-alone and 49 months for the 24 adjuvant therapy patients. Radiotherapy techniques consisted of treatment which included the regional lymphatics up to a dose of 45–50 Gy, with a final 10-Gy boost directed at the prostatic fossa. The 5- and 7-year actuarial DFS for the radiotherapy patients was 75% and 54%, respectively, and it was 43% and 24%, respectively, for the surgery-alone patients ($P = 0.043$). Clinical progression at the last follow-up was seen in one (4%) adjuvant radiotherapy-treated patient, with none showing LF. Clinical progression in the surgery-alone group was diagnosed in 22 (24%) patients, of whom 11 (12%) had LF and 11 (12%) had DF. Treatment complications of significance were seen in four (17%) patients and included two cases of urethral stricture, one of bladder neck contracture, and one of temporary lower extremity edema.

20.6.1 Management of Pathologic Stage C Tumors at USC

Treatment of patients with PS C tumors with postoperative irradiation will be presented in detail, based on the USC data (CARTER et al. 1989; PETROVICH et al. 1991; Freeman et al. 1993). Between 1972 and 1989, 221 patients with localized CaP were treated with radical retropubic prostatectomy and limited pelvic lymphadenectomy. Of these 221 patients, 114 (52%) had PS C tumors and were recommended to undergo postoperative radiotherapy. Postoperative radiotherapy was refused by 19 (17%) of these patients. Patients' ages ranged from 46 to 79 years, with a median age of 66 years. In 61 (64%) of the 95 study patients, a diagnosis of CaP was made on a routine physical examination. Obstructive signs and symptoms were present in 32 (34%) patients; in 22 cases (23%) they were due to CaP, and in ten (11%), to benign prostatic hyperplasia (BPH). The staging system used in this study was published (Gibbons et al. 1986; Freeman et al. 1993). CS in these patients was: A2 − N = 8 (8.4%), B1 − N = 34 (35.8%), B2 − N = 32 (33.7%), and C − N = 21 (22.1%). Correlations between Gleason score, CS, and PS are presented in Table 20.6. A majority (67%) of the patients had an intermediate Gleason score, while 27% had a high (8–10) score. The strength of this study is the relative uniformity of the treatment. Radical retropubic prostatectomy was performed only by two surgeons (D.G.S. and G. Lieskovsky).

Details on the surgical techniques used in this study have been published (Carter et al. 1989; Freeman et al. 1993). Postoperative radiotherapy was given within 3 months of surgery. This period was found to be optimal to permit for full postsurgical recovery, to permit for the completion of voiding training, and to minimize the probability of postradiation complications such as urethral stricture. The details of radiotherapy techniques have evolved considerably during the period of this study. The general treatment policy, however, has remained to a large extent intact. The most important principle of our treatment policy has been based on the recognition that all of the study patients have had prior radical surgery; consequently, the volume of tissue treated with radiation has been limited to the prostatic fossa and its immediate vicinity, specifically ex-

Table 20.6. Distribution of the 95 study patients by pathologic stage, clinical stage, and Gleason's score

Pathologic stage	Gleason score			Clinical stage			
	2–4	5–7	8–10	A2	B1	B2	C
C1	0	20	6	1	8	7	10
C2	4	27	6	4	18	13	2
C3	1	17	14	3	8	12	9
Total	5	64	26	8	34	32	21

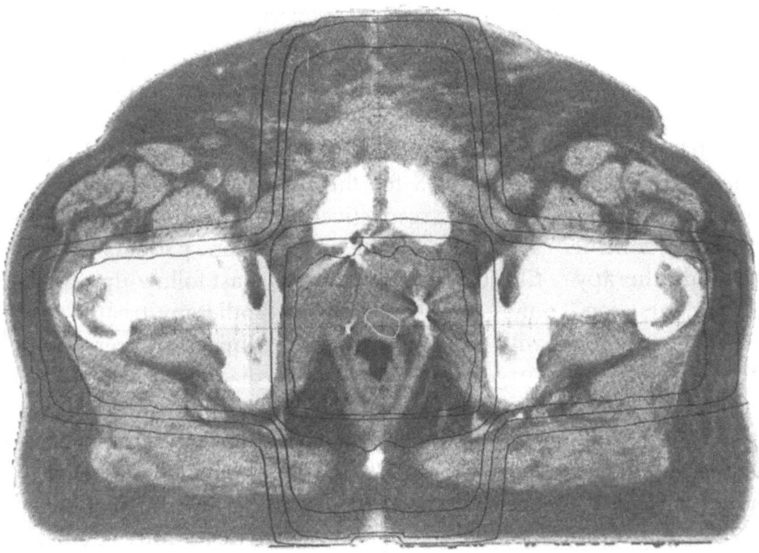

a

Fig. 20.1a–c. Reconstructed images with superposed isodose lines in the three principal orthogonal planes passing through the treatment isocenter: **a** transverse, **b** sagittal, and **c** coronal. The anterior direction is toward the top of the transverse and sagittal images, while the cephalad direction is toward the top of the coronal image. Four shaped fields with equal weights are used in this treatment plan: right and left lateral, and anteroposterior and posteroanterior. The margins of the surgically resected prostate are shown as a highlighted area in the coronal and sagittal images, and as an outlined area in the transverse plane. The isodose lines shown are the 95%, 90%, 65%, 50%, 35%, and 20%, relative to 100% as the maximum in the three-dimensional dose matrix. The prescribed daily fraction was 180 cGy to the 95% isodose surface. All four fields were treated each day (see text)

Fig. 20.1b, c

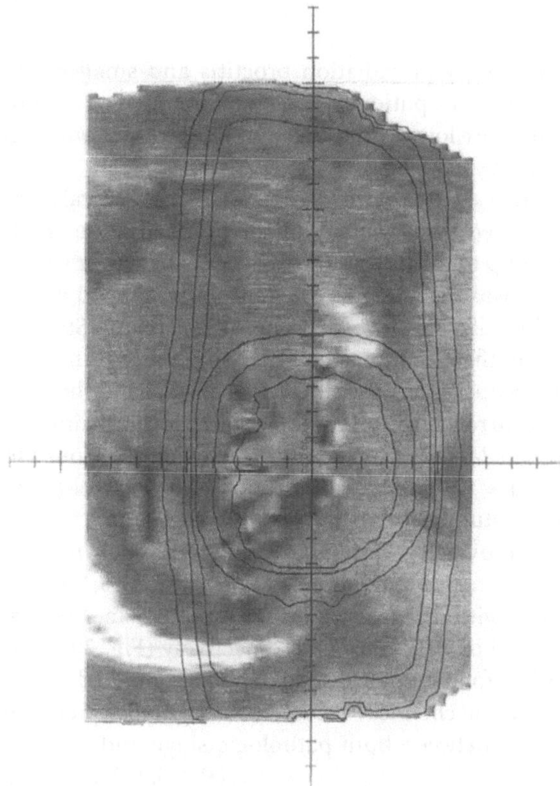

b

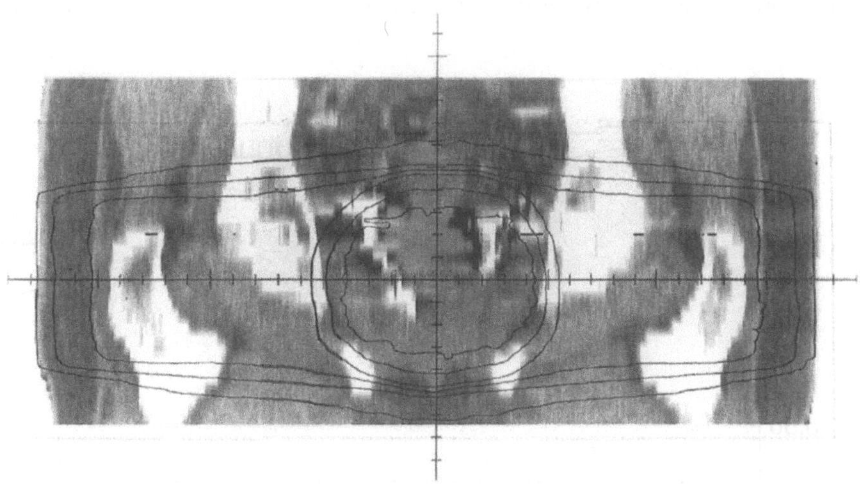

c

cluding the regional pelvic lymph nodes. Additionally, radiation doses have generally been limited to 45 Gy, given daily to the 95% isodose line at the rate of 180 cGy for a total period of 5 weeks. At the present time, the 45 Gy radiation dose remains in use for patients with PS C1 and C2 disease, while the dose is 54 Gy for those with PS C3 tumors. The daily treatments are given using the four-field "box" technique. Radiation portals are of a mean area of 100 cm^2 and are shaped in order to optimize the protection of normal tissues which are thought not to be involved by the neoplastic process, such as the small bowel or the posterior rectal wall. Typical radiation portals are shown in Fig. 20.1. The 95 study patients were treated at a 100 cm target-skin or target-axis distance. All patients but one were treated with linear accelerators of the following beam energies: 15–23 MV in 33 (35%), 4 MV in 32 (34%), and 6–10 MV in 28 (30%) patients. In one additional patient, beam energy was not specified. In an attempt to reduce the incidence and severity of radiation proctitis and small bowel irritation, the patients were recommended to temporarily use a low residue diet and were treated with full bladder.

Time up to any recurrence (PSA or clinical) was calculated from the day of the first radiation treatment up to the day when a diagnosis of tumor recurrence was made. PSA recurrence was defined as the finding of a PSA level of 0.4 ng/ml or greater. Statistical significance was calculated using the logrank test. All *P* values were two-sided and survival and the time to recurrence were estimated and plotted using the Kaplan-Meier method. Follow-up extended from 3 to 17 years, with a median duration of 6 years. None of the 95 study patients was lost to follow-up.

The overall 5- and 10-year actuarial survival for the 95 treated patients was 94% and 70%, respectively, with disease-specific 5- and 10-year actuarial survival of 99% and 78%, respectively (Fig. 20.2). At the last follow-up, 59 (62%) patients remained free of clinical or chemical recurrence. A good correlation existed between both pathologic stage and Gleason score and the disease-free status ($P < 0.0001$, logrank test). There was a progressive increase in the incidence of tumor recurrence with the increase in the Gleason score. Among the five patients with a Gleason score from 2 to 4, none had tumor recurrence, while of the 26 high (8–10) Gleason score patients, only eight (31%) remained free of tumor recurrence. Of the 64 patients with the intermediate (5–7) Gleason score, 46 (72%) remained free of PSA or clinical recurrence. These differences in the incidence of tumor recurrence based on the Gleason score had statistical significance ($P = 0.021$, logrank test). Of the 95 study patients, ten (10%) had clinical tumor recurrence. The time to clinical recurrence ranged from 1 to 9.3 years with a median time of 3.6 years and a mean time of 4 years. The time to clinical recurrence and the incidence of clinical recurrence again correlated very well with the Gleason score, with the high (8–10) Gleason score patients faring the worst ($P < 0.0001$). At the last follow-up, 56 patients were alive and free of clinical or PSA recurrence. An additional 22 (23%) patients were alive with PSA elevation (>0.3 ng/ml) and six (6%) were alive with clinical recurrence. A total of 11 (12%) patients have died, including three who died of other causes with no evidence of clinical or PSA recur-

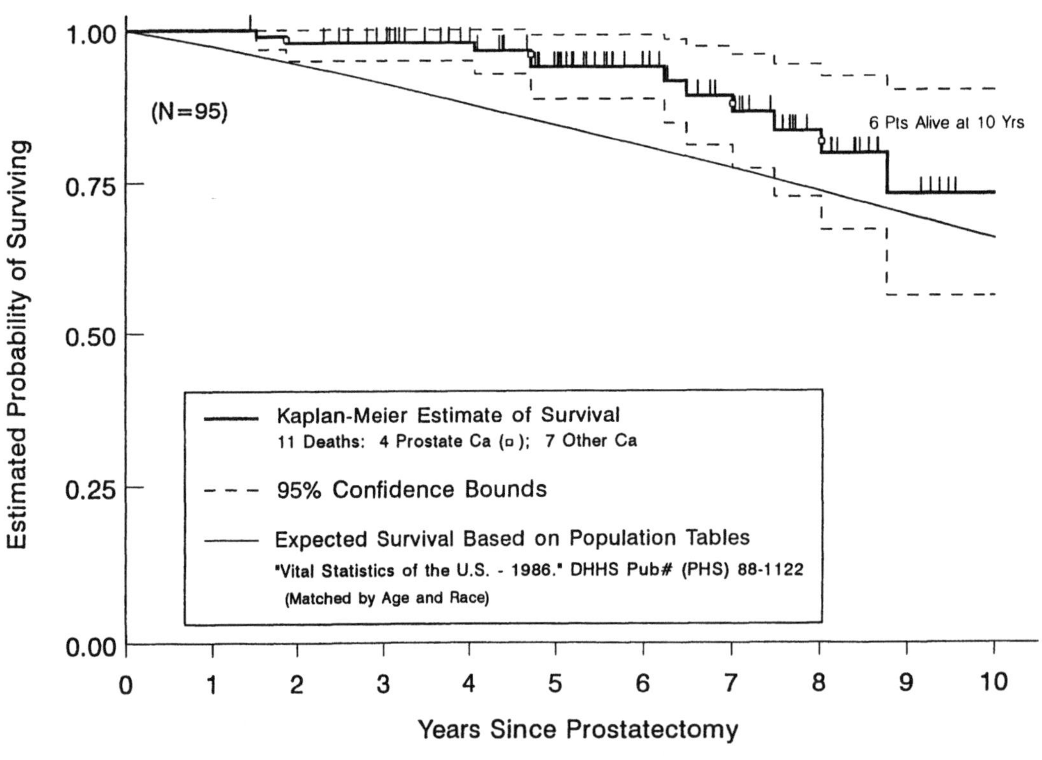

Fig. 20.2. Probability of overall survival for all 95 study patients with PS C tumors who received postoperative radiotherapy at USC. This probability of survival was compared with the expected survival based on the population tables. Bounds based on the 95% confidence intervals for the overall survival are plotted (----). Each *tick mark* represents a patient who was alive at the time of this evaluation. *Open squares* indicate a patient who was dead of prostatic carcinoma

rence, four who died of other causes with PSA >0.3 ng/ml, and four who died of CaP. Clinical failure was evident in ten (10%) patients. Of these ten, seven had distant metastases, which resulted in the death of three patients. Of the other three patients, one had DF and LF, also resulting in death, and the remaining two had LF alone and were alive at the last follow-up.

20.6.1.1 Treatment Complications in the 95 PS C Patients Treated at USC

Radical retropublic prostatectomy with pelvic lymphadenectomy resulted in no patient mortality in this group of 95 CaP patients. Major surgical complications were seen in two (2%) patients, while minor complications were recorded in five (5%). Details on surgical complications have been reported elsewhere (Freeman et al. 1993). Adjuvant postoperative irradiation was very well tolerated by the patients. A majority of these 95 patients complained during the course of treatment of mild to moderate fatigue. This problem was of no clinical significance, required no treatment, and did not persist for more than 2–3 weeks following complications of radiotherapy. Symptoms and signs of mild proctitis were seen in 34 (36%), frequency on urination in 13 (14%), dysuria in six (6%), and mild skin erythema within the posterior radiation portal in seven (8%). No acute toxicity was recorded in the 32 (32%) study patients. None of the patients developed severe or late toxicity of postoperative radiotherapy. No significant prolonged influence of postoperative radiotherapy on the degree of urinary continence was noted. Most of the patients treated experienced, during the final 2 weeks of the radiation course, a temporary decrease in the degree of continence. This typically returned to the pretreatment level within 2 weeks following the completion of radiotherapy. Continence assessment at 1 year postradical prostatectomy, followed by adjuvant radiotherapy in the 95 study patients, demonstrated the following findings: 71 (75%) patients were continent, 13 (14%) had mild stress incontinence, eight (8%) had mild to moderate (one to four pads/day) incontinence, and three had (3%) severe incontinence. It is of interest to note the degree of continence observed in 126 PS B CaP patients treated with radical prostatectomy at the same period of time by the same two surgeons (D.G.S. and G. Lieskovsky) and compare it to the incidence of continence in the 95 adjuvant radiotherapy-treated patients. There was no statistically significant difference in the continence level between these two treatment groups. Of the 126 surgery-alone PS B patients, 109 (87%) were fully continent at 1 year postoperatively, ten (8%) had mild to moderate incontinence, while seven (6%) were fully incontinent. Contrary to the popular belief, the addition of postoperative radiotherapy to radical retropubic prostatectomy in this group of 95 patients did not appreciably change patients' potency as compared to that of 126 PS B patients who were treated with surgery alone (Formenti et al. 1996).

20.7 Management of Clinical Stage C Tumors

Definitive management of CaP patients with CS C disease has usually been limited to pelvic irradiation, with or without hormonal treatment (Consensus Conference 1987). Radical prostatectomy and pelvic lymphadenectomy are generally not accepted as the treatments of choice in patients with CS C tumors, and their routine use for this stage of disease remains controversial. The main issue is the belief that definitive surgical treatment in patients with extracapsular disease is of limited clinical value. In recent years, however, this belief has been questioned; several clinical studies have examined its validity (Zincke et al. 1986; Bosch et al. 1987; Schellhammer et al. 1990; Yamada et al. 1994) and have found surgical treatment for CS C tumors, in properly selected patients, to be a safe and effective therapeutic option.

From 1966 to 1984, 1000 patients with CaP were treated with radical retropubic prostatectomy and bilateral pelvic lymphadenectomy at the Mayo Clinic (Zincke et al. 1986). Of these 1000 patients, 101 (10%) were treated for CS C tumors. Surgical candidates included: patients with extracapsular disease which was limited to the immediate periprostatic region, patients without clinical or radiographic evidence of distant metastases, and patients without apparent invasion of the trigone. Follow-up ranged from 6 months to 17 years, with a mean duration of 4.9 years. A pathologic study of prostatectomy specimens revealed 49 (49%) patients with PS C tumors and 52 (51%) patients with D1 disease. No statistically significant differences in tumor grade, incidence of seminal vesicle involvement, or tumor volume were noted between the 49 PS C and 52 PS D1 patients. There were 16 (16%) patients with documented residual tumor following radical surgery, including six in the former and ten in the latter group.

No adjuvant therapy was given to the 30 (61%) PS C and to the 17 (33%) PS D1 patients. Hormonal treatment alone was given to the 13 (13%) PS C and to the 29 (29%) PS D1 patients. A total of 12 (12%) of the 101 patients were treated with adjuvant radiotherapy, including six with additional hormonal treatment and six with radiotherapy alone. The most common (42%) hormonal treatment consisted of orchiectomy. Adjuvant irradiation was given within 6 weeks of surgery with a total dose of 50–60 Gy. Adjuvant therapy was given to 39% of PS C and to 67% of PS D1 patients. No information was provided as to the selection criteria for the use of a particular treatment. LF was diagnosed in 17 (17%) patients, of whom 13 were treated with surgery alone and four received adjuvant treatment, including one who received pelvic irradiation. Of the 47 patients who received no postoperative adjuvant therapy, 13 (28%) had LF. It is of interest to note that of the 16 patients who were known to have residual carcinoma, only two had LF including one who was treated with radiotherapy and diethylstilbestrol and one who received no adjuvant treatment. The remaining 14 patients with known residual disease received adjuvant therapy. The overall 5- and 10-year actuarial survival was 70% and 60%, respectively. There was no statistically significant difference in survival between the 49 PS C and 52 PS D1 patients. The 5- and 10-year actuarial DFS was 55% and 40%, respectively. The use of orchiectomy in the 49 patients with PS C disease did not result in significant improvement of overall and DFS, while this treatment had a major impact on DFS in patients with PS D1 tumors ($P < 0.0001$) and to a lesser degree on overall survival ($P = 0.09$). The incidence of complications was low, with one death and 2% of patients with incontinence. The authors concluded from their study that selected CaP patients with CS C tumors can be successfully and safely managed with an appropriate adjuvant therapy. Unfortunately, the authors did not recommend the criteria for the selection of this appropriate adjuvant therapy.

A study of 48 CS C patients treated with surgery was reported by Bosch et al. (1987). Radical prostatectomy with bilateral pelvic lymphadenectomy was attempted in all patients. In 23 patients there was frozen section evidence of pelvic lymph node metastases, and bilateral orchiectomy, instead of prostatectomy, was performed. Of these 23 patients, ten (43%) had tumor recurrence. The time to this tumor recurrence ranged from 6 to 61 months. The management of these ten patients with recurrent disease presented a difficult problem. They required a total of 13 surgical procedures to palliate the signs and symptoms of recurrent tumor. These 13 surgical procedures included: nine transurethral resections of the prostate (TURP), two repeated TURP, one cutaneous ureterostomy and colostomy, and one urinary diversion. Based on these data, the reported therapeutic direction in this group of 23 patients with pelvic lymphadenopathy appears not to be optimal. There was a clear need for the use of a planned adjuvant therapy. The remaining 25 patients had the planned radical prostatectomy and bilateral pelvic lymphadenectomy and no other postoperative therapy. LF was recorded in four (16%) patients, with a mean time to tumor recurrence of 9 months. It is of interest to note the major impact of seminal vesicle invasion on the incidence of LF. Of the 12 patients with seminal vesicle involvement, three (25%) had LF. This included two of five (40%) patients with positive surgical margins and one of seven (14%) of those with negative surgical margins. DF was reported in an additional four (16%); therefore, a total of eight (32%) showed tumor progression during a mean follow-up period of 43 months. No data on treatment complications were presented in this report. The authors, in spite of the treatment outcomes in the study patients, recommend this approach for (not more closely specified) selected patients presenting with CS C tumors. Schellhammer et al. (1990) reported treatment results with radical prostatectomy in 67 patients. In 50 of these 67 (75%), surgery was performed via the perineal approach. Four (6%) CS C patients were treated with surgery alone and they were followed for at least 5 years. LF was reported in three (75%) of these patients.

20.7.1 Management of Clinical Stage C Tumors at USC

From 1972 through 1989, 57 patients with CS C tumors underwent radical retropubic prostatectomy and bilateral pelvic lymphadenectomy performed by the same two surgeons (D.G.S. and G. Lieskovsky) (Yamada et al. 1994). The surgical techniques and the staging system used in the treatment of these patients have been published (Freeman et al. 1993). A Campbell's radical retropubic prostatectomy was performed in 55 (96%) patients, while two (4%) had a unilateral nerve-sparing operation. All study patients had bilateral lymphadenectomy with the preservation of lymphatics along the anterolateral aspect of the external iliac artery. Histologic examination of the surgical specimens revealed four (7%) patients with PS B2 tumors and 25 (44%) with PS C tumors which included 11 (19%) PS C1, 2 (3%) PS C2, and 12 (21%) PS C3 patients. Pelvic lymph node metastases were diagnosed in 27 (47%) of the 57 study patients. Gleason score was 2–4 in three (5%) patients, 5–7 in 31 (54%), and 8–10 in the remaining 23 (40%). Follow-up ranged from 3.5 to 19.9 years, with a median of 5.4 years.

The recommendation on the choice of adjuvant postoperative therapy depended on the stage of the disease; however, all patients were recommended to undergo postoperative irradiation. Radiotherapy techniques and radiation doses given to these patients have already been discussed in Sect. 20.6.1. Adjuvant chemotherapy consisted of cyclophosphamide (1 g/m²) either alone or combined with 5-fluorouracil (1 g) for a total treatment course of 6 months. Adjuvant hormonal treatment consisted of diethylstilbestrol (DES) given at 2–3 mg daily for a period of several months preoperatively. Statistical analysis of the data and the study end-points have already been described in Sect. 20.6.1. Distribution of patients by adjuvant therapy is shown in Table 20.7. A total of 46 (81%) patients received radiotherapy alone ($n = 21$) or in combination with systemic chemotherapy and/or hormonal treatment. Systemic chemotherapy alone or in combination with the other one or two adjuvant treatments was given to 20 (71%) of the 28 PS D1 patients, while 13 (23%) received hormonal therapy. The overall 5- and 7.5-year actuarial survival for the 57 study patients was 91% and 78%, respectively. No evidence of disease at the last follow-up, including the PSA level of 0.3 ng/ml or less, was recorded in 19 (33%) patients. The estimated probability of clinical recurrence at 5 years was 19% and, if the PSA elevation was included, this estimated probability of recurrence was 54% at 5 years posttherapy. LF was diagnosed in three (5%) patients, including two (4%) out of the 46 patients who received adjuvant irradiation. Of the 46 patients treated with adjuvant radiotherapy, two had LF in the pelvis, including one patient who had PS D1 disease. DF was recorded in nine (20%) patients and, including the PSA elevation, it was diagnosed in 18 (39%) patients. Surgical treatment was well tolerated and there was no surgical mortality. Details on surgical complications have been published (Yamada et al. 1994) and are presented in Chaps. 11 and 12. Postoperative radiotherapy was very well tolerated and there were no severe complications or complications of clinical significance. The quality of life of these 57 patients was good. In particular none of the study patients developed hematuria or required treatment for urinary tract obstruction. The degree of continence was assessed at 1 year posttreatment. Total incontinence was present in two (3%) patients, moderate (three to four pads/day) incontinence in one (2%), and mild (one to two pads/day) in seven (12%). There was no increase in the incidence of incontinence or in its severity as a result of the administration of postoperative irradiation. Based on the data from this study we recommend a judicious use of radical prostatectomy in selected patients with CS C CaP. The selection criteria include good general condition, with expected survival of 10 years or longer, and the presence of potentially resectable tumor without evidence of distant metastases.

Table 20.7. Distribution of 57 CS C patients by adjuvant therapy (modified from Yamada et al. 1994)

Therapy	Pathologic stage			Total
	B2	C	D1	
None	4	0	2	6
Radiotherapy (RT)	0	21	0	21
RT + hormonal Rx (H)	0	3	4	7
Hormonal Rx	0	1	2	3
Chemotherapy (CT)	0	0	2	2
CT + RT	0	0	15	15
CT + RT + H	0	0	3	3
Total	4	25	28	57

20.8 Management of Pathologic Stage D1 Disease

Patients suspected of having pelvic lymph node metastases are usually not being considered for radical surgical treatment as they are believed to be incurable. The patients treated with radical prostatectomy and pelvic lymphadenectomy for tumors clinically confined to the prostate, however, are not infrequently found to have pelvic lymph node metastases. The incidence of D1 disease in prostatectomy-treated patients is widely variable and depends on multiple factors including: CS, Gleason score, tumor volume, the presence or absence of extracapsular disease, and the presence of seminal vesicle involvement. The incidence of metastases in the pelvic lymph nodes in patients with CS C disease in one USC study was approximately 50% (Yamada et al. 1994). Similar data (48%) on the incidence of D1 tumors in radical prostatectomy treated patients were reported by other investigators (Bosch et al. 1987). Aggressive treatment of patients with PS D1 tumors is of importance due to the need to control the likely local relapse, which in turn is responsible for a sharp reduction in the quality of life of these patients. Very strong support for an aggressive postoperative therapy is provided in a study of 23 PS D1 patients reported by Bosch et al. (1987). These patients following pelvic lymphadenectomy were treated with bilateral orchiectomy only, with the prostate being left in situ. Of these 23 patients, ten (43%) had LF with tumor progression noted in eight patients within 5 years of lymphadenectomy. The extent of lymph node involvement correlated well with the incidence of local relapse. LF was seen in one of four (25%) patients with N1 tumors, in 5 of 13 (38%) with N2 tumors, and in four of six (67%) with N4 tumors. It is of importance to note the relatively poor quality of life of these patients. The ten patients with LF required 13 surgical procedures to control the signs and symptoms of local tumor progression. These 13 surgical procedures consisted of: TURP in nine patients, repeated TURP in two, cutaneous ureterostomy and colostomy in one, and urinary diversion in one.

20.8.1 Management of Pathologic Stage D1 Disease at USC

From 1972 to 1989, 76 CaP patients were treated with radical retropubic prostatectomy and bilateral pelvic lymphadenectomy performed by the same two surgeons (D.G.S. and G. Lieskovsky) (Freeman et al. 1994). The same treatment philosophy and similar surgical and radiotherapy treatment techniques and doses have been used in the treatment of these 76 patients as in the treatment of PS C. (Sect. 20.6.1) and CS C (Sect. 20.7.1) patients. The schedule and doses of adjuvant chemotherapy (CT) have been already discussed (Sect. 20.6.1). Histologic examination of the surgical specimens revealed only two (3%) patients with a low Gleason score (2–4); an intermediate score (5–7) was recorded in 49 (64%), and 23 (30%) patients had a high Gleason score. Similarly, most (71%) patients had large primary tumors in addition to the presence of pelvic lymph node metastases. The number of lymph nodes containing metastatic disease was: one in 28 (37%) patients, two in 11 (14%), three in 11 (14%), four to six in 15 (20%), and in 7–18 lymph nodes in the remaining ten (13%) patients. Follow-up ranged from 3 to 18 years, with a median duration of 7 years.

Of the 76 study patients, 58 (76%) received a planned course of pelvic irradiation which was initiated within 3 months of surgery (Table 20.8). The mean radiation dose was 46 Gy, given to the target volume, which included the prostatic fossa and its immediate vicinity. No attempt was made to include the regional pelvic lymphatics in the treatment volume. Adjuvant chemotherapy (CT) was given to 57 (75%) patients, with 19 (25%) patients declining to accept this therapy. Of the 57 patients treated with CT, 27 (47%) were given cyclophosphamide alone, and 30 (53%) received it in combination with 5-fluoruracil. Androgen deprivation therapy (ADT) was used in 14 (18%) patients, while bilateral orchiectomy was used in nine (12%) and DES was used in five (7%). Adjuvant therapy given to these 76 patients and the treatment outcomes are summarized in Table 20.8. At the last follow-up, 35 (46%) patients were alive with no clinical evidence of tumor recurrence or PSA elevation (PSA < 0.4 ng/ml). PSA elevation (>0.4 ng/ml) with clinical recurrence was present in 32 (42%) of these patients and three (4%) patients were alive and had PSA elevation without clinical evidence of tumor recurrence. A total of 24 (32%) patients are known to have died of CaP, while eight (11%) patients died of other causes with no evidence of tumor recurrence. Of the 32 patients with tumor recurrence, 14 (18%) had DF only, three (4%) had LF only, and two (3%) patients had LF followed

Table 20.8. Postoperative adjuvant therapy in the 76 study patients and treatment outcomes (from Freeman et al. 1994)

Treatment	Alive, NED[a]	Alive, clin. rec.	Alive, PSA >0.4 ng/ml	Dead, CaP	Dead, NED	Total
Radiotherapy	16	13	17	9	3	58
Chemotherapy	14	17	13	10	3	57
Androgen deprivation	4	2	4	2	2	14
None	1	0	1	3	0	5
Total	35	32	35	24	8	76[b]

[a] No evidence of disease with PSA <0.4 ng/ml
[b] Patients had more than one adjuvant treatment

Table 20.9. Selected results of postoperative pelvic irradiation

Investigator(s)	Year	No.	Rad. dose (Gy)	LF	%	DF	%	% Survival (years)			Complications	%	Follow-up	Comments
								5	10	15				
Ray et al.	1984	13	70	3	23			57	57		5/32	16	3–15 yrs.	Elective
		19	70	8	42									palpable tumor
Hanks	1986	11	66	0	0	1	9	86			0/21		2–11 yrs.	Elective
		10		2	20	3	30							Clinical recurrence
Bahnson et al.	1986	14	>60	1	5	5	25	75			9/20	45	Mean 55 mos.	PSC
		6						41						D1
Pilepich et al.	1984	28	>65	1	4	14	50	45			10/28	36	Mean 54 mos.	PSC
Gibbons et al.	1986	22	>63	1	5	5	23	72			7/22	32	Mean 9.2 yrs.	PSC
Jacobson et al.	1987	26	54–70	0	0	9	35	70			6/26	23	≥5 yrs.	PSC
Shevlin et al.	1989	16	>60	0	0	5	31		64		0/16		Mean 58 mos.	PSC
Anscher and Prosnitz	1987	46	>60	2	4			68	60	40	23/46	50	Mean 58 mos.	PSC
Stein et al.	1992	24	60	0	0	1	4	75	54		4/24	17	Mean 49 mos.	
Freeman et al.	1993	95	45	3	3	8	8	94	70		0/95		Median 6 yrs.	PSC
Total		330		21	6	51	15				64/330	19		

LF, Local failure; DF, distant clinical failure

by systemic tumor dissemination. It is of interest to discuss the important treatment and outcome details in the five (7%) patients who had LF. Of these five patients, two received cyclophosphamide CT alone, two received cyclophosphamide in combination with radiotherapy, and the remaining patient had ADT alone. Therefore, out of the 58 patients who received adjuvant radiotherapy, two (3%) had LF. Symptoms and signs of LF were present in only one patient with LF. This patient had PSA of <0.4 ng/ml, and an obstructing periureteral tumor. The symptoms and signs of LF were palliated with reimplantation of the ureter followed with a bilateral orchiectomy. These data on LF in patients with PS D1 disease compare favorably with other published reports on this subject (Bosch et al. 1987).

The overall 5- and 10-year actuarial survival in the 76 study patients was 88% and 66%, respectively. This survival experience was similar to that of race- and age-matched controls. The 5- and 10-year actuarial CaP-specific survival was 88% and 74%, respectively. The probability of patients developing clinical recurrence at 5 and 10 years was 29% and 62%, respectively. This treatment program was well tolerated by the study patients, with no surgical mortality and with most (91%) patients having no surgical complications. Minor surgical complications were present in two (3%) and major complications in four (5%) patients. Details on treatment complications have been presented elsewhere (Chap. 12 and Freeman et al. 1994). Full continence, which was not impacted by the administration of adjuvant radiotherapy, was recorded in 52 (68%) patients. Mild to moderate incontinence was present in eight (11%) patients, total incontinence in four (5%), and 11 (14%) patients had stress incontinence. CT was also well tolerated without major or long-lasting complications. The need for hospitalization to treat neutropenic sepsis was reported in one chemotherapy-treated patient. There was no complication reported with the use of ADT. There was good tolerance of postoperative irradiation in the 58 patients receiving this adjuvant treatment. No complications were reported in 25 (43%) patients. Mild proctitis was present in 18 (31%) patients, while six (9%) reported dysuria. An interesting and difficult to explain complication was subcutaneous fibrosis within the radiation portals in a patient who received a total of 45 Gy with the four-field technique. Based on these data we recommend adjuvant postoperative irradiation in selected patients with PS D1 tumors. No adjuvant chemotherapy for these patients is being recommended. Selected treatment results in patients receiving adjuvant postoperative radiotherapy are shown in Table 20.9.

20.9 Management of Patients with Postoperative Increase in PSA Level

Complete tumor removal following radical retropubic prostatectomy and bilateral pelvic lymphadenectomy is expected to result in the lowering of PSA, to an undetectable (<0.4 ng/ml) level. Persistent postoperative elevation of PSA is being interpreted as very important evidence for the presence of residual tumor (ABI-AAD et al. 1992). In the majority of patients with postsurgical PSA elevation the residual tumor is most likely present in the region of the prostatic fossa. The incidence of persistent PSA elevation is widely variable, and it has been reported to range from a few to more than 30% of prostatectomy patients (LINK et al. 1991; HUDSON and CATALONA 1990). In a study reported by the group from Stanford University, of 260 radical prostatectomy patients, 25 (9.6%) had detectable PSA levels without any other evidence of residual disease (LINK et al. 1991). PS in these 25 patients was: C1 in three (12%), C2 in six (24%), C3 in eight (32%), and D1 in eight (32%). Pelvic irradiation was used for the treatment of these patients, with radiation being delivered to the prostatic bed. Radiation dose was 60 Gy in 20 (80%) patients, 70 Gy in four (16%), and 54 Gy in one (4%). The treatment volume in the eight PS D1 patients and six other patients also included the entire pelvis to receive 50 Gy. Of the 25 patients treated, eight (32%) remained free of clinical or chemical recurrence for the duration of follow-up (median 18 months). PSA elevation without clinical evidence of recurrent tumor was present in eight (32%), while nine (36%) had clinical evidence of tumor progression. Following the course of radiotherapy, 15 (60%) patients had undetectable PSA, and five (20%) had a 50% PSA level reduction. Longer follow-up is necessary to assess the value of postoperative pelvic irradiation in patients with PSA elevation. In a subsequent report from the same institution, based on 39 radical prostatectomy patients including 37 with PSA elevation only and two with palpable tumor recurrence, adjuvant pelvic irradiation was given (KAPLAN and BAGSHAW 1992). All patients received radiation doses from 60 to 70 Gy, including 40–56 Gy given to whole pelvis in 19 (50%) patients. A correlation was noted between certain pathologic tumor characteristics and postoperative PSA elevations. These tumor parameters predicting postsurgical PSA elevation included positive surgical margins, high Gleason score, and seminal vesicle involvement. At the last follow-up (median 27 months), 37 of the 38 treated patients had local tumor control. PSA was undetectable at >1 year following radiotherapy in 17 (44%) patients, continued to decrease in four (10%), and was increasing in 18 (46%). Of the 18 patients with rising PSA, nine (50%) developed metastatic bone disease. Radiotherapy was well tolerated by the 38 study patients and no complications of importance were seen in this group of patients. Similar data on the effectiveness of adjuvant pelvic irradiation in prostatectomy-treated patients who show persistent PSA elevation have been reported by other investigators (HUDSON and CATALONA 1990; PEREZ et al. 1993a).

A study of 27 prostatectomy patients who had PSA elevation at months or longer since surgery was reported by the group from Mayo Clinic (SCHILD et al. 1994). PS in these 27 patients was B in ten (37%) and C in 17 (63%) patients. Radiotherapy consisted of a median dose of 64 Gy given to the prostatic fossa and its immediate vicinity. PSA initially decreased in 24 (89%) patients, including to an undetectable level in 16 (59%). The actuarial chance of maintaining undetectable PSA in these patients was 58% and 48% at 2 and 3 years, respectively. No severe or late morbidity of this pelvic radiotherapy was reported. Clearly, there is good evidence for long-term efficacy of pelvic irradiation in patients with postoperatively persisting elevation of PSA.

20.10 Management of Patients with Postoperative Clinical Local Failure

Radiation therapy to the pelvis in patients with symptomatic local recurrence following radical prostatectomy is a well-established and efficient palliative treatment modality. The incidence of major palliative benefit in these patients depends on the primary symptom(s), caused by the recurrent tumor, and ranges from a low of 50% for relieving ureteric obstruction to a high of 100% in controlling frequently distressing hematuria (PEREZ et al. 1993a). Radiotherapy portals at Mallinckrodt Institute of Radiology in St. Louis, Missouri, include the regional lymphatics (45–50 Gy) with the final boost (15–20 Gy) to a smaller volume. Of the 23 patients with postprostatectomy local tumor recurrence treated at that medical center, 17 (74%) had local tumor control. The 5- and 10-year actuarial DFS was 45% and 17%, respectively. Of these 17 patients with local tumor control, 13 subsequently developed distant metastases without local tumor recurrence. It is of importance to observe an apparent dose response in these patients. All four of the patients receiving 60–65 Gy had local control and long-term survival whereas none of the four patients who received <50 Gy had long-term tumor control or long-term survival. Of the 15 patients who received 65–70 Gy, 13 (87%) had local tumor control with 50% 5-year actuarial DFS. On the other hand the investigators found no increase in the incidence of local tumor control and DFS with increase in the volume treated. Treatment complications have been reported in seven (30%) patients and have included scrotal edema in three cases, moderate cystitis in two, small bowel obstruction in one, and urinary incontinence in one.

Achievement of local tumor control in the pelvis in patients who present with postprostatectomy relapse is of major importance. These patients tend to develop severe and difficult to control symptoms. The best policy is to offer to these patients elective adjuvant pelvic radiotherapy if, on a pathologic examination of prostatectomy specimens, there are features suggestive of high likelihood of tumor recurrence. These pathologic parameters include the presence of any of the following: D1 tumor, seminal vesicle invasion, high Gleason score, positive surgical margins, and extracapsular disease. Radiotherapy given electively has an excellent chance of preventing local recurrence. Watchful waiting does not appear to be a good management option (Bosch et al. 1987).

20.11 Conclusion

Elective adjuvant postoperative pelvic irradiation in patients with PS C disease has become an important part of the management in these patients. Although there are no prospective randomized trials to support the use of adjuvant radiotherapy in PS C patients, numerous retrospective studies strongly support its use. Moderate (45 Gy) radiation dose given to the prostatic fossa and its vicinity in patients with PS C1 and C2 tumors, as practiced at USC, is an effective therapy, controlling LD in 97% of patients. This treatment is well tolerated by the patients and results in no toxicity of clinical importance. Patients with PS C3 tumors require a more aggressive treatment which includes a higher (54 Gy) radiation dose. There is also a need to develop an effective adjuvant systemic therapy in an attempt to reduce the high incidence of DF. The management of patients with CS C disease presents a more complex problem. In carefully selected patients radical retropubic prostatectomy and bilateral pelvic lymphadenectomy followed by elective pelvic irradiation appears to produce better local tumor control rates and better overall and DFS than are obtained with the use of definitive radiotherapy or radical prostatectomy alone. Treatment strategy in patients with PS D1 tumors should include a planned use of elective postoperative pelvic irradiation to reduce the well-documented high incidence of local recurrence. Prevention of LF is of major importance in improving quality of life in these patients in addition to a probable improvement in the overall and DFS in a subset of these patients. Early elective pelvic irradiation is of importance in patients with clinical evidence of local recurrence following radical prostatectomy. In addition to major palliative benefit there appears also to be an important benefit in improvement in long-term overall and DFS. Finally, there is increasingly strong evidence to support the early use of local pelvic irradiation in patients with persistent PSA elevation following prostatectomy. The use of adjuvant radiotherapy requires careful treatment planning to prevent or minimize the probability of treatment-related complications.

References

Abi-Ada A, MacFarlane MT, Stein A, De Kernion JB (1992) Detection of local recurrence after radical prostatectomy by prostate specific antigen and transurethral ultrasound. J Urol 147:952–955

Adolfsson J (1993) Deferred treatment of low grade stage T3 prostate cancer without distant metastases. J Urol 149:326–329

American Cancer Society (1995) Cancer statistics 1995. CA Cancer J Clin 45:8–31

Anscher MS, Prosnitz LR (1987) Postoperative radiotherapy for patients with carcinoma of the prostate undergoing radical prostatectomy with positive surgical margins, seminal vesicle involvement and/or penetration through the capsule. J Urol 138:1407–1412

Babaian RJ, Dinney CPN, Ramirez EI, Evans RB (1993) Diagnostic testing for prostate cancer detection: less is best. Urology 41:421–425

Bagshaw MA, Cox RS, Ray GR (1988) Status of radiation treatment of prostate cancer at Stanford University. NCI Monogr 7:47–60

Bagshaw MA, Cox RS, Ramback JE (1990) Radiation therapy for localized prostate cancer. Justification for long-term follow-up. Urol Clin North Am 17:787–802

Bahnson RR, Garnett JE, Grayhack JT (1986) Adjuvant radiation therapy in stages C and D1 prostatic adenocarcinoma: preliminary results. Urology 27:403–406

Bosch RJLH, Kurth KH, Schroeder FH (1987) Surgical treatment of locally advanced (T3) prostatic carcinoma: early results. J Urol 138:816–822

Bostwick DG, Graham SD, Napalkow P et al. (1993) Staging for early prostate cancer: a proposed tumor volume-based prognostic index. Urology 41:403–411

Carter GE, Lieskovsky G, Skinner DG, Petrovich Z (1989) Results of local and/or systemic adjuvant therapy in the management of pathological stage C or D1 prostate cancer following radical prostatectomy. J Urol 142:1266–1270

Chodak GH, Thisted RA, Gerber G et al. (1994) Results of conservative management of clinically localized prostate cancer. N Engl J Med 330:242–248

Consensus Conference (1987) The management of clinically localized prostate cancer. JAMA 258:2727–2730
Epstein JI, Carmichael M, Walsh PC (1993a) Adenocarcinoma of the prostate invading the seminal vesicle: definition and relation of tumor volume, grade and margins of resection to prognosis. J Urol 149:1040–1045
Epstein JI, Carmichael M, Partin AW, Walsh PC (1993b) Is tumor volume an independent predictor of progression following radical prostatectomy? A multivariate analysis of 185 clinical stage B adenocarcinomas of the prostate with 5 years follow-up. J Urol 149:1478–1481
Epstein JI, Walsh PC, Carmichael M, Brendler CB (1994) Pathologic and clinical findings to predict tumor extent of nonpalpable (stage T1C) prostate cancer. JAMA 271:368–374
Fleming C, Wasson JH, Albertsen PC, Barry MJ, Wennberg JE (1993) A decision analysis of alternative treatment strategies for clinically localized prostate cancer. JAMA 269:2650–2658
Formenti S, Lieskovsky G, Simoneau A, Skinner DG, Groshen S, Petrovich Z (1996) Impact of moderate dose postoperative radiation on urinary continence and potency in patients with prostate cancer treated with nerve sparing prostatectomy. J Urol (in press)
Freeman JA, Lieskovsky G, Cook DW, Petrovich X, Chen SC, Groshen S, Skinner DG (1993) Radical retropubic prostatectomy and postoperative adjuvant radiation for pathological stage C (PCN0) prostate cancer from 1976 to 1989: intermediate findings. J Urol 149:1029–1034
Freeman JA, Lieskovsky G, Grossfeld G et al. (1994) Adjuvant radiation, chemotherapy, and androgen deprivation therapy for pathologic stage D1 adenocarcinoma of the prostate. Urology 44:719–725
Gann PH, Hennekens GH, Stampfer MJ (1995) A prospective evaluation of plasma prostate specific antigen for detection of prostatic carcinoma. JAMA 273:289–294
Garnick MB (1994) The dilemmas of prostate cancer. Do the risks of aggressive treatment for early prostate cancer outweigh the benefits? This question is one of the several unresolved issues faced by those who treat, and those who have, prostate cancer. Sci Am 270:72–81
Gibbons RP, Cole BS, Richardson RG et al. (1986) Adjuvant radiotherapy following radical prostatectomy: results and complications. J Urol 135:65–68
Gittes RF (1991) Carcinoma of the prostate. N Engl J Med 324:236–245
Hanks GE, Dawson AK (1986) The role of external beam radiation therapy after prostatectomy for prostate cancer. Cancer 58:2406–2410
Hudson MLA, Catalona WJ (1990) Effects of adjuvant radiation therapy on prostate specific antigen following radical prostatectomy. J Urol 143:1174–1177
Jacobson GM, Smith JA, Stewart JR (1987) Postoperative radiation therapy for pathologic stage C prostate cancer. Int J Radiat Oncol Biol Phys 13:1021–1024
Johansson JE (1994) Watchful waiting for early stage prostate cancer. Urology 43:138–142
Kabalin JN, Hodge KK, McNeal JE, Freiha FS, Stamey TA (1989) Identification of residual cancer in the prostate following radiation therapy: role of transrectal ultrasound guided biopsy and prostate specific antigen. J Urol 142:326–331
Kaplan ID, Bagshaw MA (1992) Serum prostate-specific antigen after post-prostatectomy radiotherapy. Urology 39:401–406
Kaplan ID, Cox RS, Bagshaw MA (1993) Prostate specific antigen after external beam radiotherapy for prostate cancer: follow-up. J Urol 149:519–522
Koch MO, Smith JA, Hodge EM, Brandell RA (1994) Prospective development of a cost-efficient program for radical retropubic prostatectomy. Urology 44:311–318
Lange PH, Narayan P (1983) Understaging and undergrading of prostate cancer. Argument for postoperative radiation as adjuvant therapy. Urology 21:113–118
Link P, Freiha FS, Stamey TA (1991) Adjuvant radiation therapy in patients with detectable prostate specific antigen following radical prostatectomy. J Urol 145:532–534
Mettlin C, Murphy GP, Menck H (1994) Trends in treatment of localized prostate cancer by radical prostatectomy: observations from the Commission on Cancer National Cancer Database, 1985–1990. Urology 43:488–492
Morton RA, Steiner MS, Walsh PC (1991) Cancer control following anatomic radical prostatectomy: an interim report. J Urol 145:1197–1200
Oesterling JE (1991) Prostate specific antigen: a critical assessment of the most useful tumor marker for adenocarcinoma of the prostate. J Urol 145:907–923
Oesterling JE, Chan DW, Epstein JI et al. (1988) Prostate specific antigen in the preoperative and postoperative evaluation of localized prostatic cancer treated with radical prostatectomy. J Urol 139:766–772
Partin AW, Yoo J, Carter HB et al. (1993) The use of prostate specific antigen, clinical stage and Gleason score to predict pathological stage in men with localized prostate cancer. J Urol 150:110–114
Perez CA, Pilepich MV, Garcia D, Simpson JR, Zivnuska F, Hederman MA (1988) Definitive radiation therapy in carcinoma of the prostate localizes to the pelvis: experience at the Mallinckrodt Institute of Radiology. NCI Monogr 7:85–94
Perez CA, Cosmatos D, Garcia DM, Eisbruch A, Poulter CA (1993a) Irradiation in relapsing carcinoma of the prostate. Cancer 71:1110–1122
Perez CA, Hanks GH, Leibel SA, Zietman AL, Fuks Z, Lee RW (1993b) Localized carcinoma of the prostate (stages T1B, T1C, T2, and T3). Review of management with external beam radiation therapy. Cancer 72:3156–3173
Petrovich Z, Lieskovsky G, Langholz B, Luxton G, Jozsef G, Skinner DG (1991) Radiotherapy following radical prostatectomy in patients with carcinoma of the prostate. Int J Radiat Oncol Biol Phys 21:949–954
Pilepich MV, Waltz BJ, Baglan RJ (1984) Postoperative irradiation in carcinoma of the prostate. Int J Radiat Oncol Biol Phys 10:1869–1873
Ray GR, Bagshaw MA, Freiha F (1984) External beam radiation salvage for residual or recurrent local tumor following radical prostatectomy. J Urol 132:926–930
Rifkin MD, Zerhouni EA, Gatsonis CA et al. (1990) Comparison of magnetic resonance imaging and ultrasonography in staging early prostate cancer. Results of a multi-institutional cooperative trial. N Engl J Med 323:621–626
Scardino PT, Frankel JM, Wheeler TM et al. (1986) The prognostic significance of post-irradiation biopsy results in patients with prostatic cancer. J Urol 135:510–515
Schellhammer PF (1988) Radical prostatectomy. Patterns of local failure and survival in 67 patients. Urology 31:191–197
Schellhammer PF, E1-Mahdi AM, Kuban DA (1990) Local failure and related complications after definitive treatment of clinical stage C carcinoma of the prostate by irradiation and surgery. Semin Urol 8:232–246

Schellhammer PF, Schlossberg SM, E1-Mahdi AM, Wright GL, Brassil DN (1991) Prostate specific antigen levels after definitive irradiation for carcinoma of the prostate. J Urol 145:1008–1991

Schild SE, Wong WW, Grado GL, Buskirk SJ, Robinow JS, Frick LM, Ferrigini RG (1994) Radiotherapy for isolated increases in serum prostate-specific antigen levels after radical prostatectomy. Mayo Clin Proc 69:613–619

Shevlin BE, Mittal BB, Brand WN, Shetty RM (1989) The role of adjuvant irradiation following primary prostatectomy, based on histopathologic extent of tumor. Int J Radiat Oncol Biol Phys 16:1425–1430

Stamey TA, Ferrari MK, Schmid HP (1993) The value of serial prostate specific antigen determinations 5 years after radiotherapy: steeply increasing value characterize 80% of patients. J Urol 150:1856–1859

Stein A, De Kernion JB, Dorey F, Smith RB (1992) Adjuvant radiotherapy in patients post-radical prostatectomy with tumor extending through capsule or positive seminal vesicles. Urology 39:59–62

Steiner MS, Morton RA, Walsh PC (1991) Impact of anatomical radical prostatectomy on urinary continence. J Urol 145:512–515

Van Poppel H, Ameye F, Oyen R, Van der Voorde W, Baert L (1994) Accuracy of combined computerized tomography and fine needle aspiration cytology in lymph node staging of localized prostatic carcinoma. J Urol 151:1310–1314

Yamada AH, Lieskovsky G, Petrovich Z, Chen SC, Groshen S, Skinner DG (1994) Results of radical prostatectomy and adjuvant therapy in the management of locally advanced, clinical stage TC, prostate cancer. Am J Clin Oncol (CCT) 17:277–285

Zagars GK, Von Eschenbach AC, Johnson DE, Oswald MJ (1987) Stage C adenocarcinoma of the prostate. An analysis of 551 patients treated with external beam radiation. Cancer 60:1489–1499

Zincker H, Utz DC, Taylor WF (1986) Bilateral pelvic lymphadenectomy and radical prostatectomy for clinical stage C prostatic cancer: role of adjuvant treatment for residual cancer and in disease progression. J Urol 135:1199–1205

21 Conformal Radiotherapy for Carcinoma of the Prostate

G. LUXTON

CONTENTS

21.1 Introduction

Although the optimum role for radiotherapy in the treatment of prostate cancer (CaP) remains controversial (e.g., STAMEY et al. 1993; KAPLAN et al. 1993; BAGSHAW et al. 1994), there is general agreement as to what the goal of radiotherapy should be when it is used. For both primary and postsurgical treatment of localized CaP a clinical target should ideally be defined three-dimensionally. This target should be treated to a therapeutic, sufficiently high radiation dose while keeping the maximum doses to the bladder, rectum, bowel, and femoral heads as low as possible. The clinical target should consist of at least the prostate gland in the case of a patient with an intact prostate or the preoperative margins of the gland in the case of a postsurgical treatment. Beyond this, the question of exactly what should be included in the clinical target and the question of what is the appropriate dose to the target for a given stage of clinical disease are issues for clinical trials.

Results from conventional radiation treatment for CaP have shown the technique to be problematic in several respects:

1. There has been a high rate of complications. The RTOG-EORTC grading criteria for lower gastrointestinal (GI) and genitourinary (GU) acute toxicity are given in HANKS et al. (1995). Of patients receiving standard field radiotherapy at one center, just prior to the commencement there of conformal field radiotherapy, acute grade GU and GI complications were observed in 57% (93/162) of patients (HANKS et al. 1995). In a small study of the treatment of locally advanced disease using conventionally shaped fields there was at least a mild transient bowel or urinary complication in most patients [75% (15/20) grade 1 GI and 60% (12/20) grade 1 GU reaction] (FORMAN et al. 1993b). The latter study involved hyperfractionated radiotherapy, i.e., more than one treatment per day, but the reported low-grade complication rates were comparable to those reviewed by VIJAYAKUMAR et al. (1993).

2. Adequacy of target coverage is questionable. In approximately one-third of cases a part of the target volume was missed in conventional radiotherapy planning for four shaped axial field irradiation based on plain film imaging and anatomic/skeletal landmarks visible on plain x-ray film alone (TEN HAKEN et al. 1989).

3. There has been a significant rate of failure to achieve local control. ZEITMAN et al. (1995) observed

G. LUXTON, PhD, Associate Professor of Radiation Oncology, Department of Radiation Oncology, University of Southern California School of Medicine, 1441 Eastlake Avenue, Los Angeles, CA 90033, USA that in a group of 504 T1–T2 patients treated by conventional radiation therapy, only 40% were disease free 10 years after treatment, as defined by a prostate specific antigen level of less than 1 ng/ml. Presumably, any local failure of radiotherapy is due to either inadequate dose or geographical miss.

Three-dimensional conformal radiotherapy is broadly defined in contemporary terminology as treatment that matches the high dose-treated volume to the three-dimensionally specified clinical target, with the dose gradient around the treatment volume sufficiently great that the dose to adjacent nontarget tissues is markedly reduced. According to LICHTER (1991), the basic 3-D hypothesis is that 3-D conformal radiotherapy allows the radiation dose level to be increased beyond standard tolerance levels without increasing complications. That is, the smaller volume treated thanks to better targeting allows treatment to proceed to higher than the standard dose. It is hoped that the increased dose made possible by conformal radiotherapy of the prostate will result in improved local control. Alternatively, it may be anticipated that complications can be reduced by the use of conformal radiotherapy, since the technique makes it possible to reduce dose to most nontarget tissues for a given dose to the prostate.

In principle, a general method for achieving an approximately conformal radiotherapy treatment plan is to craft apertures for x-ray beams originating from a number of different directions, with each field aperture conforming to the outline of the target in the beam's eye view (BEV). The concept of BEV is that of a projection of the beam aperture through the patient from the perspective of the direction of the radiation beam whether it is a near parallel beam as for proton beam irradiation or a divergent beam from the virtual point source of the x-ray beam located at the x-ray production target in the head of the accelerator (GOITEIN et al. 1983; TEN HAKEN et al. 1989; MCSHAN et al. 1990; VIJAYAKUMAR et al. 1991). The aperture could be made from standard rectangular beam collimation supplemented by a secondary blocking outline cast from a low melting point alloy (cerrobend), or alternatively, by computer-controlled multileaf secondary collimation (LOSASSO et al. 1993).

A margin around the clinical target is required to fully encompass the target while allowing for the uncertainties and variability of day-to-day patient setup, as well as the penumbra dose fall-off naturally present near the edge of a beam. The width of field margins should be informed additionally by the relative likelihood of complications resulting from excessively large margins along the different field edges. The latter are difficult to assess quantitatively, although models have been proposed for the effects of partial organ irradiation (LYMAN 1985; LYMAN and WOLBARST 1987; NIEMIERKO and GOITEIN 1991). Model parameters for different tissues (bladder, rectum, etc.) are not established. Different treatment plans can nevertheless be ordered by relative normal tissue complication probabilities (NTCPs) using best estimates for the parameters together with a model for partial volume irradiation, although the absolute NTCP values are not known. In the data reviewed by EMAMI et al. (1991) one observes a relatively higher probability of complication from partial volume irradiation of the rectum as compared to that for the bladder. This would seem to imply that equal probabilities of complication are associated with a larger margin for a treatment field edge on the side of the bladder as compared to a field edge on the side of the rectum. The rectum, moreover, tends to be in overall closer proximity to the prostate than does the bladder. Another consideration of importance, particularly for larger patients, is that a high energy x-ray beam (nominal accelerating potential 10 MeV or greater) should be used so that relatively greater tissue penetration of the high-energy beam will reduce the entrance dose required to sufficiently irradiate the target as compared to a lower energy beam.

21.2 Conventional Radiotherapy

Historically, prostate treatment has consisted of the combination of several coplanar fields, with limited field shaping. Regimens of the 1970s and early 1980s consisted of whole pelvis treatment by anteroposterior fields usually with corner blocks to limit normal tissue irradiation possibly with a component of lateral opposed fields to a dose of 40–50 Gy. Whole pelvis treatment was supplemented to a total dose of 60–70 Gy depending upon stage of disease, with fixed or arc rotation boost fields coned down to the prostate plus a small margin (PEREZ et al. 1986). The rationale for whole pelvis irradiation was that pelvic lymph nodes were thought to be a major risk for local-regional failure and therefore requiring of a treatment dose of 40–50 Gy. Furthermore, it could be argued that the prostate would safely remain within the borders of these treatment fields despite uncertainties of location associated with the modest imaging available, and uncertainties associated with organ motion and setup error. Boost treatment would consist of either fixed fields or moving arcs, to raise the total dose to the prostate to the 60–72 Gy level. In the latter half of the 1980s, whole pelvis treatment fields became less frequent, as the question of routine pelvic lymph node irradiation was challenged. In particular, postoperative fields were reduced with no apparent degradation in disease-free survival (PETROVICH et al. 1991).

21.3 Conformal Radiotherapy

21.3.1 Target Definition

Prior to the advent of whole body 3-D computerized tomographic (CT) imaging in the second half of the 1970s, it was not possible to consider conformal radiotherapy for prostate cancer, since the physical target could not be accurately identified. Target definition for conformal radiotherapy requires considerations beyond identification of the gross tumor localization as determined by CT imaging. The physician must also consider the following factors: likelihood of microscopic invasion not visible on the images, inclusion of the seminal vesicles in the target, organ motion due to variability in bladder and rectal filling, setup errors, and penumbral effects for the shaped treatment beam. A rich vocabulary for addressing these issues has been defined in report 50 of the International Commission on Radiation Units and Measurements (ICRU 1993).

ICRU 50 defines gross tumor volume (GTV) as the tumor visible on imaging or identified by clinical examination. The clinical target volume (CTV) is a clinical concept defined as the GTV with a margin added for subclinical microscopic involvement. The planning target volume (PTV) is the tissue volume designated by the clinician to require treatment, encompassing the CTV with additional margins allowing for factors such as patient motion, organ motion, patient setup uncertainties, and collimator penumbra. The additional margins introduced for the PTV (Fig. 21.1) are thus determined by geometric-physical data based on treatment methodology. In addition to these target volumes, two further volumes are defined in ICRU 50, the treatment volume (TV) and the irradiated volume (IV). The TV is the volume actually treated to the prescribed dose, and the IV is the volume irradiated to a clinically significant dose. Generally, GTV < CTV < PTV < TV < IV. Ideally, the TV would be the same as the PTV.

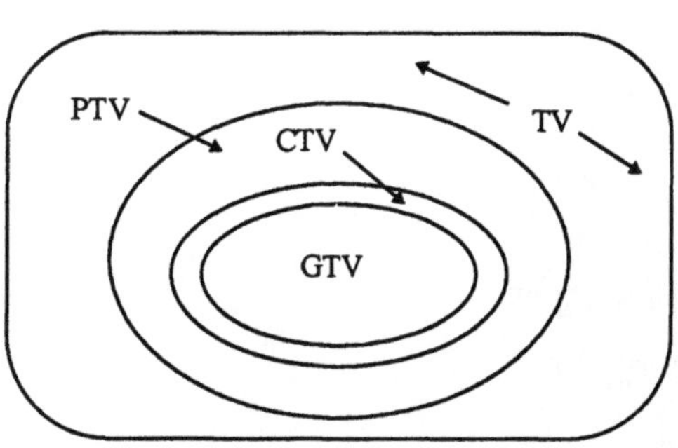

Fig. 21.1. A schematic 2-D illustration of the relationship between the gross tumor volume (*GTV*), the clinical target volume (*CTV*), the planning target volume (*PTV*), and the treated volume (*TV*). The GTV is represented by the area enclosed by the inner elliptical-shaped outline, the CTV by the next outer closed shape, and the PTV by the next. The TV is represented by the area enclosed by the outermost closed contour

21.3.2 Requirements for 3-D Conformal Radiotherapy

Successful conformal radiotherapy (C/RT) requires that the entire CTV be irradiated to a dose sufficiently high that all tumor cells are destroyed. The premise of this method is that by sharp delineation of the intended high-dose region and successful confinement of the dose to this target, it will be possible to raise the dose within the CTV to a higher level than would otherwise be possible due to the likelihood of treatment complications. The conjoint requirements of tight targeting, prescription of a high dose, and accurate dose delivery within a target in the pelvis place substantial demands on a clinical radiotherapy service. The 3D C/RT process requires systematic integration of the treatment planning and treatment processes. The following is a short list of the necessary tools.

1. A *method of placing fiducial markings on and immobilizing the patient*, so that planning information can readily and reproducibly be related to treatment setup.

2. *Three-dimensional imaging in the treatment position.* Multiplanar CT with image spacing of no more than 5 mm through the target region is the preferred data for targeting and dose calculation. CT in particular gives electron density information, and this is definitively tied to dose calculation. A retrograde urethrogram gives more consistent results than CT in determining the caudal extent of the apex of the prostate (AMES et al. 1993), and is more accurate than bony anatomy (ROACH et al. 1993).

Other imaging modalities, particularly magnetic resonance imaging (MRI), offer valuable information on underlying anatomy that, if available, should ideally be combined with the CT data to define the CTV. Precise utilization of multimodality imaging requires software tools for image registration. These tools are typically based on an assumed rigid body transformation between two image data sets, on each of which is defined a set of discrete points or contour curves representing identifiable structures. The parameters of the rigid body transformation are computed based on minimizing the sum of the squares of the differences between computed and measured coordinates (least squares fit). Methods of image registration are discussed by FRAASS et al. (1987) and KESSLER et al. (1991).

3. *Visualization software* with tools for outlining the target on each image plane and for combining the multiplanar target definition into an object that can be rendered graphically from different perspectives. The display must be able to show the target in the BEV, in conjunction with beam outlines and other points of clinical interest, such as wireframe outlines of the bladder and rectum (Fig. 21.2).

4. *Three-dimensional dose computation software.* This software is needed to provide clinical trials with accurate data. A well-designed study requires thorough characterization of patient dosimetry. In addition, dose computation and display tools are needed for evaluation of treatment plans. Examples of such tools are target and organ dose-volume histograms, and wireframe or solid surface rendering of isodose surfaces together with anatomic structures.

5. *Method of plan verification.* Simulator images can be used, for example, to verify isocenter by simple anteroposterior and lateral radiographs displaying the fiducial markers in the prescribed positions. More complex verification should include comparison of portal images taken with the treatment simulator with digitally reconstructed radiographs (DRRs) based on the treatment plan. Simulator imaging is of superior quality to that from accelerator portal images, but it is possible that this simulator imaging verification will be dispensed with in the future in the interest of cost reduction, and plan verification will be combined with treatment verification.

6. *Blocking system to implement treatment plan.* The conventional low melting point alloy

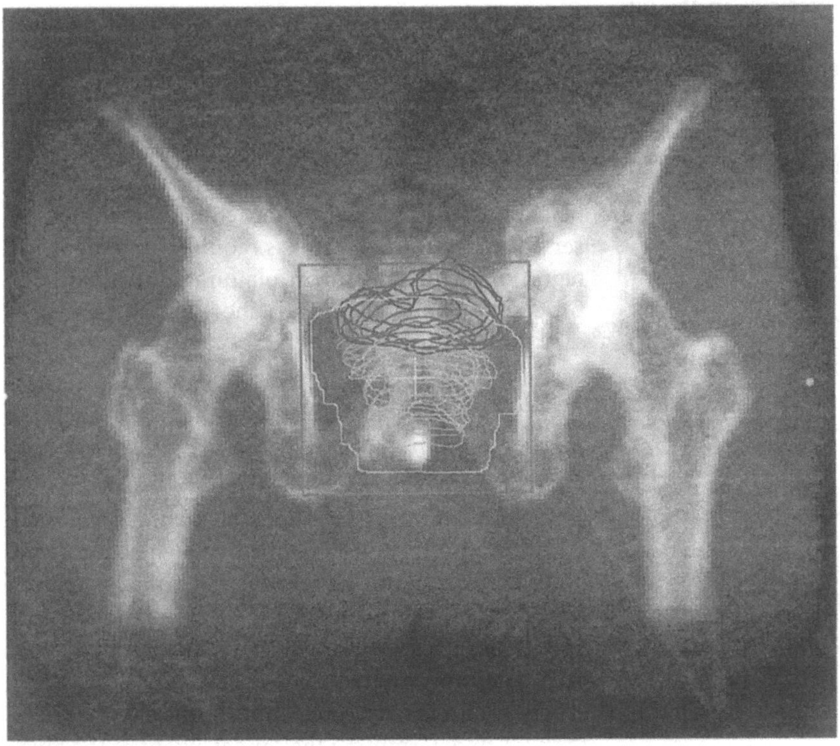

Fig. 21.2. A BEV digitally reconstructed radiograph with simulated 80-kV x-ray beam, showing wireframe graphic representations of the target and bladder. This beam is an anterior caudal oblique, directed toward the isocenter from an angle 30° caudal to the anteroposterior direction. A computer-generated outline encloses the target plus a 1.25-cm margin. Three lead shot spheres may also be seen – one on each side and the third near the midline. The lead shot appears on simulator or portal images, and can be used to verify treatment setup

(cerrobend) block casting system can be quite precise. With multiple complex customized treatment portals, however, it is more efficient to use an automatic multileaf beam-shaping system. The use of a multileaf collimator system (MLC) with finite-sized individual leafs introduces compromises in the field edge definition, but in a study by LoSasso et al. (1993) these effects were found to be negligible compared to those due to a random 5-mm setup uncertainty.

7. *Treatment verification system.* Portal films or electronic portal imaging is required to verify adherence of the treatment fields to the plan.

21.4 Uncertainties of Target Positioning

Image data that provide the basis of conformal treatment planning are obtained over a short interval at a particular moment in time at the CT scanner. While these data provide a detailed 3-D description of the patient's anatomy at the time of the imaging, many differences may be present at the time of treatment that can confound the goal of accurate dose delivery. As noted by Michalski (1994), if these uncertainties are not taken into account, a substantial fraction of the clinical target volume may be significantly undertreated, since conformal radiotherapy treatment fields tend to be small. The major sources of the misregistration of the CTV with the treatment fields are patient setup error, patient movement, and day-to-day variation in the location of the target mostly due to variable degrees filling of the bladder and rectum.

21.4.1 Patient Setup Variability

Gross patient setup errors can be prevented by use of individual patient repositioning techniques, such as foam body cradle casts, thermoplastic masks, skin marks, beam templates, and a systematic program of portal imaging. Such techniques assume great importance with the small field margins characteristic of the PTV in conformal radiotherapy. Positioning errors of greater than 5 mm were observed in 27% of pelvic fields in a port film study by Byhardt et al. (1978). The average discrepancy in each dimension between simulation and portal films for prostate treatments was found by Rabinowitz et al. (1985) to be 5.6 mm. Hanley et al. (1994) performed a study of setup accuracy of prone and immobilized casted prostate cancer patients using weekly sets of three portal images as data. Reporting on 15 patients, Hanley et al. found an average systematic error of 1.6 mm between simulation and treatment isocenters, and random setup errors in the different axes with standard deviations between 1.5 mm and 2.2 mm. The largest random setup error was in the left–right direction.

21.4.2 Variability of Location of Prostate

Several studies have appeared in the literature that document the degree of organ motion errors. Thus, Ten Haken et al. (1991) using implanted radiopaque seeds found an average motion of 5 mm, and a range extending between 0 and 20 mm. At the 1993 Annual Meeting of the American Society for Therapeutic Radiology and Oncology (ASTRO) several groups reported on similar studies. Forman et al. (1993a), using weekly CT treatment planning and image registration software in a study of ten patients, found an average maximum motion of 17 mm in the digitized prostate and seminal vesicles relative to their location with respect to the bony pelvis on the initial treatment planning CT. The maximum displacement observed was 35 mm. Beard et al. (1993a), using two CT scans 4 weeks apart in 12 patients, found average motions for the prostate relative to the bony anatomy in the anterior and lateral directions of 4 mm and 1 mm respectively (range 0–10 mm), while observing an average motion of 4.5 mm (range 0–16 mm) in the posterior aspect of the seminal vesicle. Similar differential average displacements were observed by Balter et al. (1993) and Melian et al. (1993).

21.4.3 X-ray Beam Penumbra

While megavoltage x-ray beams do provide sharper beam edge definition than cobalt-60 teletherapy units, there remains a finite transition zone between full beam intensity and the effective absence of beam. The 80%-to-20% field edge margin is dependent upon beam energy, field size, and details of collimation. For the field sizes and beam energies encountered in conformal radiotherapy of the prostate, this transition zone is typically about 8 mm. The 80%-to-50% width is typically half this size, i.e., 4 mm, while the 90%-to-50% width will be at least a few millimeters larger.

21.4.4 Impact on Treatment Margins

Margins should be designed to allow for the cumulative effect of internal organ movement (Ten Haken et al. 1991), variations in patient repositioning, and lack of certainty in field localization relative to CT (or MR) imaging. Overall clinical margins are typically in the range of 1–1.5 cm, with possibly larger margins anteriorly than posteriorly. It is generally agreed that high-dose irradiation of a portion of the rectum, for example the anterior rectal wall, is more likely to result in a complication than would low-dose irradiation of a larger volume of rectum or bladder.

21.5 Treatment Procedure

At the University of Southern California, the principles described above for conformal 3-D radiotherapy treatment of prostate cancer are implemented in the following manner.

21.5.1 Patient Preparation

Prior to CT imaging, the patient is fitted across the pelvic area with a conformal evacuated foam pellet body cast bag (Vac-Lok System, Med-Tec, Inc., Orange City, Iowa). The purpose of the cast is to provide a comfortable form for rigid and reproducible patient immobilization. The casting procedure takes less than 5 min. The procedure is performed in the radiation therapy simulator room with the patient lying comfortably supine on a plywood board (200 × 65 × 2 cm) surfaced with thin-sheeted smooth facing material. The support board is fitted with removable side rails across the region of the cast. The side rails are used as a rigid form to produce the foam casting, while the board is used to provide a reproducibly flat surface for the CT imaging. Pen marks and three self-adhesive tapes containing small (1.5-mm and 2.0-mm) lead shot spheres (Beekly Spots, Beekly Corp., Bristol, Conn.) are placed on the patient skin to serve as visual and radiopaque fiducial markers. The lead shot markers are placed in an axial plane – one on each side of the patient, and the third marker on the anterior surface, respectively horizontally and vertically offset from a tentative isocenter. Different diameter lead spherical markers are often placed on the two sides of the patient to aid in ready identification of the right and left skin markers on radiographs.

As a further aid for repositioning, the alignment is registered by skin marks on the patient that display several projections of a portable laser which may be positioned sequentially in slots in an inverted U-shaped aluminum rod that fits into positioning holes at the sides of the plywood board. The board is adjusted so that the U-shaped rod is caused to be aligned in a vertical plane perpendicular to the rotation axis of the simulator gantry, as indicated by side lasers in the room. The rod is separated a short distance caudocephalad from the foam cast.

21.5.2 CT Imaging

The patient is scanned while positioned in the foam cast on the plywood board. The various skin marks are aligned with the side light projections of the CT scanner room, so that the relationship of the patient to the scanner axis reproduces the setup on the simulator table. The patient is scanned at no more than 5-mm spacing between cuts through the pelvic region. Thirty or more cuts are taken so that the full transit of potential axial or nonaxial treatment beams can be mapped to imaged patient anatomy. Additional cuts provide useful reference anatomic imaging for comparison of DRRs with portal images. It is common practice when taking portal images to take double exposures, with the treatment field image being superimposed on a larger field second image that provides accurate anatomic identification of the portal aperture.

21.5.3 Outline Anatomy from Imaging

Critical organs, bony anatomy, and the gross target volume are now easily outlined on the set of axial CT images, using a computer input pointing device (mouse). A set of outlines defines a 3-D volume associated with an object. When a treatment plan is developed, the dose computation program can calculate treatment plan statistics, such as dose-volume histograms for the gross tumor volume, the clinical target volume, the rectum, and the bladder. Delineation of bony anatomy assists subsequent comparison of planned treatment portals with verification images.

The 3-D image set is used to define treatment fields. The isocenter, the single point of intersection of the central rays from every treatment field, is selected to be at the center of the gross tumor volume. The computer program (RT SIMULATOR) used to reformat the CT image data allows the target point to be selected to be the center of the geometric edges of the target or the target center of mass, or any other point selected by the treatment planner (Astrahan 1994).

21.5.4 Definition of Treatment Portals

The outlined structures can now be viewed in the BEV from any orientation with the central ray originating at the x-ray production target. This view is used as a tool to help select the beam direction, then to define the aperture for a treatment portal from this direction. The beam aperture is defined as a rectangle with given dimensions. The mouse is used as a freehand on-screen drawing tool to indicate field blocking if any. Alternatively, the user may instruct the software to select the aperture to automatically conform to the BEV perspective of the target plus margin of selectable size (Fig. 21.3). At the present time, a set of four or six coplanar fields is selected as a treatment plan for carcinoma of the prostate. After a beam aperture has been defined, the portal can be displayed as a DRR, modeled by beam attenuation based on 80-kVp x-rays or alternatively based on megavoltage x-rays. The latter would be potentially useful for comparison of portal images with their predicted appearance. Considerably more contrast is available at a simulated 80-kVp x-ray energy. The images are printed to paper, alternatively to transparencies as color images, with magnification selected to be the same (1.45:1) as standard simulation fields. In particular, anteroposterior (AP) and lateral DRRs with simulated 80-kVp contrast are printed out (Fig. 21.4).

21.5.5 Patient Setup on Simulator

Isocenter is now checked by setting up the patient in accordance with the displayed locations for the radiographic skin markers on the AP and lateral DRRs. Simulator films are compared with the AP, lateral,

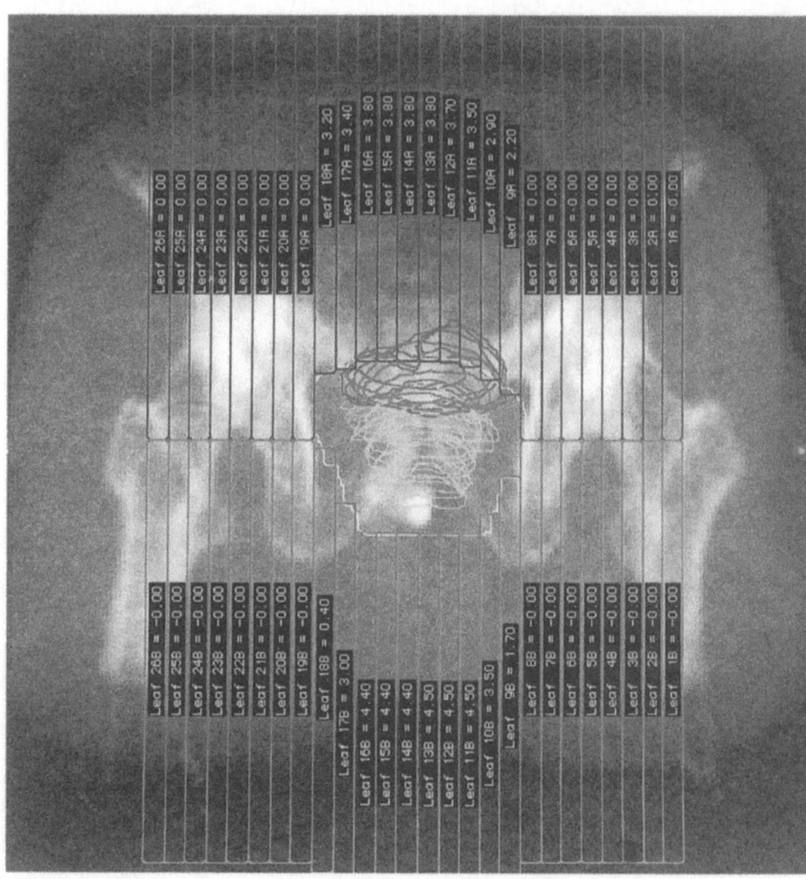

Fig. 21.3. A computer-generated multileaf collimator arrangement designed to encompass the target with a 1.25-cm margin. The beam is from the same orientation as in Fig. 21.2. Leaf coordinates are printed out for documentation and as a quality assurance measure, for comparison with treatment console readout

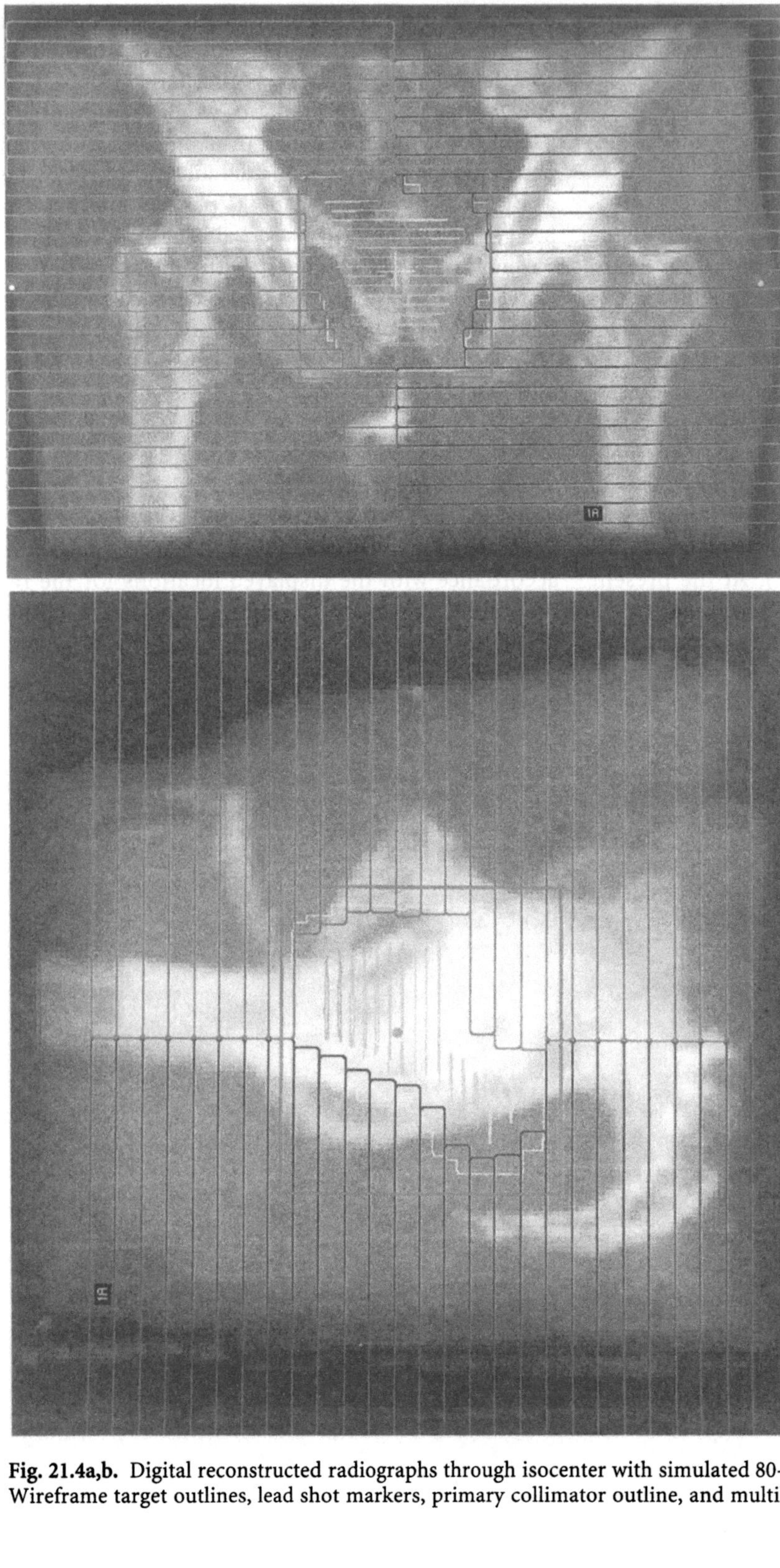

a

b

Fig. 21.4a,b. Digital reconstructed radiographs through isocenter with simulated 80-kV x-rays: **a** anteroposterior **b** left lateral. Wireframe target outlines, lead shot markers, primary collimator outline, and multileaf collimators are graphically shown and other portal BEV image prints. Not all BEV fields can be simulated owing to the interference of the image intensifier present on treatment simulators, but the AP and lateral films can be used to uniquely verify the isocenter. A third field portal image could provide data for confirmation of setup.

21.5.6 Dose Computation

Treatment fields are shaped based on the BEV. Four to six shaped fields are weighted in accordance with a trial plan and dose computation proceeds using either a commercial treatment planning system or a USC-developed 3-D dose computation algorithm. Typically, coplanar field arrangements are calculated with the commercial treatment planning system. These calculations are supplemented with full 3-D volumetric calculations based on algorithms and computer programs developed at USC over the past few years. The treatment plan is submitted to the radiation oncologist for approval.

21.5.7 Patient Treatment

The computer-simulated treatment fields are shaped on the treatment unit by uploading a number of multileaf collimator settings in the form of a computer file, with one collimator description for each of the different treatment fields. The file which is exported by RT simulator also provides useful identifying information, including the patient name and identification number. Alternatively, the DRR may be used as input data for the manufacturer's beam shaper system, which accepts digitized outlines that are usually taken from film. The monitor units are calculated for each beam and the individual fields are treated sequentially. A six-field conformal treatment can be accomplished in less than 10 min. Daily dose fraction is typically 1.8 Gy.

21.5.8 Treatment Verification

The treatment fields that are possible to be imaged are compared to DRR-predicted graphics. Portal films are taken and checked on the 1st day of treatment as well as weekly, as part of routine quality assurance. Any discrepancy is resolved, by resimulation if necessary. The availability of on-line portal imaging in our hospital allows the clinician to monitor the treatment in near real time, i.e., virtually as it occurs, although the quality of the image suffers from the inherent low contrast of megavoltage x-ray imaging.

21.6 Dosimetry Analysis – An Example

We shall illustrate the dosimetric comparison between conformal and conventional treatment planning and compare varieties of conformal radiotherapy by considering an example. We examine several treatment plans for the case of a primary radiotherapy treatment of a patient with prostate cancer. Several DRRs have already been shown for such a patient in Figs. 21.2–21.4. For each of the treatment plans described below, full 3-D dose calculations were done from which dose-volume histograms were extracted for the gross clinical target volume, the bladder and rectum, and the whole body.

21.6.1 Treatment Plans

The following plans were considered. All plans used only 20-MV x-ray beams (Varian Clinac 2300 c/d, Varian Oncology Systems, Palo Alto, Calif.).

1. Open, i.e., nonblocked, four-field pelvic treatment, consisting of A/P, P/A, and right and left lateral fields, equally weighted, and defined by the rectangular collimators built into the head of the accelerator. Field sizes were chosen so that the three-dimensionally imaged prostate gland and seminal vesicles would be approximately covered within the 90% isodose surface. The CTV was 101.4 cm^3, and 95% volume coverage by the 90% isodose surface required that the field size at isocenter be 11 cm in both the anteroposterior and the right to left lateral dimensions, and 13 cm in the caudocephalad dimension.
2. A conformally blocked four-field pelvic treatment, consisting of the same four fields as in (1), but with custom field shaping added to enclose the complete target in the BEV with a uniform margin of 1.25 cm.
3. A conformally blocked six coplanar axial field plan, with the A/P and P/A fields of (1) and (2) replaced by four beams inclined at 45° angles to the AP direction, from the right and left sides, in the form of two parallel-opposed pairs of beams. These four fields were also conformally shaped in the BEV, except that the margin around the target on the side of the rectum was reduced from 1.25 cm to 0.75 cm.

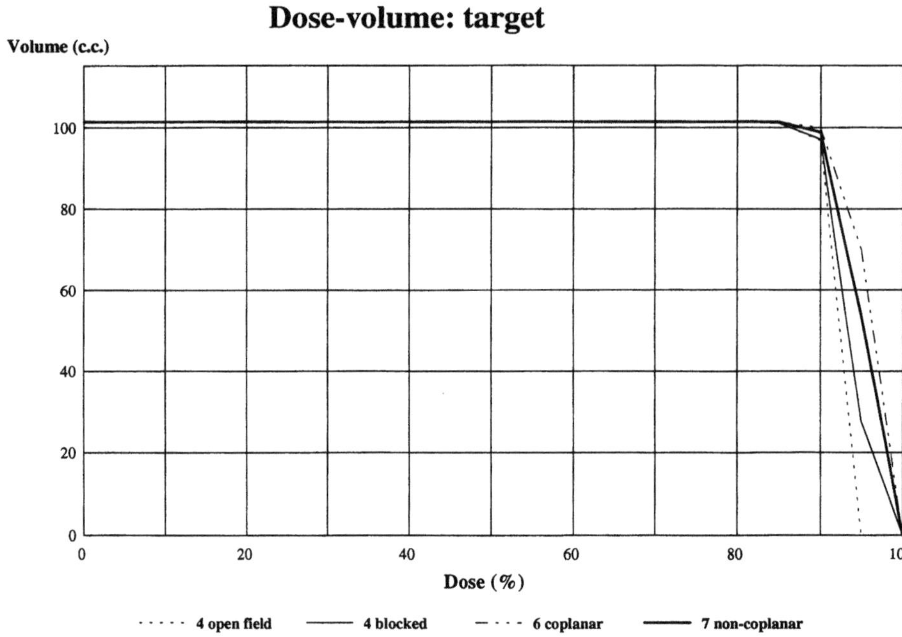

Fig. 21.5. Cumulative dose-volume histograms of dose to target from the four treatment plans discussed in the text

4. A similar plan to (3), with addition of a seventh beam, one that is not in the axial plane. The additional beam was taken to be an anterior-caudal oblique, the x-ray source originating from the direction rotated 30° inferiorly from the AP direction in the parasagittal plane (Fig. 21.2). For this seven-field plan, beam weights were modified slightly from equality: the nonaxial beam was weighted 30% higher, and the lateral beams 10% higher than the four axial oblique fields.

21.6.2 Target Coverage

The target coverage was approximately equivalent for all four treatment plans, as shown by the cumulative volume-dose distributions (similar to dose-volume histograms) in Fig. 21.5. There are minor differences among the plans in the 85%–100% dose range, where 100% refers to the maximum dose of the 3-D volume. The conformal plans show a greater volume of target receiving a dose of 95% or more, but with a reference treatment dose at the 90% level, all plans show adequate coverage of the target. Isodose distributions for the six-field plan in the sagittal, axial, and coronal planes passing through isocenter are shown in Fig. 21.6.

21.6.3 Total Volume of Nontarget Irradiation

The plans show marked differences in the total volume of nontarget tissue irradiated, as seen in the cumulative volume-dose distributions in Fig. 21.7. The major differences occur between the open field and the various conformal plans. Conformal plans reduce by 75% the volume of nontarget tissue treated to a dose that exceeds 40% of the maximum dose. This reduction persists throughout the high dose range.

The six- and seven-field plans further reduce the volume of irradiated nontarget tissue over the 35%–60% of maximum dose range, as compared to the four-field plan. The four-field plan has the best reduction of volume of nontarget tissue across the 60%–100% high dose range.

21.6.4 Volume of Bladder Irradiation

The four techniques are compared in Fig. 21.8 with respect to volume of bladder irradiated to different dose levels by the four treatment plans. Similar to the case for total nontarget tissue, one observes a major volume reduction in the high-dose region by all conformal techniques, as compared to the four open

Fig. 21.6a–c. Isodose distributions for the conformal coplanar six-field treatment plan: **a** transverse, **b** coronal, **c** sagittal. The 90%, 70%, 50%, 30%, and 10% isodose lines are shown

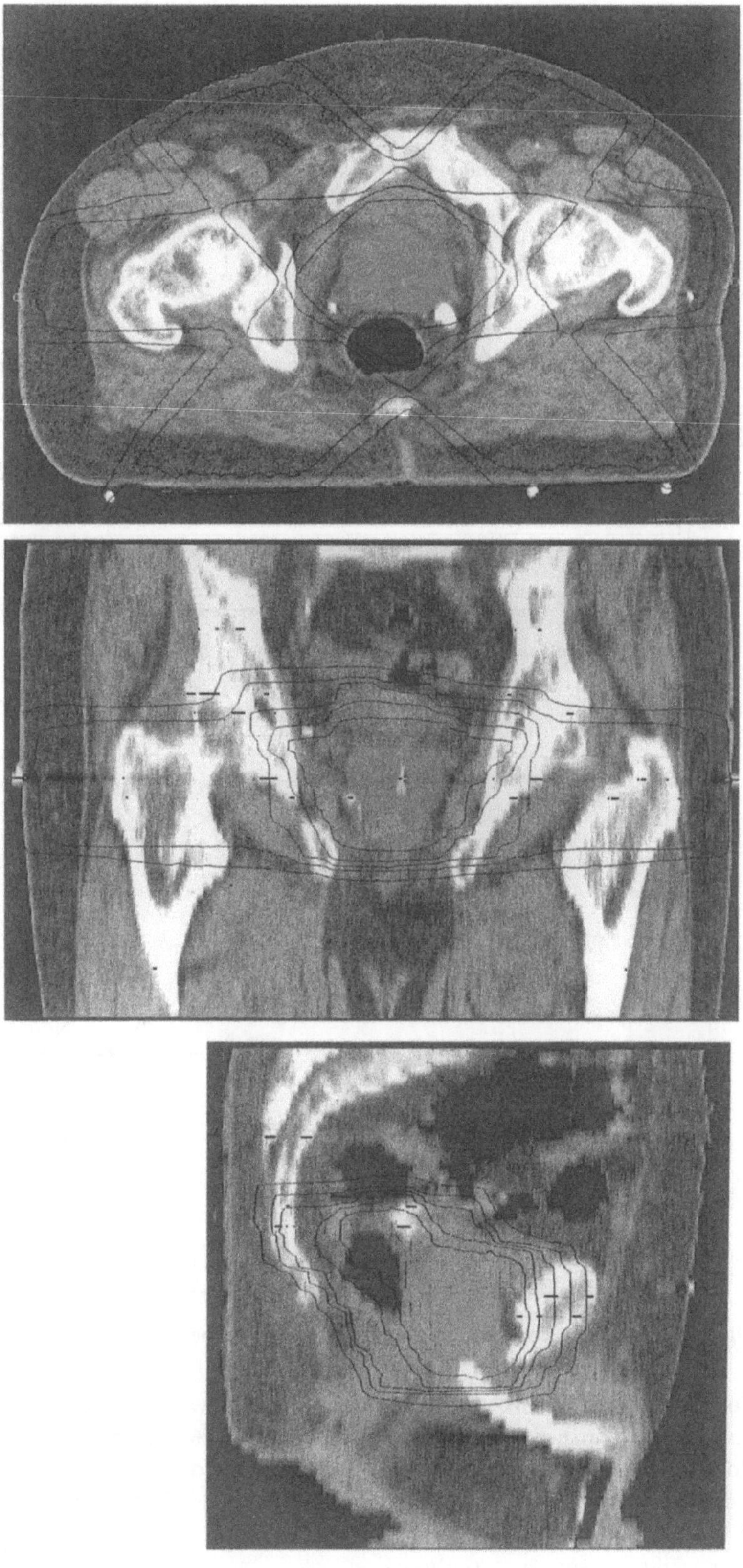

a b c

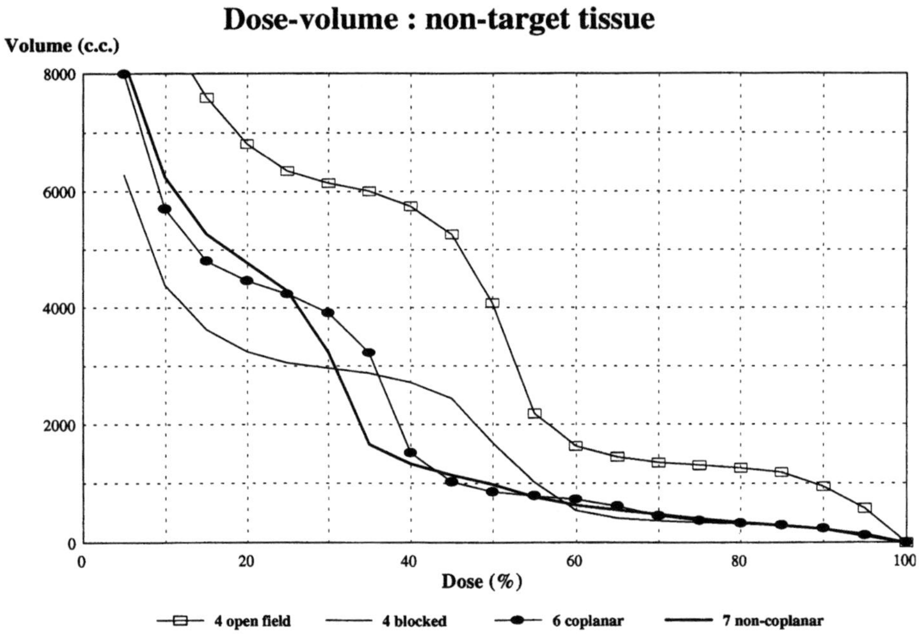

Fig. 21.7. Cumulative dose-volume histograms of dose to nontarget tisssue from the four treatment plans discussed in the text

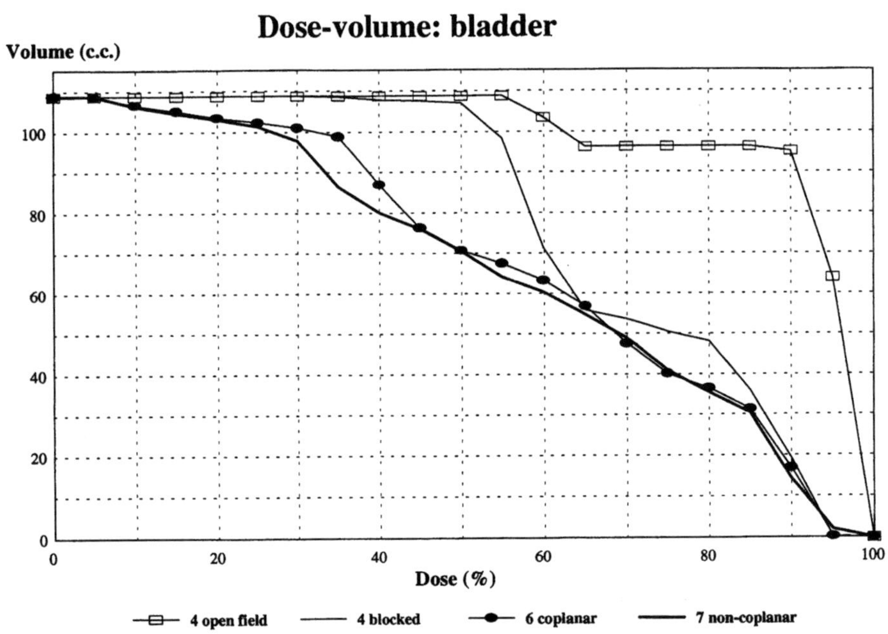

Fig. 21.8. Cumulative dose-volume histograms of dose to the bladder from the four treatment plans discussed in the text

field technique. The six- and seven-field plans show considerable further reduction across the 40%–80% dose range as compared to the conformal four-field treatment plan.

21.6.5 Volume of Rectum Irradiation

The four techniques are compared in Fig. 21.9 with respect to volume of rectum irradiated to different dose levels by the respective treatment plans. The conformal plans all are characterized by marked reduction of the volume of rectum treated to a high percentage of the treatment dose. The four shaped field technique gives the greatest rectal dose reduction, with approximately 20 cm^3 less volume of rectum irradiated to a dose level between 60% and 80%, as compared to the six- and seven-field methods. This reflects the higher relative weighting of lateral

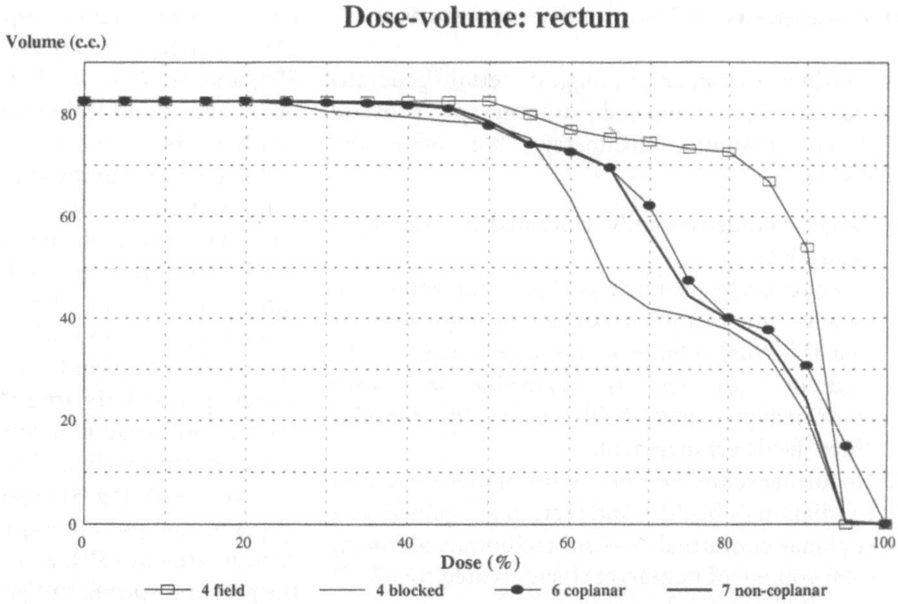

Fig. 21.9. Cumulative dose-volume histograms of dose to the rectum from the four treatment plans discussed in the text

Table 21.1. Volumes of tissues (cm^3) irradiated to certain reference doses, for the four treatment plans. The reference dose for all treatment plans is the 90% isodose surface, relative to 100% as the maximum dose. The total target volume is $101.4\,cm^3$

Tissue: dose	Four open fields	Four conformal	Six coplanar	Seven non-coplanar
Target volume: 100% ref. dose	96.9	97.3	100.0	98.9
Nontarget: 100% ref. dose	937	239	244	232
Nontarget: 80% ref.	1333	362	421	449
Nontarget: 50% ref.	5260	2440	1022	1138
Rectum + bladder: 100% ref. dose	149.1	40.4	47.7	38.5
Rectum + bladder: 80% ref.	168.0	93.7	100.9	97.5
Rectum + bladder: 50% ref.	191.3	187.2	157.4	157.5

fields for the conformal four-field plan, as compared to the six- and seven-field techniques, since the conformal lateral fields give greater protection of the rectum than do the fields from other directions.

21.6.6 Comparison of Treatment Plans

Extracting data from the dose-volume plots, we summarize in Table 21.1 the volume of nontarget tissue and the volume of rectum plus bladder combined that are irradiated to certain dose levels for the four treatment plans. Dose levels are specified relative to the reference dose, which is taken to be 90% of the maximum dose for all three treatment plans. The reference isodose surface enclosed target volumes between $97\,cm^3$ and $100\,cm^3$, the total target volume being $101.4\,cm^3$. Inspection of Table 21.1 shows that for the conformal plans, the combined volume of rectum plus bladder that is irradiated to 100% of the reference dose is decreased by 68%–74% from the open four-field technique, for which the volume is $149\,cm^3$. Total nontarget tissue irradiated to the reference dose is decreased by 75% from the $937\,cm^3$ irradiated by the four open field technique. Compared to the four-field conformal plan, the six-field plan results in 2%–17% more bladder plus rectum and total nontarget volumes irradiated to 80% and 100% of reference dose levels. At the 50% of reference dose level, however, the six-field plan results in irradiation of 58% less volume of nontarget tissue and 16% less volume of bladder plus rectum than the four-field plan. The seven-field plan lowers the irradiated volume of bladder plus rectum at the 100% level to $38.5\,cm^3$, a value slightly less than that for the four-field conformal plan. The other dose volumes for the seven-field plan are similar to those for the six-field.

21.7 Dosimetry of Conformal Treatment Plans

The dosimetry comparison suggests certain generalizations in 3-D conformal radiotherapy prostate treatment planning dosimetry. We offer the following:

1. Target volume is readily irradiated to a homogeneous dose.
2. A reduction by as much as 75% in the volume of bladder and rectum irradiated to high dose, as well as in total volume of nontarget tissues irradiated to high dose is achievable with four conformally shaped fields, using the familiar "box" fields arrangement.
3. No further reductions in volume of high dose level irradiation of bladder and rectum are gained by a coplanar conformal six-field technique, although total volume of nontarget tissue treated to 50% is reduced by more than half.
4. Addition of non-coplanar fields can reduce by a limited amount the bladder and rectum volumes in the intermediate-to-high dose range.
5. In all conformal plans there will be a volume of bladder or rectum that will be irradiated to the reference dose or higher, because portions of these organs are contiguous to the clinical target.

21.8 Reported Results of Conformal Treatment

The paradigm of 3-D conformal radiotherapy for prostate cancer is relatively recent. It is therefore not surprising that current reports from clinical trials give information about acute effects and short-term response, and do not yet provide the long-term follow-up data that will be required to establish efficacy of this approach.

An important clinical measure of the conformal 3-D technique is the incidence of acute complications from conformal treatment, as compared to conventional treatment. Since the 3-D technique treats a smaller volume, one would expect that complication rates would decrease. This has been observed. In an early report, Soffen et al. (1992) compared treatment-related morbidity for 26 patients treated with conformal radiotherapy (C/R) with 20 patients treated with standard radiotherapy (SR) immediately prior to the group's implementation of the 3-D technique. Thirty-one percent (8/26) of C/R patients had acute symptoms that required physician intervention (grade 2 or higher complications), as compared to 60% (12/20) in the SR group. In a more recent report from the same group, Hanks et al. (1995) showed acute complications for 84/247 (34%) of C/R patients and for 93/162 (57%) of the preceding SR patients ($P < 10^{-5}$). In a multivariate analysis, only volume and technique (C/R vs SR) were significantly related to incidence of morbidity.

In a study comparing the week-by-week acute complications of radiotherapy treatment Vijayakumar et al. (1993) reported on 116 patients, 16 of whom were treated by conventional treatment (group A), 57 with CT-based manual beam shaping (group B), and 43 with computer-BEV techniques (group C). Significantly lower toxicity rates were observed, particularly after the 2nd week of treatment, for the conformal BEV group C compared to groups A and B, separately and collectively.

Corn et al. (1995) report improved effectiveness of conformal radiotherapy (C/R) compared to standard treatment (SR), as measured biochemically by the prostate-specific antigen (PSA) response at 1 year following treatment. Ninety-six percent (95/99) of C/R patients had PSA levels <4 ng/ml versus 85% (28/33) of SR patients. For PSA levels <1.5 ng/ml, the corresponding numbers are 76% (75/99) and 55% (18/33) for C/R and SR patients respectively. Both PSA levels have statistical significance with P values less than 0.03 and 0.02, respectively. The authors point out that this measure of outcome appears to be of clinical importance, noting that in a review by Russell et al. (1991) it was observed that the end point of normalization of PSA at 6–12 months following radiotherapy corresponds to a 4%–18% adverse clinical outcome, much better than the 42%–100% adverse clinical outcome for those with an abnormal PSA.

21.9 Future Directions

In conformal radiotherapy of the prostate, there will continue to accrue technological improvements in both treatment planning and treatment delivery. Computer-controlled dose delivery increases the relevance of new software developments in treatment planning by providing a means for executing increasingly complex treatments. Software developments in the form of 3-D visualization and planning tools already implemented at a limited number of centers will become widely implemented. Further software development will include the following areas:

1. *Increased treatment automation.* This is needed to keep complex treatments affordable and to

make it feasible to prescribe more complex treatments. An example of complex treatment is the long-anticipated programmed dynamically varying multileaf collimators during arc therapy.

2. *Automatic optimization in treatment planning.* A most straightforward application of this technology would be automatic selection of optimum weights of a preselected set of trial beams. Computer-assisted treatment planning would also be used to optimize selection of gantry angles from among a preselected set of fixed and moving beams. Optimization would be based on using mathematical scoring functions for organ and target irradiation. In the long term, optimization will most likely include computer calculation of normal tissue complication probability (NTCP), with its minimization as an optimization criterion. Standardization of 3-D techniques will undoubtedly be developed in clinical trials. There will be great interest in the near term in the clinical results of escalated treatment, with target doses increased because of the dose-volume reduction of the nontarget tissue. The long-term value of conformal radiotherapy will have to await well-understood long-term results.

21.10 Summary

Conformal radiotherapy of the prostate is a 3-D treatment planning methodology that offers a major dose-volume reduction to the bladder, rectum, and other nontarget tissue, as compared to conventional treatment. This method is expected to reduce complications of treatment, and early indications are that it does (Vijayakumar et al. 1993; Hanks et al. 1995). Averaged over five patients, C/R with a four-field box technique was found by Soffen et al. (1991) to reduce average bladder and rectum dose by 14% each. Dose escalation studies are now underway, and preliminary indications are that the increased doses are well tolerated by patients (Leibel et al. 1994a). There are early reports of a measure of increased effectiveness of C/R (Corn et al. 1995). C/R requires patient immobilization and reproducible setup and software for 3-D perspective of beams in relation to the imaging and outlining of target and organs. Target motion relative to the bony anatomy and limitations of setup accuracy must be considered in defining field margins. Several conformal treatment plans have been compared, and their main characteristics with respect to nontarget tissue irradiation have been described. Automated beam-shaping equipment permits rapid execution of the complex conformal treatment plans. Finally, a look to the near future glimpses increased automation and computer-assisted treatment plan optimization.

References

Ames JW, Hartz W, Litwin S, Hanks GE (1993) The retrograde urethrogram is more accurate than CT in identifying the caudal prostate margin for conformal treatment planning, (Abstr). 35th Annual Meeting of the American Society for Therapeutic Radiology and Oncology. New Orleans, October 1993. Int J Radiat Oncol Biol Phys 27 S1:137–138

Astrahan MA (1994) CT based 3D radiation therapy simulation and treatment planning on the Macintosh, (Abstr). 36th Annual meeting of the American Association of Physicists in Medicine (AAPM), Anaheim, July 1994. Med Phys 21:913

Bagshaw MA, Cox RS, Hancock SL (1994) Control of prostate cancer with radiotherapy: long-term results. J Urol 152:1781–1785

Balter J, Sandler HM, Lam K, Bree RL, Lichter AS, Ten Haken RK (1993) Measurement of prostate motion over the course of radiotherapy, (Abstr). 35th Annual Meeting of the American Society for Therapeutic Radiology and Oncology. New Orleans, October 1993. Int J Radiat Oncol Biol Phys 27 S1:223

Beard CJ, Bussiere MR, Plunkett ME, Coleman CN, Kijewski PK (1993a) Analysis of prostate and seminal vesicle motion, (Abstr). 35th Annual Meeting of the American Society for Therapeutic Radiology and Oncology, New Orleans, October 1993. Int J Radiat Oncol Biol Phys 27 S1:136

Beard CJ, Kaplan ID, Coleman CN (1993b) The challenge for conformal therapy for prostate cancer (editorial). Int J Radiat Oncol Biol Phys 26:705–707

Byhardt RW, Cox JD, Hornburg A, Liermann G (1978) Weekly localization and detection of field placement error. Int J Radiat Oncol Biol Phys 4:881–887

Corn BW, Hanks GE, Schultheiss TE, Hunt MA, Lee WR, Coia LR (1995) Conformal treatment of prostate cancer with improved targeting: superior prostate-specific antigen response compared to standard treatment. Int J Radiat Oncol Biol Phys 32:325–330

Diaz A, Roach M 3rd, Marquez C et al. (1994) Indications for and the significance of seminal vesicle irradiation during 3D conformal radiotherapy for localized prostate cancer. Int J Radiat Oncol Biol Phys 30:323–329

Emami B, Lyman J, Brown A et al. (1991) Tolerance of normal tissue to therapeutic irradiation. Int J Radiat Oncol Biol Phys 21:109–122

Forman JD, Mesina CF, He T et al. (1993a) Evaluation of changes in the location and shape of the prostate and rectum during a seven week course of conformal radiotherapy, (Abstr). 35th Annual Meeting of the American Society for Therapeutic Radiology and Oncology. New Orleans, October 1993. Int J Radiat Oncol Biol Phys 27 S1:222

Forman JD, Orton C, Ezzell G, Porter AT (1993b) Preliminary results of a hyperfractionated dose escalation study for locally advanced adenocarcinoma of the prostate. Radiother Oncol 27:203–208

Fraass BA, McShan DL, Diaz RF, Ten Haken RK, Aisen A, Gebarski G, Lichter AS (1987) Integration of magnetic resonance imaging into radiation therapy treatment planning: I. Technical considerations. Int J Radiat Oncol Biol Phys 13:1897–1908

Goitein M, Abrams M, Rowell D, Pollari H, Wiles J (1983) Multidimensional treatment planning. II. Beam's eye-view, back projection, and projection through CT sections. Int J Radiat Oncol Biol Phys 9:789–787

Hanks GE, Schultheiss TE, Hunt MA, Epstein B (1995) Factors influencing incidence of acute grade 2 morbidity in conformal and standard radiation treatment of prostate cancer. Int J Radiat Oncol Biol Phys 31:25–29

Hanley J, Mageras GS, Sun J, Leibel SM, Fuks Z, Kutcher GJ (1994) The use of port films from multiple projections to determine the spatial distribution of setup errors for prostate cancer patients (Abstr). 36th Annual Meeting of the American Society for Therapeutic Radiology and Oncology. San Francisco, October 1994. Int J Radiat Oncol Biol Phys 30 S1:175

ICRU Report No. 50 (1993) Prescribing, recording, and reporting photon beam therapy. International Commission on Radiation and Measurements, Bethesda, MD

Kaplan ID, Cox RS, Bagshaw MA (1993) Prostate specific antigen after external beam radiotherapy for prostatic cancer: followup. J Urol 149:519–522

Kessler ML, Pitluck S, Petti P, Castro JR (1991) Integration of multimodality imaging data for radiotherapy treatment planning. Int J Radiat Oncol Biol Phys 21:1653–1667

Leibel SA, Heimann R, Kutcher GJ et al. (1994a) Three-dimensional conformal radiation therapy in locally advanced carcinoma of the prostate: preliminary results of a phase I dose-escalation study. Int J Radiat Oncol Biol Phys 28:55–65

Leibel SA, Zelefsky MJ, Kutcher GJ et al. (1994b) The biological basis and clinical application of three-dimensional conformal external beam radiation therapy in carcinoma of the prostate. Semin Oncol 21:580–597

Lichter AS (1991) Three-dimensional conformal radiotherapy: a testable hypothesis. Int J Radiat Oncol Biol Phys 21:853–855

LoSasso T, Chui CS, Kutcher GJ, Leibel SA, Fuks-Z, Ling CC (1993) The use of a multi-leaf collimator for conformal radiotherapy of carcinomas of the prostate and nasopharynx. Int J Radiat Oncol Biol Phys 25:161–170

Lyman JT (1985) Complication probability as assessed from dose volume histograms. Radiat Res 104:S13–S19

Lyman JT, Wolbarst AB (1987) Optimization of radiation therapy. III. A method of assessing complication probabilities from dose-volume histograms. Int J Radiat Oncol Biol Phys 13:103–109

Mageras GS, Fuks Z, Obrien J et al. (1994) Initial clinical experience with computer-controlled conformal radiotherapy of the prostate using a 50-MeV medical microtron. Int J Radiat Oncol Biol Phys 30:971–978

McShan DL, Fraass BA, Lichter AS (1990) Full integration of the beam's eye view concept into computerized treatment planning. Int J Radiat Oncol Biol Phys 18:1485–1494

Melian E, Kutcher G, Leibel S, Zelefsky M, Baldwin B, Fuks Z (1993) Variation in prostate position: quantitation and implications for three-dimensional conformal radiation therapy, (Abstr). 35th Annual Meeting of the American Society for Therapeutic Radiology and Oncology. New Orleans, October 1993. Int J Radiat Oncol Biol Phys 27 S1:137

Michalski JM (1994) Accounting for localization and organ motion uncertainty in treatment planning In: Purdy JA, Fraass BA (eds) A categorical course in physics: three-dimensional treatment planning. Radiological Society of North America, Chicago, p 41

Niemierko A, Goitein M (1991) Calculation of normal tissue complication probability and dose-volume histogram reduction schemes for tissues with a critical element architecture. Int J Radiat Oncol Biol Phys 20:166–176

Perez CA, Pilepich MV, Zivnuska F (1986) Tumor control in definitive irradiation of localized carrcinoma of the prostate. Int J Radiat Oncol Biol Phys 12;523–531

Petrovich Z, Lieskovsky G, Langholz B, Luxton G, Jozsef G, Skinner DG (1991) Radiotherapy following radical prostatectomy in patients with carcinoma of the prostate. Int J Radiat Oncol Biol Phys 21:949–954

Prostate (1992) In: Beahrs OH, Henson DE, Hutter RVP, Kennedy BJ (eds) Manual for staging of cancer, 4th edn. American Joint Committee on Cancer. J.B. Lippincott, Philadelphia pp 181–183

Rabinowitz I, Broomberg J, Goitein M, McCarthy K, Leong J (1985) Accuracy of radiation field alignment in clinical practice. Int J Radiat Oncol Biol Phys 11:1857–1867

Roach M 3rd, Pickett B, Holland J, Zapotowski KA, Marsh DL, Tatera BS (1993) The role of the urethrogram during simulation for localized prostate cancer. Int J Radiat Oncol Biol Phys 25:299–307

Roach M 3rd, Pickett B, Rosenthal SA, Verhey L, Phillips TL (1994) Defining treatment margins for six field conformal irradiation of localized prostate cancer. Int J Radiat Oncol Biol Phys 28:267–275

Russell KJ, Dunatov C, Hafermann MD et al. (1991) Prostate specific antigen in the management of patients with localized adenocarcimoma of the prostate treated with primary radiation therapy. J Urol 146:1046–1052

Sandler HM, Perez-Tomayo C, Ten Haken RK, Lichter AS (1992) Dose escalation for stage C (T3) prostate cancer: minimal rectal toxicity observed using conformal therapy. Radiother Oncol 23:53–54

Soffen EM, Hanks GE, Hwang CC, Chu JCH (1991) Conformal static field therapy for low volume low grade prostate cancer with rigid immobilization. Int J Radiat Oncol Biol Phys 20:141–146

Soffen EM, Hanks GE, Hunt MA, Epstein BE (1992) Conformal static field radiation therapy treatment of early prostate cancer versus non-conformal techniques: a reduction in acute morbidity. Int J Radiat Oncol Biol Phys 24:485–488

Stamey TA, Ferrari MK, Schmid HP (1993) The vaue of serial prostate specific antigen determinations 5 years after radiotherapy: steeply increasing values characterize 80% of patients. J Urol 150:1856–1859

Ten Haken RK, Perez-Tomayo C, Tesser RJ, McShan DL, Fraass BA, Lichter AS (1989) Boost treatment of the prostate using shaped, fixed fields. Int J Radiat Oncol Biol Phys 16:193–200

Ten Haken RK, Forman JD, Heimburger DK et al. (1991) Treatment planning issues related to prostate movement in response to differential filling of the rectum and bladder. Int J Radiat Oncol Biol Phys 20:1317–1324

Vijayakumar S, Low N, Chen GTY et al. (1991) Beam's eye view-based photon radiotherapy. I. Int J Radiat Oncol Biol Phys 21:1575–1586

Vijayakumar S, Awan A, Karrison T et al. (1993) Acute toxicity during external-beam radiotherapy for localized prostate cancer: comparison of different techniques. In J Radiat Oncol Biol Phys 25:359–371

Zeitman AL, Coen JJ, Dallow KC, Shipley WU (1995) The treatment of prostate cancer by conventional radiation therapy: an analysis of long-term outcome. Int J Radiat Oncol Biol Phys 32:287–292

22 Systemic Therapy for Carcinoma of the Prostate

E. Mazeman and P. Bertrand

CONTENTS

22.1 Introduction

Recent years have witnessed a significant effort to improve the screening and the treatment of localized prostate cancer. However, 30%–40% of newly diagnosed cases are already at an advanced stage for which only medical treatment can be considered. Hormonal treatment has its limitations and since its discovery, there have been no spectacular therapeutic advances: life expectancy of patients with advanced prostate cancer has not changed. Systemic treatment is the subject of a wide variety of research from clinical trials to ultra-sophisticated scientific investigations. Various therapeutic modalities, some well documented and commonly used, others more recent or simply experimental, are discussed below to illustrate current and possible future treatment options in advanced prostate cancer.

E. Mazeman, MD, PhD, Professor, Department of Urology, Hôpital Claude Huriez, Centre Hospitalier Regional, 59037 Lille, France

P. Bertrand, MD, Department of Urology, Hôpital Claude Huriez, Centre Hospitalier Regional, 59037 Lille, France

22.2 Hormonal Treatment

22.2.1 Why and When to Treat Advanced Prostate Cancer?

When Huggins and Hodges in 1941 documented the beneficial impact of bilateral orchiectomy on metastatic prostate cancer, the first question was whether this form of treatment increased patient survival. The studies of Vest and Frazier (1946) and Nesbit and Plumb (1946), comparing hormonally treated patients with those not hormonally treated, concluded that the former group appeared to exhibit a definite trend toward improved survival. These reports were legitimately criticized because of their retrospective nature, the lack of randomization, and the introduction of antibiotics, such as sulfonamide, at about the same time as endrocrine therapy.

The Veterans Administration Cooperative Urological Group (VACURG 1967) studied about 4000 patients in two historical prospective and randomized trials. In the first trial patients were divided into four treatment groups: (a) placebo, (b) bilateral orchiectomy, (c) diethylstilbestrol (DES) 5 mg/day, and (d) DES plus orchiectomy. In the second trial the treatment groups were: (a) placebo, (b) DES 0.2 mg/day, (c) DES 1 mg/day, and (d) DES 5 mg/day. As soon as cancer progression was noted in patients in the placebo group, hormonal therapy was begun. In these series, delaying hormonal therapy did not appear to compromise overall survival and so the question of the timing of androgen suppression was posed. In 1982 Lepor et al. reported on the longevity of 200 patients with stage C and D prostate cancer, diagnosed between 1937 and 1943. Although the patients in the hormonal therapy group had an estimated survival of 709 days versus 550 days for the control group, statistically this difference is explained by a lower mortality in the patients who entered the study late rather than by the effect of hormonal treatment, thereby raising the question of the usefulness of endocrine therapy. The VACURG conclusions gave rise to controversy for various reasons: the patients in the placebo group were sometimes later hormonally treated, lymph node dissection and bone scanning were not included in the patient's workup, and the number of patients included in the studies was too small to allow for statistically significant conclusions.

A later update of the VACURG survival data by BYAR and CORLE (1988) demonstrated that early androgen withdrawal prolonged survival in younger patients with high-grade tumor (Gleason score 7–10) and stage D disease, but this was not so evident for older patients or for patients with low-grade and lower stage disease. In addition, experimental studies of ISAACS and COFFEY (1981) using the Dunning R-3327-H rat prostatic carcinoma model demonstrated that the cause of androgen resistance was the intrinsic heterogeneity of the tumor and not castration-induced adaptation.

In conclusion, there is no valid reason for delaying treatment in advanced prostate carcinoma. Starting hormonal treatment might have some influence on survival, and it is probably better to treat a small tumor rather than a large one. In this decision-making process the quality of life has to be considered in a patient who knows he has a cancer which is progressing and who may develop symptomatic bone metastases, and one must also bear in mind that it has not been demonstrated that the hormone-sensitive part of the tumor may keep its sensitivity as the tumor progresses. On the other hand, the patient who really has a choice must be informed that hormonal treatment will make him impotent.

22.2.2 Endocrine Regulation of Prostate Growth

Androgens are derived from two sources: the testis and the adrenal cortex. Both are under the control of the hypothalamus and the anterior pituitary gland: Luteinizing hormone-releasing hormone (LHRH) and corticotropin-releasing factor (CRF) are released by the hypothalamus and transported to the anterior pituitary gland, where LHRH stimulates the production of luteinizing hormone (LH) and follicle-stimulating hormone (FSH) and CRF stimulates the production of adrenocorticotropin hormone (ACTH). LH stimulates testosterone production by the Leydig cells of the testis, which accounts for approximately 90% of the total testosterone in circulation. ACTH stimulates adrenal androgen production of androstenedione and dehydroepiandrosterone, the precursors of testosterone and dihydrotestosterone (DHT). Feedback inhibition modulates these secretions. Testosterone and, to some degree, adrenal androgens are converted into DHT in the prostatic cells by 5α-reductase. DHT is bound to a nuclear receptor and this complex interacts with specific DNA sequences to increase the transcription and production of RNAs.

The concept of endocrine management of prostate cancer is based on the suppression of androgen production or on the neutralization of androgens' effects at target cells.

22.2.3 Hormonal Therapies

22.2.3.1 Surgical Castration, Estrogens, and LHRH Analogues

Bilateral orchiectomy definitively reduces circulating testosterone to the castrate range in 24 h. Complications of this procedure are minimal, with side-effects including loss of libido and impotence, as always with androgen deprivation. Some of the psychological impact can be reduced with a subcapsular orchiectomy which leaves the tunica as a structure in the scrotum.

Until recently estrogens were, along with surgical castration, the most common form of endocrine therapy in advanced prostate cancer. Primarily they suppress pituitary gland secretion of LH by a negative feedback on the hypothalamic-pituitary-gonadal axis. They also increase testosterone-binding globulin and thereby decrease bioavailable testosterone levels. Furthermore they have a direct action on prostatic cells. DES has been the most commonly used: the first VACURG study has shown that a dose of 5 mg/day results in effective medical castration but with an excessive cardiovascular complication rate. In the second VACURG trial it was demonstrated that the 1 mg dose was as effective as the 5 mg dose while being associated with fewer cardiovascular complications. With the emergence of LHRH analogues, estrogens have nevertheless been abandoned.

Since the discovery by SCHALLY et al. in 1971 of the LHRH amino acid sequence, several studies have shown that LHRH agonists produce responses and survival rates similar to DES or surgical castration.

The first injection causes a stimulatory effect with increasing testoterone and LH that results in what is called "flare phenomenon." This side-effect occurs during the first week of therapy and even if the complications are rare, it is advisable to prescribe an antiandrogen before the first analogue depot injection. Testosterone levels reach their castrate value within the first 4 weeks and those levels are maintained for the duration of the treatment. Side-effects are primarily the symptoms due to androgen withdrawal. Four molecules are available: leuprolide, triptoreline, goserilin in monthly injections, and buserilin as an injection every 2 months.

22.2.3.2 Antiandrogens

Antiandrogens block the action of androgens at their target cells. They may be divided into two types: steroidal with progestational effects and nonsteroidal or pure antiandrogens.

The three pure antiandrogens currently used (nilutamide, flutamide, and casodex) are associated with a rise in testosterone and LH levels resulting from the inhibition of the negative feedback of androgens at the hypothalamic-pituitary level. Their difference resides in their pharmacokinetics and toxicities.

Nilutamide has a half-life of about 40 h, allowing once a day administration of 150 mg. The side-effects include alcohol intolerance, light-dark adaptation disorders, and acute interstitial pneumonia. Flutamide is given three times per day. Gynecomastia and diarrhea are the most common side-effects. Casodex is given in a daily dose of 50 mg; gynecomastia and diarrhea are again the most common side-effects.

Steroidal antiandrogens differ from pure antiandrogens because, in addition to the blockade of androgen receptors, they also have a progestational effect that partially inhibits the release of LH and thereby the testosterone production of the testis. The two current molecules are cyproterone acetate (CPA) and megestrol acetate (MGA). In a phase III trial by the genitourinary group of the European Organization for Research on the Treatment of Cancer (EORTC), MGA appeared to be of less efficacy than either CPA or DES in terms of progression-free survival and overall survival. A 250 mg/day dose of CPA produced identical results with significantly less cardiovascular side-effects than 3 mg/day of DES (Pavone-Malacuso et al. 1986). Steroidal antiandrogens suppress libido and cause impotence but can be used to reduce the troublesome hot flushes after orchiectomy or LHRH analogue treatment. The small number of trials and the risk of a gradual rise in plasma testosterone concentration after 6–10 months limit the use of these drugs as monotherapy.

22.2.3.3 5α-Reductase Inhibitors

The effect of finasteride on stage D prostate cancer was reported in a randomized, double-blind, placebo-controlled study and suggested the minor activity of this drug. It was noted that patients with bone metastases at the onset of the study failed to show a decrease of PSA in contrast to those without bone disease. The variation of 5α-reductase activity among metastatic sites and the importance of 5α reduced androgen metabolites in the maintenance of prostatic cancer growth remain unclear (Presti et al. 1992).

22.2.3.4 Ketoconazole

Ketoconazole is widely used as an antifungal agent. In high doses (400 mg three times a day) it inhibits the biosynthesis of testicular and adrenal androgens and castration levels can be achieved within 24–48 h. Therapy with ketoconazole is limited by its side-effects but the prompt decrease in plasma testosterone and the reversibility of androgen withdrawal can be useful in some particular indications. There is limited response in hormonally resistant prostate cancer.

22.2.3.5 Aminoglutethimide

Aminoglutethimide blocks the production of adrenal androgens. Given in combination with hydrocortisone to prevent adrenal insufficiency, it is rarely used in androgen-resistant cancer and the objective response rate is low.

22.2.4 Total Androgen Ablation

The concept of total androgen ablation is based on the neutralization of adrenal androgens as well as those of testicular origin. After medical or surgical castration, adrenal androgens are responsible for maintaining intraprostatic DHT levels, and it was postulated that these low levels of DHT continue to stimulate androgen-sensitive cells. HUGGINS and SCOTT were the first in 1945 to use a surgical adrenalectomy as a second-line treatment for patients with a hormone-refractory tumor. Then medical adrenalectomy was performed using cortisone, aminoglutethimide, or ketoconazole but always as a second-line treatment. Compared to adrenalectomy, antiandrogens offered a simple means of counteracting adrenal androgens. In 1985 LABRIE et al. published encouraging results from a phase 2 trial, using antiandrogens in combination with castration as first-line hormonal therapy for advanced prostate cancer. Multiple randomized studies have since been performed.

The results of a study including 600 patients and comparing leuprolide and flutamide versus leuprolide and placebo were reported by CRAWFORD et al. (1989). Both median progression-free survival (16.5 months vs 13.9 months) and overall survival (35.6 months vs 28.3 months) were greater in the combination arm. Patients with minimal disease (metastases in pelvis or axial skeleton or soft tissue nodal involvement) and good performance status had a more significant benefit.

A recent update at 60 months after registration confirmed these data and showed a 29-month difference in progression-free survival and a 19-month difference in survival for patients with good prognostic factors (EISENBERGER et al. 1994).

In 1990 the EORTC presented the analysis of a study with 327 patients randomized as orchiectomy or goserilin and flutamide. With a median follow-up of 18 months there was no difference in survival (DENIS et al. 1990). An update with the mean follow-up at 4 years showed a statistical advantage lengthening the time before subjective or objective cancer progression and decreasing the incidence of cancer deaths in the goserilin–flutamide combination. The difference seemed to be more pronounced in patients with good prognostic factors but the results were not statistically significant (DENIS et al. 1993).

JANKNEGT et al. (1993) published an update of a study which randomized 457 patients to receive orchiectomy or orchiectomy and nilutamide. The mean time or progression was 20.8 months in the nilutamide group compared to 14.9 months in the placebo group. Mean time to death was 37.1 months in the nilutamide group compared to 29.8 months in the placebo group.

An overview by DALESIO (1992) of 25 randomized trials with 5425 available patients showed a 5-year survival rate of 19.7% for the treatment group compared to 16.7% for the control group. The annual death hazard ratio was variable in the subgroups, showing a reduction of 10% with flutamide, 6% with nilutamide, and 0% with CPA.

These recent data suggest that maximal androgen ablation is superior to standard castration, especially for patients with good prognostic factors. However, the benefit is not very important, and survival was improved only by 6–8 months except in the study of Crawford and co-workers [an update of the first report by CRAWFORD et al. in 1989 showed improvement in survival by 19 months in patients with good prognostic factors (EISENBERGER 1994)]. The challenge remains to define the subgroups that may benefit to a greater extent (DENIS and MURPHY 1993).

22.2.5 Intermittent Androgen Suppression

GLEAVE et al. (1994) have tested the effects of intermittent androgen withdrawal in the LNCaP prostate tumor model and it was suggested that this therapeutic modality could delay progression to androgen independence. The feasibility of this procedure was evaluated by GOLDENBERG et al. (1995) on 47 patients. The first period of treatment was about 36 weeks and it was started again when serum PSA levels increased, approximately 30 weeks after the interruption. If PSA levels did not fall into the normal range, patients were not included. No adverse consequences of this procedure were demonstrated and patients' quality of life increased. However, randomized studies are needed to evaluate the effect on progression-free survival and overall survival.

22.3 Chemotherapy

If hormonal ablation remains the standard therapy for advanced prostate cancer, the majority of treated patients will relapse, given time, into a hormonally unresponsive state. Experimental studies have demonstrated the initial heterogeneity of prostate cancer cells including androgen-dependent and androgen-independent clones (ISAACS and COFFEY 1981). Cytotoxic chemotherapy has been used to eliminate the non-androgen-dependent tumor after failure of hormonal treatment but the current results obtained with single agents and multidrug regimens remain disappointing and might lead one to consider prostate cancer as a chemoresistant tumor. The reason for these findings could be that chemotherapeutic agents usually lead to cancer cell death after cell division, yet 90% of prostatic cancer cells are in interphase and thus resistant to standard cytotoxic chemotherapy (KYPRIANOU et al. 1991).

Many comments have been made about the difficulties in interpreting the value of chemotherapy in hormonally resistant prostate cancer. The usual response criteria of oncologic trials are inapplicable because most of the patients have no measurable disease due to the predominance of bone metastases. The criteria used in the trials can vary considerably (cf. for example, the introduction of the term "stable disease" by the National Prostatic Cancer Project). This may explain the sometimes contradictory results, even when the same drug is tested. The introduction of PSA, as a response criterion, in the more recent studies does not solve this problem, because the level of this marker fluctuates widely and is not always correlated with regression of measurable disease.

22.3.1 Phase II Studies

In a recent analysis by YAGODA and PETRYLAK (1993) of 26 clinical trials conducted between 1987 and 1991 and using a single chemotherapeutic agent, only six drugs showed an objective response rate [complete response (CR) plus partial response (PR)] greater than 10%. The best results were obtained with vinblastine in continuous infusion, with 21% CR + PR; trimetrexate showed some promise, with 17% CR = PR.

The use of drug combinations does not enhance the response rate. In an overview by EISENBERGER (1990) the association of cisplatin and doxorubicin yielded 23% CR + PR, and YAGODA and PETRYLAK (1993) mentioned the combination of estramustine plus vinblastine as yielding a 14% CR + PR. All these trials require confirmation.

22.3.2 Prospective Randomized Studies

Two studies conducted by the NPCP must be cited because patients were randomized either to single-agent arm (various agents were used) or to a no chemotherapy control arm. In neither study was there a significant survival advantage between treatment arms (EISENBERGER 1990).

Obviously the results obtained with chemotherapy are not encouraging but, as mentioned by EISENBERGER (1990), one must consider that urologic oncologists usually still reserve this treatment for those patients who have become refractory to endocrine treatment and who are unlikely to respond to any other therapy. Moreover, as with hormonal treatment, cytotoxic chemotherapy may be less efficient in previously treated advanced cancers. In that case, no benefit from androgen deprivation can be expected, which justifies the continuing research to develop nonhormonal treatments able to act on hormonally independent cell clones.

22.4 New Approaches to Therapy

During the five past decades no therapy has clearly demonstrated an ability to increase patient survival in advanced prostate cancer. The disappointing results of hormonal treatment are due to the initial presence of androgen-independent cells. These androgen-independent clones represent the main challenge for researchers, there being a need to understand their origin and to find curative therapeutic modalities. One of the most important developments in cancer research is based on the identification of a genetic basis for malignant transformation. Carcinogenesis is considered as a multistep process of accumulated damage in specific genes concerned in cellular growth and differentiation. These specific genes include oncogenes, tumor suppressor genes, growth factors, and their receptors. For example about 100 oncogenes have been identified but only four (c-*myc*, c-*sis*, c-*ras*, and c-*erb*B-2/*neu*) have been studied in prostate cancer and their role is not well established. Growth factors are proteins whose overexpression can confer a malignant potential on a cell. Epidermal growth factor, fibroblast growth factor, and insulin growth factor have been identified in the normal growth and differentiation of the prostate. Experimental studies have suggested that some of these factors could play a major role in the progression from androgen-dependent to androgen-independent cancer growth even if no clear pattern has emerged. The activation of oncogenes in carcinogenesis is accompanied by loss of the function of the tumor suppressor genes. P53 suppressor gene has been the most studied in prostate cancer and compared with other neoplasms, its alteration seems to occur less frequently. P53 gene mutation is probably a late event in the progression of prostate cancer indicating an increasing cellular proliferation rate, grade, stage, and androgen independence (NETTO and HUMPHREY 1994). Although there are limitations to all these experimental studies, this pathway represents the only future for a curative therapy of advanced prostate cancer. Using previous experimental results, new treatments have been proposed.

22.4.1 Suramin

Suramin is a polysulfonated naphthylurea that was originally used for the treatment of trypanosomiasis and onchocerciasis and has been investigated for a possible role in HIV patients. In addition, suramin has been documented to have antitumor effects in vitro in a variety of neoplasms, including prostate cancer. It has been demonstrated that suramin is able to block the activity of several growth factors, including those involved in prostatic carcinogenesis. Finally, this drug also has an adrenocorticolytic effect, thereby lowering adrenal androgen levels.

These observations led MYERS et al. (1992) to test suramin in 38 patients with metastatic androgen-resistant prostate cancer. Among the 17 evaluable patients, only six had an objective PR and in none of them did the bone lesions resolve. Just one of the remaining 21 patients with only bone metastases experienced resolution of more than 50% of the lesions. A more than 50% decrease in the PSA levels was observed in 21 of the 38 patients. Median survival was 42.3 weeks, which is approximately the survival time of patients with hormone-refractory cancer.

A difficult issue with suramin is its toxicity, directly associated with plasma level above 350 μg/ml, which unfortunately is the level required to obtain a therapeutic response. As there is a large individual variation in suramin blood levels for a given dose, monitoring of the drug level is of critical importance and requires the use of complex nomograms. Suramin-related toxicity includes hematologic disorders, peripheral neuropathy, infections, coagulopathy, hyperglycemia, skin rash, serum creatinine elevation, and nonspecific fatigue syndrome.

For the time being, suramin can be considered a possible agent in the treatment of advanced prostate cancer but its toxicity and the difficulties with its management compared to the objective response rate preclude its current use. Research must continue to optimize its administration or to find a new form with better tolerance.

22.4.2 Gene Therapy

Gene therapy may be defined as the introduction of new genetic material into a patient, with therapeutic intent. Usually protocols involve transfer of DNA using viruses such as a retrovirus or an adenovirus. In cancer the most developed gene therapy strategy is the use of a gene-modified tumor vaccine: tumor cells are extracted from a patient with metastatic disease and modified with immunomodulatory genes; these irradiated cells are then reinjected into the patient (GLODE 1994). Gene therapy in prostate cancer is at its beginning. SANDA et al. (1994) have shown the benefit of using a tumor vaccine consisting of granulocyte macrophage colony stimulating factor (GM-CSF) transduced irradiated Mat-ly-lu cells in the Dunning rat model of prostate cancer. An evaluation of its clinical feasibility based on these experimental findings is proposed, utilizing retroviral transduction of GM-CSF into tumor cells from radical prostatectomy specimens. Other techniques for gene therapy are under evaluation but, whatever the strategy used, the main problem is the choice of gene to transfer, and in the prostate many genes seem capable of altering the biologic behaviour of the tumor cells.

22.5 Systemic Radionuclide Therapy

Bone metastases are common in advanced prostate cancer. They cause deep pain, pathologic fractures, and spinal cord compression, compromising the patient's quality of life. Hormonal therapy can have a beneficial impact on these symptoms but in patients with a hormone-refractory tumor these complications often represent the main clinical problem. The pain can be managed with narcotic analgesics, local radiotherapy for well-defined sites, and hemibody radiation in patients with diffuse disease. More recently the delivery of radiation by injection of a radioisotope has been used. The first radionuclide tested in this indication was phosphorus-32 with a subjective response rate of 60%–70% in terms of pain relief. However, the injection of this molecule was associated with a high incidence of myelosuppression due to the incorporation of phosphorus-32 into marrow elements, limiting its clinical use (SILBERSTEIN et al. 1992). Strontium-89 is a beta-emitting isotope with a half-life of 50.5 days which localizes preferentially at metastatic sites, sparing healthy bone and bone marrow. It is the most studied radioisotope, but others, including rhenium and samarium, are now available.

22.5.1 Clinical Use of Strontium-89

When using strontium-89, a single dose is administered intravenously on an outpatient basis. The dose used varies in the different reported trials. A randomized study of the Radiation Therapy Oncology Group was performed to determine the maximum safe dosage, testing 4.0, 6.5, 9.0, and 11.5 mCi of strontium-89. The 4.0 mCi dose was the maximum tolerated, while with higher doses there was little analgesic improvement (PORTER and VAISHAMPAYAN 1994). The major side-effect is hematologic dose-dependent toxicity, particularly thrombocytopenia occurring 4–8 weeks after injection. Recovery is gradual and often incomplete. Another side-effect is an increase in the pain (flare response) beginning 1–2 days after injection and lasting 2–4 days. Higher doses of pain medication or administration of a short course of steroids can be recommended in such cases (ROBINSON 1993).

22.5.2 Strontium-89 After Failure of Conventional Radiotherapy

Robinson initiated the first evaluation of strontium-89 in patients with osteoblastic metastatic disease. An 80% response rate was reached in terms of decrease in pain, reduced need for pain medication, and improved quality of life (ROBINSON et al. 1989). These data were confirmed by LAING et al. (1991) in a study concerning the use of strontium-89 after failure of hormonal therapy and conventional radiotherapy. At 3 months, 75% of patients experienced partial pain relief and 22% had become pain free. Another series by LEVINGTON et al. (1991) comparing the injection of strontium-89 and stable strontium-85 as placebo demonstrated that the therapeutic effect of strontium-89 was effective and due to its radiation.

22.5.3 Strontium-89 as an Adjuvant to External Beam Radiotherapy

The role of external beam radiotherapy in pain control remains important but after local treatment new sites of pain frequently develop. It was thought that strontium-89 might prevent the development of such painful new locations. A randomized phase III Canadian trial evaluated 124 patients receiving radiotherapy and either strontium or a placebo. Progression as measured by the appearance of new sites of pain or the requirement for radiotherapy showed a statistical difference in favor of strontium-89. However, the 10.8 mCi dose used produced severe hematologic toxicity (PORTER et al. 1993). Another study by BOLGER et al. (1993) compared strontium-89 against conventional radiotherapy: pain response at the initial sites of pain was similar in the two groups but patients receiving strontium-89 were less likely to experience new sites of pain.

In conclusion, the primary role of strontium-89 lies in the palliation of pain in patients with metastatic disease. Favorable results are obtained with acceptable side-effects in about 80% of patients, but for a short average period of 6 months. It is as effective as conventional radiotherapy and seems to delay pain progression. Therefore systemic radionuclide therapy could be proposed early in the evolution of painful bone metastases.

22.6 Conclusion

Androgen deprivation therapy remains the gold standard in the treatment of advanced prostate cancer but sooner or later patients will relapse into a hormonally unresponsive state, which is one of the major problems facing urologists today. Hormonal treatment has clearly shown its limits whatever the method employed. Research aiming to increase the efficacy and reduce the side-effects of currently used treatments, such as chemotherapy, must be continued. At the same time the development of new approaches is critically needed. In the immediate future, gene therapy, which is still at an experimental stage, probably represents one of the most important challenges facing urologic oncology.

References

Bolger JJ, Dearnaley DP, Kirk D (1993) Strontium-89 (Metastron) versus external beam radiotherapy in patients with painful bone metastases secondary to prostate cancer: preliminary report of a multicenter trial. Semin Oncol 20 (Suppl 2):32–33

Byar DP, Corle DK (1988) Hormone therapy for prostate cancer: results of the VACURG studies. NCI Monogr 7:165–170

Crawford ED, Eisenberger MA, McLeod D, Spaulding JT, Benson R, Dorr FA (1989) A controlled trial of leuprolide with and without flutamide in prostatic carcinoma. N Engl J Med 321:419–424

Dalesio O (1992) Complete androgen blockade in prostate cancer: an overview of randomized trials. Prostate 4 (Suppl):111–114

Denis L, Murphy GP (1993) Overview of phase III trials on combined androgen treatment in patients with metastatic prostate cancer. Cancer 72 (Suppl):3888–3895

Denis L, Smith P, Carneiro de Moura JL et al. (1990) Orchiectomy versus goserilin plus flutamide in patients with metastatic prostate cancer. Eur Urol 18:34–40

Denis L, Carneiro de Moura JL, Bono A et al. (1993) Goserilin acetate and flutamide versus bilateral orchiectomy: a phase III EORTC trial, (30853). Urology 42:119–130

Eisenberger MA (1990) Chemotherapy for endocrine resistant cancer of the prostate. In: EORTC genitourinary group monograph 8. Treatment of prostatic cancer-facts and controversies. Wiley-Liss, New York, pp 155–164

Eisenberger MA, Crawford ED, Wolf M et al. (1994) Prognostic factors in stage D2 prostate cancer; important implications for future trials: results of a cooperative intergroup study (Int 0036). Semin Oncol 21:613–619

Gleave ME, Bruchovsky N, Bowden M, Goldenberg SL, Sullivan LD (1994) Intermittent androgen suppression prolongs time to androgen independent progression in the LNCaP prostate tumor model. J Urol 151:457A

Glode LM (1994) The molecular bridge to gene therapy. Urology 44:81–88

Goldenberg SL, Bruchovsky N, Gleave ME, Sullivan LD, Akakura K (1995) Intermittent androgen suppression in the treatment of prostate cancer; a preliminary report. Urology 45:839–845

Huggins C, Hodges CV (1941) Studies on prostatic cancer: effects of castration, of estrogen and androgen injection on serum phosphatase in metastatic carcinoma of the prostate. Cancer Res 1:293–297

Huggins C, Scott WW (1945) Bilateral adrenalectomy in prostate cancer. Ann Surg 122:1031–1041

Isaacs JT, Coffey DS (1981) Adaptation versus selection as the mechanism responsible for the relapse of prostatic cancer to androgen ablation therapy as studied in the Dunning R-3327-H adenocarcinoma. Cancer Res 41:5070–5075

Janknegt RA, Abbou CC, Bartoletti R et al. (1993) Orchiectomy and nilutamide or placebo as treatment of metastatic prostatic cancer in a multinational double blind randomized trial. J Urol 149:77–83

Kyprianou N, Martikainen P, Davis L, English HF, Isaacs JT (1991) Programmed cell death as a new target for prostate cancer therapy. Cancer Surv 11:265–275

Labrie F, Dupont A, Belanger A et al. (1985) Combination therapy with flutamide and castration (LHRH agonist or orchiectomy) in advanced prostate cancer: a marked improvement in response and survival. J Steroid Biochem 23:833–841

Laing AH, Ackery DM, Bayly RJ et al. (1991) Strontium-89 chloride for pain palliation in prostatic skeletal malignancy. Br J Radiol 64:816–822

Lepor H, Ross A, Walsh PC (1982) The influence of hormonal therapy on survival of men with advanced prostatic cancer. J Urol 128:335–340

Levington VJ, McEwan AJ, Ackery DM et al. (1991) A prospective, randomized, double blind crossover study to examine the efficacy of strontium-89 in pain palliation in patients with advanced prostate cancer metastatic to bone. Eur J Cancer 27:954–958

Myers C, Cooper M, Stein C et al. (1992) Suramin: a novel growth factor antagonist with activity in hormone-refractory metastatic prostate cancer. J Clin Oncol 10:881–889

Nesbit RM, Plumb RT (1946) Prostatic carcinoma: a follow-up on 795 patients treated prior to endocrine era and comparison of survival rates between these and patients treated by endocrine therapy. Surgery 20:263–272

Netto GJ, Humphrey PA (1994) Molecular biologic aspects of human prostatic carcinoma. Am J Clin Pathol 102 (Suppl 1):S57–S64

Pavone-Malacuso M, De Voogt HJ, Viggiano G et al. (1986) Comparison of diethylstilbestrol, cyproterone acetate and medroxyprogesterone acetate in the treatment of advanced prostate cancer. J Urol 136:624–630

Porter AT, Vaishampayan N (1994) Strontium-89 in metastatic prostate cancer. Urology 44:75–80

Porter AT, McEwan AJB, Powe JE et al. (1993) Results of a randomized phase III trial to evaluate the efficacy of strontium-89 adjuvant to local field external beam irradiation in the management of endocrine resistant metastatic prostate cancer. Int J Radiat Oncol Biol Phys 25:805–813

Presti JC, Fair WR, Andriole G et al. (1992) Multicenter randomized, double blind, placebo controlled study to investigate the effect of finasteride (MK-906) on stage D prostate cancer. J Urol 148:1201–1204

Robinson RG (1993) Strontium-89. Precursor targeted therapy for pain relief of blastic metastatic disease. Cancer 72 (Suppl):3433–3435

Robinson RG, Preston DF, Spicer JA, Martin NL, Schiefelbein M (1989) Strontium-89: improved clinical response with increasing dose in patients with painful metastatic prostate and breast cancer in bone. J Nucl Med 30:843

Sanda MG, Ayyagari SR, Jaffee E et al. (1994) Demonstration of a rational strategy for human prostate cancer gene therapy. J Urol 151:622–628

Schally AV, Arimura A, Baba Y et al. (1971) Isolation and properties of FSH and LH-releasing hormone. Biochem Biophys Res Comm 43:393–399

Silberstein EB, Algazzar AH, Kapilivsky A (1992) Phosphorus 32 radiopharmaceuticals for the treatment of painful osseous metastases. Semin Nucl Med 21:17–27

Vest SA, Frazier TH (1946) Survival following castration for prostate cancer. J Urol 56:97–102

Veterans Administration Cooperative Urological Research Group (1967) Treatment and survival of patients with cancer of the prostate. Surg Gynecol Obstet 124:1011–1017

Yagoda A, Petrylak D (1993) Cytotoxic chemotherapy for advanced hormone-resistant prostate cancer. Cancer 71 (Suppl):1098–1109

23 Hyperthermia for Carcinoma of the Prostate

S. Szmigielski, B. Stawarz, H. Goethuys, L. Baert, H. Van Poppel, H. Zielinski, N. Piotrkowicz, A.M. Nissar Syed, and Z. Petrovich

CONTENTS

S. Szmigielski, MD, PhD, Professor of Pathophysiology, Center for Radiobiology and Radiation Safety, Military Institute of Hygiene and Epidemiology, 128 Szaserow, 00-909 Warsaw, Poland

B. Stawarz, MD, PhD, Professor and Chairman, Department of Urology, uL. Listopada 15-10, Warsaw 03446, Poland

H. Goethuys, MD, Senior Resident, Department of Urology, St. Pieter's Hospital, Catholic University of Leuven, Brusselsestraat 69, 3000 Leuven, Belgium

L. Baert, MD, Professor and Chairman, Department of Urology, St. Pieter's Hospital, Catholic University of Leuven, Brusselsestraat 69, 3000 Leuven, Belgium and Clinical Professor, Department of Urology and Radiation Oncology, University of Southern California School of Medicine, 1441 Eastlake Avenue, Los Angeles, CA 90033, USA

H. Van Poppel, MD, PhD, Professor, Department of Urology, St. Pieter's Hospital, Catholic University of Leuven, Brusselsestraat 69, 3000 Leuven, Belgium

H. Zielinski, MD, PhD, Center for Radiobiology and Radiation Safety, Military Institute of Hygiene and Epidemiology, 128 Szaserow, 00-909 Warsaw, Poland

N. Piotrkowicz, MD, PhD, Center for Radiobiology and Radiation Safety, Military Institute of Hygiene and Epidemiology, 128 Szaserow, 00-909 Warsaw, Poland

A.M. Nissar Syed, MD, Clinical Professor of Radiation Oncology, University of Southern California School of Medicine and Medical Director, Radiation Oncology Memorial Medical Center, Long Beach, CA 90801, USA

Z. Petrovich, MD, Professor of Radiation Oncology and Urology, Chairman, Department of Radiation Oncology, University of Southern California School of Medicine, 1441 Eastlake Avenue, Los Angeles, CA 90033, USA

23.1 Introduction

More than 85 years have elapsed since, in 1910, the German physician Carl Muller first described the potential for using hyperthermia (HT) as a new adjuvant to radiotherapy (RT) in the management of patients with advanced malignant neoplasms. In empiric studies of the first 100 patients with superficial tumors, Muller used high-frequency electromagnetic fields generated by a medical diathermy apparatus (Muller 1912). Despite poor control of his HT parameters during these early clinical trials, a significant improvement of the expected radiation effect in HT-treated patients was noted.

Subsequently, for many years, sporadic reports from a few radiation oncology centers enthusiastically confirmed the benefit of adjuvant HT in various superficial malignant tumors treated with RT. However, it was not until the early 1970s that broad scientific efforts were focused on the elucidation of mechanisms leading to selective killing of neoplastic cells by HT and on the potential of increasing the radiosensitivity of tumors by means of HT. Numerous experimental studies undertaken in the past two decades have resulted in a better understanding of basic mechanisms of hyperthermic cytotoxicity and radiosensitization at the cellular level. There has also been considerable progress in clinical HT, including better definition of indications for HT in curative and palliative treatments of cancer patients. This has in turn resulted in the development of a new generation of HT equipment which allows for more precise and better controlled heating of tumors. In spite of the major improvements in the available HT equipment, much work needs to be done in this area. The clinical results obtained so far support the general opinion that HT alone has no role or only a very limited role in the curative treatment of cancer. It may be useful, however, as a palliative treatment in highly selected patients such as those who have contraindications to RT. The use of HT alone in these selected patients is frequently effective in the relief of pain and is able to control bleeding from ulcerative tumors; generally, HT may provide an improved quality of life in patients with locally advanced and severely symptomatic tumors. The optimal role for HT appears to be in combination with RT or chemotherapy. A combination of these modalities offers better control of the disease process by increasing the incidence of local tumor control (GERWECK 1985). This, however, depends on our ability to homogeneously heat tumors. At the present time no available HT equipment is capable of homogeneously heating large superficial or deep-seated tumors. The current common use for adjuvant HT is in the palliative treatment of locally advanced and/or recurrent superficial neoplasms. The widely accepted indications for curative application of HT as an adjuvant to RT include: head and neck tumors, locally advanced breast neoplasms, adenocarcinoma of the rectum and esophagus, carcinoma of the cervix and vagina, soft tissue sarcomas, cutaneous melanomas, and primary tumors of the eye (OVERGAARD 1989). Phase I–II clinical trials of RT-HT combination in the above tumors have consistently shown promising results (BERDOV and MENTESHASHVILI 1990; KAKEHI et al. 1991; MATSUI et al. 1991; PETROVICH et al. 1989; SAPOZINK et al. 1986). The enhancement of the radiation effect on neoplastic tissue by HT is expressed by the thermal enhancement ratio (TER). The TER varies considerably, from a low of 1.1 to a high of 4, and depends on multiple factors, including tumor histology, tumor volume, and the timing of HT treatments (OVERGAARD 1989).

Adenocarcinoma of the prostate (CaP) is the most common human malignancy (see Chap. 20 for details) and frequently (61% of cases) presents a problem as a result of local tumor recurrence (KAPP 1986; PETROVICH and BAERT 1993). In 1995, it is anticipated that 24644 patients with CaP will die because of the presence of recurrent or persistent locoregional disease (KAPP 1986 and Chap. 20). This tumor is therefore a good candidate for HT-RT clinical trials. Several reported phase I–II clinical trials have shown good treatment tolerance and strong evidence of therapeutic activity (PETROVICH and BAERT 1993).

Important and strong evidence for the effectiveness of the RT-HT combination was recently provided in a report of a phase III, prospective randomized trial in patients with recurrent melanoma (OVERGAARD et al. 1995). This study was conduced in several major medical centers in Europe. A total of 134 patients with a diagnosis of recurrent melanoma were randomly assigned to receive RT alone ($n = 65$), consisting of three fractions of 8 or 9 Gy each, given in 8 days, or the same RT combined with HT, consisting of three sessions ($n = 63$) of 43°C, applied for 60 min. Superficial HT was used for the treatment of these patients with and without skin cooling, at 433 or 915 MHz. In multivariate analysis, the addition of HT to RT was the most important ($P = 0.0015$) factor influencing tumor response, followed by tumor diameter ($P = 0.0048$), radiation dose ($P = 0.049$), and sex (female) of the patient ($P = 0.018$). The probability of tumor control at 5 years for patients treated with RT alone was approximately 28%, while it was 45% for those in the combined treatment group ($P = 0.0056$). The addition of HT in this study did not significantly increase the incidence or severity of acute or late radiation complications.

23.2 Strategies for Synergistic Killing of Cancer Cells

Adenocarcinoma of the prostate belongs to a group of slowly proliferating neoplasms and irrespective of the degree of cell differentiation is relatively resistant to chemotherapy and only moderately sensitive to radiotherapy (FAUL 1992). The treatment decision for the individual patient with CaP should be based on numerous factors, including the extent of local disease, histologic grade, performance status of the patient, patient age, etc. The aim of effective treatment should be maximal lowering of tumor burden followed by procedures which can restrain or delay the regrowth of the surviving fraction of tumor cells. Selective cytoreduction of malignant cells with limited injury to surrounding normal tissues can be obtained by conventional techniques of surgery and/or RT (Fig. 23.1). These treatment modalities are the first choice for effective curative therapy of localized CaP (FAUL 1992; PETROVICH et al. 1993). For patients with more advanced disease the main cytoreductive procedures include hormonal treatment aimed at eliminating the androgenic stimulus for the androgen-dependent CaP cells to proliferate (ALTWEIN and FAUL 1990) and combinations of hormonal treatment with radio- or chemotherapy (BENSON and GILL 1986).

Hyperthermia at a temperature of 43°–44°C leads to killing of neoplastic cells and therefore may be considered as one of the cytoreductive treatments. Hyperthermic cytotoxicity for neoplastic cells was well characterized in vitro by GERWECK (1985). This cytotoxicity of HT appears to be dependent not only on the proliferation rate and DNA-ploidy of heated

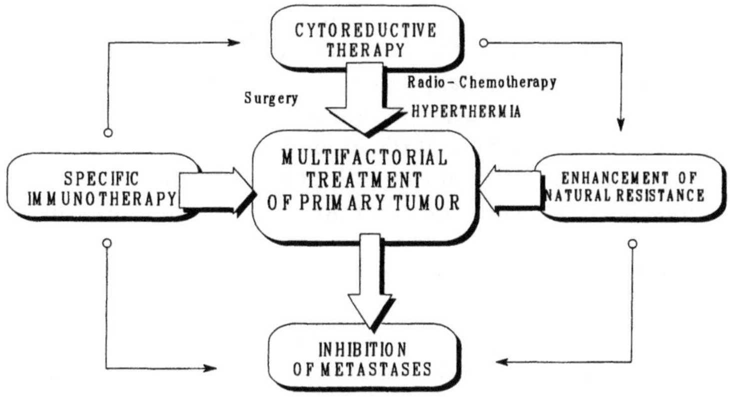

Fig. 23.1. Multimodality treatment of primary tumor with a combination of cytoreductive techniques and various forms of immunotherapy

cells, but also on environmental conditions such as oxygenation of the medium, acidity, availability of nutritional elements in the medium, and accumulation of lactic acid and other acidic products of anaerobic metabolism in the heated cells (HAHN 1982). A similar dependence of hyperthermic cytotoxicity on the environmental conditions has also been found for HT in vivo (OVERGAARD 1977). Based on the above data it may be concluded that neoplastic cells situated in hypoxic, ischemic, and generally acidified (due to shift of neoplastic cells to anaerobic metabolism and subsequent accumulation of lactic acid) regions of the tumor are more sensitive to HT and can be killed even by moderate heating. All cytoreductive techniques used for the treatment of cancer lead to more or less selective killing of neoplastic cells. This in turn leads to formation in the tumor of necrotic foci, injury to blood vessels, and appearance of hypoxic regions in the treated tissues. The surviving neoplastic cells localized in these regions seem to be a good target for HT treatment. It is therefore reasonable to plan application of HT as an adjuvant cytoreductive treatment at a certain period *after* completion of treatment with radiotherapy or chemotherapy. Surprisingly, such a schedule of combined treatment has never been systematically used in clinical trials. Support for the performance of such clinical trials is provided by animal experiments. For example, FABRICIUS et al. (1992) transplanted EW, human hormone-dependent undifferentiated CaP subcutaneously into nude mice and during the logarithmic phase of growth of these cells, treated them with 2 mg/kg 4-epirubicin. Following the administration of this chemotherapy, some of the transplanted tumors were additionally treated with a single session of 920-MHz HT. Effects of the therapy were assessed by measurement of tumor volume, serum levels of prostate specific antigen (PSA) and histologic examination of treated tumors. Both HT and 4-epirubicin applied alone led to partial reduction of tumor size, appearance of necrotic foci, and lowering of serum PSA. The neoplastic cells, however, were still present on histologic examination, and following a brief period of stabilization of tumor mass, the surviving cancer cells started to regrow. A combination of 4-epirubicin followed by HT showed a synergistic effect of the two modalities, manifested by a more profound reduction of tumor size, confirmed microscopically by nearly total tumor destruction and only trace levels of serum PSA. Nevertheless, small foci of cancer cells were still surviving following the therapy with HT and chemotherapy. In another study BLOCH et al. (1994) found that lonidamine and HT tested on the Dunning R3327G rat CaP show a synergistic action. There was a considerable enhancement of the cytotoxicity of lonidamine by fractionated HT; this was primarily manifested by considerably reduced tumor growth rate after application of the combined treatment.

The strategy for employing HT in combined treatment for CaP following application of other treatment modalities such as RT, chemotherapy, or hormonal treatment is aimed at achieving the optimal cytotoxic potential of HT. This in turn will lead to further cytoreduction by killing the cells suppressed by the prior application of anticancer therapy. Enhancement of sensitivity of cancer cells to radiation or chemotherapy requires simultaneous application of HT and RT or chemotherapy (HAHN 1982; OVERGAARD 1989). Despite these general guidelines for the use of HT as a cytotoxic or sensitizing factor in combined treatment of CaP, detailed timing and optimization of schedules of combined treatments should be established based on the available experimental models of CaP (e.g., Dunning R3327G rat CaP or transplantable CaP EW in mice) and subsequently tested in well-controlled clinical trials. At the present time, there is still a scarcity of convincing data on optimal timing of HT when added to the conventionally accepted treatment options for CaP. This appears to be one of the main factors limiting wider use of HT in the treatment of CaP and placing HT treatment still among the experimental treatment modalities for use in CaP patients.

Another modality that contributes to the multidisciplinary approach to the primary tumor, resulting in local tumor response and consequently in reduction of the tumor burden, appears to be specific immunotherapy. Immunotherapy works primarily to enhance the natural resistance of the host (Fig. 23.1). Convincing data which have accumulated over the years indicate that patients with advanced CaP tend to develop suppression of various cell-mediated immune responses (HADDEN and SPREAFICO 1985; SCHULTZE and SOMMERFELD 1993). The increased activity of suppressor T lymphocytes and lowered natural killer (NK) cytotoxicity are the most frequently observed phenomena (OKABE et al. 1979; KASTELAN et al. 1992; TARLE et al. 1993). This in turn lowers the natural nonspecific resistance of the host and increases the risks for development of bacterial and viral infections, particularly if antineoplastic treatment consists of chemotherapy which is likely to be responsible for depressing further the immune reactions of the host. A number of different forms of nonspecific and specific immunotherapy have been proposed as adjuvant treatment in curative and palliative therapy of neoplasms (HADDEN and SPREAFICO 1985; SCHULTZE and SOMMERFELD 1993). The treatment aim was to stimulate the immune system and regulate the reaction depressed by the neoplastic process and by the therapeutic intervention. In general, the enhancement of natural resistance, either passive (administration of immunologically active substances, including interferons, interleukins, and growth and differentiation factors) or active (administration of macrophage activators, inducers of interferon synthesis, or lymphocyte system stimulators), has weak, if any, *direct* antineoplastic activity. This direct antineoplastic activity is expressed in terms of inhibition of proliferation of cancer cells or direct killing of the cells. The indirect effects of immunotherapy may, however, considerably improve the final outcome of therapy.

SZMIGIELSKI et al. (1992) treated a group of 30 patients with advanced (stage C and D) CaP with six sessions of transrectal HT followed by a series of intratumoral injections of a potent activator of macrophage function – an immunomodulating biosubstance *Propionibacterium granulosum*. Assessment of the oncologic and urologic status of the patients revealed that the combination of HT and nonspecific immunomodulation resulted in local remission of prostatic tumors. In addition there was an improvement in urination in a considerably larger number of patients when compared to the group of patients treated with HT alone. These preliminary clinical observations need to be confirmed in additional clinical trials. These trials should include a combination of cytoreductive HT and procedures leading to the enhancement of natural resistance of the host. There is laboratory evidence indicating that local HT leads to transient enhancement of NK cytotoxic activity in mice (YOSHIOKA et al. 1990).

Specific immunotherapy is an attractive, although as yet not fully proven, method of cytoreduction in the treatment of CaP. In the near future, however, specific immunotherapy may be added to the treatment modalities available for the management of CaP patients. The specific immunotherapy techniques include the use of monoclonal antibodies, the use of various tumor vaccines, recombinant bacterial toxins coupled to antineoplastic antibodies, activated autologous lymphocytes, or genetically modified neoplastic cells (SCHULTZE and SOMMERFELD 1993; VIEWEG et al. 1994). Most of these specific immunotherapy modalities are at present in the process of being tested in the laboratory and this field has been experiencing very rapid growth. Unfortunately, it appears that CaP is more resistant to these forms of therapy than some other human tumors in which specific immunotherapy is effective. The first preliminary clinical trials of the use of specific immunotherapy in patients with advanced CaP did not yield encouraging results (SCHULTZE and SOMMERFELD 1993). Nevertheless, the antineoplastic efficacy of specific immunotherapy depends to some extent on the general immune status of the host and, therefore, the killing potential of "immunologic bullets" may be increased after enhancement of the nonspecific resistance of the host. This stimulates interest in experiments evaluating the efficacy of specific immunotherapy in heat-suppressed CaP cells and testing the antineoplastic potential of combined HT and specific immunotherapy.

A review of the available data on applications of HT in laboratory and clinical trials of CaP clearly indicates a role for HT in the multidisciplinary management of patients with advanced disease (FAUL 1992). The rationale for the use of HT in the management of CaP is based on two distinct and well-documented mechanisms: direct hyperthermic cytotoxicity and hyperthermic sensitization of neoplastic cells to ionizing radiation and to certain cytostatics (Hahn 1982; Overgaard 1989).

The efficacy of HT treatments depends on the ability to uniformly heat the prostate infiltrated with cancerous cells. Major progress in HT equipment development is needed before we can meet this essential requirement of uniform heating of the volume of interest. Progress may come from the application of new HT systems allowing for reasonably uniform heating of the whole prostate using two applicators (transrectal and transurethral) with phase steering (Debicki et al. 1992, 1995). Phase I clinical trials on the use of transrectal HT in patients with advanced CaP (Douwes et al. 1992; Servadio and Leib 1984; Szmigielski et al. 1988) generally lack control of temperature distribution inside the heated prostate and thus cannot provide convincing evidence of the cytotoxic potential of HT in CaP. Nevertheless, virtually all such studies have reported improvement in symptoms and a temporary decrease in tumor volume. Local remissions in a few HT-treated CaP patients have been reported (Stawarz et al. 1993). At this time there is a real need for well-controlled phase II and III randomized studies on the use of HT and other antineoplastic modalities in the treatment of less advanced (stage C) CaP. The present state of knowledge on the biologic rationale for the use of HT with RT indicates that the first choice for randomized studies should be a combination of HT with RT (Fig. 23.1). The aim of these proposed studies must be to assess the ability of HT to sensitize neoplastic cells in order to enhance the cytotoxic effect of radiation or cytostatics and to assess the direct cytotoxic potential of HT against neoplastic cells suppressed by other treatments. The schedule of such studies has to include proper timing of the treatment, with the first sessions of HT applied simultaneously with the tested cytoreductive modality (e.g., radiotherapy), followed by a second course of HT some time later. Certainly, a properly planned randomized study for comparison of important variables is needed.

23.3 Clinical Results

Hyperthermia of the prostate for CaP has been applied using deep regional, interstitial, and intracavitary HT modes. Multiple phase I–II clinical trials have clearly demonstrated beneficial effects of HT in terms of improved incidence of local tumor controls in patients with locally advanced and/or recurrent CaP (Petrovich et al. 1993; Petrovich and Baert 1993; Prionas et al. 1994). Prostatic HT for CaP has usually been applied in combination with RT, while several reports have shown good treatment results with HT alone (Servadio and Leib 1984, 1991; Stawarz et al. 1993; Yerushalmi et al. 1982). Increased incidence of local tumor control which may be obtained with the use of adjuvant HT is of major importance since it is likely to influence survival and to improve the quality of life of these patients (Kapp 1986; Petrovich et al. 1993).

23.3.1 Deep Regional Hyperthermia

The use of deep regional HT has been shown to be of major palliative benefit in patients with deep-seated locally advanced and/or recurrent tumors (Petrovich et al. 1989, 1991; Sapozink et al. 1986). Some of the published reports have included treatment results in patients with locally advanced CaP (Petrovich et al. 1991). In the aforementioned report, from 1982 to 1988, 53 patients with advanced genitourinary tract malignancy were treated with deep regional HT in phase I clinical trials. This group of 53 patients included 20 with locally advanced and/or recurrent CaP. Most of these 20 patients had recurrent tumors and were not expected to be responders to standard management such as RT alone, systemic chemotherapy, or hormonal management. All patients received deep regional HT with a BSD-1000 annular phased array (BSD Medical Corporation, Salt Lake City, Utah, USA). The mean HT frequency used in the treatment of these of 20 patients was 60 MHz with a mean of four HT sessions being given. HT treatments were scheduled once or twice a week together with RT. Interstitial thermometry was required to monitor temperature throughout all treatments. Manual or automated thermal mapping was used in all patients. The aim of HT was to elevate the target tissue temperature to a T_{mean} of 42.5°C for a period of about 45 min. Due to the technical difficulties this target temperature was only infrequently obtained and a formula for computation of temperatures lower than the desired 42.5°C was used (Petrovich et al. 1989). In fact, in just over 50% of the patients, T_{mean} exceeded 40°C for the duration of HT treatments. The 20 study patients received pelvic irradiation with 4- to 25-MV photon beams. Multiple shaped radiation portals were used for the daily radiation treatments. The total radiation dose depended on the extent of prior irradiation, with only seven (35%) patients receiving >50 Gy. A majority (60%) of these patients received lower radiation doses. None, however, received <20 Gy. A standard radiation daily dose of 180 cGy was used to treat these 20 patients. No concomitant hormone therapy was given to any of the patients.

The 1-, 2-, and 3-year actuarial survival was 82%. Complete tumor regression (CR) was recorded in four (20%) patients and partial response (PR) in an additional four (20%). The remaining 12 (60%) patients had a lesser degree of response or no response. It is of interest to note that all patients with major response (CR + PR) received a radiation dose >50 Gy. Deep regional HT was well tolerated by most (80%) of the treated patients. Major palliative benefit was obtained in two-thirds of the patients. Pain in the treated region was the most common problem experienced by these patients. In nearly 50% of the treated patients, pain during HT was a power-limiting factor. The most frequently relieved symptom was pelvic pain, followed by relief of signs and symptoms of bladder outlet obstruction.

The main advantage of the use of deep regional HT is its potential ability to treat relatively noninvasively deep-seated pelvic tumors. This treatment is performed on an outpatient basis and does not require the use of sedation and anesthesia. Major limitations to the widespread use of deep regional HT in patients with CaP include the need for complex and relatively expensive equipment, the need for a well-trained treatment team (physician, physicist, and nursing staff), and the need for careful patient selection. Patients who are generally not considered to be good candidates for deep regional HT are those with moderate to severe cardiovascular disease and severe hypertension. This patient selection is necessary in order to minimize the probability of adverse reactions. Based on the above, at the present time, the use of other HT modes for patients with CaP appears more appealing.

23.3.2 Interstitial Hyperthermia

In an attempt to increase and maintain intraprostatic $T_{mean} > 42.5°C$ and reduce the probability of systemic stress which may be associated with the use of deep regional HT, in the early 1980s interstitial HT began to be investigated. The interstitial technique requires intraprostatic placement of several miniaturized antennas. These antennas should be distributed evenly through the volume of interest. The spacing between individual antennas and separate planes should generally not exceed 15 mm.

The group from Stanford University reported treatment results in patients with recurrent and previously untreated, locally advanced CaP (Kaplan et al. 1991; Bagshaw et al. 1991; Prionas et al. 1994). The treatment protocol in the group of patients managed with curative intent included approximately 50 Gy external beam radiotherapy, given in 180-cGy daily increments. This was followed 3 weeks later by exploratory laparotomy with pelvic lymph node sampling and intraoperative interstitial implant giving 20–30 Gy over a period of 2–3 days. Radiofrequency interstitial HT was given immediately prior to iridium-192 therapy, which was followed by radioactive isotope removal. In contrast to the patients treated with deep regional HT, intraprostatic temperatures >42°C were easy to obtain and easy to maintain throughout each interstitial HT session in all patients treated. This thermoradiotherapy program was well tolerated by the patients. Early treatment results showed good tumor regressions, which the investigators felt to be better than those obtained in T3 tumors managed with pelvic irradiation alone.

Dr. Syed of the Memorial Medical Center in Long Beach, California has the widest experience with the use of interstitial thermoradiotherapy in patients with recurrent and/or locally advanced CaP (Syed et al., unpublished data). The essential components of Dr. Syed's treatment protocol include staging laparotomy with pelvic lymph node sampling and simultaneous interstitial iridium-192 implant. The total radiation dose from this implant is approximately 35 Gy, given at a rate of 40–50 cGy per hour. There is a single interstitial localized current field (500 kHz) HT. Treatment temperature is carefully monitored with multiple thermocouples and maintained at a $T_{mean} > 42°C$. In all study patients this therapeutic temperature has proved easy to obtain and easy to maintain for 60 min of treatment. External beam pelvic irradiation is started approximately 3 weeks following the exploratory laparotomy. The total radiation dose from external beam RT is 35 Gy given at a daily dose of 180 cGy. A total of 80 patients were treated with this protocol, including 55 previously untreated patients with clinical stage (CS) C tumor and 25 patients with recurrent CaP. With a median follow-up of more than 3 years, clinical local control was obtained in 50 (91%) primarily treated patients and in 21 (84%) of those with recurrent CaP. Disease-free survival was 70% for the 55 CS C patients and 76% for the 25 patients with recurrent

Table 23.1. Treatment complications in interstitial thermoradiotherapy-treated patients (from SYED et al., unpublished data)

Complications	Clinical stage C		Recurrent CaP		Total	%
	No.	%	No.	%		
Proctitis	5	9	5	20	10	12
Cystitis	0	0	1	4	1	1
Incontinence	2	4	1	4	3	4
Bowel fistula	1	2	1	4	2	2
Temporary colostomy	1	2	2	8	3	4
Permanent colostomy	1	2	1	4	2	2
Total	10[a]	18	11[b]	44	21	26

[a] Two patients had more than one complication
[b] Three patients had more than one complication

tumors. It is of interest to note the treatment outcome in the 25 patients with recurrent disease. Rapid (2–3 month) tumor regression was seen in 23 (92%) patients, with PSA returning to normal levels in 18 (72%). PSA began to increase again in four of these patients. Two patients are known to have died of CaP, including one with local and distant failure and one of an unrelated cause. The complication rate was 15% for the 55 CS C patients and 32% for the 25 recurrent disease patients (Table 23.1).

Major benefits of the use of interstitial HT include (a) predictable power deposition within the prostate, (b) a good temperature distribution throughout the volume of interest, (c) easy achievement of a $T_{mean} >$ 42°C, and (d) ability to use interstitial multiple thermometry points, which is very difficult with the two alternative HT modes, i.e., deep regional and intracavitary HT.

Disadvantages of the use of interstitial HT include the need for general anesthesia, the need for up to several days of hospitalization, which sharply increases the cost of treatment, and the use of an invasive treatment technique, which may result in a greater probability of treatment complications than is seen with the other two HT modes.

23.3.3 Intracavitary Hyperthermia

Intracavitary HT alone or combined with RT has been used in the management of thousands of cancer patients worldwide, yet there are very few reports of phase III prospective randomized trials.

An important study to evaluate efficacy of intracavitary HT was reported by BERDOV and MENTESHASHVILI (1990). A total of 115 patients with T4N0M0 adenocarcinoma of the rectum were randomized to receive preoperative irradiation alone (n = 59) or the same RT combined with intracavitary HT (n = 56). RT consisted of 40 Gy delivered in ten equal fractions of 4 Gy each, given 3 times per week. Intracavitary HT was given 4–5 times at a frequency of 915 MHz. The intracavitary applicator was not described in this report. A temperature of 42°–43°C was maintained for 60 min during each HT session. CR was obtained in 9 (16%) of the 56 HT-RT patient and PR in 30 (54%) patients. This compared with one (2%) patient showing CR and 20 (34%) patients PR among the 59 preoperative RT-alone patients (P = 0.05). The 5-year survival rate was 36% in the former and 7% in the latter group (P = 0.05). Following the combined treatment 31 (55%) patients had sufficient tumor volume reduction to perform the planned radical surgery, as compared to 16 (27%) patients in the RT-alone group. Postoperative complications were reported in 38 (68%) RT-HT patients and in 27 (46%) of the RT-alone group. This incidence of postoperative complications appears high by Western standards, but the investigators failed to make any comments regarding this problem.

Successful use of intracavitary HT in patients with genitourinary tumors has been reported by several investigators. Preoperative treatment with external beam RT (40 Gy in 4 weeks) and intravesical HT (42°–43°C) with a warm water intravesical solution containing 30 μg/ml bleomycin was used in the management of 56 patients with carcinoma of the bladder (KAKEHI et al. 1991; MATSUI et al. 1991). CR was noted in 25 (45%) and PR in 21 (38%) study patients (Table 23.2). CR was 62% in T1 tumors and 39% in T2 and T3 tumors. The 38 patients with T2 and T3 tumors had a combined CR and PR of 84%, as compared with a figure of 56% among patients treated for

Table 23.2. Treatment response in patients with bladder carcinoma treated with thermochemoradiotherapy (From MATSUI et al. 1991)

Tumor stage	CR	%	PR	%	NR	%	Total	%
T1	10	62	4	25	2	12	16	100
T2 + T3	15	39	17	45	6	16	38	100
T4	0	0	0	0	2	100	2	100
Total	25	45	21	38	10	18	56	100

CR, Complete response; PR, partial response; NR, no response similar tumors with RT alone (50–70 Gy). This treatment was very well tolerated with only minimal toxicity being reported.

The first transrectal intracavitary antenna for patients with CaP was described by MENDECKI et al. (1980). This antenna was noncooled and was designed to operate at 2450 MHz. The problem with the use of a noncooled microwave antenna lies in its pattern of power deposition, which is greatest in the rectal mucosa, next to the applicator (ASTRAHAN et al. 1989; ASTRAHAN and DEBICKI 1994; DEBICKI et al. 1992, 1995). Rectal mucosa is also relatively sensitive to acute and late heat injury (LI et al. 1989). This sensitivity of rectal mucosa to HT precludes the effective use of uncooled rectal applicators in patients with CaP.

Results of the first phase I clinical trial with the use of a transrectal antenna was reported by YERUSHALMI et al. (1982). These investigators used an uncooled transrectal antenna, operated at 2450 MHz, in the treatment of 15 patients with locally advanced CaP. A mean of 12 intracavitary treatments was given without providing temperature data or other important HT parameters. Most of these 15 CaP patients were also receiving RT and/or hormonal therapy, making evaluation of treatment results difficult. Good treatment tolerance and a lack of major toxicity was reported. Substantial tumor regression was noted in all 15 treated patients. The authors reported improvement in quality of life in these patients, with excellent and long-lasting palliative benefit being noted.

A similar treatment outcome was reported in a study of 44 patients with advanced CaP and treated with intracavitary HT alone (SERVADIO and LEIB 1984, 1991). The 44 patients treated included 17 (39%) with severely symptomatic locoregional disease and widespread metastases. The remaining 27 (61%) patients had unresectable and severely symptomatic locally advanced tumors. Transrectal HT consisted of six to ten 1-h treatments, given twice per week with a water-cooled applicator at 915 MHz. The temperature was monitored with multiple sensors placed on the rectal mucosa and in the prostatic urethra. The temperature ranged from 41° to 44°C. Unfortunately, the authors did not provide important details on the temperature monitoring and the number of patients treated at a higher (44°C) or lower (41°C) temperature. The outcome of this study is rather difficult to evaluate since of the 27 patients with locally advanced tumors, eight (30%) also received full-dose (70 Gy) pelvic irradiation and an unspecified subset of patients was also treated with hormonal therapy. Of the 17 patients with widespread metastases, 12 (71%) had major objective improvement, including six (35%) who had relief of severe pelvic pain. All of the 27 patients with symptomatic locoregional disease showed objective and subjective improvement. It is of interest to note that a needle biopsy was obtained in 11 of these patients and revealed no evidence of carcinoma in nine (82%). HT was very well tolerated by the 44 study patients and there were no complications of clinical importance. The 44 study patients were treated on an outpatient basis without sedation or anesthesia. The authors concluded that transrectal microwave HT is an efficient and effective treatment modality in patients with symptomatic locoregional CaP (SERVADIO 1992).

MONTORSI et al. (1992) reported treatment results with transrectal microwave HT in 46 patients with CS D1 and D2 CaP. All patients had moderate to severe symptoms of their disease. Pelvic pain was reported by 38 (83%), signs and symptoms of bladder outlet obstruction were seen in 22 (48%), and 24 (52%) patients presented with retention. All study patients failed total androgen ablation therapy, which was given for a period of at least 3 months. HT was given twice a week for a total of ten sessions of 60 min each, using an intracavitary HT system, Prostathermer 99D (Biodan Medical Systems, Rehovot, Israel). A water-cooled applicator was used for the treatment of these 46 patients. Three thermocouples were used to measure the temperature of the anterior rectal wall and in the prostatic urethra. Prostate temperature was estimated at 43.5°C with 0.5°C variation being permitted. It is unfortunate that this prostate temperature was estimated rather than measured directly with the use of an interstitial thermometry system. Based on interstitial temperature measurements in the prostate, we found the temperature estimation method based on a special formula to be grossly inaccurate, making it unsuitable for use in clinical practice (ASTRAHAN and DEBICKI 1994). The majority of the 46 treated patients reported substantial improvement of their symptoms, resulting in an improvement in quality of life. Objective parameters such as postvoiding residual volume (PRV) were measured at 2 years following the administration of HT and there was significant improvement in PRV ($P = 0.05$), but not in flow rates. Prostatic HT was found to be a safe and effective treatment, with only one (2%) patient having a rectal fistula. This problem responded well to conservative treatment. Similar conclusions were reported in a study of 14 CS C CaP patients (LOTTI et al. 1990).

In contrast to the good results reported in the above studies a less optimistic treatment outcome was noted by FLUCHTER et al. (1992). These investigators used similar treatment instrumentation to that of SERVADIO and LEIB (1991) and treated 11 patients with metastatic, hormone-refractory CaP. The patients received eight 1-h HT sessions given once a week and preceded by intravenous infusion of 50 mg Epirubicine (Farmitalia, Carlo Erba GmbH). Of the 11 treated patients, six (55%) showed disease progression while five (45%) had minor responses or stable disease. No objective decrease in the size of the treated tumor was noted in these five patients; there was only a temporary decrease in the serum PSA levels. The authors concluded a lack of therapeutic activity in the 11 patients treated with a combination of intracavitary HT and chemotherapy.

All of the above studies used transrectal applicators for the treatment of CaP patients. Transurethral HT (TUHT), on the other hand, has been extensively tested in many trials in patients with benign prostatic hyperplasia but has infrequently been used in patients with CaP (PETROVICH et al. 1993). A study of 38 CaP patients treated with a combination of TUHT, chemotherapy, and hormonal therapy was reported by DOUWES et al. (1992). The 38 study patients included 18 (47%) with CS A2 or B and 20 (53%) with CS C or D1. HT was administered in two or three sessions of 3 h each, using a radiofrequency from 500 kHz to 100 MHz. Temperature was controlled at 44.5°C. Six weeks following completion of the HT treatment program, the 18 patients with less advanced tumors underwent radical prostatectomy and pelvic lymphadenectomy. Surgery was in turn followed by a course of pelvic irradiation. In the group of 20 patients with more advanced tumors no surgery was attempted. No response to the treatment or progressive disease was noted in the majority (60%) of these patients; CR was seen in two (10%) and PR in six (30%) patients. The follow-up period was only 6 months. The authors concluded that TUHT enhanced the therapeutic effectiveness of chemotherapy or hormonal therapy. Objectively, this conclusion is not warranted based on the presented data. In fact one can conclude that the authors used a complex multimodality treatment program and the evaluation of tumor response in this study is impossible.

A very interesting and intriguing study was reported on the treatment of 15 advanced CaP patients (SZMIGIELSKI et al. 1991, 1994; STAWARZ et al. 1993). Of particular interest are cell-mediated immunologic responses, which will be addressed in detail later in this chapter. During a 15-month period, 15 symptomatic patients with progressive, hormone-nonresponsive CaP were treated with transrectal HT. Severe symptoms were present in eight (53%) patients while seven (47%) had moderately severe symptoms due to the presence of extensive locoregional disease. According to the UICC staging system there were ten (67%) T3 and five (33%) T4 patients. Extensive metastatic bone disease was present in six (40%) patients. The mean prostate volume was 51 cc. Transrectal HT (TRHT) was given with an intracavitary applicator driven at 2450 MHz. Temperature during each treatment was measured on the rectal mucosa and interstitially in the prostate. The temperature was controlled in the prostate at 43.5°C with miniaturized thermistors YSI-400 (Yellow Spring, Colorado, USA). Each patient received TRHT alone, twice a week, for a total of six treatments. Cell-mediated immune studies were performed in all patients. Of the 15 patients treated, three (20%) had CR, including one who presented with bone metastases. PR was obtained in five (33%) patients, including one who had complete regression of bone metastases. The 5-year actuarial survival was 51%, with a median survival of 42 months. With a minimum follow-up >5 years, three (20%) were free of disease with normal PSA values. Major long-term palliative benefit was seen in eight (53%) patients. This treatment program was very well tolerated, with mild toxicity (proctitis) recorded in three (20%) patients. This appears to be a very important study; it should, however, be interpreted cautiously, since it is based on a relatively small number of patients treated in a single medical center.

An interesting phase I study utilizing intracavitary HT with ultrasound in 14 patients was recently reported (FOSMIRE et al. 1993). Fourteen CS C2 and D1 patients were treated with thermoradiotherapy. RT was given in a standard fashion using the four-field technique. The total RT dose ranged from 67 to 70 Gy, given at a daily rate of 180–200 cGy. A total of 22 HT treatments were given with eight patients receiving two treatments. Interstitial prostatic temperature was measured with two or three probes containing seven thermocouples each. Temperature >42.5°C for 30 min was recorded by 36% of the thermometry points and T_{mean} was 41.9°C.

T_{max} outside of the prostate did not exceed 41.1°C. Generally, the treatment was well tolerated by the study patients: in 17 (77%) treatments they showed good tolerance, in three (14%) fair tolerance, and in two (9%) treatments pain or other discomfort was a power-limiting factor. Mild hematuria was recorded in five (23%) treatments and moderate hematuria in two treatments. This problem was most likely due to the interstitial probe placements. The investigators concluded that with appropriate instrument modifications, a uniform temperature of >42.5°C is obtainable throughout the prostate.

23.3.3.1 Intracavitary Hyperthermia with Phase Steering

All HT modes suffer as a result of insufficient and nonuniform power deposition in the prostate. The highest temperature has always been measured next to a noncooled intracavitary applicator (Astrahan and Debicki 1994; Debicki et al. 1992, 1995). It was apparently shown that power deposition was modified with the use of coolant, and depending on the temperature of this coolant the highest temperature was closer or further away from the antenna. The transurethral applicator was capable of heating to >42°C a cylindrical volume of periurethral prostate measuring approximately 12 mm in diameter and 4–5 cm in length. The transrectal applicator with cooling was capable of heating to >42°C the posterior part of the prostate, up to 2 cm anterior to the anterior rectal wall (Debicki et al. 1992; Astrahan and Debicki 1994). None of the available intracavitary applicators when used individually were capable of homogeneously heating the entire prostate, particularly its anterior lobe. Simultaneous use of transrectal and transurethral antennas produced an entirely different heating pattern to that obtained with individual applicators when they were separately energized. Heating of almost any part of the prostate could be selectively enhanced by changing phase relationship between the two applicators. These data, which were obtained through computer modeling and phantom measurements, were confirmed by prostatic intraoperative temperature measurements in five male dogs. Subsequently, detailed temperature measurements which were performed intraoperatively in six patients confirmed these findings (Debicki et al. 1992). It was established that the highest temperatures could be obtained in the center of the prostate rather than, as would have been expected, close to the surface of each intracavitary antenna. In these intraprostatic temperature measurements, therapeutic (>42°C) temperatures could be obtained in any part of the prostate.

Based on the above data, it was felt justified to begin phase I–II clinical trials in patients with locally advanced CaP. The first clinical trial was simultaneously phased in at the Catholic University of Leuven and at USC in 1991. The eligibility criteria were: (a) histologically confirmed CaP, (b) absence of previous treatment with surgery or RT, and (c) CS B2, C, D1, or locally symptomatic D2 disease refractory to hormonal management. RT consisted of pelvic irradiation using the four-field "box" technique with >10-MV photon beams. The total radiation dose was >66.6 Gy given daily at 180 cGy. All portals were to be treated on a daily basis and the radiation dose was prescribed to the 95% isodose line. A USC-developed transurethral applicator and a water-cooled transrectal applicator were used simultaneously with an appropriate phase adjustment for the treatment of patients. The transrectal antenna was designed to limit its radiation to a cross-sectional angle of 150°, facing the prostate. HT treatments were scheduled twice a week for a total of six treatments, given for 45 min, at a steady state, after RT, during the first 3 weeks of the radiation course. Temperature was measured interstitially in the center of the prostate using a Bowman-type thermistor. This thermistor was introduced under local anesthesia using the perineal approach with ultrasound guidance. An intraprostatic temperature >42°C was obtained in all treatments. T_{mean} in the prostate measured interstitially was 43°C. In addition, the temperature was measured on the anterior rectal wall and in the prostatic urethra. T_{mean} was 44.8°C in the prostatic urethra and 37°C on the anterior rectal wall, with T_{max} in the rectum not exceeding 40°C.

A total of 13 patients were treated: three B2, eight C, and two D1 patients. The mean Gleason's score was 6.4. Follow-up extended from 3 to 48 months with a mean of 18 months. Symptom score (on the Food and Drug Administration recommended symptom score scale) increased from a mean of 12 before the treatment to a mean of 19 during the treatment course. At 6 months posttreatment the score had decreased to a mean of 6. PSA decreased from a mean of 11.9 ng/ml before the treatment course to a mean of 1.9 ng/ml at 6 months posttreatment. Treatment complications consisted of one case of urethral stricture and two cases of retention which required temporary placement of a suprapubic catheter. More patients with longer follow-up are needed to evaluate late treatment toxicity as well as the degree of therapeutic activity.

Based on the temperature data obtained clinically at the Catholic University of Leuven and USC, the temperature distribution in the prostate with simultaneous use of two antennas and phase steering was superior than that obtained in published reports with single intracavitary applicators. It is apparent that more clinical experience with the use of dual applicators system is needed to complete the evaluation as to their usefulness in the clinic.

23.4 Clinical Effects of HT in Advanced CaP

Transrectal HT of the prostate with water-cooled applicators allows for safe heating of the glandular tissues to 42°–44°C with a rapid drop of temperature at a distance of 1–1.5 cm from the surface of the radiator. This implies that only a relatively small part of tumor, particularly that located close to the radiating antenna, may be directly affected during the HT session. A major part of the tumor volume, however, will be exposed to temperatures of 41°–43°C and may become heat-suppressed. These heat-suppressed tumor cells may develop the well-known phenomenon of thermotolerance (Overgaard and Nielsen 1983) and express a temporary resistance to subsequent heating. On the other hand, they may attract infiltration with immunocompetent mononuclear cells (Fig. 23.2) and, as a consequence, trigger the stimulation of certain cell-mediated immune responses (Szmigielski et al. 1992). Over many years a great amount of experimental data have been accumulated indicating a diversity of symptoms of immune stimulation following HT treatment of animal tumors (Dickson and Shah 1980; Szmigielski and Janiak 1977). Using the model of rabbit VX2 tumors treated with local HT, Shah and Dickson (1978) showed that the immunocompetence of the tumor-bearing host is related to effects of the thermotherapy. Animals responding to HT treatment with regression of primary tumors showed marked and sustained enhancement of delayed hypersensitivity in skin tests and increased levels of antitumor antibodies. On the other hand, those rabbits which were not cured by HT showed a progressive decrease of response in skin tests and trace titer of the antibodies. A similar relation between HT-evoked tumor regression and the immune status of the tumor-bearing host was observed in rats bearing the syngeneic MC7 sarcoma (Dickson and Shah 1980). In view of the data available at that time, Dickson and Shah (1980) concluded that "... an increase in host immunocompetence has accompanied the tumor regression that followed curative heating. The data indicate that an intact immune system is necessary not only for tumor regression, but also for maintenance of the host anti-tumor immunity that subsequently develops." This statement remains valid today and thus more interest should be directed toward in-depth study of the mechanisms of the immune responses triggered by HT treatment of neoplasms (Fig. 23.2) and ways of augmenting immune responses that may increase the efficacy of HT treatment.

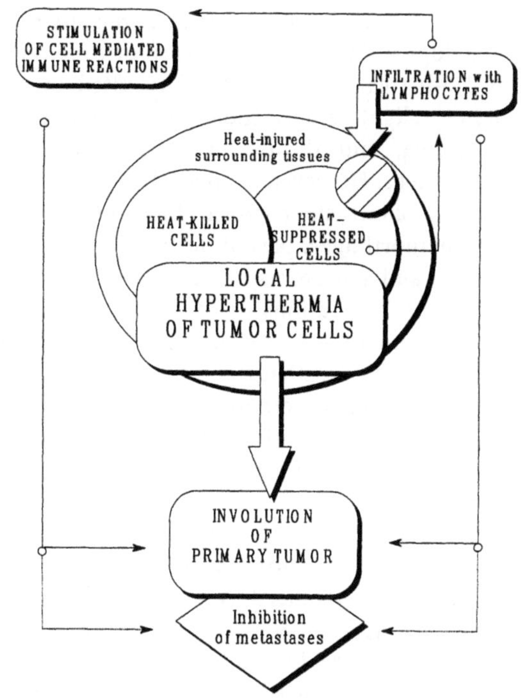

Fig. 23.2. Possible mechanisms leading to regression of primary tumor after local hyperthermia. Note that local hyperthermia kills only some neoplastic cells, suppresses other cancer cells, and produces thermal injury to the surrounding normal cells. An inflammatory response developing in the thermally damaged region attracts lymphocytes. This in turn results in stimulation of cell-mediated immune reactions that lead to regression of the primary tumor and inhibition of metastases

Histologic examinations of prostatic tissues after transrectal HT to 42°–44°C have been performed both in dogs and in patients. These histologic studies have confirmed the opinion that at lower temperatures the direct thermal killing of cells resulting in necrotic foci is weakly expressed and the thermal damage is mostly limited to edema and diffuse interstitial inflammation. Leib et al. (1986) and

Servadio et al. (1990) heated transrectally prostates of 20 dogs to 42°–44°C under various time regimens. Six 1.5-h treatments at 42.5°C resulted in prostate edema, slight enlargement of glandular tissue, hyperemia, and diffuse infiltrations with mononuclear cells. However, no necrotic foci were identified. By contrast, necrotic foci, in addition to microhemorrhages, partial destruction of glandular tubules, and symptoms of acute inflammation with large, focal infiltrations, were observed following six 1.5-h treatments at 44.5°C. In view of these results the authors concluded that the HT range of 42°–44°C is safe and unable to permanently damage normal tissue, while heating at 44.5°C or above causes necrosis and may destroy the prostate tissues (Leib et al. 1986).

Histologic results of HT treatment in human CaP were reported by Strohmaier et al. (1992). Twenty patients with advanced (CS C and D) CaP were treated with four 60-min HT sessions using a transrectal 915-MHz applicator. The intraprostatic temperature during HT sessions was fixed at 42°–43°C. One or two weeks after the last session of HT, samples of prostatic tissue were taken for microscopic examination following surgery (radical prostatectomy or transurethral resection in stage C CaP patients, punch biopsy in stage D patients). Histologic examination revealed that several days after heating the prostatic stroma still showed marked edema and diffuse interstitial inflammation with massive infiltration with lymphocytes, plasma cells, and, to a lesser degree, mononuclear macrophages. Hyperemic capillaries and interstitial bleeding, visible in parts of the heated prostate, completed the picture of persistent diffuse inflammation. No signs of destruction of tumor cells could be found in these studies. From the obtained results the authors concluded that transrectal HT at 42°–43°C did not cause significant necrosis of CaP cells (Strohmaier et al. 1991, 1992), and thus the possible reduction of tumor mass in HT-treated patients has to be based on some other causes. This again cells attention to the possible role of heat-suppressed cells (Fig. 23.2), infiltrating lymphocytes, and heat-evoked diffuse inflammation of the cancerous prostate that may cause modulation of cell-mediated immunity, which may be responsible for the final outcome of the HT treatment.

Increase of the temperature to above 44°C resulted in more damage to the prostatic tissue and production of necrotic foci. Lauweryns et al. (1991) studied histologic changes in four patients with urinary outflow obstruction due to BPH. These patients were treated with transurethral HT and the temperature was controlled on the urethral surface at 45° ± 1°C. Due to the sharp radial temperature gradient of the antenna used for HT, thermal damage of periurethral tissues was most pronounced 6 mm radially and 4–5 cm longitudinally around the radiator. Acute changes observed 24–48 h following a single 70-min HT session consisted of periurethral edema, parenchymal hemorrhages, and occasional, partial small-vessel thrombosis. Selective coagulation necrosis of the parenchymal smooth muscles with sparing of smooth muscle fibers in the vessel walls was also noted. Histopathologic changes found in patients 7 days following the administration of ten HT treatments showed even more severe and deeper lesions (Lauweryns et al. 1991). Four weeks following the administration of a series of ten HT treatments the reparative processes of injury to periurethral tissues predominated. It was represented by ingrowing granulation tissue with its organization and, lastly, fibrosis. This sequence of histopathologic changes indicated a predominance of irreversible thermal cell injury and death over suppression and reversible damage (Fig. 23.2) upon repeated heating to 44°–45°C. Such thermal injury of neoplastic cells would be greater than that obtained in the published clinical trials of CaP treatment with transrectal HT, where the intraprostatic temperatures do not exceed 43°–44°C (Servadio and Leib 1984; Szmigielski et al. 1988; Strohmeier et al. 1992). In these transrectally treated prostates the histologic lesions were limited to diffuse inflammation and infiltrations with immunocompetent cells. It is apparent that uniform heating of the cancerous prostate to 44°–45°C is essential to obtain the desired effects. There is a need to improve the design of rectal applicators and to improve on temperature monitoring during HT sessions.

23.4.1 Assessment of Tumor Response, Survival, and Quality of Life

As diffuse interstitial inflammation of the prostatic stroma predominates in patients with CaP treated with transrectal HT, we concluded that the involution of tumors observed in some treated patients may have resulted from their immune responses, which were stimulated by the inflammation- and tumor-infiltrating lymphocytes and by the heat-suppressed, but not killed cancer cells (Fig. 23.2) (Szmigielski et al. 1987). This hypothesis was subsequently subjected to a phase I clinical trial. From

1985 through 1987 15 patients with advanced CaP received transrectal HT at the Department of Clinical Urology, MMA Postgraduate Medical School in Warsaw Poland (SZMIGIELSKI et al. 1988). This study was repeated in 1989–1990 using another group of 15 patients with advanced CaP (SZMIGIELSKI et al. 1991) and a third group of 22 patients received HT treatments from 1991 to 1993, making a total of 52 patients (Table 23.3). The period of observation from application of the HT treatments in these patients ranged from 2.5 to 7 years (Table 23.3). All treatments were given using a water-cooled microwave applicator at 434 or 2450 MHz. Local transrectal HT was given twice a week for a total of six sessions. Each HT session lasted for 30 min at steady-state temperature, controlled on the rectal mucosa at 45°C. This resulted in an intraprostatic temperature of 42°–43°C at a distance of 1–1.5 cm from the radiating applicator. A number of biochemical tests (including measurement of serum levels of PSA, PAP, carcinoembryonic antigen, and alkaline phosphatase), ultrasonographic imaging of the prostate, and scintigraphic and radiographic examinations of the skeleton and internal organs were applied for assessment of general clinical status and primarily for the evaluation of locoregional tumor and to search for distant metastases. Additionally, in these patients studies of immune reactions were performed before HT, upon the completion of six HT sessions, and at 1–4 months following this therapy (SZMIGIELSKI et al. 1991, 1994).

Evaluation of the results of treatment (Table 23.3) revealed that about 40% of patients responded to the administered HT therapy, but in the remaining 60% of patients no tumor inhibition could be documented. Of the 22 responders observed in the three studies, the majority (15 patients) had transient partial remission of the primary tumor with lowering of the serum levels of tumor markers (PSA, PAP) and an improvement in the local and general condition, while complete response with disappearance of all symptoms of the disease was noted only in seven patients. Furthermore, the remissions observed in HT-treated responders were only transient and following 6–18 months some symptoms or signs of CaP could again be found in most of the responders (e.g., increase of PSA and/or PAP, palpable nodules in the prostate and periprostatic region, positive pelvic lymphography). The benefits of HT-evoked responses became apparent during analysis of survival of HT-treated CaP patients (Table 23.3). Patients who responded to HT with remissions survived significantly longer (about 73% of these patients survived 3 years) than did nonresponders (10% with 3-year survival), the difference being significant at $P < 0.01$ (Table 23.3). Among the respond-

Table 23.3. Treatment response to transrectal HT in patients with advanced CaP treated in Warsaw

Phase I Study	Study I	Study II	Study III	Total
No. of patients	15	15	22	52
Period of observation (years)	>7.0	4.5–5.2	2.5–3.5	2.5–7.0
Treatment response				
Complete response	3 (20)[a]	2 (13)	2 (9)	7 (13)
Partial response	5 (33)	4 (26)	6 (27)	15 (28)
Total major response	8 (53)	6 (40)	8 (36)	22 (42)
Survival among responders (years)				
1	8 (53)	6 (40)	7 (32)	21 (40)
2	7 (47)	5 (33)	7 (32)	19 (37)
3	6 (40)	5 (33)	5 (23)	16 (31)
5	3 (20)	1 (7)	–	–
Survival among nonresponders (years)				
1	7 (47)	7 (47)	12 (55)	26 (50)
2	5 (33)	4 (27)	8 (36)	17 (33)
3	1 (7)	0 (0)	2 (9)	3 (6)
Overall survival (years)				
1	15 (100)	13 (87)	19 (86)	47 (90)
2	12 (80)	9 (60)	15 (68)	36 (69)
3	7 (47)	5 (33)	7 (32)	19 (37)
5	3 (20)	1 (7)	–	–

[a] Percentages are shown within parentheses

ers from the first and second studies (Table 23.3) there were several patients who survived 5 years or longer and were still free of symptoms of the disease or had mild symptoms of CaP (e.g., elevated PSA levels, enlarged prostate) with a generally good health status. At the present time, we cannot offer a reasonable explanation for the difference in responses to HT treatments among our CaP patients, though there is the earlier discussed concept of a possible relation of treatment responses to reactions of the host's immune system. No method was found to predict in advance the response to HT in individual cases of advanced CaP. Nevertheless, it is our feeling that with progress in hyperthermic instrumentation which will allow uniform heating of cancerous prostate to cytotoxic temperatures, the efficacy of HT treatment may be further increased.

23.4.2 Immune Reactions in Patients Undergoing Hyperthermia

Histologic evidence of inflammation in a considerable part of the prostate heated with transrectal applicators suggests that a reaction may be triggered by the host's immune system. This is particularly so in view of the fact that most of the HT treatment protocols for CaP include repeated heating sessions. Surprisingly, the present knowledge concerning immune reactions to local heating of tissues, both normal and neoplastic, is very limited. Earlier studies revealed that local HT of experimental tumors stimulated cell-mediated immune reactions and enhanced immunogenicity of HT-suppressed cancer cells (Dickson and Shan 1980). Until recently, however, no systematic studies have been undertaken on this subject. A review of the literature revealed that most of the investigations on the effects of HT on the immune system were devoted either to whole-body hyperthermia or to in vitro studies of immunocompetent cells exposed to elevated temperatures. Whole-body HT at core body temperatures of 38.5°–40°C caused only minimal effects on the immune responses of normal mice after 2–4 h exposure to radiant heat (Greeley et al. 1992). Under these conditions whole-day HT did not influence the absolute number of peripheral blood lymphocytes, although the proportion of lymphocyte subsets was temporarily changed, with an immediate increase in splenic CD4+ (helper) cells. This was followed within 18 h by an overall decrease in Lyt-2+ and Thy-1.2+ cells and an increase in the fraction of mature T lymphocytes in the thymus (Greeley et al. 1992). More intensive whole-body HT (core body temperature 40°–41.5°C) induced in mice by exposure in microwave chambers (Szmigielski and Janiak 1977) or by conventional heating stimulated cell-mediated immunity in normal mice with a transient increase in lymphocytosis. There was also enhanced reactivity of blood lymphocytes to mitogens [phytohemagglutinin (PHA) and concanavalin A (Con-A)] and stimulation of cytotoxicity. The above signs of immune stimulation were demonstrated after a single 2-h exposure to microwave HT. Similar responses of the immune system were observed in mice treated with daily 2-h HT sessions for 4 days. A prolonged exposure to daily HT sessions (e.g., for 7–11 days), however, gradually diminished the intensity of immune stimulation and finally led to signs of suppression of lymphocyte function (Szmigielski and Janiak 1977). The analysis of immune reactions in normal mice exposed to whole-body HT suggested that the observed phenomena may be mediated by an altered distribution of lymphocyte pools in the heated organs (homing of lymphocytes) and by circulating factors rather than by some heat-induced alterations in the cells themselves (Greeley et al. 1992).

Immunocompetent cells, including macrophages, T-lymphocytes, and natural killer (NK) lymphocytes, are among the cells most sensitive to temperature elevation (Yoshioka et al. 1990). In vitro studies revealed a biphasic reaction of lymphocytes to HT, showing stimulation of physiologic functions (e.g., transformation rates in PHA/Con-A microcultures, release of cytokines) at 38°–39°C, followed by a rapid inhibition of these functions as the temperature was increased to 41°–42°C (Izumi et al. 1983; Yoshioka et al. 1989). NK cells isolated from murine or rat spleen lost their lytic activity following exposure to 41°–42.5°C for 30 min, but this activity was partially recovered after reincubation at 37°C (Yang et al. 1992). Exposure to temperatures exceeding 43°C inhibited irreversibly the lytic activity of NK cells (Greeley et al. 1992).

Reaction of the immune system to local HT may result both from thermal injury of immunocompetent cells in the heated tissues and from factors released from the areas where temperatures do not reach the levels inhibiting lymphocyte functions (Yoshioka et al. 1990). Hind limbs of normal mice heated locally in hot water after maintaining the temperature of muscles at 43°C for 45 min showed a biphasic reaction of the NK cytotoxic activity. The NK activity was noted to be suppressed 2 days following a single session of local HT and significantly enhanced (by 25%–30%) 7 days following the heat exposure. The authors concluded that this enhancement of NK cytotoxic activity following local HT may play an important role in the antitumor effect of heat therapy. They were, however, not able to provide direct evidence to support their hypothesis, particularly in view of the fact that the mice used in the study did not bear tumors (Yoshioka et al. 1990). Mice bearing transplanted Lewis lung carcinoma also showed stimulation of cell-mediated cytotoxicity in response to local HT with circulating hot water. Two sessions of local HT applied 6 and 10 days after the implantation of cancer cells resulted in inhibition of growth of the primary tumor and lowering of the number of lung metastases, accompanied by enhanced activity of splenic granulocyte-macrophage progenitor cells. The authors concluded that the antimetastatic effect in HT-treated tumor-bearing mice reflected the immune-associated responses, including activation of cytotoxic mechanisms.

23.4.2.1. Function of Granulocytes in Hyperthermia-Treated Patients

Evaluation of the function of granulocytes in HT-treated CaP patients was performed in 30 subjects from the second and third Warsaw studies (Table 23.3) (Szmigielski et al. 1992). In this group of patients HT treatment resulted in 14 complete or partial local responses (responders in Table 23.4), while the remaining 16 patients did not respond to HT with a detectable change in the course of disease (nonresponders). The ratio of responders to nonresponders was similar to that observed in the three studies of CaP patients treated with HT (Table 23.3).

Function of the granulocyte system was investigated before HT treatment, upon the completion of six sessions of transrectal HT, and 1 week, 1 month, and 2 months following the therapy. For assessment of the granulocyte system, granulocytosis, percentage of polymorphonuclear leukocytes reducing nitro-BT, the size of the blood and bone marrow reserve pools of mature granulocytes (released after administration of epinephrine or hydrocortisone), phagocytosis, and serum levels of muramidase (lysozyme) were investigated.

Twenty-two of the 30 investigated patients (73%) showed stimulation of function of mature blood granulocytes (increased index of phagocytosis and number of nitro-BT-reducing polymorphonuclear leukocytes) with faster turnover of phagocytizing cells (increased serum levels of muramidase) upon the completion of HT treatment (Table 23.4). These signs of stimulation of the function of peripheral granulocytes were accompanied in nine patients (30%) by an increase in the bone marrow reserve pool. This was a consequence of faster kinetics of granulopoiesis and stimulated maturation of the progenitors. One week after completion of HT treatments all signs of stimulation of the function of granulocytes still remained at the same level as during the treatment (Table 23.4), but 1 and 2 months later stimulation of the granulocyte function was no longer present and in the majority of patients the tests were within normal limits (Table 23.4). At all times when these studies were performed (before HT, upon completion of HT treatment, and 1 week, 1 month, and 2 months thereafter) no difference in test results regarding granulocyte function was found between responders and nonresponders to HT. In view of this finding, the whole group of a 30 CaP patients treated with transrectal HT was analyzed as a single entity. The number of granulocytes in the peripheral blood rose from a mean of 4800 cells/mm^3 before HT to about a mean of 6600 cells/mm^3 upon the completion of therapy ($P < 0.05$). This was accompanied by increases in the fraction of nitro-BT-

Table 23.4. Stimulation of the granulocyte system in the 30 patients with advanced CaP treated with transrectal HT

	Responders ($n = 14$)				Nonresponders ($n = 16$)			
	After HT	1 week	1 month	2 months	After HT	1 week	1 month	2 months
Granulocytosis (increment >30%)	9	7	2	1	13	13	4	3
Nitro-BT reduction (>10% positive cells)	7	6	2	1	14	15	3	2
Phagocytosis index (score >240)	6	6	1	0	12	11	2	2
Serum muramidase (>10 mg/l)	8	5	1	0	11	12	2	3
Bone marrow granulocyte reserve pool increment (>120%)	3	5	2	0	6	4	3	1

reducing granulocytes from 6.43% ± 1.82% to 10.42% ± 2.71% ($P < 0.01$) and in the serum level of muramidase lysozyme) from 6.12 ± 2.31 mg/L to 9.86 ± 4.11 mg/L ($P < 0.01$) Additionally, the phagocytic index of granulocytes rose from 198 ± 26 before HT treatment to 259± 52 ($P < 0.05$) after completion of the therapy. Similarly, the bone marrow reserve pool of granulocytes released after administration of hydrocortisone was significantly larger in nine of the 30 HT-treated patients (increment of granulocytosis about 80% before HT treatment and 112%–146% after completion of the therapy; the sum of individual differences was significant at $P < 0.05$).

On the basis of all these results we concluded that application of transrectal HT in patients with advanced CaP evokes rapid stimulation of the granulocyte (and probably also macrophage) system, probably in response to diffuse inflammation of the prostatic stroma. Stimulation of the phagocytic cell system appeared early during HT therapy and was clearly demonstrable after completion of the six treatment sessions. The analysis of the appearance of granulocyte stimulation in HT-treated CaP patients failed to show any difference between patients who responded to the therapy with remissions and those who failed the treatment (nonresponders). This suggested that the stimulation of function of the granulocyte (macrophage) system is a transient, nonspecific reaction to thermal damage of the prostate and periprostatic region (e.g., the rectal wall) during repeated sessions of transrectal HT. There was no indication that this stimulation contributed to the treatment outcome.

23.4.2.2 Function of T Lymphocytes and NK Cytotoxic Cells

Evaluation of the function of peripheral blood T lymphocytes and NK cytotoxic cells was performed in the 30 advanced CaP patients treated with transrectal HT in the first and second Warsaw studies (Table 23.3) and in the 30 healthy men (aged 62–76 years) without neoplastic diseases. Monitoring of T and NK cell functions included assessment of subsets of peripheral blood lymphocytes. They were identified by an indirect immunofluorescence staining technique using CD3 (pan-T), CD4 (T helper-inducer), and CD8 (T suppressor-cytotoxic) mouse monoclonal antibodies. The mitogenic responses of isolated peripheral blood mononuclear cells (PBMCs) to PHA and Con-A in 72-h microcultures and the NK cytotoxic activity of PBMCs against a ^{51}Cr-labeled target K-526 erythroleukemic cell line were also studied. Details of the techniques used for monitoring of T and NK cell functions have been published elsewhere (Szmigielski et al. 1991). The mean values and range of the values for the tested parameters in the group of the 30 men without neoplastic disease are presented in Table 23.5. Prior to the HT treatment, at least two of the five tested parameters of T and NK cell function were below the range for the control group in 24 (80%) of the CaP patients, while three or more of the parameters were similarly lowered in 16 (53%). Mean values for the group of CaP patients and other results (Table 23.5) were compared to the control group. This comparison showed that all parameters were significantly lower ($P < 0.01$) in patients suffering from advanced CaP.

Table 23.5. Evaluation of T lymphocytes and NK cytotoxicity in peripheral blood of 30 patients (aged 58–74 years) with advanced (stage C and D) CaP

	Control group (n = 30) men, aged 62–76 years without neoplastic disease		Cancer of the prostate (n = 30) before HT		
			Below range	In the range	Above range
	Mean ± SD	Range			
T lymphocytes (CD3+) (cells per mm³ × 10³	1.93 ± 0.26	1.72–2.24	12 (40%)	16 (53%)	2 (7%)
T helper cells (CD4+) (cells per mm³ × 10³	0.34 ± 0.11	0.26–0.48	14 (47%)	12 (40%)	4 (13%)
CD4+/CD8+ ratio (T helper/T suppressor)	2.68 ± 1.12	1.67–4.14	19 (63%)	11 (37%)	0 (0%)
PHA transformation index (transformation rate induced/spontaneous)	12.1 ± 5.7	8.4–22.6	7 (23%)	17 (57%)	6 (20%)
NK cytotoxicity rate [% ^{51}Cr released from K-562 cells by lymphocytes at E (effector): T (target) cell ratio of 50:1]	26.4 ± 11.8	14.3–44.8	9 (30%)	20 (67%)	1 (3%)

Table 23.6. Stimulation of the lymphocyte system in the 30 patients with advanced CaP treated with transrectal HT

	Responders (n = 14)				Nonresponders (n = 16)			
	After HT	1 mos.	2 mos.	3 mos.	After HT	1 mos.	2 mos.	4 mos.
T lymphocytes (CD3+) (>150% pretreatment)	2	3	8	4	1	2	4	2
T helper cells (CD4+) (>200% pretreatment)	1	4	9	6	1	3	4	2
CD4+/CD8+ ratio (increment >1.50)	0	3	8	5	1	4	5	3
Transformation in vitro (2× pretreatment transformation ratio)	0	4	6	3	0	2	3	2
NK cytotoxicity (>150% pretreatment)	2	7	13	6	2	3	6	3

Decreased cell-mediated immunity in patients with genitourinary cancers had previously been reported by other investigators (HERR 1980; WIRTH et al. 1985; ZEMBALA et al. 1977). These studies suggested a relationship between the intensity of immunosuppression, stage of disease, and prognosis for survival. In patients treated for CaP with radiotherapy, chemotherapy, or hormonal therapy, NK-mediated cytotoxic activity has been shown to be inversely related to tumor mass and tumor extent (KASTELAN et al. 1992). No such correlation has been found between tumor grade and NK-mediated cytotoxic activity (KASTELAN et al. 1992; TARLE et al. 1993). In the Warsaw studies of CaP patients a wide range of NK cytotoxic activity was noted. Admittedly, only nine of the 30 CaP patients (30%) had an NK cytotoxicity rate below the bottom level of the range established for the control group (Table 23.5). In the control group, however, there were two patients with low levels of NK cytotoxicity, expressed as release of only 14.3% and 15.2% of chromium from prelabeled target cells, with the majority of other values ranging at about 20%–40%. Therefore, a more convincing decrease in the NK cytoxicity in CaP patients is revealed by comparison of mean values and standard deviations for the two groups: 26.4 ± 11.8 for the control group and 17.3 ± 13.2 for the CaP patients ($t = 2.77$, $P < 0.05$).

Analysis of the results for the investigated parameters of function of T lymphocytes and NK cytotoxicity in CaP patients after transrectal HT revealed that the tested functions were also stimulated in some of the treated patients (Table 23.6). The kinetics of stimulation of these cell systems were, however, different from those reported previously for granulocytes. Upon completion of six sessions of transrectal HT and 1 week following the treatment, when stimulation of granulocyte function was evident, the individual results of all investigated lymphocytic parameters (subsets of T lymphocytes, T helper/T suppressor ratio, transformation rates in vitro, NK cytotoxic activity) did not differ from the pretreatment values. At 1 and 2 months after HT, a considerable number of CaP patients responded with significant increases in the investigated parameters when compared to the pretreatment values. These increases included the number of T lymphocytes and T helper cells in peripheral blood [12 (40%) of the 30 HT-treated CaP patients], in turn resulting in an increase in the T helper/T suppressor ratio (13 patients, i.e., 43.3%), and activation of NK-mediated cytotoxicity (19 patients, 63%). The peak effect of the individual stimulation was noted at 2 months after HT (Table 23.6), after which a decrease occurred. The analysis of expression of the stimulation of cell-mediated immune reactions in relation to clinical response to HT therapy (responders vs nonresponders) (Table 23.6) did not show a correlation between the degree of stimulation of T lymphocytes (increment of T lymphocyte and T helper cell number, CD4+/CD8+ ratio, and transformation rate) and the appearance of remission of the primary tumor. In contrast to T lymphocyte function, NK-mediated cytotoxicity of PBMCs showed a correlation with the clinical results of HT in the investigated group of CaP patients. The patients who responded to HT with enhancement of NK activity (when compared to the individual pretreatment values) more frequently had tumor remissions (responders) than did those patients with unchanged NK activity following the treatment (Table 23.6). Of the 30 patients treated with transrectal HT, 19 (63%) responded with significant enhancement of NK activity (at least by 150% of individual pretreatment values) at 2 months after therapy. Most of the 19 patients with enhancement of NK activity were among those with treatment response (13 of 14 responders); only six patients in the group of 16 nonresponders showed enhancement of NK activity ($\chi^2 = 9.85$, $P < 0.01$). This confirmed the recent finding that the assessment of NK activity of PBMCs may be a useful test in advanced CaP for predicting the individual reaction of the patient to the applied therapy (Tarle et al. 1993).

23.5 Conclusions

In one phase III prospective randomized trial in patients with cutaneous melanoma, the use of an HT-RT combination has been shown to be more effective than RT alone in terms of local tumor control and long-term survival (Overgaard et al. 1995). Two additional, prospective, multi-institutional randomized trials have demonstrated a similar HT efficacy and are currently in the process of being published. No such strong data showing the effectiveness of adjuvant HT exist in patients with locally advanced CaP. The use of HT alone in patients with CaP has been shown to be effective in achieving good to excellent palliation in some phase I–II studies. The existing HT instrumentation is not capable of consistently and homogeneously heating the entire volume of interest, which is a necessary requirement for HT in cancer therapy. There is an urgent need to develop HT antennas which are specifically designed for the treatment of patients with CaP. The use of a dual antenna system with phase steering to a certain extent may be able to meet this requirement (Debicki et al. 1992; Astrahan and Debicki 1994). Studies with the use of HT alone in patients with CaP, as reported by Szmigielski et al. (1992) and Szmigielski et al. (1994), and particularly the immunologic hypothesis of these authors, are very interesting and intriguing. There is, however, a need to confirm these interesting findings in clinical trials in other medical centers. Generally, there is a need to activate well-designed, phase II–III, prospective clinical trials using an HT-RT combination. These trials *must* use interstitial intraprostatic temperature measurements in addition to intracavitary ones in *all* treatments.

Acknowledgements. This work was partly supported by reseach grant 4/4018/91/02 from the Polish Committee of Scientific Research (KBN) in Warsaw, Poland.

References

Altwein JE, Faul P (1990) Probleme und Prinzipien der Hormontherapie des fortgeschrittenen Prostatakarzinoms. Klin Wochenschr 68:347–358

Astrahan MA, Debicki PS (1994) Physical principles of microwave hyperthermia of the prostate. In: Petrovich Z, Baert L (eds) Benign prostatic hyperplasia. Innovations in management. Springer, Berlin Heidelberg New York, pp 205–237

Astrahan MA, Sapozink MD, Cohen D, Luxton G, Kampp T, Boyd S, Petrovich Z (1989) Microwave applicator for transurethral hyperthermia of benign prostatic hyperplasia. Int J Hyperthermia 5:283–296

Bagshaw MA, Prionas SD, Goffinet DR et al. (1991) External beam irradiation combined with the use of Iridium-192 implants and radiofrequency-induced hyperthermia in the treatment of prostatic carcinoma. In: Smith PH, Pavone-Macaluso M (eds) EORTC Genitourinary Group Monograph 10. Urological oncology: reconstructive surgery, organ conservation and restoration of function. Wiley-Liss, New York, pp 275–279

Benson RC, Gill GM (1986) Estramustin phosphate compared with diethylstibestrol. A randomized, double-blind, crossover trial for stage D prostate cancer. Am J Clin Oncol 9:341–351

Berdov BA, Menteshashvili GZ (1990) Thermoradiotherapy of patients with locally advanced carcinoma of the rectum. Int J Hyperthermia 5:881–890

Bloch WE, Lokeshwar BL, Ferrel SM, Block NL (1994) Enhancement of hyperthermic toxicity by lonidamine in the Dunning R3327G rat prostatic adenocarcinoma. Prostate 24:131–138

Debicki P, Astrahan MA, Ameye F, Oyen R, Baert L, Haczewski A, Petrovich Z (1992) Temperature steering in prostate by simultaneous transurethral and transrectal hyperthermia. Urology 40:300–307

Debicki P, Okoniewski M, Okoniewska E, Shrivastava PN, Debicka AM, Baert L, Petrovich Z (1995) Cooled microwave transrectal applicator for adjustable directional beam for prostate treatment. Int J Hyperthermia 11:95–108

Dickson JA, Shah SA (1980) Hyperthermia and the immune response in cancer therapy. Cancer Immunol Immunother 9:1–10

Douwes FR, Moschutz HR, Pontiggia P (1992) Local hyperthermia in the treatment of prostate cancer. In: Bichler K-H, Strohmaier WL, Wilbert DM (eds) Hyperthermia of the prostate – state of the art. PMI, Frankfurt, pp 53–58

Fabricius PG, Issels R, Schmitz C, Hofer C, Permanetter W (1992) Efficacy of thermochemotherapy in PC EW tumor model in nude mice. In: Bichler K-H, Strohmaier WL, Wilbert DM (eds) Hyperthermia of the prostate – state of the art. PMI, Frankfurt, pp 29–35

Faul P (1992) Prostatic cancer – what to do? Eur Urol 22:89–98

Fluchter SH, Bichler K-H, Strohmaier WL, Nelde J, Wilbert DM (1992) Epirubicin and hyperthermia in metastasizing prostatic cancer in hormonal relapse. In: Bichler K-H, Strohmaier WL, Wilbert DH (eds) Hyperthermia of the prostate – state of the art. PMI, Frankfurt, pp 36–42

Fosmire H, Hynynen K, Drach GW, Strea B, Swift P, Cassady JR (1993) Feasibility and toxicity of transrectal ultrasound hyperthermia in the treatment of locally advanced adenocarcinoma of the prostate. Int J Radiat Oncol Biol Phys 26:253–259

Gerweck LE (1985) Hyperthermia in cancer therapy. The biological basis and unresolved questions. Cancer Res 45:3029–3032

Greeley EH, Helfrich BA, Feuermann LL (1992) Radiant heat-induced hyperthermia in mice: in vivo effects on the immune system. Int J Hyperthermia 8:209–220

Hadden JW, Spreafico F (1985) New strategies of immunotherapy. Semin Immunopathol 8:321–333

Hahn GM (1982) Hyperthermia and cancer. Plenum Press, New York

Herr HW (1980) Suppressor cells in immunodepressed bladder and prostate cancer patients. J Urology 123:635-639

Izumi A, Koga S, Maeta M (1983) Effect of in vitro hyperthermia on murine and human lymphocytes. Cancer 51:2061-2065

Kakehi Y, Nishio Y, Yoshida O (1991) Multidisciplinary treatment of invasive bladder cancer. Urol Int 47:120-122

Kaplan J, Kapp DS, Bagshaw MA (1991) Secondary external-beam radiotherapy and hyperthermia for local recurrence after iodine-125 implantation in adenocarcinoma of the prostate. Int J Radiat Oncol Biol Phys 20:551-554

Kapp DS (1986) Sites and disease selection for hyperthermia clinical trials. Int J Hyperthermia 2:139-156

Kastelan M, Kraljic I, Tarle M (1992) NK cell activity in treated prostate cancer patients as a probe for circulating tumor cells: hormone regulatory effects in vivo. Prostate 21:111-120

Lauweryns J, Baert L, Vandenhove J, Petrovich Z (1991) Histopathology of prostatic tissue after transurethral hyperthermia. Int J Hyperthermia 7:221-230

Leib Z, Rathem A, Lev A, Servadio C (1986) Histopathological observations in the canine prostate treated by local microwave hyperthermia. Prostate 8:93-102

Li DJ, Qiu SL, Zhou SL (1989) Late heat damage in normal swine rectum: a comparison of thermosensitivity of rectum and oesophagus. Int J Hyperthermia 5:717-724

Lotti T, Altieri V, Mirone V, Ottaviano N, Russo A (1990) Local hyperthermia for treatment of advanced prostatic carcinoma: preliminary results. In: Bichler HI (ed) Consensus on hyperthermia for the 1990s. Plenum Press, New York, pp 525-529

Matsui K, Takebayashi S, Watai K, Kakehi M, Kubota Y, Yao M, Shui T (1991) Combination radiotherapy of urinary bladder carcinoma with chemohyperthermia. Int J Hyperthermia 7:19-26

Mendecki J, Friedenthal E, Botstein C, Paglione R, Sterzer F (1980) Microwave applicators for localized hyperthermia of cancer of the prostate. Int J Radiat Oncol Biol Physics 6:1583-1588

Montorsi F, Guazzoni G, Colomo R, Galli L, Bergamaschi F, Rigatti P (1992) Transrectal microwave hyperthermia for advanced prostate cancer: long-term clinical results. J Urol 148:342-345

Muller C (1910) Eine neue Behandlungsmethode bosartiger Geschwulste. Munchener Med Wochenschr 29:1490-1493

Muller C (1912) Therapeutische Erfahrungen an 100 mit Kombination von Rontgenstrahlen und Hochfrequenz, resp. Diathermie behandelten bosartigen Neubildungen. Munchener Med Wochenschr 29:1546-1549

Okabe T, Ackerman R, Wirth M, Frohmuller HGW (1979) Cell-mediated cytotoxicity in patients with cancer of the prostate. J Urology 122:628-632

Overgaard J (1977) Effect of hyperthermia on malignant cells in vivo. A review and hypothesis. Cancer 37:2637-2648

Overgaard J (1989) The current and potential role of hyperthermia in radiotherapy. Int J Radiat Oncol Biol Phys 16:535-549

Overgaard J, Nielen OS (1983) The importance of thermotolerance for the clinical treatment with hyperthermia. Radiother Oncol 1:167-171

Overgaard J, Gonzalez Gonzalez D, Hulshof MCCM, Arcangeli G, Dahl O, Mella O, Bentzen SM (1995) Randomised trial of hyperthermia as adjuvant to radiotherapy for recurrent or metastatic malignant melanoma. Lancet 345:540-543

Petrovich Z, Baert L (1993) Intracavitary thermoradiotherapy for various tumor sites. In: Seegenschmiedt MH, Sauer R (eds) Interstitial and intracavitary thermoradiotherapy. Springer, Berlin Heidelberg New York, pp 311-317

Petrovich Z, Langholz B, Gibbs FA et al. (1989) Regional hyperthermia for advanced tumors: a clinical study of 353 patients. Int J Radiat Oncol Biol Phys 16:601-607

Petrovich Z, Emami B, Kapp D et al. (1991) Regional hyperthermia in patients with recurrent genitourinary cancer. Am J Clin Oncol 14:472-477

Petrovich Z, Ameye F, Baert L et al. (1993) New trends in the treatment of benign prostatic hyperplasia and carcinoma of the prostate. Am J Clin Oncol 16:187-200

Prionas SD, Kapp DS, Goffinet DR, Ben-Yosef R, Fesseden P, Bagshaw MA (1994) Thermometry of interstitial hyperthermia given as an adjuvant to brachytherapy for the treatment of carcinoma of the prostate. Int J Radiat Oncol Biol Physics 28:151-162

Sapozink MD, Gibbs FA Jr, Egger MJ, Stewart JR (1986) Regional hyperthermia for clinically advanced deep-seated pelvic malignancy. Am J Clin Oncol 9:162-169

Schultze H, Sommerfeld HJ (1993) Immunotherapie beim Prostatakarzinom. Urologie 32:382-289

Servadio C (1992) Local hyperthermia for the treatment of diseases of the prostate. In: Bichler K-H, Strohmaier WL, Wilbert DM (eds) Hyperthermia of the prostate - state of the art. PMI, Frankfurt, pp 7-14

Servadio C, Leib Z (1984) Hyperthermia in the treatment of prostate cancer. Prostate 5:205-211

Servadio C, Leib Z (1991) Local hyperthermia for prostate cancer. Urology 38:307-309

Servadio C, Leib Z, Lev A (1990) Local hyperthermia to canine prostate. A pilot study. Urology 35:156-164

Shah SA, Dickson JA (1978) Effect of hyperthermia on the immunocompetence of VX2 tumor bearing rabbits. Cancer Res 38:3523-3528

Stawarz B, Zielinski H, Szmigielski S, Debicki P, Petrovich Z (1993) Transrectal hyperthermia as a palliative treatment for advanced adenocarcinoma of the prostate and a study of cell-mediated immunity. Urology 41:548-553

Strohmaier WL, Bichler KH, Bocking A, Fluchter St H (1991) Histological effects of local microwave hyperthermia in prostatic cancer. Int J Hyperthermia 7:27-33

Strohmaier WL, Bocking A, Bichler K-H (1992) Histological results of hyperthermia treatment in prostate cancer. In: Bichler K-H, Strohmaier WL, Wilbert DM (eds) Hyperthermia of the prostate - state of the art. PMI, Frankfurt, pp 15-19

Szmigielski S, Janiak M (1977) Reaction of cell mediated immunity to local hyperthermia of tumors and its potentiation by immunostimulation. In: Streffer C (ed) Cancer therapy by hyperthermia and radiation. Urban and Schwarzenberg, Baltimore, pp 80-92

Szmigielski S, Jeljaszewicz, J, Pulverer G (1987) Thermoimmunotherapy of advanced neoplasms - a concept and preliminary results. Biomed Pharmacother 41:132-138

Szmigielski S, Zielinski H, Stawarz B et al. (1988) Local microwave hyperthermia in treatment of advanced prostatic adenocarcinoma. Urol Res 16:1-7

Szmigielski S, Sobczynski J, Sokolska G, Stawarz B, Zielinski H, Petrovich Z (1991) Effects of local prostatic hyperthermia on human NK and T cell function. Int J Hyperthermia 7:869-880

Szmigielski S, Stawarz B, Sobczynski J, Sokolska G, Jeljaszewicz J, Pulverer G (1992) Thermoimmunothrapy of advanced prostate cancer with intrarectal microwave hyperthermia and intraumoral injections of Propionibacterium granulosum KP-40. A concept and preliminary results with monitoring of the immune system. In: Bichler K-H, Strohmaier WL, Wilbert DM (eds) Hyperthermia of the prostate - state of the art. PMI, Frankfurt, pp 20–28

Szmigielski S, Stawarz B, Petrovich Z (1994) Cell-mediated immune response in patients undergoing prostatic hyperthermia. In: Petrovich Z, Baert L (eds) Benign prostatic hyperplasia. Springer, Berlin Heidelberg New York, pp 275–289

Tarle M, Kraljic I, Kastelan M (1993) Comparison between NK cell activity and prostate cancer stage and grade in untreated patients. Urol Res 21:17–21

Vieweg J, Rosenthal FM, Bannerji R, Heston WD, Fair WR, Gansbacher B, Gilboa E (1994) Immunotherapy of prostate cancer in the Dunning rat model: use of cytokine gene modified tumor vaccine. Cancer Res 54:1760–1765

Wirth M, Schmitz-Drager BJ, Ackerman R (1985) Functional properties of natural killer cells in carcinoma of the prostate. J Urology 133:973–978

Yang H, Lauzon W, Lemaire I (1992) Effect of hyperthermia on natural killer cells: inhibition of lytic function and microtubule organization. Int J Hyperthermia 8:87–97

Yerushalmi A, Servadio C, Leib Z, Fisheloitz Y, Rokovsky E, Stein J (1982) Local hyperthermia for treatment of carcinoma of the prostate. Prostate 6:623–630

Yoshioka A, Miyachi Y, Imamura S (1989) Immunological effects of in vitro hyperthermia. J Clin Lab Immunol 29:95–97

Yoshioka A, Miyachi Y, Toda K, Imamura S, Hiraoka M, Abe M (1990) Effects of local hyperthermia on natural killer activity in mice. Int J Hyperthermia 6:261–267

Zembala M, Mytar B, Popiela T, Asherson GL (1977) Depressed in vitro peripheral blood lymphocyte response to mitogens in cancer patients: the role of suppressor cells. Int J Cancer 19:605–609

24 Cryotherapy for Carcinoma of the Prostate

J.D. SCHMIDT

CONTENTS

24.1 Background

The use of low temperature of subzero modalities for medical treatment dates back to the mid-nineteenth century. Initially the agents used included liquid gases such as air, oxygen, nitrogen, and hydrogen. Around the turn of the century ether spray, ethyl chloride spray, and solidified carbon dioxide were introduced. The modern era of cryosurgery began following World War II, when liquid nitrogen at a temperature of −190°C became available. Liquid nitrogen was used commonly for the treatment of various skin lesions and was later employed to destroy some brain tumors as well as the lesions of parkinsonism and other neuromuscular disorders.

The first urologic uses of liquid nitrogen cryosurgery were made in the mid 1960s by GONDER et al. (1964), who demonstrated that freezing produced adequate tissue destruction in the canine prostate. In 1966 GONDER et al. (1966) performed prostate cryosurgery in humans, treating bladder outlet obstruction from both carcinoma and benign prostatic hyperplasia. The technique was accomplished transurethrally using a cryoprobe that was shaped like a urethral sound. Advantages ascribed to this technique included its rapid completion with the patient under a spinal anesthesia and minimal blood loss. Transurethral cryotherapy also provided effective local tumor control for patients who were poor open surgical candidates (SOANES and GONDER 1968). Initial reports of metastases regressing after repeat prostate freezing raised the issue of an associated immunologic mechanism but this hypothesis has never been substantiated (SOANES et al. 1970; ABLIN et al. 1971; GURSEL et al. 1972).

Complications of the transurethral technique of prostatic cryosurgery included urethral sloughing of necrotic tissue causing urinary obstruction and repeated manipulations. Also the monitoring of the procedure was imprecise, with rectal palpation mainly being employed. Modifications of the procedure, including perineal exposure to dissect off the rectum and monitoring by open cystostomy (REUTER 1972), were still insufficient to prevent cryodestruction of adjacent normal structures.

The procedure was modified in the late 1960s by FLOCKS et al. (1972), who used open perineal exposure of the prostate, similar to radical perineal prostatectomy or simple perineal prostatectomy for BPH, for placement of the cryoprobe directly into the malignancy. In this fashion, the tumor was destroyed directly with less urethral sloughing. However, the control of the cryoablation, entirely visual, was still inadequate, and local complications were common, including both urethral–rectal and urethral–cutaneous fistulas in a total of approximately 12% of patients. The majority of patients treated by FLOCKS et al. (1972) and O'DONOGHUE et al. (1975) were those who required local control of extensive lesions; however, a smaller number of patients had this same treatment instead of standard radical prostatectomy or irradiation techniques.

J.D. SCHMIDT, MD, Professor and Head, Division of Urology, University of California San Diego Medical Center, 200 West Arbor Drive, San Diego, CA 92103-8897, USA

Of interest, however, were the results of open perineal cryosurgery as summarized by LOENING et al. (1980), LOENING and LUBAROFF (1984), BONNEY et al. (1982), and BONNEY et al. (1983). Their results at 10 years' follow-up showed that on a stage-by-stage basis, patients treated with open perineal cryosurgery had progression-free survival and overall survival rates equal to those treated with standard techniques. However, because at that time few urologists were interested in performing radical prostatectomy and the technique of perineal prostatectomy was confined to only a few centers, the utilization of open perineal cryosurgery never became particularly popular.

A further modification of the technique occurred in 1974, when MEGALLI et al. (1974) used the closed perineal approach with a single percutaneous probe positioned and monitored via rectal palpation. This modification avoided the open incision and resulted in less urethral sloughing. However, the placement of the probe and monitoring of the cryoablation was strictly by rectal palpation and empirical.

In the mid and late 1980s, two important breakthroughs in technicological development, now very common to urologists, occurred that renewed interest in prostate cryosurgery. These two technicological advances were (a) transrectal ultrasound monitoring of the prostate, and (b) improved percutaneous access to structures such as the kidney, liver, and prostate. In 1988 ONIK et al. (1988) showed that real-time ultrasound was useful in monitoring prostate cryosurgery. ONIK et al. (1991) carried out a pilot study using transrectal ultrasound-guided cryoablation of the dog prostate, revealing that precise probe positioning and accurate regulation of the freezing process could be achieved in this fashion. ONIK et al. (1993) then transferred this technique to the treatment of prostate carcinoma in humans. Their preliminary findings indicated that the technique improved the control of freezing, which in turn decreased local complications. The problem of urethral sloughing was decreased further with the use of an investigational intraoperative urethral warming device. The procedure could be completed reasonably quickly with the patient under regional or general anesthesia and was associated with minimal blood loss and a very brief hospitalization, generally 2 days.

Since this author (SCHMIDT 1973) had considerable experience with the open perineal approach for prostate cryosurgery, the transition to transperineal cryoablation using ultrasound guidance was relatively smooth and occurred at the University of California San Diego Medical Center in early 1993. Our technique and experiences will be included later in this chapter.

24.2 Mechanisms of Action

Cryosurgery can be defined as the in situ freezing and devitalization of malignant tissues. The freezing process must be applied and precisely controlled to produce a predictable zone of necrosis that will destroy the target lesion as well as an appropriate margin of surrounding tissue. The various well-recognized mechanisms of action in cryotherapy are listed in Table 24.1.

Since temperature is a measure of the kinetic energy of molecular motion, as the temperature is lowered, molecular processes slow and can be arrested. Using a rapid freeze and slow thaw technique, two primary effects are noted, comprising direct and indirect cryodestruction. During the period of direct damage, the tissue goes through both hypothermia and true freezing. Hypothermic effects are divided into two types: metabolic uncoupling and compromise of structural integrity. Freezing begins in both the extracellular compartments and the microvascular network. As ice is formed of pure solid water by the exclusion of electrolytes and organic chemicals, the cells become exposed to an extremely hyperosmotic environment. This extracellular hyperosmotic fluid draws water out of the cell, resulting in increased tissue ice content plus shrinkage of cells which then damages cell membranes and causes protein denaturation. At a temperature of $-15°C$, the majority of the extracellular environment is frozen causing trapping of tissue and production of shearing forces which disrupt the cellular structure.

The slow process of thawing is also a damaging environment for cells. As ice melts, any remaining intact cells are exposed to a hypotonic environment.

Table 24.1. Mechanisms of action of cryoablation

1. Protein denaturation via dehydration
2. Transfer of water from intracellular to extracellular space
3. Rupture of cell membrane from ice crystal expansion
4. Toxic concentrations of cellular constituents
5. Thermal shock from rapid supercooling
6. Slow thawing
7. Vascular stasis
8. Variable tissue and cellular responses to subzero temperatures

This water returns to within the remaining cells, causing cellular bursting.

The delayed or indirect ablative effects of cryosurgery continue mostly due to destruction of the microvasculature that results in tissue anoxia and thrombosis. This process includes local edema with activation of the inflammation cascade. Tissue microphages invade, resorbing the lesion.

Further information on the cryobiology related to this treatment is beyond the scope of this chapter but interested readers are encouraged to pursue the writings of GAGE (1992).

24.3 Indications

At the University of California San Diego Medical Center, indications for prostate cryosurgery fall into three broad categories. The first and the largest of the three groups is that of patients who have localized disease without prior treatment and who are either offered or elect to undergo this technique rather than radical prostatectomy or irradiation. This group of patients was the smaller group in the series of FLOCKS et al. (1972). The second category includes those patients who have had recurrent or relapsing local prostate cancer following irradiation techniques, whether external beam radiation therapy, brachytherapy, or a combination of the two. The third and smallest group includes those patients who have large local lesions, often in the presence of metastatic disease, where the procedure is indicated for the control and prevention of local complications such as repeated hematuria, urinary obstruction, and retention. This group was the larger category of patients treated by the open perineal approach by FLOCKS et al. (1972).

24.4 Current Techniques and Patient Follow-up

24.4.1 Single Freeze

Preoperatively patients undergo digital rectal examination of the prostate, prostate biopsy, urinalysis, chest x-ray, standard bone scan and measurement of complete blood count, chemistry panel, and determination of alkaline phosphatase levels, prostate-specific antigen (PSA), and prostatic acid phosphatase. Pelvic magnetic resonance imaging and/or computerized tomography is performed on selected patients looking either for extra-prostatic extension or for regional pelvic lymph node involvement. Patients with prostate glands of more than 40–45 g are placed on preoperative endocrine therapy usually consisting of luteinizing hormone-releasing hormone agonists (LHRH agonists) and/or antiandrogen therapy for a minimum of 3 months.

The goal of prostate cryotherapy is the ablation of the entire gland and in some cases ablation of areas of local tumor extension. The procedure is performed using the Accuprobe system cryosurgery instrument from Cryomedical Sciences Inc., which employs cryoprobes 3 mm in diameter, and the transrectal ultrasound apparatus of Bruel and Kjaer employing the 7.5-MHz transducer.

Patients receive perioperative antibiotics for 24 h and undergo either general, spinal, or epidural anesthesia. The patient is placed in the dorsal lithotomy position and cystoscopy is performed to determine the local anatomy and pathology as well as to rule out any unrecognized lesions that must be dealt with. A percutaneous suprapubic cystostomy catheter is inserted under cystoscopic guidance, and a large-caliber Foley catheter is placed per urethra. Sterile saline at approximately 40°C is infused to irrigate the lower urinary tract, with the inflow via the suprapubic tube and the outflow via the urethral catheter. This warm irrigation is employed to prevent urethral freezing and subsequent necrosis and stricture.

If needed, the scrotum is sutured to the anterior abdominal wall to allow access to the perineum. Ultrasound monitoring of the prostate is then carried out looking for asymmetry, overall dimensions and volume, and any evidence of extraprostatic extension. Typically five cryoprobes are used with the probe pattern of placement consisting of two probes anterolaterally, two probes posterolaterally, and one probe in a suburethral location. Additional probes can be placed in an extraprostatic position such as in the seminal vesicles should there be evidence of disease in that area.

During the visualization via ultrasound, 18 gauge needles are positioned percutaneously in the prostate down to the prostatovesical junction using a perineal biopsy guide. The stylets are withdrawn and replaced with a 0.038-inch J-tip guide wire which is inserted through the needle and the needle removed. Small skin incisions are made at the perineal skin level to allow the entry of the dilators and cannulas over the guide wires. After tract dilation is complete to the level of the prostatovesical junction, the guide wires and dilators are removed, leaving typically five cannulas in place. The cryoprobes are inserted through the cannulas under ultrasound monitoring, and the proximal insulating ends of the cannulas pulled back over the cryoprobes. With the position of the cryoprobe tips verified via ultrasound, the cryoprobes are activated and fixed to the tissue at a temperature of −50° to −70°C.

Freezing is then carried out by quickly decreasing the probe temperatures to approximately −196°C for 5–10 min; this freezing is begun anteriorly to prevent the freeze zone from interfering with the ultrasound imaging of the yet unfrozen gland. The cryoablation is frequently expanded beyond the prostate to reach areas of local tumor extension such as the seminal vesicle. During the entire procedure, ultrasonic visualization continues to determine adequate ablation of the gland and tumor as well as to prevent injury to surrounding tissues such as the anterior rectal wall, the bladder neck, and the trigone.

After satisfactory cryoablation is accomplished, the cryoprobes are thawed slowly and withdrawn. The small perineal incisions are closed with interrupted fine chromic sutures; the suprapubic and urethral catheters are irrigated and placed to straight drainage.

24.4.2 Double Freeze

Since there is evidence from the cryobiology literature that a repeat or second or double freeze-thaw cycle will provide more complete destruction should any cellular elements remain, selected patients may be treated with this modification. The double freeze technique is more typically performed in patients with larger glands or larger tumors. In this technique, the cryoprobes are thawed slowly and when the prostatic tissue image begins to reconstitute on ultrasound, the cryoprobes are kept in their initial position and reactivated similar to the first freeze. The second freeze-thaw cycle then proceeds with monitoring via transrectal ultrasound. In this fashion, theoretically, any surviving cancer cells will be both prefreeze and freeze sensitized and then forced to undergo an additional destructive cycle of freezing (von Eschenbach et al. 1994).

24.4.3 Pull-back Freeze

In larger prostate glands, the apex of the gland may not be ablated sufficiently with the initial placement of the five cryoprobes. To insure cryoablation of the apical area, after the cryoprobes are thawed and the prostate gland reconstitution occurs on ultrasound, the cryoprobes are repositioned in a more distal fashion and fixed to the tissue at −50° to −70°C with another cycle of freeze-thaw occurring in that area.

24.4.4 Follow-up

During the first 24 h following cryosurgery, the urethral Foley catheter is removed, a PSA level is obtained, and the patient usually discharged home to take 2 weeks of oral antibiotics, typically 500 mg ciprofloxacin orally b.i.d. The patient is instructed to clamp his suprapubic cystostomy tube after about 1 week and to begin voiding trials with measurement of residual urine volumes. When the postvoid residual volumes are less than 50–100 ml, the suprapubic cystostomy is removed. Patients are typically followed at 1, 3, and 6 months and then at 6-month intervals thereafter. In addition to a full history of voiding habits and sexual function, digital rectal examination is performed along with urinalysis and PSA determinations. Follow-up ultrasound-guided biopsy of the area is recommended at between 3 and 6 months and then again at either 1 year or 2 years. Patients who were placed on endocrine therapy prior to the cryoablation have this treatment stopped postoperatively.

24.4.5 Retreatment

As patients are followed postoperatively with both serum PSA determinations and one or more biopsies, there will exist a cadre of patients who do have evidence of persistent, if not recurrent, prostate carcinoma. Among other alternative therapies at that point, a second attempt at cryotherapy is included. The technique of the retreatment is very similar to the initial treatment, with the exception that the target (gland and tumor) is generally much smaller than at the time of the initial treatment and thus requires either fewer cryoprobes or a shorter duration of freezing. In the University of California San Diego Medical Center experience, retreatment cryosurgery has been performed on 20 patients in a series of 292 men for a total retreatment of 6.8%. Post-cryotherapy follow-up is similar to that in individuals having only a single session of cryosurgery.

24.5 Results

24.5.1 University of California San Diego

Since March 1993, 292 men with prostate cancer have received prostatic cryoablation with a total of 312 procedures. Their clinical stages have included T1–T4, N0–N1, M0–M1. Their average age has been 68 years. Cryoablation has been accomplished with five cryoprobes in 80% of men. Most men voided spontaneously with removal of their suprapubic cystoscopy tube by 10–14 days. One hundred and thirty-seven men have had a follow-up biopsy with negative biopsies occurring in 118 (86%) and with persistent cancer documented as a positive biopsy in 19 (14%) (Fig. 24.1). However, since nine of the positive biopsies occurred in patients with extensive disease (T3–T4, M1), the negative biopsy rate in localized disease (stages T1–T2) is 92%.

Typically PSA levels rise initially, likely secondary to extreme prostatic infarction, but then fall subsequently. Normal range PSA levels have occurred in 83% of patients (75 of 90 followed) and one-half of these are in the near nondetectable range of less than 0.5 ng/ml. Figure 24.2 compares the results of post-cryotherapy biopsies with the preoperative serum PSA levels in 83 patients. Thus far there seems to be no statistical difference relating the pretreatment PSA level to the biopsy outcome.

In a smaller group of 21 patients receiving prostate cryoablation for relapses to prior irradiation, postoperative biopsies have been negative in 18 (86%). PSA Levels have been in the normal range in 10 of 15 (67%) with six of the ten (40% of the total) in the near nondetectable range. Figure 24.3 compares the results of post-cryosurgical biopsies in patients who have had prior radiotherapy (21 patients) with the results in those who have not had irradiation (116 patients). The biopsy-negative and -positive rates are equal in both groups.

Of the patients having retreatment cryosurgery, one has had a second post-cryosurgery biopsy and is now biopsy-negative with a PSA of less than 0.2 ng/ml. In the entire series, no perioperative deaths have occurred and no patients have required transfusion.

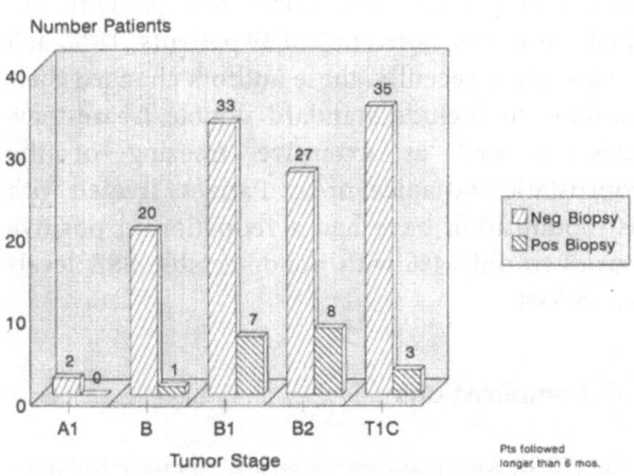

Fig. 24.1. Comparison of results of post-cryotherapy biopsies to preoperative clinical stage in 137 patients

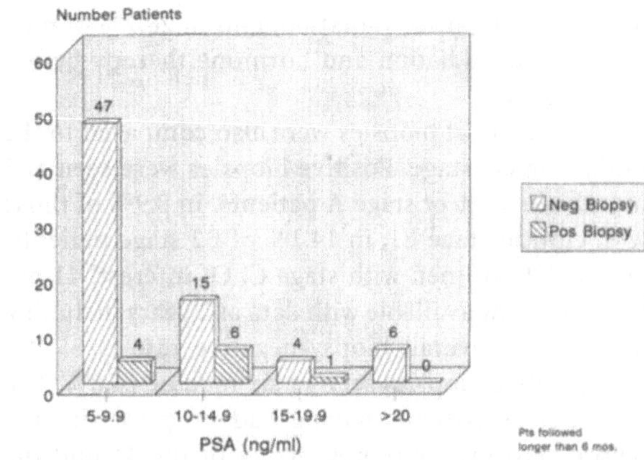

Fig. 24.2. Comparison of results of post-cryotherapy biopsies to preoperative serum prostate-specific antigen (*PSA*) levels in 83 patients

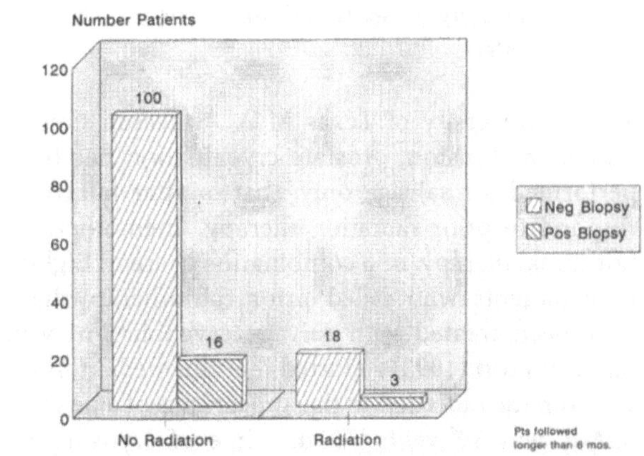

Fig. 24.3. Comparison of results of post-cryotherapy biopsies to presence (21 patients) or absence (116 patients) of prior radiotherapy for prostate cancer

24.5.2 Allegheny General Hospital

As stated earlier, the first use of transperineal cryoablation using ultrasound guidance for prostate cryosurgery was performed at the Allegheny General Hospital in Pittsburgh, Pennsylvania by ONIK et al. (1991). MILLER et al. (1994) and COHEN (1995) have recently updated results on 383 patients who underwent 443 cryosurgical procedures. Clinical stages included 33 men with stage A1, 41 with A2, 45 with B1, 75 with B2, 100 with stage C, 30 with stage T0, and 17 with stage D1 disease. Of the 354 men biopsied at 3 months, 53 or 15% were positive for persistent carcinoma. Positive biopsies at 3 months were seen in 11.3% of patients who had no prior therapy, in 18.3% of men who had received hormone therapy, in 27.3%

of men having prior radiation, and in 26.7% of men having both radiation and hormone therapy before cryosurgery.

The results of biopsies were also compared to the initial clinical stage. Positive biopsies were seen at 3 months in 8.5% of stage A patients, in 8.9% of those with clinical stage B1, in 14.7% of B2 stage patients, and in 22% of men with stage C. Of interest, 41 patients are now available with data at 2 years including biopsy. The overall biopsy-negative rate is 85.4%, with positive biopsies seen in six men or 14.6%. The subgroup of patients having had no prior therapy before cryosurgery represents 24 of the 41 and the positive biopsy rate at 2 years in this subgroup is 16.7%.

24.5.3 University of Texas M.D. Anderson Cancer Center

At the University of Texas M.D. Anderson Cancer Center in Houston, prostate cryoablation has been performed for salvage only, that is after failure to respond to prior radiation therapy, chemotherapy, hormonal therapy, or a combination thereof. Eighty-nine patients who failed prior radiotherapy have only been treated with salvage cryoablation. von Eschenbach (1995) reported that the median interval from the radiation to the appearance of a positive biopsy was 3.5 years. At the time of cryosurgery, more than half of the patients had biopsies showing Gleason scores 8 through 10. Forty-seven of the 89 patients underwent a single freeze-thaw cycle with the remaining 42 undergoing a double freeze-thaw cycle.

Sixty-seven patients have been monitored with biopsies at 6 months. Fifty-two or 78% of the biopsies have been negative. The biopsy-negative rate was only 69% in those patients having the single freeze but increased to 92% in the 25 patients having the double freeze-thaw cycle. Most patients experienced a fall in PSA following cryotherapy. Overall, 25% of the patients have undetectable PSA levels, the results being similar in both the single and double freeze groups. However, to date none of the patients undergoing a second freeze thaw cycle have had a subsequent increase in PSA.

24.5.4 Crittenton Hospital (Rochester, Michigan)

The results of prostate cryotherapy have been recently reported by Bahn et al. (1994) and Lee et al. (1994). These authors have treated patients with combined antiandrogen therapy usually consisting of an LHRH agonist and an antiandrogen for a minimum of 3 months prior to performing cryoablation. They reported residual cancer, that is positive biopsies, at 3 months in only 2 of 134 patients (1.5%) who were clinically stage T2 or less pretreatment. At 1 year follow-up, the positive biopsy rate in 34 patients is 3.9%, for an overall residual cancer rate of 3%.

In patients with clinical stage T3, the positive biopsy rate at 3 months is 11.3%; none of 15 patients followed for 1 year have had a positive biopsy. The overall positive biopsy rate in their clinical stage T3 group is 14.1%.

Bahn et al. (1994) and Lee et al. (1994) also pointed out that the post-cryosurgery PSA levels were significantly lower in patients having negative biopsies. They report PSA levels averaging 0.4 ng/ml at 1 year in patients with negative biopsies.

24.5.5 Others

Long et al. (1995a) recently reported on 84 cryoablation procedures in 80 patients with clinical stage T1–T3 prostate carcinoma. Of their last 50 procedures, they found undetectable PSA levels in 90% of men at 3–6 months. These authors report a 15% positive biopsy rate.

Long et al. (1995b) also have performed 23 cryosurgical procedures on 21 patients with prostate cancer relapsing after radiation. Thus far only ten patients have been studied with post-cryosurgical biopsies, and three of the ten showed tumor. In each case, the positive biopsies were noted only in seminal vesicle tissue. Undetectable PSA levels have been reported in two-thirds of their patients at last follow-up.

Shinohara and Carroll (1995) reported on 70 cryosurgical prostate procedures in 65 patients. Residual cancer was noted in 9 of 49 patients (18%) at 3 months. More recently, these authors changed their technique to include standard double freeze-thaw cycles as well as extensive freezing of the periprostatic and apical areas. Patients treated with this modification have had a reduction in positive biopsies to only 4% with nondetectable PSA levels seen in 64%

24.6 Complications

In the UCSD Medical Center series, 169 patients have been evaluated by Weider et al. (1995) for complica-

Table 24.2. Complications of prostate cryosurgery: University of California San Diego program (169 patients)

Complication	No.
None	91
Impotence	34
Incontinence	11
Bladder neck obstruction requiring surgery	7
Urethrorectal fistula	7
Urethral stricture	7
Hematuria	3
Thrombosis hemorrhoids	2
Urethritis	1
Epididymitis	1
Urinary tract infection	1
Penile numbness	1
Unknown	4

tions (Table 24.2). Note that more than one-half of the patients reported no problems. The 34 patients reporting impotence represent approximately one-half of those who had reasonably normal sexual function prior to the cryoablation. Thus far, complications requiring operative management have occurred in 6.3% of all patients treated. In the immediate postoperative interval, perineal ecchymosis, urinary stress or urge incontinence, and genital edema are seen but are almost always transient. The rate of significant complications including urinary incontinence, urethral stricture, bladder neck contracture, and rectourethral fistula is higher in the group of patients having had relapse of prostate cancer following prior radiotherapy.

A greater number of complications including persistent cancer requiring radical prostatectomy have been reported by Cox and Crawford (1995) and Grampsas et al. (1995) However, these authors' series included many clinical stage T3 patients and patients with carcinoma recurring post-irradiation.

24.7 Pathologic Changes

Histologic findings following prostate cryosurgery were first reported by Hansen and Wanstrup (1973). These authors reported on mostly early histologic findings, stating that the epithelial elements seen on these biopsies represented the initial or pre-cryosurgery morphology. Later, Petersen et al. (1978) reported on post-cryosurgery prostate biopsies, emphasizing cancer recurrences but not other histologic changes.

More recently, Shabaik et al. (1995) have reported on 64 patients from the UCSD Medical Center series in whom biopsies were performed at any time from 5 to 48 weeks following cryosurgery. Their significant findings in the stroma and epithelial components are listed in Table 24.3. The earliest and most frequent changes noted were stromal fibrosis, basal cell proliferation and regenerating acini, and the presence of hemosiderin granules in the stroma. Eight patients showed persistent carcinoma, and these recurrences correlated with higher initial grade and stage but did not correlate with baseline PSA levels. Significantly, six of the eight (75%) positive post-cryosurgery biopsies showed no evidence of the cryoablation background of the stroma and epithelium as was seen in the 56 patients (87.5%) with negative post-cryosurgery biopsies. Shabaik et al. reported that these post-cryosurgical histologic changes were consistent and easily recongnized.

24.8 Conclusions

Ultrasound-guided percutaneous transperineal prostate cryosurgery can be performed rapidly, usually in a period of 2 h or less, with the patient under regional or general anesthesia and with minimal blood loss. The results of transrectal ultrasound-guided transperineal percutaneous prostate cryoablation in the treatment of prostate cancer appears promising. The technique, with short follow-up, is an effective modality for the eradication of localized prostate cancer in as many as 92% of patients.

Improved results in post-cryosurgery PSA levels and negative biopsies may be achievable with modifications such as double freezing and pull-back freezing at the apex, although the complication rate may also increase with the increased destruction of tissue. Thus far most complications that have occurred have been relatively minor and required limited intervention. With limited short-term follow-up from our series as well as other series, transrectal ultrasound-

Table 24.3. Prostate cryotherapy: histopathologic findings

Stromal:	Fibrosis
	Hemosiderin pigment deposits
	Chronic inflammation
	Hyalinization
	Necrosis
	Hemorrhage
	Calcification
Epithelial:	Basal cell hyperplasia
	Squamous metaplasia
	Residual carcinoma

guided transperineal percutaneous cryoablation of the prostate appears to be effective in eradicating local prostate cancer with minimal morbidity.

Although longer follow-up is essential, prostate cryosurgery can be considered as: (a) a primary treatment alternative to radical prostatectomy or irradiation techniques, or (b) a treatment for salvage of men having recurrent cancer following irradiation, whether external beam or interstitial, or (c) a treatment for debulking of large primary tumors.

References

Ablin RJ, Soanes WA, Gonder MJ (1971) Prospects for cryoimmunotherapy in cases of metastasizing carcinoma of the prostate. Cryobiology 8:271–279

Bahn DK, Lee F, Solomon MH, Gontina H, Klionsky DL, Lee FT Jr (1994) Prostate cancer: US-guided percutaneous cryoablation. Radiology 194:551–556

Bonney WW, Fallon B, Gerber WL et al. (1982) Cryosurgery in prostatic cancer: survival. Urology 19:37–42

Bonney WW, Fallon B, Gerber WL et al. (1983) Cryosurgery in prostatic cancer: elimination of local lesion. Urology 22:8–15

Cohen JK (1995) Cryosurgical ablation of the prostate: patterns of failure and two year post treatment data as compared to external beam radiation therapy. J Urol 153:503A

Cox RL, Crawford ED (1995) Complications of cryosurgical ablation of the prostate to treatment localized adenocarcinoma of the prostate. Urology 45:932–935

Flocks RH, Nelson CMK, Boatman DL (1972) Perineal cryosurgery for prostatic carcinoma. J Urol 108:933–935

Gage AA (1992) Workshop report: progress in cryosurgery. Cryobiology 29:300–304

Gonder MJ, Soanes WA, Smith V (1964) Experimental prostate cryosurgery. Invest urol 1:610–619

Gonder MJ, Soanes WA, Shulman S (1966) Cryosurgical treatment of the prostate. Invest Urol 3:372–378

Grampsas SA, Miller GJ, Crawford ED (1995) Salvage radical prostatectomy after failed transperineal cryotherapy: histologic findings from prostate whole-mount specimens correlated with intraoperative transrectal ultrasound images. Urology 45:936–941

Gursel E, Roberts M, Veenema RJ (1972) Regression of prostatic cancer following sequential cryotherapy to the prostate. J Urol 108:928–932

Hansen RI, Wanstrup J (1973) Cryoprostatectomy: histological changes elucidated by serial biopsies. Scand J Urol Nephrol 7:100–104

Lee F, Bahn DK, McHugh TA, Onik GM, Lee FT Jr (1994) US-guided percutaneous cryoablation of prostate cancer. Radiology 192:769–776

Loening S, Lubaroff D (1984) Cryosurgery and immunotherapy for prostate cancer. Urol Clin North Am 11:327–336

Loening SA, Hawtrey C, Bonney W, Narayana A, Culp DA (1980) Cryotherapy of prostate cancer. Prostate 1:279–286

Long JP, Fallick MF, Layne J (1995a) Cryoablation of the prostate in the treatment of patients with localized disease following radiotherapy. Presented at Cryosurgery Symposium, San Antonio, TX, 18–19 March 1995

Long JP, Fallick MF, Larock D (1995b) Cryoablation of the prostate in patients with stages T1-T3 adenocarcinoma of the prostate. Presented at Cryosurgery Symposium, San Antonio, TX, 18–19 March 1995

Megalli MR, Gursel EO, Veenema RJ (1974) Closed perineal cryosurgery in prostatic cancer. Urology 4:220–222

Miller RJ, Cohen JK, Merlotti LA (1994) Percutaneous transperineal cryosurgical ablation of the prostate for the primary treatment of clinical stage C adenocarcinoma of the prostate. Urology 44:170–174

O'Donoghue EPN, Milleman LA, Flocks RH, Culp DA, Bonney WW (1975) Cryosurgery for carcinoma of prostate. Urology 5:308–316

Onik G, Cobb C, Zabkar J, Porterfield B (1988) Ultrasound characteristics of frozen prostate. Radiology 168:629–631

Onik G, Porterfield B, Rubinsky B, Cohen J (1991) Percutaneous transperineal prostate cryosurgery using transrectal ultrasound guidance: animal model. Urology 37:277–281

Onik G, Cohen JK, Reyes GD, Rubinsky B, Chang Z, Baust J (1993) Transrectal ultrasound-guided percutaneous radical cryosurgical ablation of the prostate. Cancer 72:1291–1298

Petersen DS, Milleman LA, Rose EF, Bonney WW, Schmidt JD, Hawtrey CE, Culp DA (1978) Biopsy and clinical course after cryosurgery for prostatic cancer. J Urol 120:308–311

Reuter HJ (1972) Endoscopic cryosurgery of prostate and bladder tumors. J Urol 107:389–393

Schmidt JD (1973) Cryosurgical prostatectomy. Cancer 32:1141–1144

Shabaik A, Wilson S, Bidair M, Masson D, Schmidt J, Parsons CL (1995) Pathologic changes in prostate biopsies following cryoablation therapy of prostate carcinoma. J Urol Pathol 3:183–193

Shinohara K, Carroll PR (1995) Improved results of cryosurgical ablation of the prostate. Presented at Cryosurgery Symposium, San Antonio, TX, March 18–19, 1995

Soanes WA, Ablin RJ, Gonder MJ (1970) Remission of metastatic lesions following cryosurgery in prostatic cancer: immunologic considerations. J Urol 104:154–159

Soanes WA, Gonder MJ (1968) Use of cryosurgery in prostatic cancer. J Urol 99:793–797

von Eschenbach AC (1995) Results of a phase I/II study of cryoablation for recurrent carcinoma of the prostate: the University of Texas M.D. Anderson Cancer Center experience. J Urol 153:503A

von Eschenbach AC, Babaian RJ, Evans RB (1994) Technique of cryosurgery of the prostate. Atlas Urol Clin North Am 2:184–191

Weider J, Schmidt JD, Casola G, vanSonnenberg E, Stainken BF, Parsons CL (1995) Transrectal ultrasound-guided transperineal cryoablation in the treatment of prostate carcinoma: preliminary results. J Urol 154:435–441

Subject Index

List of Contributors

Thomas E. Ahlering, MD
Associate Professor of Surgery
Division of Urology
University of California, Irvine
101 The City Drive
Orange, CA 92668
USA

Luc Baert, MD
Professor and Chairman
Department of Urology
St. Pieter's Hospital
Catholic University of Leuven
Brusselsestraat 69
B-3000 Leuven
Belgium

and

Clinical Professor Department of Urology
and Radiation Oncology
University of Southern California
School of Medicine
1441 Eastlake Avenue
Los Angeles, CA 90033
USA

Malcolm A. Bagshaw, MD, FACR
Professor of Radiation Oncology, Emeritus
Department of Radiology (A-097)
Stanford University Medical Center
Stanford, CA 94305–5105
USA

Patrick Bertrand, MD
Department of Urology
Hôpital Claude Huriez
Centre Hospitalier Regional
F-59037 Lille
France

Luther W. Brady, MD
Professor and Chairman
Department of Radiation Oncology
and Nuclear Medicine
Medical College of Pennsylvania
and Hahnemann University
230 N. Broad Street
Philadelphia, PA 19102-1192
USA

SU-Chiu Chen, PhD
School of Public Health
Chung-Shan Medical and Dental School
113 Ta-Ching Street
Section 2
Taichung
Taiwan 402

Gerhard A. Coetzee, PhD
Associate Professor, Department of Urology
USC School of Medicine
Kenneth Norris Jr. Cancer Hospital
and Research Institute
Los Angeles, CA 90033-0804
USA

Brian J. Costleigh, MD
Clinical Instructor of Radiation Oncology
Medical College of Pennsylvania and Hahnemann University
230 N. Broad Street
Philadelphia, PA 19102-1192
USA

Richard S. Cox, PhD
Senior Scientist, Radiation Oncology
Department of Radiology, Room S-044
Stanford University Medical Center
Stanford, CA 94305-5105
USA

Paola Dal Cin, PhD
Center for Human Genetics
University of Leuven
Herestraat 49
B-3000 Leuven
Belgium

Dirk De Ridder, MD
Consultant Urologist, Department of Urology
St. Pieter's Hospital
Catholic University of Leuven
Brusselsestraat 69
B-3000 Leuven
Belgium

Aziz A. Elgamal, MD
Consultant Urologist and Research Fellow
Department of Urology
St. Pieter's Hospital
Catholic University of Leuven
Brusselsestraat 69
B-3000 Leuven
Belgium

John A. Freeman, MD
Assistant Professor of Urology
Division of Urology
University of North Carolina
Burnett-Womack Building CB#7235
Chapel Hill, NC 27599
USA

Jorge E. Freire, MD
Assistant Professor
Department of Radiation Oncology
and Nuclear Medicine
Medical College of Pennsylvania
and Hahnemann University
230 N. Broad Street
Philadelphia, PA 19102-1192
USA

Hans Goethuys, MD
Senior Resident, Department of Urology
St. Pieter's Hospital
Catholic University of Leuven
Brusselsestraat 69
B-3000 Leuven
Belgium

Gary D. Grossfeld, MD
Department of Radiation Oncology
University of Southern California School of Medicine
1441 Eastlake Avenue, G-34
Los Angeles, CA 90033
USA

Steven L. Hancock, MD
Associate Professor of Radiation Oncology,
Department of Radiation Oncology (A-097)
Stanford University Medical Center
Stanford, CA 94305-5105
USA

Becki S. Hill, MD
Resident, Department of Radiation Oncology
Medical College of Pennsylvania and Hahnemann University
230 N. Broad Street
Philadelphia, PA 19102
USA

Daniel Kahn, MD
Associate Professor, Department of Radiology
The University of Iowa and
Veterans Administration Medical Center
200 Hawkins Drive
Iowa City, IA 52242-1089
USA

Wim J. Kirkels, MD, PhD
Department of Urology
Erasmus University and Academic Hospital Dijkzigt
Dr. Molewaterplein 40
NL-3015 GD Rotterdam
The Netherlands

Gary Lieskovsky, MD
Professor of Urology and Radiation Oncology
University of Southern California
School of Medicine
2025 Zonal Avenue, GH5900
Los Angeles, CA 90033
USA

Mary Ann Lockett, MBA
Radiation Oncology Center
Mallinckrodt Institute of Radiology
Washington University School of Medicine
4939 Children's Place
St. Louis, MO 63110
USA

Wallace A. Longton, MD
Resident, Department of Radiation Oncology and Nuclear Medicine
Medical College of Pennsylvania and Hahnemann University
230 N. Broad Street
Philadelphia, PA 19102-1192
USA

Gary Luxton, PhD
Associate Professor of Radiation Oncology
Department of Radiation Oncology
University of Southern California School of Medicine
1441 Eastlake Avenue
Los Angeles, CA 90033
USA

Etienne Mazeman, MD, PhD
Professor, Department of Urology
Hopital Claude Huriez
Centre Hospitalier Regional
F-59037 Lille
France

Bizhan Micaily, MD
Associate Professor
Department of Radiation Oncology and Nuclear Medicine
Medical College of Pennsylvania and Hahnemann University
230 N. Broad Street
Philadelphia, PA 19102-1192
USA

Jeff Michalski, MD
Radiation Oncology Center
Mallinckrodt Institute of Radiology
Washington University School of Medicine
4939 Children's Place
St. Louis, MO 63110
USA

Curtis T. Miyamoto, MD
Assistant Professor
Department of Radiation Oncology and Nuclear Medicine
Medical College of Pennsylvania and Hahnemann University
230 N. Broad Street
Philadelphia, PA 19102-1192
USA

Paolo Montemaggi, MD
Visiting Scientist
Department of Radiation Oncology and Nuclear Medicine
Medical College of Pennsylvania and Hahnemann University
230 N. Broad Street
Philadelphia, PA 19102-1192
USA

and

Assistant Professor
Institute of Radiology
Department of Radiation Therapy
Catholic University of the Sacred Heart
Rome
Italy

A.M. Nissar Syed, MD
Clinical Professor of Radiation Oncology
University of Southern California School of Medicine
and Medical Director, Radiation Oncology Memorial Medical Center
Long Beach, CA 90801
USA

Bo-Johan Norlén, MD, PhD
Associate Professor and Head
Department of Urology
University Hospital
S-75185 Uppsala
Sweden

Brian Norouzi, MD
Division of Urology
University of California, Irvine
101 The City Drive
Orange, CA 92668
USA

Raymond H. Oyen, MD, PhD
Professor, Department of Radiology
University Hospitals
Catholic University of Leuven
Herestraat 49
B-3000 Leuven
Belgium

Carlos A. Perez, MD, FACR
Professor of Radiation Oncology
Director, Radiation Oncology Center
Mallinckrodt Institute of Radiology
Washington University School of Medicine
4511 Forest Park
St. Louis, MO 63108
USA

Zbigniew Petrovich, MD, FACR
Professor, Department of Radiation Oncology and Urology
Chairman, Department of Radiation Oncology

University of Southern California School of Medicine
1441 Eastlake Avenue
Los Angeles, CA 90033
USA

Norbert Piotrkowicz, MD, PhD
Center for Radiobiology and
Radiation Safety
Military Institute of Hygiene and Epidemiology
128 Szaserow
00-909 Warsaw
Poland

Ronald K. Ross, MD
Professor, Department of Preventive Medicine
USC School of Medicine
Kenneth Norris Jr. Cancer Hospital
and Research Institute
Los Angeles, CA 90033-0804
USA

Joseph D. Schmidt, MD
Professor and Head, Division of Urology
University of California San Diego Medical Center
200 West Arbor Drive
San Diego, CA 92103-8897
USA

Donald G. Skinner, MD
Professor and Chairman, Department of Urology
University of Southern California School of Medicine
2025 Zonal Avenue, GH5900
Los Angeles, CA 90033
USA

Bronislaw Stawarz, MD, PhD
Professor and Chairman
Department of Urology
ul. Listopada 15-10
Warsaw 03446
Poland

Stanislaw Szmigielski, MD, PhD
Professor of Pathophysiology
Center for Radiobiology and Radiation Safety
Military Institute of Hygiene and Epidemiology
128 Szaserow
00-909 Warsaw
Poland

Wim M. Van de Voorde, MD, PhD
Professor, Department of Pathology
University Hospitals (K.U. Leuven)
Minderbroedersstraat 12
B-3000 Leuven
Belgium

Herman Van Den Berghe, PhD
Professor and Chairman
Department of Human Genetics
Head of Center for Human Genetics
University of Leuven
Herestraat 49
B-3000 Leuven
Belgium

Hein Van Poppel, MD, PhD
Professor, Department of Urology
St. Pieter's Hospital
Catholic University of Leuven
Brusselsestraat 69
B-3000 Leuven
Belgium

Richard D. Williams, MD
Rubin H. Flocks Chair
Professor and Head
Department of Urology, 3 RCP
The University of Iowa
200 Hawkins Drive
Iowa City, IA 52242-1089
USA

Henryk Zielinski, MD, PhD
Center for Radiobiology and
Radiation Safety
Military Institute of Hygiene and Epidemiology
128 Szaserow
00-909 Warsaw
Poland

MEDICAL RADIOLOGY – Diagnostic Imaging and Radiation Oncology

Titles in the series already published

Diagnostic Imaging

Innovations in Diagnostic Imaging Edited by J.H. ANDERSON

Radiology of the Upper Urinary Tract Edited by E.K. LANG

The Thymus – Diagnostic Imaging, Functions, and Pathologic Anatomy Edited by E. WALTER, E. WILLICH and W.R. WEBB

Interventional Neuroradiology Edited by A. VALAVANIS

Radiology of the Pancreas Edited by A.L. BAERT, co-edited by G. DELORME

Radiology of the Lower Urinary Tract Edited by E.K. LANG

Magnetic Resonance Angiography Edited by I.P. ARLART, G.M. BONGARTZ and G. MARCHAL

Contrast-Enhanced MRI of the Breast S.H. HEYWANG-KÖBRUNNER and R. BECK

Radiation Oncology

Lung Cancer Edited by C.W. SCARANTINO

Innovations in Radiation Oncology Edited by H.R. WITHERS and L.J. PETERS

Radiation Therapy of Head and Neck Cancer Edited by G.E. LARAMORE

Gastrointestinal Cancer – Radiation Therapy Edited by R.R. DOBELBOWER, Jr.

Radiation Exposure and Occupational Risks Edited by E. SCHERER, C. STREFFER and K.-R. TROTT

Radiation Therapy of Benign Diseases – A Clinical Guide S.E. ORDER and S.S. DONALDSON

Interventional Radiation Therapy Techniques – Brachytherapy Edited by R. SAUER

Radiopathology of Organs and Tissues Edited by E. SCHERER, C. STREFFER and K.-R. TROTT

Concomitant Continuous Infusion Chemotherapy and Radiation Edited by M. ROTMAN and C.J. ROSENTHAL

Intraoperative Radiotherapy – Clinical Experiences and Results Edited by F.A. CALVO, M. SANTOS and L.W. BRADY

Radiotherapy of Intraocular and Orbital Tumors Edited by W.E. ALBERTI and R.H. SAGERMAN

Interstitial and Intracavitary Thermoradiotherapy Edited by M.H. SEEGENSCHMIEDT and R. SAUER

Non-Disseminated Breast Cancer Controversial Issues in Management Edited by G.H. FLETCHER and S.H. LEVITT

Current Topics in Clinical Radiobiology of Tumors Edited by H.-P. BECK-BORNHOLDT

Practical Approaches to Cancer Invasion and Metastases
A Compendium of Radiation Oncologists Responses to 40 Histories Edited by A.R. KAGAN with the assistance of R.J. STECKEL

Radiation Therapy in Pediatric Oncology Edited by J.R. CASSADY

Radiation Therapy Physics Edited by A.R. SMITH

Late Sequelae in Oncology Edited by J. DUNST and R. SAUER

Mediastinal Tumors. Update 1995 Edited by D.E. WOOD and C.R. THOMAS, Jr.

Thermoradiotherapy and Thermochemotherapy
Volume 1: Biology, Physiology, and Physics
Volume 2: Clinical Applications
Edited by M.H. SEEGENSCHMIEDT, P. FESSENDEN and C.C. VERNON

Carcinoma of the Prostate. Innovations in Management Edited by Z. PETROVICH, L. BAERT, and L.W. BRADY

Springer-Verlag and the Environment

We at Springer-Verlag firmly believe that an international science publisher has a special obligation to the environment, and our corporate policies consistently reflect this conviction.

We also expect our business partners – paper mills, printers, packaging manufacturers, etc. – to commit themselves to using environmentally friendly materials and production processes.

The paper in this book is made from low- or no-chlorine pulp and is acid free, in conformance with international standards for paper permanency.

MIX
Papier aus verantwortungsvollen Quellen
Paper from responsible sources
FSC® C105338

If you have any concerns about our products,
you can contact us on
ProductSafety@springernature.com

In case Publisher is established outside the EU,
the EU authorized representative is:
Springer Nature Customer Service Center GmbH
Europaplatz 3, 69115 Heidelberg, Germany

Printed by Libri Plureos GmbH
in Hamburg, Germany